MW00844953

Sandlin's Textbook of
HEARING AID AMPLIFICATION

Technical and Clinical Considerations

Third Edition

Editor-in-Chief for Audiology
Brad A. Stach, PhD

Sandlin's Textbook of
HEARING AID AMPLIFICATION
Technical and Clinical Considerations

Third Edition

Michael J. Metz, PhD

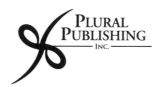

PLURAL
PUBLISHING
INC.

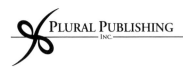

5521 Ruffin Road
San Diego, CA 92123

e-mail: info@pluralpublishing.com
Website: http://www.pluralpublishing.com

FSC
www.fsc.org
MIX
Paper from
responsible sources
FSC® C011935

Copyright © by Plural Publishing, Inc. 2014

Typeset in 10/12 Palatino by Flanagan's Publishing Services, Inc.
Printed in the United States of America by McNaughton & Gunn, Inc.

All rights, including that of translation, reserved. No part of this publication may be
reproduced, stored in a retrieval system, or transmitted in any form or by any means,
electronic, mechanical, recording, or otherwise, including photocopying, recording, taping,
Web distribution, or information storage and retrieval systems without the prior written
consent of the publisher.

For permission to use material from this text, contact us by
Telephone: (866) 758-7251
Fax: (888) 758-7255
e-mail: permissions@pluralpublishing.com

*Every attempt has been made to contact the copyright holders for material originally printed in
another source. If any have been inadvertently overlooked, the publishers will gladly make the
necessary arrangements at the first opportunity.*

Library of Congress Cataloging-in-Publication Data

Sandlin's textbook of hearing aid amplification : technical and clinical considerations /
[edited by] Michael J. Metz.—Third edition.
      p. ; cm.
  Textbook of hearing aid amplification
  Hearing aid amplification
  Preceded by Textbook of hearing aid amplification / edited by Robert E. Sandlin. 2nd ed.
2000.
  Includes bibliographical references and index.
  ISBN-13: 978-1-59756-563-9 (alk. paper)
  ISBN-10: 1-59756-563-6 (alk. paper)
  I. Metz, Michael J., editor of compilation. II. Title: Textbook of hearing aid amplification.
III. Title: Hearing aid amplification.
  [DNLM: 1. Hearing Aids. 2. Hearing Impaired Persons--psychology. 3. Hearing Loss—
rehabilitation. WV 274]
  RF300
  617.8'9—dc23
                         2013042554

Contents

Preface

Bob and I discussed a third edition to his 1990 and 2000 textbook during a many lunches while overlooking the boats and the harbor in Oceanside, California. Having known, travelled, and taught with Dr. Sandlin for many years, I never ceased to be amazed at his inquiring mind, and his insight into matters both professional and clinical. Most of all, I was overwhelmed by his commitments and his humanity. After all, it's not many who, having passed their 80th birthday, would still feel compelled to contribute to his profession by preparing a third edition textbook. Robert E. Sandlin, PhD, my friend and business partner, died on May 3rd in 2012. He would have been 85 in June that year. He died peacefully with his family by his side, and he displayed the same dignity in passing as he did during his entire life. I have never known anyone quite like Bob, and most who knew him no doubt feel the same way. He was a very special person. And, he was a dedicated audiologist throughout his entire life. His death left me with the task of finalizing his last contribution, and I offer it to his memory.

Editing a text is sort of like directing an orchestra. If the performance is terrible, the conductor rightfully bears the brunt of the criticism. If the performance goes off without a hitch and the arrangement is reasonable, the contributors, be they strings and horns or virtuoso audiologists, should get the credit. Lots of exceptional audiologists, engineers, and clinicians contributed again to this third edition and, if this production is successful, the credit belongs to them.

Some of the chapters in this third edition have not been revised to any extent. Likely, we would all agree that the rules of physics and acoustics, the history of amplification efforts, and so on have not changed all that much in the past 25 years. Also, some of the second edition chapters are no longer in the text. Some of the past contributors are no longer practicing, and some have died. Some chapters have simply been updated, while others have undergone major revision. Even though physics and acoustics have changed little, the technology and clinical approaches to understanding and aiding hearing loss have changed dramatically. There are added chapters that discuss amplification with children, new and future technologies, and practices recommended by professional organizations. We have shortened some chapters that we believe are better managed in topic-specific texts and writings. Overall, we have attempted to gather old and new authors who can address some of the relevant topics (circa 2013) concerning the clinical application of hearing amplification.

It is tempting to think that the entire topic of amplification for the hearing impaired can be covered in one textbook. In practice, and in discussions over our lunches, we found it necessary to eliminate many topics of considerable interest in order to keep the text at a weight that could be managed by most adults using a backpack. I am not so sure we succeeded because, as we reviewed our decisions, we were dismayed in that many topics seem missing. But, we have given it a good start, and the invitation is open to those who follow to fill in the voids we missed.

This preface to the third edition is intentionally short in the hope that its shortness will inspire some to remember the contributions Sandy made to audiology in general and hearing aid practices specifically. My hope, and I believe it was Bob's hope also, is that all readers will find knowledge in the text that will help them deliver better care to their hearing-impaired patients. All of these writers offer their contributions as a tribute to Bob. My gratitude goes to all of them. Finally, it has been my privilege to have been associated with my long-time friend and colleague, Sandy. I hope that all you who read this text will find a similarly rewarding friend and collaborator.

Mike Metz
Irvine, California
Summer, 2013

Introduction

The first edition of *Textbook of Hearing Aid Amplification* was compiled by contributors to represent the state of the art and science of dispensing hearing aids in the 1980s. The second volume brought much of the science up to the mid-1990s. This third edition again renews the views of experienced contributors as held at the end of the first decade of the 21st century.

The processes involved in dispensing hearing aids have changed markedly in the past 15 years, and the revision of this text reflects much of those changes. However, there are some major changes in the text that deserve mention. The reader familiar with the prior editions will recall that the majority of the contributions dealt with fitting amplification to adults, and there was a bit more emphasis on the therapeutic aspects of amplification that lead to successful use of hearing aids. There have been some major changes in the organization of this third edition.

The first major change is that of overall organization. The text now consists of five overlapping sections. The first chapter—Historical Overview—consists of the overview from pioneers in the field of hearing aid design. As history seldom undergoes substantial changes, one will note that this overview is essentially the same as it appeared in the second edition.

Section Two, consisting of five chapters, is dedicated to an increased understanding of the acoustics encountered in the fields of speech and hearing. In this section, general principles of sound, resonances, and the influences of couplers are discussed in detail. Also in this section, one will find in-depth discussions of high fidelity amplifying and compression, as well as the use of directional microphones in hearing aid applications. The contributors of this section are considered among the premier authorities in the field.

Section Three consists of only two chapters, Chapters 7 and 8, contributed by research and technical people associated with two major hearing aid manufacturers. These chapters lean heavily on the math and science that should underlie the fitting of modern hearing aids. The upper division or graduate student will find these chapters challenging and rewarding. They will constitute an important part of the foundation of understanding the complexity and capabilities of today's hearing aids.

Section Four, four chapters, consists of the contributions of six experienced clinicians who discuss the considerations that go into the decisions of selection of hearing instruments for hearing impaired adults and children.

Section Five contains seven chapters. The general direction of these eleven clinicians concerns the fitting and use of appropriate amplification and assistive devices to various types and degrees of hearing loss. The considerations surrounding cochlear implants and single-sided hearing loss are of particular interest as are the considerations involving fitting formulae. The use of real ear measures is discussed in nice detail.

The fitting of hearing aids to varying types, patterns, and degrees of hearing loss is considered by many to be more of an art than a science. However, as with any health field evolving through this age of increasing technology, it behooves the astute clinician to be well-versed in the science underlying the use of amplification for hearing loss. This third edition is more heavily based in science that it is in art. While it is not all inclusive, it certainly will benefit the advanced student as well as the experienced clinician to become better equipped to manage a patient's hearing loss.

Contributors

Hanne Pernille Andersen, PhD
Evidence Researcher
Widex A/S
3540 Lynge
Denmark
Chapter 8

Kristian T. Andersen, MscEE
Widex A/S
3540 Lynge
Denmark
Chapter 8

Lars Bækgaard, MScEng
Team Leader
Research and Development Department
Widex A/S
3540 Lynge
Denmark
Chapter 8

Ruth A. Bentler, PhD
Professor
Department of Communication Sciences
    and Disorders
University of Iowa
Iowa City, Iowa
Chapter 6

**Julie Bier, AuD, F-AAA,
Board Certified in Audiology**
Clinical Audiologist
The Audiology Center
Fletcher Allen Health Care
Colchester, Vermont
Chapter 10

Jergen Cederberg, MScEng
Widex A/S

3540 Lynge
Denmark
Chapter 8

George Frye, MSEE
President
Frye Electronics
Tigard, Oregon
Chapter 14

Inga Holube, Dr.rer.nat.
Professor
Institute of Hearing Technology and
    Audiology
Jade University of Applied Sciences
Oldenburg, Lower Saxony
Germany
Chapter 7

Judy L. Huch, AuD
Founder
Oro Valley Audiology and Tanque Verde
    Audiology
Founding Member, Section Editor
*Hearing Health and Technology Matters
    (HHTM)*
Associate Professor
Speech and Hearing Department
University of Arizona
Tucson, AZ
Chapter 16

Anders Holm Jessen
Evidence Researcher
Widex A/S
3540 Lynge
Denmark
Chapter 8

Andrew B. John, PhD
Assistant Professor
Department of Communication Sciences
    and Disorders
University of Oklahoma Health Sciences
    Center
Oklahoma City, Oklahoma
Chapter 17

Patricia A. Johnson, AuD
Audiologist
Etymotic Research, Inc.
Elk Grove Village, Illinois
Chapter 4

Mead C. Killion, PhD, ScD (hon)
Chief Technology Officer
Etymotic Research, Inc.
Elk Grove Village, Illinois
Chapter 4

Dawn Burton Koch, PhD
Director
Collaborative Research
Advanced Bionics LLC
Valencia, California
Chapter 18

Brian M. Kreisman, PhD
Associate Professor
Department of Communication Arts and
    Sciences
Director
Center for Amplification, Rehabilitation and
    Listening (CARL)
Calvin College
Grand Rapids, Michigan
Chapter 17

Edward H. Lybarger, BA
President
Arden Communications Group, Inc.
Meadows Lands, Pennsylvania
Chapter 1

Samuel F. Lybarger, BS
Retired
Chapter 1

Robert L. Martin, PhD
Author of "Nuts & Bolts"

The Hearing Journal
Audiologist
La Mesa, California
Chapter 15

Phillip T. McCandless, PhD
Owner
Quiet Technologies, Inc., Manufacturing
    Research of Communication Products
Ridgeland, Mississippi
Chapter 13

William H. McFarland, PhD
Veterans Administration Hospital
Helena, Montana
Chapter 2

Michael J. Metz, PhD
Retired
Irvine, California
Chapter 20

Morton Agerbaek Nordahn, MSc, PhD
Head of Audiological Research and
    Innovation
Head of Evidence
Widex A/S
3540 Lynge
Denmark
Chapter 8

Robert E. Novak, PhD, CCC-A
Professor
Otolaryngology-Head and Neck Surgery
Director
Center of Excellence in Communication
    Sciences and Disorders
University of Texas Health Sciences Center
Clinical Research Scientists and Audiologist
Geriatric Research Education and Clinical
    Center (GRECC) and Audiology Services
Audie L. Murphy VA Hospital
San Antonio, Texas
Chapter 11

Sara Neumann, AuD
Clinical Audiologists and Deaf Education
    Consultant
Hearts for Hearing Foundation
Oklahoma City, Oklahoma
Chapter 12

Mary Jo Osberger
Retired
Former Director of Clinical Research
Advanced Bionics, LLC
Valencia, California
Chapter 18

Chester Z. Pirzanski, BSc
Research and Development Process
    Engineer
Custom ITE Development
Unitron, HQ
Canada
Chapter 3

Henning Puder, Dr-Ing
Group Head of Research and Development
    "Signal Processing"
Siemens Audiology Solutions
Erlangen, Bavaria
Associate Professor
Research Group "Adaptive Systems of
    Speech and Audio Signal Processing"
Institute of Telecommunications
Darmstadt University of Technology
Darmstadt, Hesse
Germany
Chapter 7

Mike Lind Rand, PhD, MScEE
Research and Development
Widex A/S
3540 Lynge
Denmark
Chapter 8

The late Robert E. Sandlin, PhD
San Diego, California
Chapter 20

Joseph J. Smaldino, PhD
Professor
Department of Communication Sciences
    and Disorders
Illinois State University
DeKalb, Illinois
Chapter 17

Karen Spayd, Aud, F-AAA
Chief of Audiology
Department of Communication Disorders
    and Sciences

California State University North Ridge
Northridge, California
Chapter 2

Robert W. Sweetow, PhD
Professor
Department of Otolaryngology-Head and
    Neck Surgery
University of California San Francisco
San Francisco, California
Chapter 10

Thilo Thiede, PhD
Research and Development
Widex A/S
3540 Lynge
Denmark
Chapter 8

Thomas Troelsen, MSc
Widex A/S
3540 Lynge
Denmark
Chapter 8

Michael Ungstrup
Research and Development
DSP Features
Widex A/S
3540 Lynge
Denmark
Chapter 8

L. Maureen Valente, PhD
Director of Audiology Studies
Program in Audiology and Communication
    Sciences
Associate Professor
Department of Otolaryngology
Washington University St. Louis School of
    Medicine
St. Louis, Missouri
Chapter 19

Michael Valente, PhD
Director of Adult Audiology
Professor of Clinical Otolaryngology
Division of Adult Audiology
Department of Otolaryngology-Head and
    Neck Surgery
Washington University St. Louis School of
    Medicine

St. Louis, Missouri
Chapter 19

Therese M. Velde, PhD
Oticon A/S
2765 Smørum
Denmark
Chapter 7

Theodore H. Venema, PhD
Clinical Audiologist and Owner
NexGen Hearing, Inc. (University Heights)
Victoria, British Columbia
Canada
Chapter 5

Gary Walker, PhD
National Acoustics Laboratories of Australia
Sydney, New South Wales
Australia
Chapter 9

**Søren Westermann, EVP,
MSc, Electronics**
Widex A/S
3540 Lynge
Denmark
Chapter 8

Jace Wolfe, PhD
Hearts for Hearing Foundation
Oklahoma City, Oklahoma
Chapter 12

Yu-Hsiang Wu, PhD
Assistant Professor
Department of Communication Sciences
and Disorders
University of Iowa
Iowa City, Iowa
Chapter 6

This text really represents the work of Robert E. Sandlin, with whom I shared a business and educational relationship for over 20 years. I have never met a person more dedicated to his field than Bob. It is also worth noting that most of us will not ever meet a person who has more integrity and honesty than Sandy had. I recall that he disliked only three people he had ever met, none of whom contributed to this text, and none of whose identities he ever revealed.

Thanks, Bob, for being our colleague.

CHAPTER 1

A Historical Overview

SAMUEL F. LYBARGER
EDWARD H. LYBARGER

Hearing impairment has been recognized as a handicap for many centuries. Amplification devices to ameliorate its effects date back at least several centuries, with their effectiveness increasing rapidly when electrical and electronic technologies became available. This chapter outlines some general history and gives a number of specific examples.

The authors acknowledge Dr. Kenneth W. Berger's book, *The Hearing Aid—Its Operation and Development* (1984), as one of the primary sources of historical material for this chapter. No material in the first edition was dated later than about 1987, and many important developments related to hearing aids have occurred since then. Although it will be possible to mention only a limited number of these in this new edition, it is hoped that those selected will illustrate the important advances in technology and the tremendous reduction in size of today's hearing aids.

The authors received help from many sources, and particularly want to thank Elmer Carlson, Mead Killion, George Frye, Wayne Staab, and Dave Preves for their assistance. The 50th anniversary issue of *The Hearing Journal*, current issues of it and *The Hearing Review*, and our file of back issues of *Hearing Instruments* provided much help.

THE TIME FRAME

Hearing aid technology to date may be divided roughly into five main periods. The first is the acoustic era, during which devices such as horns, trumpets, and speaking tubes were utilized to amplify sound. The second is the carbon hearing aid era, during which telephone technology was adapted to hearing aid construction. The third is the vacuum tube era, which made possible greater amplification, wider response range, and reduced internal noise. The fourth era is the transistor era, and the fifth has been designated as the microelectric/digital era. Figure 1–1 illustrates these periods.

The Acoustic Era

Perhaps the first acoustic hearing aid was simply the hand cupped behind the ear. Berger (1984) noted that it has been recorded that the Roman emperor Hadrian (AD 117–135) used this method. There is considerable benefit from this universally available aid, which collects and reflects sound toward the pinna. Figure 1–2 shows curves of cupped-

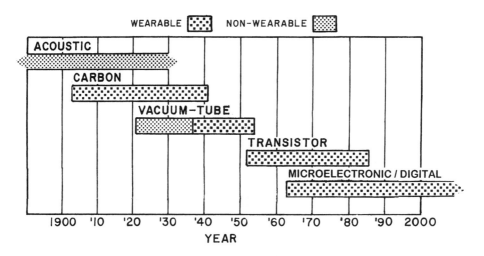

Figure 1–1. Principal hearing aid technology eras.

hand insertion gain. The solid curve is from de Boer (1982), who made the test on a manikin. The dotted curve was derived from data in a report by Filler, Ross, and Wiener (1945). It can be seen that there is quite useful amplification in the 1000 to 3000 Hz range.

According to Berger (1984), animal horns were used to aid hearing as early as the 13th century. De Boer (1982) measured the insertion gain of the horn shown in Figure 1–3 on a manikin and obtained the gain curve shown in Figure 1–4. Useful amplification is indicated between 250 and 2000 Hz.

References to man-made trumpets to aid hearing appeared in the 17th century. The idea of devices with a large opening tapering down to a small exit hole at the ear canal became well established in that century. Berger (1984) reported that the earliest illustration of a trumpet, a relatively simple funnel device, appeared in a book by Dekkers in 1673. In 1692, Nuck showed a rather complex trumpet, with a coiled section between a horn and the eartip.

Further development of ear trumpets took place in the 1700s and particularly in the

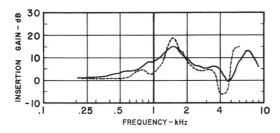

Figure 1–2. Insertion gain from a cupped hand. Solid curve from de Boer, 1982; dotted curve from Filler, Ross, and Wiener, 1945.

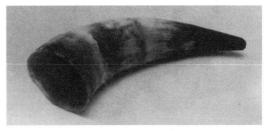

Figure 1–3. Antique animal horn. Reprinted from de Boer, 1982, with permission.

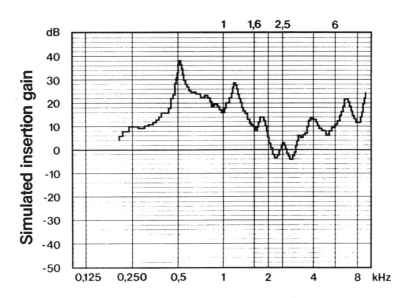

Figure 1–4. Insertion gain of animal horn. Reprinted from de Boer, 1982, with permission.

1800s. These trumpets included, in addition to conical trumpets, "ladle" trumpets, pipe-shaped trumpets, and "dome" trumpets. The speaking tube long remained a standard item.

A "tin trumpet" illustrated in a catalog of William V. Willis & Co. (ca. 1930) was stated to be "the best known and most used of all hearing devices" (Figure 1–5). Cone diameters available ranged from 3¾ to 6 inches. Figure 1–6 shows a "London trumpet" from the same catalog. It was a folded horn to reduce length. Many other acoustic devices appeared in this catalog. One of them was called "auricles" (Figure 1–7). Not only was this a wearable acoustic device, but it was also binaural.

De Boer (1982) measured the insertion gain of several antique trumpets on a KEMAR manikin. One type is shown in Figure 1–8. The average insertion gain of four trumpets tested by de Boer is shown in Figure 1–9, along with curves for two transistor aids.

Acoustic devices are still being patented and used today (e.g., Goode, 1985). They have had the longest history by far of any form of hearing aid. Although not very acceptable cosmetically, the larger acoustic devices actually provided a great deal of gain and were of real benefit when no other means of amplification was known.

The Carbon Era

The telephone, invented by Alexander Graham Bell in 1876, used a magnetic micro-

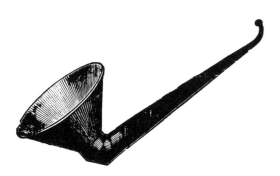

Figure 1–5. Tin trumpet from V. Willis & Co. catalog (ca. 1930).

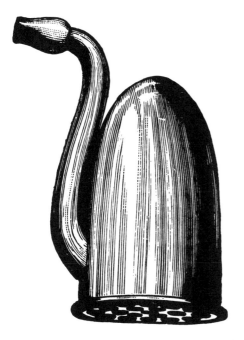

Figure 1–6. London trumpet from V. Willis & Co. catalog.

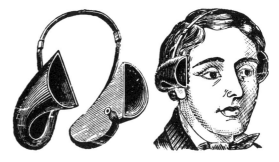

Figure 1–7. Auricles from Willis & Co. catalog.

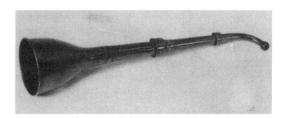

Figure 1–8. Antique trumpet. Reprinted from de Boer, 1982, with permission.

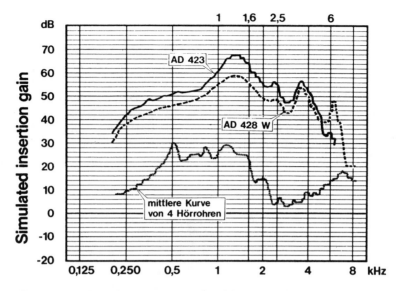

Figure 1–9. Average insertion gain of four antique trumpets (*bottom curve, compared with two transistor curves above*) from de Boer, 1982, with permission.

phone, which did not amplify sound. The invention of carbon transmitters by Blake and by Hughes in 1878 provided the amplification capability that made telephone technology adaptable to hearing aids.

The first practical commercially available wearable carbon hearing aid in the United States was made by Miller Reese Hutchinson in 1902, although Hutchinson had received a patent as early as 1899. His invention became the basis for "Acousticon" hearing aids. Berger (1984) gave excellent historical information on the adaptation of telephone techniques to hearing aids.

Construction

The simple carbon hearing aid consisted of three elements: a sensitive carbon microphone, a magnetic receiver, and a battery, plus necessary connecting cords. An example of a simple but quite sensitive hearing aid microphone of 1930 is shown in Figure 1–10. The cover and diaphragm have been taken off to show the carbon backplate with eight pockets, each containing four highly polished 1.0-mm diameter carbon spheres (term-

ed *globules*). With the 2¼-inch diameter by 0.015-inch-thick carbon diaphragm held in place a few thousandths of an inch from the backplate, by screwing on the cover and with the microphone in a vertical position, the carbon globules rest gently against the diaphragm and the sloping sidewalls of the pockets. Vibration of the diaphragm produces relatively large variations in the microphone resistance and the battery current passing through the magnetic receiver winding is modulated correspondingly.

Instead of globules, some microphones used carbon granules similar to those used in telephone transmitters. These were held in a shallow cylindrical pocket between the diaphragm and a backplate. A washer of felt or similar material held the granules in place. The surface areas of the diaphragm (if metal) and the back electrode were often gold-plated.

Figure 1–11 shows some of the types of carbon used. In the left ring is carbon granule material, which was used in both microphones and carbon amplifiers, particularly by Western Electric. In the center ring are small highly polished carbon globules, typically 0.5

or 0.6 mm in diameter, used mainly in carbon amplifiers. In the right ring are the larger 1.0-mm polished carbon globules used in microphones such as that in Figure 1–10.

Magnetic receivers, either bipolar or monopolar, were used with carbon aids. Early receivers were of the large "watch-case" size; miniaturized receivers followed in the 1920s. An open view of a 1930 miniature receiver is shown in Figure 1–12. Three permanent magnets were used. A coil on the central soft iron core was wound to give the desired electrical impedance. The diaphragm, which has a soft iron armature attached, was clamped in the receiver cap. Accurate adjustment of the air gap was made by screwing the cap on the case to the correct position.

Batteries for carbon hearing aids were of the carbon-zinc type, mostly two or three cell. Batteries usually were custom made,

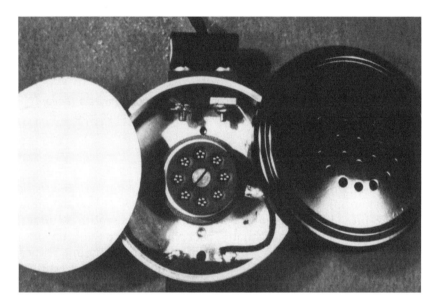

Figure 1–10. 1930 carbon microphone with cover removed.

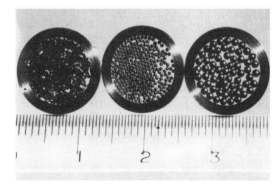

Figure 1–11. Types of carbon. Left: carbon granules. Center: 0.5-mm polished globules. Right: 1.0-mm polished globules.

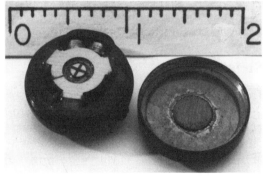

Figure 1–12. 1930 miniature magnetic receiver.

with sockets to fit a particular manufacturer's hearing aids. Some hearing aids could use flashlight batteries.

The microphone shown in Figure 1–10 is of the "direct" type, with sound impinging directly on the diaphragm through holes in the cover. "Indirect" microphones had the diaphragm facing away from the talker and into a dish-shaped reflector-resonator. The sound entered the reflector through openings surrounding the basic microphone case. The indirect construction is shown later in Figure 1–22. Microphone output could be increased by 5 or 10 dB by the reflector, mostly in the 1000 to 3500 Hz range.

Multiple microphones, both direct and indirect, were used in an effort to increase gain and output. Hearing aids with two microphones were extensively used.

Carbon Amplifiers

Because of the limited gain of the simple carbon hearing aid, carbon amplifiers were developed. Similar devices, called microphonic relays, had been used in telephony. An early carbon amplifier was invented by Sell (1925) for Siemens hearing aids (Figure 1–13). Carbon amplifiers, or "boosters," were used widely in the 1930s.

The principle of the carbon amplifier is simple. The vibration of the receiver diaphragm, instead of producing amplified sound in the ear canal, is used to drive another microphone, or carbon cell, that further increases the signal delivered to the receiver. In Figure 1–13, the magnetic system, receiving the energy from the microphone, causes a diaphragm (35) to vibrate. The opposite side of the diaphragm forms one electrode of a shallow cylindrical carbon cell in which there are carbon granules (41). The back of the carbon cell is formed by electrode 43.

Another type of carbon amplifier is shown in Figure 1–14. In this design, a vibrating reed carries a carbon electrode spaced a small distance from an insulating block in which there is a shallow cylindrical carbon cell. Carbon globules rather than granules were used in this device. A second carbon electrode closed the cell.

Figure 1–15 shows a circuit for an amplified carbon hearing aid. One battery current loop includes the microphone and the

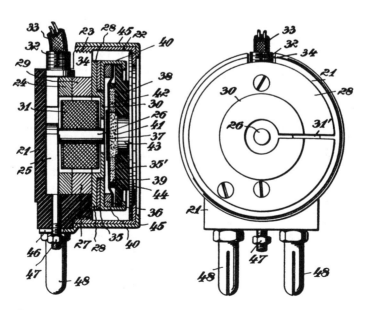

Figure 1–13. Carbon amplifier. Reprinted from Sell, 1925, with permission.

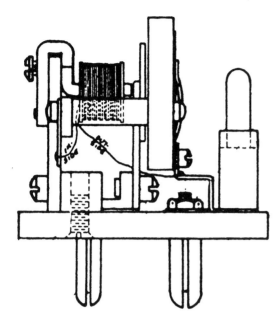

Figure 1–14. Carbon amplifier—vibrating reed type. (ca. 1934).

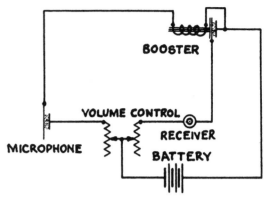

Figure 1–15. Circuit for an amplified carbon hearing aid.

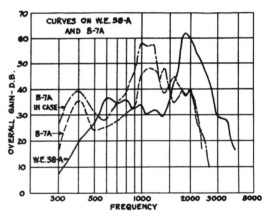

Figure 1–16. Response curves of an amplified and unamplified carbon aid.

amplifier winding; a second loop includes the carbon cell and the receiver. Note the two variable resistance sections in the volume control, necessary to prevent common impedance in the loops from causing "motorboating." Even internal resistance in the batteries sometimes can cause oscillation. It is interesting to note that the motorboating problem, which has plagued hearing aid engineers for decades, was present even in amplified carbon hearing aids.

Although not standardized, acoustical measurements that gave some idea of carbon hearing aid performance were being made by 1932. Figure 1–16 shows response curves for two hearing aids as given in a 1932 engineering report. A large condenser microphone was used to measure the sound pressure level in both the field and in the coupler (see Figure 1–50), which had a volume of about 0.5 cc. The solid curve is for an amplified Western Electric Model 38-A. The dotted curve is for an unamplified Radioear Model B-7A. The dash-dot curve shows the useful increased gain when the B-7A was placed in its small carrying case.

Figure 1–17 shows the gain of the 38-A amplifier alone. Gain up to 1500 Hz averages about 12 dB; peak gain is about 26 dB. Figure 1–18 indicates 1937 gain curves for a Radioear model. This model had three available microphones, four amplifiers, one flat and three miniature air receivers, and three bone receivers.

Figure 1–18 shows the gain using a #1 microphone and a #2 miniature air receiver in combination with four different amplifiers and without any amplifier (lowest dotted curve). These tests would have been made with a coupler employing a half-inch microphone.

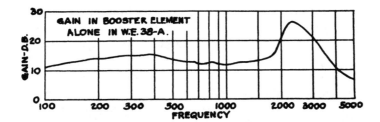

Figure 1–17. Gain of amplifier alone (Western Electric model 38-A carbon hearing aid).

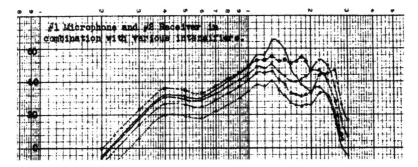

Figure 1–18. Gain curves of a Radioear carbon hearing aid model.

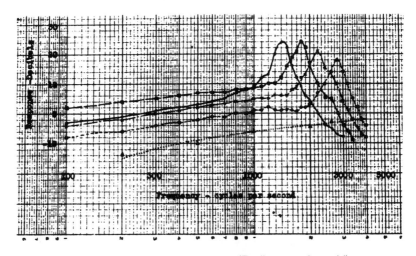

Figure 1–19. Amplifier response curves (Radioear carbon aid).

Figure 1–19 shows response curves for the carbon amplifiers. The amplified gain is the response curve minus the lowest dotted curve, which was made without any amplifier in the test circuit. Gain ranged from about 8 to 17 dB in the low frequencies to about 21 to 29 dB at the peaks.

It will be noted that the high frequency cutoff of carbon hearing aids generally was below 3000 Hz.

Some Special Features of Carbon Hearing Aids

Selective Amplification

The idea that different amplification patterns were needed for different types of hearing losses originated during the carbon era. Miller Reese Hutchinson, in 1905, Hincks (England), in 1913, Lybarger, in 1938, and others patented devices to select combinations of carbon hearing aid components.

Bone Conduction

The first wearable bone conduction hearing aid was introduced by Sonotone Corporation in 1932. The bone receiver (Lieber, 1933) had a small projecting gold-plated button attached to a vibrating strip driven by a magnetic system. It was held against the mastoid by a headband. A regular amplified carbon hearing aid was used to drive the receiver. According to an available engineering report, this early bone conduction hearing aid produced a somewhat lower sensation level on a normal ear than would be produced by direct

listening in a sound field. Thus, the gain for a normal ear was negative. However, if a large air-bone gap existed, the gain could be substantial. Figure 1–20 is a graph from the report.

The pressure of the small button of the receiver against the head made it uncomfortable to wear. Also, the air gap, and thus the sensitivity, changed with static force. One later receiver (Lybarger, 1941) distributed the static force over a much larger smooth receiver face and also kept the air gap nearly constant with respect to static force.

A major improvement in bone receiver construction was made by Greibach of Sonotone, a construction that is the principal one in use today. After long patent interference litigation with Koch of Acousticon, Greibach (1939) was granted a patent on a "reaction" type bone receiver. Its magnetic air gap was unaffected by external force against the case, which was completely closed. A floating mass inside the case, actually that of the magnetic driving system, was vibrated by the magnetic driving system through a spring attached to the case. The reaction force developed was transmitted to the mastoid by the case. Figure 1–21 shows a form of the device.

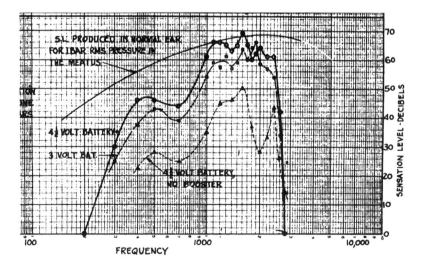

Figure 1–20. Sensation levels for normal ears with and without the first Sonotone bone conduction carbon aid. Reprinted from Lieber, 1933, with permission.

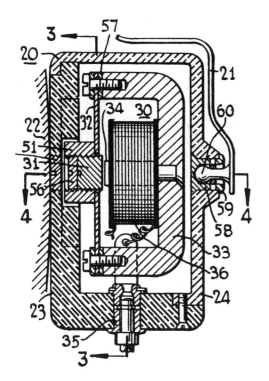

Figure 1–21. Diagram of Greibach bone vibrator.

Telephone Use

Using the telephone with a carbon hearing aid was a problem. The direct type hearing aid shown in Figure 1–10 had a raised ring on the front cover to center the telephone receivers of that day. With indirect carbon microphones, the diaphragm faced the wrong way and was inside the reflector. One solution to this problem is shown in Figure 1–22. Holes were put in the back of the microphone (now facing forward) to allow sound from the telephone receiver to enter the microphone case and reach the diaphragm. A shutter arrangement was provided to close the holes when the telephone was not in use to prevent a serious loss of low-frequency response.

Summary

During its approximately four-decade duration, the carbon era, in spite of its many limitations, contributed much to the well-being of the hearing impaired. During this era, many

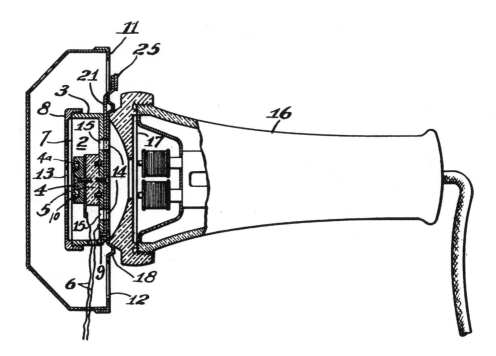

Figure 1–22. Telephone shutter device, indirect carbon microphone.

techniques and concepts were developed that enhanced later hearing aid technologies.

The Vacuum Tube Era

Lee DeForest invented the triode vacuum tube in 1907. It was quickly adapted to radio and telephone applications. The first hearing aid using a vacuum tube was the "Vactuphone," invented by Hanson (1920). It was made by Western Electric Company and distributed by Globe Phone Company starting in October 1921. It used a carbon microphone and one Western Electric type 215 "peanut tube" (Figure 1–23).

Patents issued to Tillyer (1923) and Kranz (1928) showed carbon microphones and vacuum tube amplifiers and were primarily concerned with adjusting the frequency response to meet the characteristics of hearing impairment. Berger (1984) mentioned several other early vacuum tube hearing aids that presumably used carbon microphones.

In 1924, a large multitube hearing aid was developed by E. A. Myers. It became available as the Radioear hearing aid in about 1925. It employed a moving coil microphone, which was superior to a carbon microphone because of its amplitude linearity and freedom from internal noise. A rubber diaphragm was used in an effort to obtain a smoother response. Figure 1–24 shows the interior of an early battery-operated Radioear (ca. 1926). Five Daven triodes were used. A six-volt storage battery supplied the filaments and the magnetizing winding of the microphone. Three large "B" batteries supplied 135 volts (V) for the plate circuits. The Myers device is further described by Lybarger (1987).

The Rochelle salts crystal microphone appeared in nonwearable vacuum tube hearing aids as early as 1936. A Tel-audio table model appeared that year. The Sonotone "Perceptron," a carryable crystal microphone vacuum tube hearing aid, was introduced in 1937.

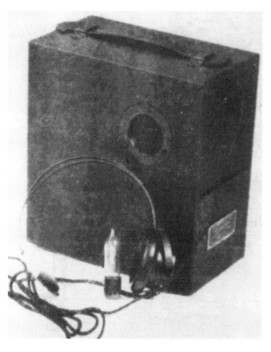

Figure 1–23. Hanson "Vactuphone" from V. Willis & Co. catalog.

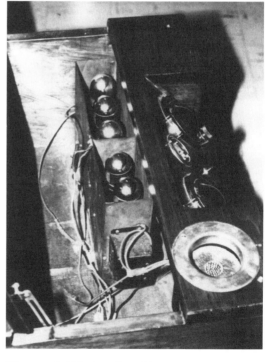

Figure 1–24. Interior of battery-operated vacuum tube Radioear that used a moving coil microphone (ca. 1926).

Truly wearable vacuum tube hearing aids did not appear in the United States until 1937 and were preceded by such hearing aids in England, where initial production of small battery-operated vacuum tubes took place. The High Vacuum Valve Co. of London (Hyvac) produced "midget" triodes, pentodes, triode-diodes, and variable-μ tubes. They ranged from ⅝ to ²⁵⁄₃₂ inches in diameter and from 2 inches to 2½ inches long. Battery drains were somewhat high for wearable hearing aids. Hyvac's 1938 book of specification sheets included quite a number of hearing aid circuit diagrams. Among them were diagrams for automatic gain control (AGC) aids, using the diode section of a triode output tube to supply the rectified voltage to control the gain of the variable-μ amplifier stages.

The bimorph Rochelle salts crystal microphone was of equal importance to small vacuum tubes in developing wearable vacuum tube hearing aids. Invented by Sawyer of Brush Development Company, this type of microphone had small size, high output, good frequency response, and high impedance well suited to work into the grid of a vacuum tube. Figure 1–25 is a diagram of a typical hearing aid crystal microphone construction. The twister type of crystal was supported on three corners by viscous pads to reduce the sharpness of the resonant peak. The thin aluminum diaphragm was fastened to the fourth corner.

Crystal receivers, notably the Brush DJ, had the advantages of light weight and wider frequency response than most magnetic receivers. However, both crystal microphones and receivers were affected by humidity and by temperatures exceeding about 110°F.

Probably the earliest wearable vacuum tube hearing aid made in the United States was Arthur Wengel's "Stanleyphone," available in 1937 and 1938 according to Watson and Tolan (1949). This hearing aid used Hyvac tubes, as did an early Telex hearing aid. It is likely that the earliest hearing aid using United States-made vacuum tubes was the Aurex, developed by Walter Huth and introduced in May of 1938. Figure 1–26 shows the interior of this hearing aid. It used four small triode tubes made by Aurex and had a large Brush crystal microphone. The case was 5 inches long, but thinner at the edges to fit comfortably in a pocket.

The Aurex hearing aid had low clothing rub noise, much better than the Wengel hear-

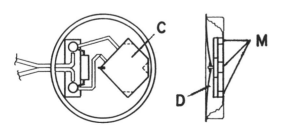

Figure 1–25. Hearing aid type crystal microphone. *C*: Rochelle salts crystal. *M*: viscous mounts. *D*: aluminum diaphragm.

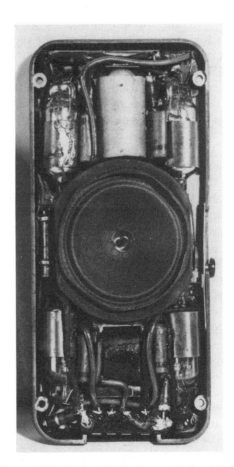

Figure 1–26. Four-triode Aurex aid (ca. 1938).

ing aid, in which the microphone was firmly attached to the case. The favorable clothing noise condition of the Aurex was achieved by a soft rubber microphone mounting, plus a lead mass attached to the microphone. Cubert of Aurex applied for a patent on this arrangement. Carlisle of Sonotone and Lybarger of Radioear filed patent applications on vibration mounts at about the same time, and a patent interference case resulted. The interference was won by Cubert; the others received royalty-free licenses by prior agreement.

In 1938, the Raytheon Company released its first series of subminiature pentode vacuum tubes and became the predominant supplier of hearing aid tubes. Interestingly, Raytheon's subminiature tube production (in later years for purposes other than hearing aids) continued until January of 1986.

The first Raytheon types were the CK501X voltage amplifier and the CK502X and CK503X output tubes. They were slightly over ½ inches in diameter and were 1½ inches long. Figure 1–27 is an inside view of a 1939 Radioear aid that used these early tubes. A crystal microphone and either a crystal or magnetic receiver could be used with this hearing aid.

A problem with early tubes was vibration of the filament when the tube received a tap. This microphonic effect created an objectionable ringing sound in the output. Tubes, particularly those used in the early amplifier stages, were inspected for this characteristic and rejected if the microphonics were too strong. Improved tube construction and shorter filaments of later voltage amplifier tubes eventually eliminated the problem.

By 1942, Raytheon's change to a flat tube shape (0.285 × 0.385 inches) allowed hearing aids to be made thinner. Another important development was the 0.625 V filament voltage amplifier tube. Two filaments could now be connected in series to reduce "A" battery current drain. Figure 1–28 shows the interior of a 1942 hearing aid using flat tubes. The filament drain was 60 mA total. By 1947, filament drain for three tubes was down to

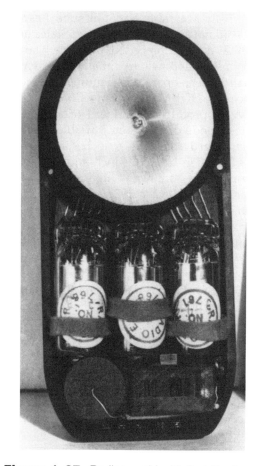

Figure 1–27. Radioear aid with first Raytheon subminiature tubes (1939).

40 mA and further reductions followed. In 1949, tube size again dropped to 0.220 × 0.285 inches in section and to a shorter length.

One-Piece Hearing Aids

Until 1944, vacuum tube hearing aids required large external "A" and "B" batteries. Two battery developments changed the picture. The RM-4 Ruben mercury battery, originally made by Mallory for military applications, made an excellent "A" battery. It was much smaller than a carbon-zinc battery of equal capacity and had a much flatter discharge curve. The other development was a small layer type "B" battery made by Eveready

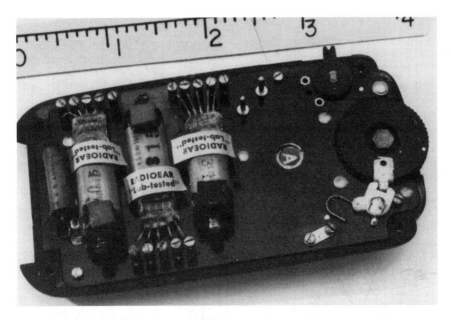

Figure 1–28. 1942 hearing aid using Raytheon flat tubes.

that had good capacity. Using these batteries, Beltone introduced a one-piece vacuum tube hearing aid in July 1944 that received immediate acceptance. Only one cord, from the hearing aid to the receiver, was needed. Within 2 or 3 years, most hearing aids used the one-piece construction and further reductions in size continued.

Performance

Vacuum tube hearing aids had higher gain, wider frequency range, and lower distortion than carbon hearing aids. Figure 1–29 shows full-on gain curves for some 1940 hearing aids. The solid curves are for full "A" and "B" voltages; the dashed curves are for both batteries at the end of useful life. Note that frequency response extends up to about 4000 Hz, some 1000 Hz higher than that typical of carbon hearing aids. Saturation output was typically around 120 dB SPL, but well over 130 dB in powerful hearing aids. At least one powerful hearing aid had six vacuum tubes. Extensive detail on vacuum tube hearing aids is found in Watson and Tolan (1949). Hector, Pearson, Dean, and Carlisle (1953)

give information on vacuum tube hearing aid technology just prior to the introduction of transistors.

Special Features

Adjustment

Many innovations took place during the vacuum tube era. With electronic circuitry, it became easy to cut lows or highs and to limit maximum gain and output. Thus, the flexibility of control was much greater than for carbon hearing aids.

Telephone Use

An innovation that has remained important is the telephone induction coil. In 1936, Tel-Audio introduced an AC-operated desk aid that had a large external telephone induction pickup coil, as shown in Figure 1–30. In 1946, a wearable Radioear vacuum tube aid with a built-in telephone pickup coil was introduced. Within a few years, other manufacturers adopted the idea and today nearly all moderate-to high-gain aids have built-in "telecoils."

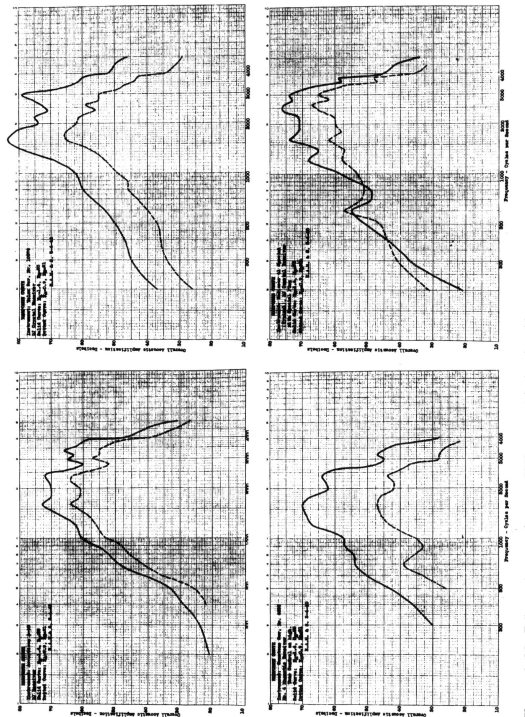

Figure 1–29. Full-on gain curves for some 1940 vacuum tube hearing aids.

Magnetic Microphone

Another 1946 innovation was the introduction of the magnetic microphone, primarily by one manufacturer. An input transformer was used between the microphone and the grid circuit of the first tube. The magnetic microphone had a big advantage over the crystal microphone: It was not damaged by temperature or humidity conditions normally encountered. It also turned out that the magnetic microphone was exceptionally well suited for use with transistors. Figure 1–31 shows a cross section of the 1946 Radioear magnetic microphone. Note the horizontally spaced sound entrance slots that make the microphone directional. This was probably the first hearing aid with this feature (Lybarger, 1947). The position of the telephone pickup coil can also be seen in this figure.

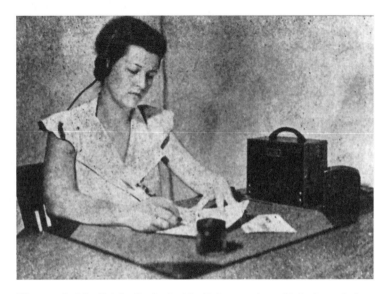

Figure 1–30. Tel-Audio desk aid with large external telephone induction pickup coil (1936).

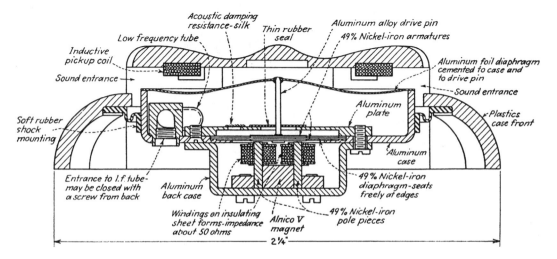

Figure 1–31. Cross section of a magnetic microphone used in a 1946 vacuum tube hearing aid.

Earmold Venting

Grossman (1942) invented earmold venting. Its initial use was with the "button" type receivers on vacuum tube aids. Grossman had an adjustable vent opening in a short tube between the receiver and a shallow earmold. Venting, in many forms, has become a standard fitting technique when needed.

Summary

The vacuum tube era served the needs of the hearing impaired extremely well. Many technological advances were made. It should also be mentioned that it was during this era that the birth of audiology took place.

The Transistor Era

The transistor era started late in 1952 and produced dramatic improvements in hearing aid technology. Invented at Bell Telephone Laboratories, the transistor was first described in a 1948 article in the *Physical Review*. The first transistor was a "point-contact" type,

possibly never used in hearing aids. Late in 1952, Raytheon Company released their CK718 PNP alloy junction germanium transistor for hearing aid use. The change from vacuum tubes to transistors did not significantly change acoustical performance, but did vastly reduce the cost of operation and the size of the battery supply; only a single low voltage battery was needed. There was about a 100 to 1 reduction in battery power requirements.

The input impedance of early transistor amplifiers was about 1000 ohms, much too low for the generally used crystal microphone. Three solutions were developed: a "hybrid" amplifier with two vacuum tube stages preceding a current saving output stage, a step-down transformer coupling the crystal microphone to the first transistor stage, or a magnetic microphone with impedance matching that of the transistor input stage. The latter approach became the standard method for many years.

Figure 1–32 shows a magnetic microphone all-transistor hearing aid released early in 1953. Three transistors were used. The receiver was a magnetic type with impedance

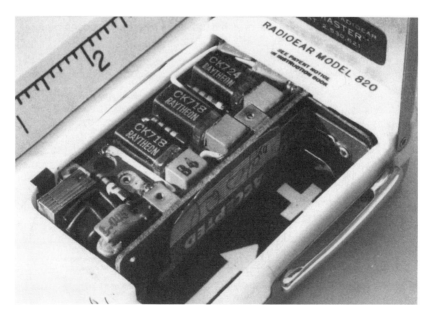

Figure 1–32. 1953 hearing aid that used three Raytheon CK718 transistors and a magnetic microphone.

suitable for direct series connection from the battery to the collector of the transistor output stage. One, two, or three RM-1 mercury batteries could be used, or, for extremely long life, a single RM-12 battery could give some 2,000 hours of operation.

Several improvements and size reductions were made in germanium transistors by Raytheon. Planar silicon transistors replaced the germanium types about 1960. In addition to providing high reliability and low noise, these also greatly reduced the number of components needed. The higher input impedance of the silicon transistors proved valuable when ceramic and electret microphones became available. Figure 1–33 compares the size of the early germanium transistor with that of a tiny discrete silicon transistor later available.

During 1953, miniaturized balanced-armature magnetic microphones for hearing aids appeared. One early unit was made by Shure Brothers (Bauer, 1953). It was about 1 inch in diameter and ⅜ inches thick. In 1953, Knowles Electronics began to produce small, rectangular shaped balanced-armature microphones. As a result of continued research and development, Knowles improved performance and reduced the size of balanced armature transducers, becoming the primary supplier to the hearing aid industry for these devices.

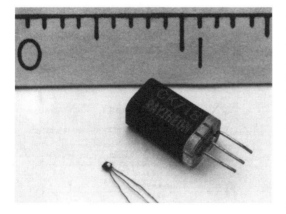

Figure 1–33. Size of Raytheon CK718 transistor compared with later Raytheon planar silicon transistor.

With increased transistor and component availability, a wide variety of transistorized body aids was produced. Size dropped as smaller microphones, batteries, and other components became available. The hearing aid industry and the hearing impaired are heavily indebted to the foresight and competence of component suppliers, who have made continued size reduction and improved acoustical performance possible.

By 1955, the size of body aids had come down significantly. That year is important, however, because it marked the beginning of ear level hearing aid development with the introduction of the eyeglass aid by Otarion. In this aid, the components were built into the two eyeglass temples and connected by wiring across the fronts. The receiver, a rectangular balanced armature unit, was in the temple opposite that containing the microphone and had a sound outlet projecting toward the ear canal. A flexible plastic tube carried the sound to an earmold. The temples of this aid were heavy and bulky, and some manufacturers thought the eyeglass aid was too large to be successful. However, eyeglass aid construction improved rapidly and by 1959 constituted about 50% of U.S. hearing aid sales. In due course, it became possible to put all the components in one temple.

The eyeglass aid made practical the utilization of the CROS (Contralateral Routing of Signals) concept, originated by Harford and Barry (1965). The original concept was to put a microphone on the side of the head with the bad ear and "inject" the sound picked up there into the canal of the good ear on the other side of the head. By eliminating head shadow, excellent results were obtained for unilateral hearing losses. The eyeglass hearing aid was ideally suited for CROS, because concealed wires could be carried across the eyeglass fronts. It turned out that the frequency response characteristics resulting from the venting action of the small tubing in the open ear canal were extremely beneficial for the large number of persons with "ski-slope" type hearing loss who had previously had poor results from hearing aids. The "open canal" fitting has remained very important.

The ear level concept had many advantages. It eliminated clothing noise, put the microphone in a more favorable location near the ear, eliminated cords, and made binaural hearing with hearing aids truly significant.

The behind-the-ear (BTE) aid was an outgrowth of the eyeglass aid. As components became smaller, they could all be put into the portion of the eyeglass temple behind the pinna. When this was done, it was quite logical to remove the front portion of the eyeglass temple, leaving a BTE hearing aid. By 1959, BTE aids constituted 25% of U.S. hearing aid sales; by 1962, they exceeded eyeglass hearing aid sales. They remained the dominant type of aid until they were overtaken by the in-the-ear (ITE) type in 1985. A wide variety of amplification characteristics has been available in BTE aids.

In 1964, a BTE aid introduced by Zenith was the first to use an integrated circuit (IC) amplifier, the latter made by Texas Instruments. Since then, improvements in IC technology to reduce size and expand functions have made ICs very desirable for use in all forms of hearing aids.

The Microelectronic/ Digital Era

The invention of the field effect transistor (FET) made possible microphone developments in the late 1960s that have had a profound influence on the performance and size of hearing aids. The frequency response advantages of a medium-size ceramic microphone over a magnetic microphone were realized in a 1967 body aid that used a separate FET with its characteristic very high input impedance.

A landmark advance took place in 1968, when a ceramic element and an FET with its associated circuitry were enclosed in a tiny metal case (Killion & Carlson, 1970). This microphone gave much smoother and wider response than magnetic microphones and was much more rugged. Figure 1–34 shows a diagram of one type of ceramic/FET microphone.

The excellent low frequency response of the ceramic/FET microphone made practical the miniature directional microphone in 1969. The first of these was made in Germany using U.S.-made ceramic/FET microphones and were incorporated in U.S. hearing aids made by Maico. Microphones made in the United States followed (Carlson & Killion, 1974). The directional microphone has remained an available feature in a number of BTE aids and in some ITE aids.

An even more dramatic development in 1971 was the very tiny electret/FET microphone (Killion & Carlson, 1974). This microphone was capable of very smooth and wide band response. A very important feature was its far lower sensitivity to mechanical vibration than either the magnetic or ceramic/FET microphones. This was of great importance in any type of aid in which the microphone and receiver were in the same small case, such as BTE, ITE, and in-the-canal (ITC) aids. Figure 1–35 shows the construction of one type of electret/FET microphone. Intensive

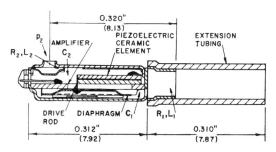

Figure 1–34. One type of Knowles ceramic/FET microphone. Courtesy of Knowles Electronics, Inc.

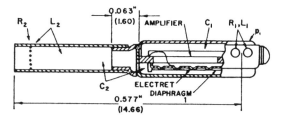

Figure 1–35. One type of Knowles electret/FET microphone. Courtesy of Knowles Electronics, Inc.

development of this type of microphone has reduced its size significantly. Figure 1–36 shows a tiny 1986 Knowles electret/FET microphone alongside an early Knowles magnetic microphone.

To illustrate the remarkable reduction in size that has occurred in very recent years, Figure 1–37 shows a Knowles FI amplified microphone in actual size, with amplification information to its right. Figure 1–38 shows the Etymotic D-Mic, which has two ports for its directional operation and a third port for

nondirectional operation. The D-Mic is only ¼ inches in diameter and fits easily on an ITE faceplate.

As late as 1961, hearing aids were considered by some to be "low fidelity" devices (Harris, Haines, Kelsey, & Clark, 1961). Not everyone agreed with this, of course. It has been demonstrated that almost any desired degree of "high fidelity" can be achieved in hearing aids, were it to be found useful. Whereas the upper frequency limit for carbon aids was typically 3000 Hz or less and about

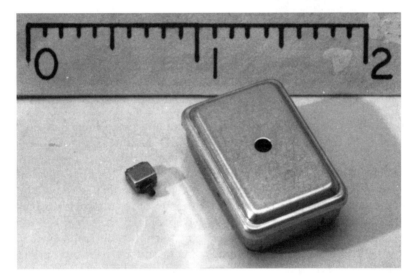

Figure 1–36. Comparison of early Knowles magnetic microphone (ca. 1953) with a tiny 1986 Knowles electret/FET microphone.

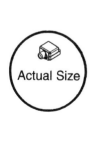

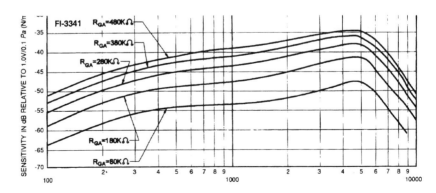

Figure 1–37. Ultra-small Knowles Electronics FI Series electret microphone with self-contained amplifier providing up to 30 dB of gain (*per curves at right*) 1998.

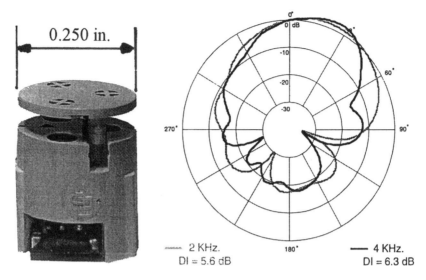

Figure 1–38. Extremely small D-MIC directional microphone with polar curves. Courtesy of Etymotic Research.

4000 Hz for most vacuum tube aids, major advances in receiver design and in "earmold plumbing" raised the upper limit to almost any desired useful value in the transistor era. Knowles and Killion (1978) described the performance of the BP-1817 receiver, which, when used with appropriate tubing connections, was capable of delivering good response to 9000 Hz. Killion (1981) summarized earmold options for wideband hearing aids. Many receiver designs became capable of wideband response.

The Knowles Amplified Receiver

This very small, highly efficient device, released in October 1988, has contributed tremendously to the development of very tiny hearing aids, even those that fit completely in the ear canal (CIC). By having the output-stage electronics within the receiver, space is released in the hearing aid electronics area to make the aid smaller. The use of a Class D amplifier stage reduces size and battery current and increases output power with low distortion.

The production development of the amplified receiver was accomplished by the joint efforts of Elmer Carlson (Knowles) and Mead Killion (Etymotic Research). It was designated as the Knowles EP Receiver. It is only 0.250 inches long, 0.171 inches wide, and 0.119 inches thick, as shown in Figure 1–39.

In order to provide room for the microelectronic Class D amplifier inside the receiver case, a new transduction mechanism arrangement is used, as shown in Figure 1–40. The smaller coil-winding space suitable for the Class D circuit provides space within the receiver housing for the amplifier. To keep battery current as low as possible for the amount of output power needed, three models of the EP receiver were made available.

The operation of the Class D amplifier is explained in detail in an article by Carlson (1988). The concept of including the Class D amplifier in the receiver case was covered in patents by Killion (1983, 1987).

The K-Amp

An article by Mead C. Killion entitled "An Acoustically Invisible Hearing Aid" appeared in *Hearing Instruments* magazine in October 1988. The article was a progress report on a "K-AMP" integrated circuit amplifier then under development. Actual delivery of K-AMP amplifiers began in about 1989.

The K-AMP concept originated following Mead Killion's (1979) doctoral studies at Northwestern University. It was based on the idea that high fidelity amplification for persons with hearing impairment was beneficial and could be provided. A first consideration was that the input/output curve of a hearing aid should be modified to reduce overloading of the ear at high levels. Figure 1–41 shows a more desirable situation (Killion, 1993).

A second consideration was that distortion for high level input signals should be reduced. This was achieved by the use of the Class D amplified receiver.

A third consideration was that the frequency response of a hearing aid should change with the input sound pressure level, as shown in Figure 1–42 (Killion, 1993).

Other features of the K-AMP amplifier further increased its flexibility (Kruger & Kruger, 1993).

The circuitry required to achieve these desirable amplifier objectives was necessarily complex, but achieved in a remarkably small size. The size was later reduced sufficiently to fit into small ITC aids. Figure 1–43 shows one type of 1998 K-AMP. It is extremely tiny, considering the complex circuitry provided, and has received wide industry acceptance.

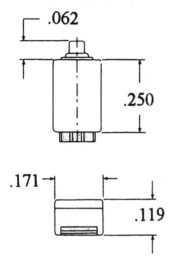

Figure 1–39. Dimensions of Knowles Electronics EP Amplified Receiver (inches).

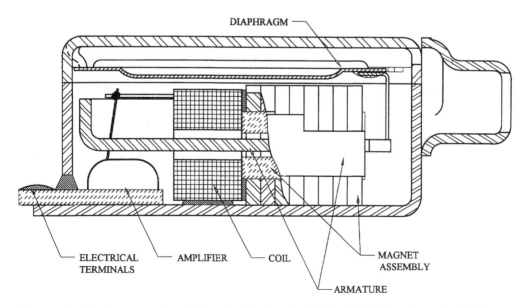

Figure 1–40. Cross-section of Knowles Electronics EP Amplified Receiver, about 15 times actual size. Courtesy of Elmer V. Carlson.

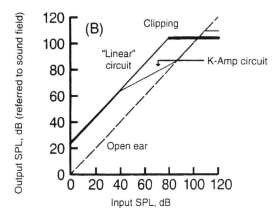

Figure 1–41. Preferred input-output characteristics for a high-fidelity hearing aid.

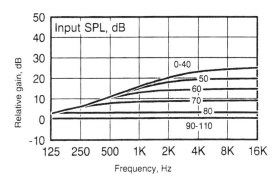

Figure 1–42. Relative gain vs. frequency for increasing input levels with K-AMP.

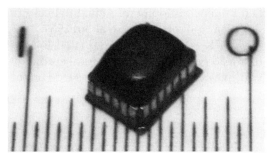

Figure 1–43. Enlarged photograph of a 1998 Etymotic Research K-AMP. Scale divisions under it are ½ millimeter apart. The complex amplifier measures only 0.132 × 0.181 × 0.100 inches.

and other components, ITE technology took on new life and by 1975 had captured 18% of the market. A decade later, the ITE market share was approximately 65%, including the relatively new ITC instruments introduced in 1983. By 1989, ITC aids were a full 20% of the total ITE market. Further size reductions became possible in the 1990s, beginning with the Siemens XP peritympanic model that sat almost at the eardrum and required a fairly complex impressioning procedure to insure complete safety.

CIC Instruments

The development of new silicone impression materials led to more easily obtainable deep canal impressions that did not impinge on the tympanic membrane. In 1993–1994, Starkey and Argosy introduced CIC instruments in which the shells terminated some 5 to 7 mm beyond the second bend of the canal, and the microphones sat 1 to 2 mm inside the aperture. By seating these instruments into the bony portion of the canal, it was possible to reduce significantly (and in some cases eliminate) the occlusion effect, allowing unvented instruments—almost a necessity when working with the available space in the canal.

Because of the microphone location and the smaller cavity adjacent to the eardrum, the actual performance of a CIC aid is considerably higher than indicated by a 2 cc coupler

In 1998, a programmable version of the K-AMP became available.

Further Size Reductions

In-the-ear (ITE) aids started to appear statistically in 1961 and puttered along at a low market percentage through 1974. Early ITE aids were sometimes more out-of-the-ear than in-the-ear. However, as a result of major reductions in the size of microphones, receivers, batteries (a significant development in 1977 was the zinc-air battery, which has about double the capacity of a mercury or silver oxide battery of the same size and does not require relatively scarce materials),

test. Preves and Leisses estimate that that the microphone inlet location could increase gain by about 7 dB, and that the deep canal placement of the receiver might result in a further gain of about 6 dB, compared with a full-shell ITE aid (Preves & Leisses, 1995).

Because of relative inaccessibility of the CIC instrument, the usual type of volume control cannot be used. Various means of handling this problem have been devised, such as a magnetic control or signals from a handheld control.

Not all hearing losses can be fit with ITE products, and BTE instruments continue to represent almost one-fifth of all hearing aid sales. The evolution of extremely soft silicone earmolds in 1989–1990 allowed the BTE style to replace most body instruments by providing a better seal within the canal to reduce the incidence of acoustic feedback.

In 1997, more than 1.8 million hearing aids were sold in the United States, with 64% of all fittings involving binaural amplification. The 1997 breakdown by style follows:

ITE (Full Shell)	37.2%
ITC	23.8%
BTE	18.8%
CIC	11.8%
Half-shell	7.2%

Programmable Hearing Aids

A programmable aid is one in which the gain, output, and frequency response can be set to meet requirements indicated by the user's audiogram, using a computer in which the output is connected to a multiple contact terminal on the hearing aid by a cable from the computer. Various fitting systems in the computer program are available.

The earliest date for the availability of programmable aids may have been 1988 (3M, Widex), followed in 1989 by Maico and in 1991 by Siemens.

The subject of digitally programmable hearing aids was extensively discussed by Staab in a review article in the *British Journal of Audiology* (Staab, 1990).

In 1992, the Hi-Pro standard interface for programmable instruments became available and is still in use.

In 1995, the first programmable CIC was introduced by Maico. Siemens introduced a programmable CIC in 1996.

The availability of programmable hearing aids has increased significantly in recent years. Many manufacturers currently utilize the "NOAH" system for programming, available through the Hearing Instrument Manufacturers Software Association (HIMSA).

Digital Hearing Aids

The earliest wearable digital hearing aid was made in experimental form in 1983 by Audiotone. It had a behind-the-ear portion that contained the analog-to-digital (A/D) converter, the digital signal processing (DSP), and the digital-to analog (D/A) converter. It was described fully in the October 1983 *Hearing Aid Journal* under the title "A Wearable Digital Hearing Aid." The authors were James Nunley, Wayne Staab, John Steadman, Perry Wechsler, and Bonnie Spencer. In addition, David Egolf and Robert Brechbiell participated in the project (Nunley, Staab et al., 1983).

The digital processing used in this device (and in most later wearable hearing aids) is described as follows:

1. The hearing aid microphone picks up airborne speech signals.
2. These analog speech signals are digitized in real time by the A/D converter.
3. The central processing unit (which is a very small computer or microprocessor) mathematically manipulates these digitized data according to programmed instructions. For example, the central processing unit may be programmed to change the frequency pattern to increase the high frequencies and reduce the low frequencies of the incoming signal. This would be a relatively simple operation. On the other hand, the ability to adapt to

changing environments and to suppress noise is much more difficult.

4. The resulting output sequence is changed to analog form by the D/A converter.
5. The analog output signal is used to drive the hearing aid receiver.

Several benefits from the digital processing are mentioned in the article, including reduction of feedback, adjustment of programming to meet user requirements, improving signal-to-noise ratio, and more precise and adjustable response characteristics.

A comprehensive article by Wayne J. Staab, entitled "Digital Hearing Instruments" shows the basic circuitry in a digital hearing aid (Staab, 1987). An analog input portion precedes the digital portion, which is followed by an analog output portion, as shown in Figure 1–44.

According to the *Hearing Journal's* 50th Anniversary issue, the first digital ear level aids were introduced in 1995, by both Oticon and Widex.

An open platform digital hearing aid was introduced by Philips in 1997. In this instrument, the user can select any one of four different algorithms in the hearing aid (an algorithm is a prescribed set of well-defined rules or processes for the solution of a problem in a finite number of steps). A DSP chip developed by Philips manages all aspects of signal processing. BTE or ITE units on each ear are operated by a remote controller using infrared signals.

The handheld remote controller turns the aid on or off, switches to telephone mode if desired, controls gain, and has push buttons that select one of the four algorithms available, as follows:

1. Single-channel broadband input and output audio gain control (AGC), maximizing fidelity.
2. Two-channel TILL (treble increases at low level) input and output AGC, emphasizing comfort.
3. Two-channel BILL (bass increases at low level) input and output AGC, emphasizing clarity.
4. Four-channel input and output AGC having independent control of performance in each channel to allow equalizing.

In a paper given at the 1998 American Auditory Society meeting, Staab reported on

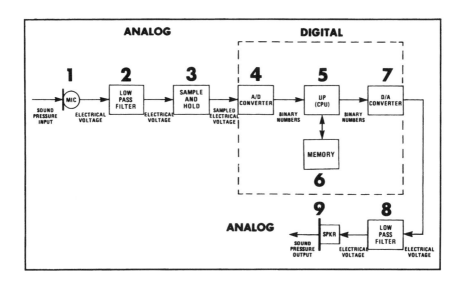

Figure 1–44. Block diagram of a digital hearing instrument. (From "Digital Hearing Instruments," Wayne J. Staab, 1987. *Hearing Instruments, 38*. Reprinted with permission.)

a study made on 14 subjects using open platform digital hearing aids. The conclusions reached were:

■ Signal processing preferences by hearing aid users do change over time.
■ Patients indicate a desirability to have multiple signal processing schemes at their disposal.
■ Patient-preferred signal processing preferences bear little resemblance to recommendations made by audiologists.
■ An "open platform" system allows multiple signal processing approaches to satisfy patient preferences.

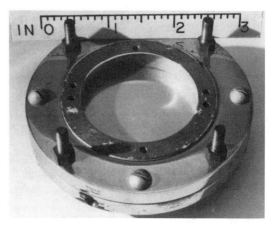

Figure 1–45. Large condenser microphone (1932).

HEARING AID MEASUREMENT

The earliest measurement tool for hearing aid testing was the human ear. Engineers and technicians tested hearing aids by listening to them or by having someone with a hearing impairment listen and report the results. An experienced listener could do much better than one might expect; some very good hearing aids were developed with this still-useful technique.

To measure any acoustical device accurately requires the measurement of sound pressure or intensity. The first accurate device for this was the Rayleigh disk (Rayleigh, 1882), a small, light disk supported by an easily twisted suspension. In a strong sound field, the disk turned an amount proportional to the sound intensity. It was used as a primary standard well into the 1930s, and possibly longer (Ballantine, 1932; Beranek, 1949; Inglis, Gray, & Jenkins, 1932; Olson & Massa, 1934).

In 1917, Wente of Bell Telephone Laboratories invented the condenser microphone (Wente, 1917). This device, in improved forms, has remained the most important means of sound pressure measurement. Early condenser microphones were large and heavy. Figure 1–45 shows a large microphone that was used by the author for hearing aid measurement as early as 1932. Its diaphragm

diameter was 1.687 inches and its outside diameter 3³⁄₁₆ inches. It weighed 1¼ pounds without its preamplifier.

Although the Rayleigh disk or thermophone (see Beranek, 1949) was useful for calibration, the electrostatic grille, or actuator, described by Ballantine (1932) was preferable. A carefully machined metal grille having alternate bars and slots was placed a small, accurately known distance from the microphone diaphragm. The open slots prevented acoustic loading of the diaphragm. The edge of the grille was insulated from the microphone by a thin mica sheet. A DC polarizing and a sine wave voltage were applied. The diaphragm was vibrated by electrostatic attraction and the equivalent sound pressure calculated. A grille used by the author in 1932 is shown in Figure 1–46. The cavity in front of the diaphragm and diffraction effects had to be taken into account to derive the free field calibration from the grille calibration (Ballantine, 1932).

Descriptions of smaller condenser microphones appeared in 1932 (Hall, 1932; Harrison & Flanders, 1932). In the 1930s, the Western Electric 640-A, predecessor of the well-known 640-AA, was developed.

Smaller companies frequently did not have funds for expensive state-of-the-art devices and had to make their own equipment. Figure 1–47 shows a 1932 half-inch

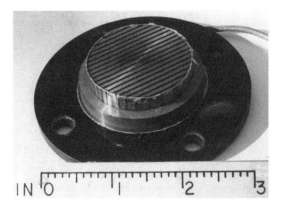

Figure 1–46. Electrostatic grille for condenser microphone calibration (1932).

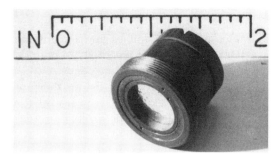

Figure 1–47. Half-inch diaphragm condenser microphone (1932).

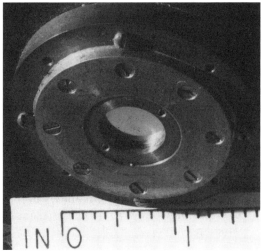

Figure 1–48. Half-inch condenser microphone used in coupler (ca. 1937).

diaphragm condenser microphone used by the author. It was patterned somewhat after the Hall design, but used a prestretched 0.0005-inch aluminum diaphragm. This microphone was used for both field and coupler measurements. It appears first to have been calibrated by comparison with a grille-calibrated large condenser microphone. A later (ca. 1937) in-house half-inch condenser microphone, made for coupler use, is shown in Figure 1–48. A small electrostatic grille was used to calibrate this and subsequent in-house half-inch microphones.

Cook (1940) reported on a new and precise primary method of calibrating condenser microphones, the reciprocity method. This method was further developed by DiMattia and Wiener (1946), and was fully described by Beranek (1949). It remains the basic precision method of microphone calibration.

Another device for moderately accurate primary calibration at low frequencies is the pistonphone. A piston-phone calibration at a low frequency plus an electrostatic grille frequency response curve can provide satisfactory accuracy for many purposes.

A large step forward in sound pressure measurement was made in 1943 with the introduction of the Western Electric 640AA condenser microphone. By making the entire metal structure out of stainless steel, including the 0.00025-inch-thick diaphragm, excellent stability was achieved. This microphone soon became the preferred sound pressure measurement device. An exploded view of the 640-AA from Beranek (1949) is shown in Figure 1–49. The outside diameter is 0.936 inches and the free diaphragm diameter 0.726 inches.

Some years after the introduction of the 640-AA, a series of measurement condenser microphones was developed by Bruel and Kjäer that included nominal diameters of 1 inch (Type L, similar to the 640-AA), ½ inches, ¼ inches, and ⅛ inches. In addition to the 1-inch, the ½-inch microphone is of particular interest for hearing aid measurements. It is useful for measuring input sound pressure levels and sound pressure levels in ear simulators, such as the Zwislocki coupler. It has good characteristics to at least 20 kHz.

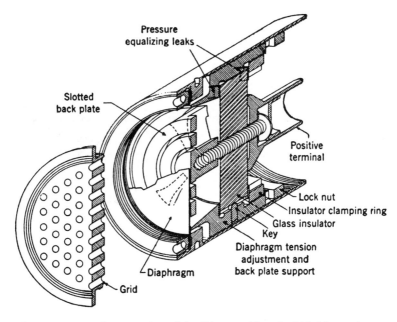

Figure 1–49. Construction of the Western Electric 640-AA condenser microphone. (From *Acoustic Measurements*, by L. L. Beranek, 1949. p. 217. Copyright 1949 John Wiley and Sons. Reprinted with permission.)

Couplers

The use of couplers for measuring earphone performance dates back at least to the 1920s. A simple coupler consists of a cylindrical cavity of chosen volume, with a calibrated condenser microphone diaphragm forming all or part of an end wall. According to Inglis and colleagues (1932), couplers had been used for some years.

The earliest coupler located in the elder author's 1932 records used a large condenser microphone. The cavity was very thin and had a volume of about 0.5 cc, as shown in Figure 1–50. The smaller volume would have given higher SPLs than a 2 cc coupler. Another coupler from the author's 1933 records used a half-inch microphone. It had a tube ¼ inches in diameter and ¹¹/₁₆ inches long to simulate the earmold hole and a volume of 0.5 cc beyond that.

West (1930) described an artificial ear that added an acoustic resistance element to a coupler for measuring supra-aural earphones. This was based on measurements of

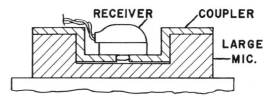

Figure 1–50. Insert earphone coupler using a large condenser microphone (1932).

the impedance of real ears (West, 1929). The design had a long acoustic transmission line leading out of the coupler cavity.

About 1936, the author adapted the acoustic line idea for measuring insert earphones. A half-inch in-house condenser microphone was used (see Figure 1–48). The coupler or "artificial ear" arrangement is shown in Figure 1–51. A tube about ⅛ inches in diameter and ¹/₁₆ inches long led from the receiver nub to a 0.75 cc cavity. A ¼ inches in diameter acoustic line about 8 feet long led out of the cavity and provided about 128 acoustic ohms of resistance. Graduated

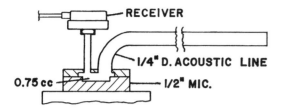

Figure 1–51. 1937 coupler with acoustic line.

amounts of yarn were placed at the far end of the line to minimize reflection. This device was used for testing both carbon and vacuum tube hearing aids until general acceptance of the 2 cc coupler.

The 2 cc coupler was first described by Romanow at a 1940 meeting of the Acoustical Society of America. Publication followed as *Bell Telephone System Monograph B-1314* and then in the *Journal of the Acoustical Society* (Romanow, 1942). Figure 1–52 shows the form of the 2 cc coupler used by Romanow. Romanow's paper has been the foundation on which hearing aid test standards have been based. The 2 cc coupler has proved to be an accurate and reproducible device for comparing hearing aid performance. Results obtained with it can be processed to estimate insertion gain for typical average situations. It is not useful for measuring the effects of earmold venting because it lacks acoustic damping. West (1929) and Inglis and colleagues (1932) made ear impedance measurements applicable for supra-aural earphones. Zwislocki (1971) measured ear canal and eardrum impedance on human ears and invented an earlike coupler well suited for measuring insert earphones. The Zwislocki coupler, slightly modified (Sachs & Burkhard, 1972), was employed in the Knowles Electronics Manikin for Acoustic Research (KEMAR). It is shown in Figure 1–53. It has an ear canal simulating section terminated by a half-inch Bruel & Kjär (B&K) condenser microphone. Four tuned acoustic networks are coupled to the central hole to produce the desired acoustic impedance characteristics.

The KEMAR manikin (Burkhard & Sachs, 1975) simulates the head and torso of an average human adult. It has made possible

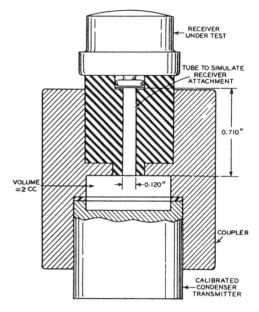

Figure 1–52. Romanow 2 cc coupler.

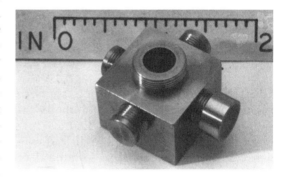

Figure 1–53. Knowles DB100 ear simulator—Zwislocki type.

more realistic overall measurement of hearing aid performance and takes into account the acoustic effects of the body, head, pinna, and ear canal. Tests on the manikin with and without a hearing aid provide a measure of typical insertion gain.

Prior to the early 1970s, the measurement of hearing aid performance was limited to manufacturing and repair facilities due to the extent and cost of the equipment required for it. In 1973, B&K introduced a test system designed to be used in dispensers' offices, but it was quickly eclipsed in the same year by

Frye Electronics' first digital hearing aid analyzer. That device featured automatic readout of amplitude and distortion, and was the forerunner of all automated in-office hearing aid test gear (Skafte, 1990). Frye and others continually have developed and further automated their systems for both the manufacturer and dispenser.

As hearing aids have been reduced further in size to fit entirely within the ear canal, yet another coupler has evolved (Figure 1–54) to take into account the smaller volume of air through which the amplified sound passes. The HA-1 coupler may understate at-the-eardrum gain by as much as one-half (Figure 1–55), due to its large physical volume relative to that of the unfilled canal between the tip of the hearing aid and the tympanic

membrane, and the frequency-dependent impedance changes of the TM itself.

Although not yet conforming to any standard, the CIC coupler (in conjunction with correction factors built into the test gear) will provide much more accurate gain and output curves than will a standard HA-1 unit (Frye, 1996).

Bone Conduction Couplers

A mechanical coupler for bone receivers was described by Hawley (1939). It used a vibration pickup to measure the vibration at a central point of the bone receiver face. A leather load simulated the headbone impedance. Carlisle and Pearson (1951) described a very practical strain gauge type artificial mastoid that integrated the vibration of the bone receiver surface. An IEC standard, *Publication 373*, defines a mechanical coupler that can be used for audiometer or hearing aid bone vibrator measurements.

Probe Tube Measurements

Probe tube measurement of hearing aid performance on the ear of the person being fitted, employing computerized leveling, programming, and display is becoming widespread. The concept of using a probe tube to measure sound pressure in the ear canal dates back at least to Inglis and colleagues (1932). They placed a very small probe tube coupled to a condenser microphone in the open ear canal to measure the SPL produced by a sound source. Then they derived the SPL produced by a supra-aural earphone by loudness comparison. The probe tube was calibrated by a Rayleigh disk.

Filler, Ross, and Wiener (1945) reported their historic study on the pressure distribution in the auditory canal in a progressive sound field. They used a small metal probe tube (i.d. = 0.025 inches) coupled to a Western Electric 640-AA microphone. A soft plastic tube (i.d. = 0.038 inches) was added for insertion into the ear canal to avoid possible

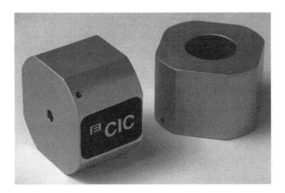

Figure 1–54. CIC coupler. Courtesy of Frye Electronics, Inc.

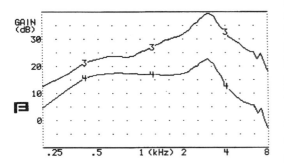

Figure 1–55. Comparison of same hearing aid measured through both CIC (*Curve 3*) and HA-1 (*Curve 4*) couplers. Courtesy of Frye Electronics, Inc.

damage. Their comprehensive study of the acoustic properties of the ear canal was published by Wiener and Ross (1946).

The first reported direct use of a probe tube for measuring hearing aid performance is believed to have been by Nichols and colleagues (1945) in *OSRD Report 4666*. A probe tube was run through the earmold to its tip, as shown in Figure 1–56, and the sound pressure in the ear canal was measured. The purpose was to compare real-ear SPLs with those measured in a 2 cc coupler to correct coupler measurements accordingly. Real-ear versus 2 cc coupler corrections measured by Nichols and colleagues for various receivers were shown in Beranek (1949).

More recently, the use of probe tubes in earmolds to measure insertion gain was described by Dalsgaard and Jensen (1976), and has had considerable influence in stimulating the insertion gain concept.

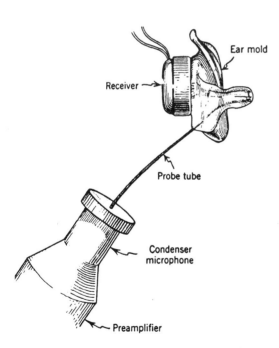

Figure 1–56. Probe tube in earmold (From Electro-acoustical Characteristics of Hearing Aids [*OSRD Report 4666*], by R. H. Nichols, R. J. Marquis, W. G. Wiklund, A. S. Filler, D. B. Feer, and P. S. Veneklasen, 1945. Copyright 1949 by Harvard University Electro-Acoustic Laboratory.)

Hearing Aid Test Standards

The paper by Romanow and work by others that started as early as 1935 or 1936 formed a basis for standardizing methods of hearing aid measurement. In 1944, under the auspices of the American Hearing Aid Association, the first U.S. hearing aid measurement standard, "Tentative Code for Measurement of Performance of Hearing Aids," was completed. Dr. Fred W. Kranz was chairman of the committee that developed the standard. It was later published in the *Journal of the Acoustical Society of America* (Kranz, 1945). Since that time, a number of hearing aid or related standards have been published by the American Standards Institute or its predecessors. An article on the history of hearing aid measurement standards has been accepted for publication by the *American Journal of Audiology* in the near future. It lists ANSI standards of interest. Also, a complete series of International Electrotechnical Commission (IEC) hearing aid measurement standards have been published. Brief descriptions of ANSI and IEC standards were given by Lybarger and Olsen (1983).

Development of new hearing aid standards and updating of existing standards in the United States is being continued by working groups of ANSI Committee S3 on Bioacoustics.

REVIEW QUESTIONS

1. What acoustic aids were used prior to the introduction of electrical hearing aids?

2. What were the first electrical hearing aids?

3. When were vacuum tube aids first introduced?

4. When were magnetic microphones first used in wearable hearing aids?

5. Who invented the transistor and when?

6. What was the first ear level type hearing aid?

7. When were CIC hearing aids introduced?

8. When did programmable hearing aids become available?

9. Who introduced wearable digital hearing aids?

10. When was the 2 cc coupler first described?

REFERENCES AND SUGGESTED READINGS

Ballantine, S. (1932). Technique of microphone calibration. *Journal of the Acoustical Society of America, 25*, 319–360.

Bauer, B. B. (1953). A miniature microphone for transistorized amplifiers. *Journal of the Acoustical Society of America, 25*, 867–869.

Beranek, L. L. (1949). *Acoustic measurements.* New York, NY: Wiley.

Berger, K. W. (1984). *The hearing aid—Its operation and development.* Livonia, MI: National Hearing Aid Society.

Burkhard, M. D., & Sachs, R. M. (1975). Anthropometric manikin for acoustic research. *Journal of the Acoustical Society of America, 58*, 214–222.

Carlisle, R. W., & Pearson, H. A. (1951). A strain gauge type artificial mastoid. *Journal of the Acoustical Society of America, 23*, 300–302.

Carlson, E. V. (1988). An output amplifier whose time has come. *Hearing Instruments, 39*, 30–32.

Carlson, E. V., & Killion, M. C. (1974). Subminiature directional microphones. *Journal of the Acoustical Society of America, 22*, 92–96.

Cook, R. K. (1940). Absolute pressure calibration of microphones. *Journal of Research of National Business Standards, 28*, 489–503.

Cook, R. K. (1941). *Journal of the Acoustical Society of America, 12*, 415–420.

Dalsgaard, S. C., & Jensen, O. D. (1974). Measurement of insertion gain of hearing aids. *Proceedings of the Eighth ICA Congress,* London, UK.

Dalsgaard, S. C., & Jensen, O. D. (1976). Measurement of the insertion gain of hearing aids. *Journal of Audiologic Technology, 15*, 170–183.

de Boer, B. (1982). *An investigation into the performance of antique hearing aids from the pre-electric era.* [Private publication of Mr. de Boer].

de Boer, B. (1984). Performance of hearing aids from the pre-electronic era. *Audiologic Acoustics, 23*, 34–55.

DiMattia, A. L., & Wiener, F. M. (1946). On the absolute pressure calibration of condenser microphones by the reciprocity method. *Journal of the Acoustical Society of America, 18*, 344.

Filler, A. G., Ross, D. A., & Wiener, F. M. (1945). *The pressure distribution in the auditory canal in a progressive sound field (Report No. PNR 5).* Cambridge, MA: Harvard University, Psycho-Acoustic Laboratory.

Frye Electronics. (1996). *Operator's Manual for FONIX FP-40 Hearing Aid Analyzer.*

Goode, R. L. (1985). *Ear acoustical hearing aid.* U.S. Patent 4,556,122.

Greibach, E. H. (1939). *Bone conduction hearing device.* U.S. Patent 21,030. Filed November 11, 1933; issued March 14, 1939.

Griffing, T. S., & Heide, J. (1983). Custom canal and mini in-the-ear hearing aids. *Hearing Instruments, 34*, 31–32.

Grossman, F. M. (1942). *Electrically and acoustically excited hearing aid.* U.S. Patent 2,363,175. Filed August 26, 1942; issued November 21, 1944.

Hall, W. M. (1932). Miniature condenser transmitter for sound field measurements. *Journal of the Acoustical Society of America, 4*, 83.

Hanson, E. G. (1920). *Telephone apparatus for the deaf.* U.S. Patent 1,343,717. Filed June 11, 1919; issued June 15, 1920.

Harford, E., & Barry, J. (1965). A rehabilitative approach to the problem of unilateral hearing impairment: Contralateral routing of signals (CROS). *Journal of Speech and Hearing Disorders, 30*, 121–138.

Harris, J. D., Haines, H. L., Kelsey, P. A., & Clark, T. D. (1961). The relation between speech intelligibility and the electroacoustic characteristics of low fidelity circuitry. *Journal of Auditory Research, 1*, 357–381.

Harrison, H. C., & Flanders, P. B. (1932). Efficient miniature condenser microphone system. *Journal of the Acoustical Society of America, 4*, 51(S).

Hawley, M. S. (1939). An artificial mastoid for audiphone measurements. *Bell Laboratories Record, 18*, 73–75.

Hector, L. G., Pearson, H. A., Dean, N. J., & Carlisle, R. W. (1953). Recent advances in hearing aids. *Journal of the Acoustical Society of America, 25*, 1189–1194.

Hincks, E. T. (1913). British Patent 10,000.

Hutchinson, M. R. (1905). U.S. Patent 789,915.

Inglis, A. H., Gray, C. H. G., & Jenkins, R. T. (1932). A voice and ear for telephone measurements. *Bell System Technical Journal*, 293–317.

Killion, M. C. (1979). *Design and evaluation of high-fidelity hearing aids.* Unpublished doctoral dissertation, Northwestern University, Evanston, IL.

Killion, M. C. (1981). Earmold options for wideband hearing aids. *Journal of Speech and Hearing Research, 46*, 10–20.

Killion, M. C. (1983). U.S. Patent 4,592,087.

Killion, M. C. (1987). U.S. Patent 4,689,819, show concept of including amplifier in receiver case.

Killion, M. C. (1993). The K-AMP hearing aid: An attempt to present high fidelity for persons with impaired hearing. *American Journal of Audiology, 2,* 52–74.

Killion, M. C., & Carlson, E. V. (1970). A wideband miniature microphone. *Journal of the Audiologic Engineering Society, 18,* 631–635.

Killion, M. C., & Carlson, E. V. (1974). A subminiature electret-condenser microphone of new design. *Journal of the Audiologic Engineering Society, 22,* 237–243.

Knowles, H. S., & Killion, M. C. (1978). Frequency characteristics of recent broad band receivers. *Journal of Audiologic Technology, 17,* 86–99.

Kranz, F. W. (1928). *Apparatus for aiding hearing.* U.S. Patent 1,679,532. Filed October 10, 1921; issued August 7, 1928.

Kranz, F. W. (1945). Tentative code for measurement of performance of hearing aids. *Journal of the Acoustical Society of America, 17,* 144–150.

Kruger, B., & Kruger, F. M. (1993). The K-AMP hearing aid: A summary of features and benefits. *Hearing Instruments, 44/1,* 30–35; *44/2,* 26–28.

Lieber, H. (1933). U.S. Patent 1,940,533.

Lybarger, S. F. (1938). *Method and apparatus for selecting and prescribing audiophones.* U.S. Patent 2,112,560.

Lybarger, S. F. (1941). *Bone conduction receiver.* U.S. Patent 2,230,499. Filed October 5, 1938; issued February 4, 1941.

Lybarger, S. F. (1947, November). Development of a new hearing aid with magnetic microphone. *Electrical Manufacturing.*

Lybarger, S. F. (1987). An early auditory training system. *Journal of the Audiologic Engineering Society, 35,* 270–275.

Lybarger, S. F., & Olsen, W. O. (1983). Hearing aid measurement standards: An update and bibliography. *Hearing Journal, 36,* 19–20.

Nichols, R. H., Marquis, R. J., Wiklund, W. G., Filler, A. S., Feer, D. B., & Veneklasen, P. S. (1945). *Electro-acoustical characteristics of hearing aids* (OSRD Report 4666). Cambridge, MA: Harvard University, Electro-Acoustic Laboratory. (Library of Congress, Order No. PB 143405)

Nunley, J., Staab, W., Steadman, J., Wechsler, P., & Spencer, B. (1983). A wearable digital hearing aid. *Hearing Journal, 36,* 29–31.

Olson, H. F., & Massa, F. (1934). *Applied acoustics.* Philadelphia, PA: P. Blakiston's Son & Co.

Preves, D. A., & Leisses, M. E. (1995). Some questions about CIC hearing aids. *Audecibel, 44,* 10–16.

Rayleigh, L. (1882). On an instrument capable of measuring the intensity of aerial vibrations. *Phil. Magazine, 14,* 186–187.

Romanow, F. F. (1942). Methods for measuring the performance of hearing aids. *Journal of the Acoustical Society of America, 13,* 294–304.

Sachs, R. M., & Burkhard, M. D. (1972). *Zwislocki coupler evaluation with insert earphones* (Report No. 20022–1). Franklin Park, IL: Knowles Electronics.

Sell, H. (1925). *Microphonic relay.* U.S. Patent 1,624,511. Filed May 6, 1925; issued April 12, 1927.

Skafte, M. D. (1990). 50 years of hearing health care. *Hearing Instruments, 4.*

Staab, W. J. (1987). Digital hearing instruments. *Hearing Instruments, 38.*

Staab, W. J. (1990). Digital/programmable hearing aids—An eye toward the future. *British Journal of Audiology, 24,* 243–256.

Tillyer, E. D. (1923). *Ear trumpet.* U.S. Patent 1,659,965. Filed May 7, 1923; issued February 21, 1928.

Walker, G., & Dillon, H. (1982). *Compression in hearing aids: A review and some recommendations* (NAL Report No. 90). Canberra: Australian Government Publishing Service.

Watson, L. A., & Tolan, T. (1949). *Hearing tests and hearing instruments.* Baltimore, MD: Williams & Wilkins.

Wente, E. C. (1917). A condenser transmitter as a uniformly sensitive instrument for the absolute measurement of sound intensity. *Physics Revue, 10,* 39–63.

West, W. (1929). Measurements of the acoustical impedance of human ears. *Post Office Electrical Engineering Journal, 21,* 293–300.

West, W. (1930). An artificial ear. *Post Office Electrical Engineering Journal, 22,* 260–263.

Wiener, F. M., & Ross, D. A. (1946). The pressure distribution in the auditory canal in a progressive sound field. *Journal of the Acoustical Society of America, 18,* 401–408.

Zwislocki, J. J. (1971). *An earlike coupler for earphone calibration.* (Report No. LSC-S-9). Syracuse, NY: Syracuse University, Laboratory Sensory Communication.

CHAPTER 2

Speech Perception and Hearing Aids

WILLIAM H. MCFARLAND
KAREN SPAYD

INTRODUCTION

The most important goal in fitting hearing aids to the hearing-impaired is the restoration of speech understanding. Although for any one individual there may be some other requirement that takes precedence (Kochkin, 2007).

Advances in hearing aid technology over the last 20 years have improved the ability of hearing health care professionals to provide better hearing of speech by people with hearing impairment, especially in quiet. Patient performance in noise, however while improving, still falls short of the ideal.

Part of the dilemma is most likely related to the diverse needs of people with hearing losses, both personal and physiological, and to the almost impossible task that hearing aids are assigned. Conversational speech sounds vary from an average of 65 to 75 dB sound pressure level (SPL) for the low-frequency vowels and diphthongs, while the consonants may be as much as 30 dB lower in intensity (Fletcher, 1953). Although the long-term speech spectrum or conversational average intensity is 65 to 75 dB SPL, the intensity of vowels and consonants can drastically vary from syllable to syllable. Consonants have a more significant variation compared with vowels, both in intensity and duration. This enormous variation in syllables continues to plague and challenge the hearing aid compressors and amplifiers that must make split-second to second decisions. Furthermore, speech may be embedded in a background of noise as much as 20 to 30 dB higher. The net result must be amplified to audibility,

yet many impaired ears will not have enough residual hearing to detect, let alone recognize, many of the high-frequency consonants that are processed. In ears with enough residual hearing, there still may be poor discrimination of a variety of speech cues.

Finally, there remains the possibility that the hearing aid itself may eliminate important speech sound information due to its inherent limitations in algorithm processing, necessary adjustments by the audiologist, or limitations of advanced circuits that may enhance speech in some situations, but make speech perception worse in others.

THE ACOUSTICAL NATURE OF SPEECH

Speech sounds have a wide range of intensities. Fletcher (1953) described a range of 680 to 1 in the power of the strongest vowel /ɔ/ to the weakest consonant /θ/. This can result in a range of almost 30 dB between different sounds in the same utterance. In general, vowels and diphthongs are the most intense sounds and carry the least amount of information for recognition and understanding of ongoing speech, while the consonants are the weakest of speech sounds and yet carry the most importance for the correct understanding of speech.

The sensation level of speech is also important with regard to understanding. Figure 2–1 illustrates the performance/intensity function for listeners with normal hearing when processing monosyllabic words.

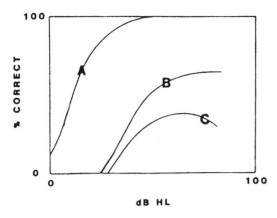

Figure 2–1. Performance-intensity functions. **A.** Normal hearing. **B.** Sensorineural hearing loss. **C.** Retrocochlear disorder. (From Hodgson, W. R. (1988). Discrimination of acoustic signals. In R. E. Sandlin (Ed.), *Handbook of hearing aid amplification, Volume I* (p. 290). Copyright 1995 by Singular Publishing Group. Reprinted with permission.)

Note that, to achieve 100% understanding, the words must be presented at least 25 dB above threshold for the same words (threshold being defined as the level at which 50% of the words are understood) or as much as 40 dB above speech detection level (the level at which the presence of speech is noted, but discrimination may not exist). The performance/intensity function for hearing impaired listeners with cochlear hearing loss shown in the same figure varies significantly from patient to patient but is notably different from that for listeners with normal hearing in that:

■ The range of intensities at which any speech understanding is possible is much reduced;

■ Maximum understanding is often less than 100% and in some instances may be very poor;

■ Understanding may get worse as the intensity of speech increases beyond a certain level.

The intelligibility of individual speech sounds is enhanced by a complex interaction of the frequency, intensity and temporal characteristics of each sound. In addition, speech sound spectra vary considerably from the effect of coarticulation. Amazingly speech sounds still retain their identity at least to listeners with normal hearing, in spite of a wide variety of speakers and adjacent speech sounds. Resonance in the vocal tract results in formant patterns that represent various positions of the tongue, lips, and oral cavity as they create vowels and diphthongs. These formants also provide some information as to the following consonant sounds (Danaher, Osberger, & Pickett, 1973; Martin, Pickett, & Coltin, 1972). So then, some speech sounds are naturally enhanced by the vocal tract whereas others are dampened. Their ability to retain their "identity" in some conditions and not in others remains the focus on hearing aid algorithms, particularly during the "release from masking" methods employed during noise algorithms as described later on in this chapter.

Temporal resolution is also important in speech sound recognition. Changes in duration, pausing, and syllable-rate tempo provide some assistance in speech understanding (Minifie, 1973). Minifie also stated that absolute prediction of intelligibility cannot be made solely on the basis of the spectral characteristics of speech sounds in relation to the configuration of the hearing loss. It is clear, however, that speech spectra are of primary importance in this process. Case in point, some hearing aid fittings and particularly some protocols for children, now demand SII indices to be reported along with prescriptive targets in order to obtain this desired level of prediction of intelligibility. The SII represents the proportion of the speech spectrum that is audible for a given speech material (Moore & Malicka, 2013). The SII is calculated from the spectrum of the speech signal and the subject's hearing thresholds (Moore & Malicka, 2013). Although there may be other cognitive and psychoacoustic overlays in the ultimate understanding of speech, the speech spectra and its potential for its modification continues to be the blueprint for hearing aid analysis and programming.

Figure 2–2 represents the results of a study by Hirsh, Reynolds, and Joseph in 1954.

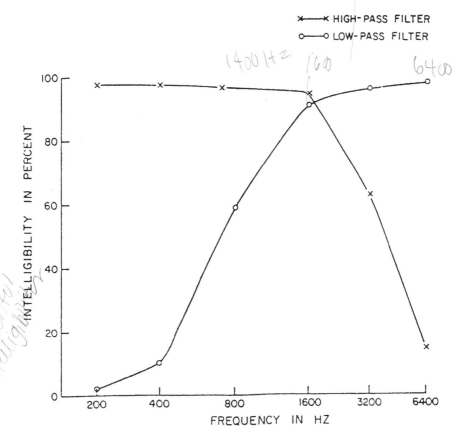

Figure 2–2. Relationship between high- and low-pass filtering and intelligibility of speech. (From Hirsch, I., Reynolds, E., & Joseph, M. (1995). *Speech acoustics and intelligibility.* In R. E. Sandlin (Ed.), *Handbook of hearing aid assessment and use in audiologic habilitation* (p. 95). Copyright 1986 by Williams & Wilkins. Reprinted with permission.)

They measured the intelligibility of monosyllabic words in the Central Institute for the Deaf Auditory Test W22. These investigators examined the effect of various band-pass filter settings on speech intelligibility. The authors found that for low-pass filtering, there was little loss of information with filter cutoffs as low as 1600 Hz. Performance did begin to decline below this, however, and dropped by 25% when the low-pass cutoff reached 800 Hz. High-pass filtering had little effect until 1600 Hz. Above this frequency, performance began to decrease markedly. Clinical guidelines from studies such as this have led to the belief that intact hearing between the frequencies of 500 and 2000 Hz is necessary for relatively normal speech understanding.

How hearing loss configuration degrades speech understanding, given these important speech frequencies, and how the use of hearing aids recovers this lost function is still of utmost importance to the audiologist.

Hearing Loss Configuration and Speech Perception with Hearing Aids

Hodgson (1997) offered the following generalizations about speech intelligibility and hearing loss configuration:

Persons with flat loss will probably have better discrimination than those with sloping high-frequency hearing loss.

Individuals with good low-frequency hearing and a high-frequency loss will hear vowels well and consonants poorly.

There is no impressive evidence that persons with profound loss, fragmented audiograms, and no measurable sensitivity over the speech range (500–2000 Hz) can learn to discriminate speech independent of visual clues.

Perhaps the most commonly used theory in calculating speech perception loss due to hearing loss or speech perception gain after amplification is the Articulation Index (Fletcher, 1929; Fletcher & Galt, 1950, Kryter, 1962a, 1962b.) The standardized version (ANSI S 3.5-1969) identifies the long-term speech spectrum and its overall bandwidth, divides this bandwidth into 20 narrower contiguous bands of different widths but of equal weighting with regard to the contribution toward intelligibility. The standard also incorporates the amplitude fluctuations that contribute to the understanding of speech. The important amplitudes cover a 30 dB range across the range of frequencies included in the index (200–6100 Hz). This 30 dB range is asymmetrically distributed around the rms value of the average long-term speech spectrum. The resolution of the amplitude fluctuations in each band is 1 dB. Thus, this method is more accurate if smaller increments are used in testing than the typical 5 dB increment.

Once pure-tone thresholds are known, the number of decibels of speech above threshold in each band and the weight of each band are calculated to give the total proportion of the speech spectrum that is audible. For example, if all of the spectrum is audible, the articulation index would be 1.0. If only one-half was audible, it would be 0.5, and so on. Clinical measures of pure-tone thresholds typically provide frequency information at only 6 to 9 points across the frequency range. Thus the use of 20 bands may be more appropriate to the researcher than the clinician. Popelka and Mason (1987) described a nine-band method

that would conform better to the octave and half-octave frequencies available to the clinician. The Articulation Index focuses on hearing sensitivity across frequencies. It can give an estimate of the loss of speech intelligibility as a result of hearing loss and also help the clinician calculate the amount of gain needed across the frequency range to elevate the speech spectrum above threshold. Popelka and Mason (1987) cautioned that the Articulation Index only quantifies audibility but does not predict the actual speech recognition performance an individual might have. With complete audibility of the speech spectrum, many individuals with hearing loss still have difficulty understanding speech. This may be a result of suprathreshold auditory processing deficits inherent in the impaired auditory system, limitations of hearing aid processing, or both.

Suprathreshold Considerations in Hearing Loss of Cochlear Origin

A common complaint of people with sensorineural hearing loss is: "Even with my hearing aid(s), I can hear but I can't understand." Moore (1996) stated that, for hearing losses up to 45 dB, audibility is the most important factor. But for losses greater than 45 dB, poorer discrimination of suprathreshold stimuli is also of major importance. This belief is also an extension of another belief that the larger the dB loss, the more inner hair cell damage and involvement, thus creating poorer discrimination. This concept is critical when hearing aids are considered as a way of improving speech intelligibility. Take, for example, a patient who is encouraged to spend significantly more money than he or she has previously spent for advanced programmable digital technology, yet misunderstands important speech information frequently enough to cause dissatisfaction with the hearing aids. The potential for improvement may have been compromised by the poorer suprathreshold processing related to cochlear dysfunction. If there are additional processing difficulties at higher levels of the nervous system (Stach, 1995), the potential for improvement becomes even more restricted.

Hodgson (1995) reported average speech discrimination scores for normal hearers and persons with acquired sensorineural hearing losses (Table 2–1). It should be noted that these results were obtained at suprathreshold levels with amplification deemed enough to provide the best speech understanding. The results show a steady deterioration of speech understanding from 97% for borderline-normal hearing losses to 26% for severe losses (poorer than 66 dB).

A wide body of research has identified several suprathreshold processing skills that are diminished by cochlear loss.

Cochlear Damage and Frequency Selectivity

Frequency selectivity refers to the ability of the auditory system to separate or resolve the components of a complex sound (Moore, 1996). It has been demonstrated that psychophysical tuning curves obtained on animals with cochlear damage are markedly broader than those obtained from animals with normal hearing. Figure 2–3 reveals the wider tuning curve associated with sensorineural hearing loss. Broader psychophysical tuning curves have been found on humans with cochlear losses in studies that used notched-noise maskers (Dubno & Dirks, 1989; Leek & Summers, 1993; Stone, Glasberg, & Moore, 1992). These studies agree that the auditory filters in persons with cochlear loss are broader than normal, and that the degree of broadening increases with increasing hearing loss (Moore, 1996).

A behavioral consequence of these broader tuning curves may result in poorer frequency discrimination. Hodgson (1995) stated that difference limen for frequency (DLF) is increased on individuals with sensorineural hearing loss; that is, they require a greater change in

Table 2–1. Auditory Discrimination Scores of Patients with Acquired Sensorineural Hearing Loss

Thresholds (db re: ANSI 1969 norm)	Age	Number of Ears	Mean Score (%)
Normal (0–10 dB)	Under 65	175	97.31
	Over 65	5	96.40
Borderline normal (11–25 dB)	Under 65	75	97.07
	Over 65	15	94.67
Mild loss (26–45 dB)	Under 65	55	88.36
	Over 65	57	83.12
Moderate loss (46–65 dB)	Under 65	12	63.83
	Over 65	24	66.33
Severe loss (66–85 dB)	Under 65	2	26.00
	Over 65	4	26.50
Profound loss (86+ db)	Under 65	2	2.00

Source: From Hodgson, W. R. 1980. *Basic audiologic evaluation.* Baltimore, MD: Williams & Wilkins. Copyright 1980 by Williams & Wilkins. Reprinted with permission.

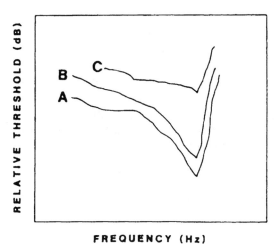

RELATIVE THRESHOLD (dB)

FREQUENCY (Hz)

Figure 2–3. Tuning curves. **A.** Idealized tuning curve on an auditory neuron. **B.** Idealized psychological tuning curve. **C.** Psychophysical tuning curve of an individual with sensorineural hearing loss. (From Hodgson, W. R. (1988). Discrimination of acoustic signals. In R. E. Sandlin (Ed.), *Handbook of hearing aid amplification, Volume I* (p. 284). Copyright 1995 by Singular Publishing Group. Reprinted with permission.)

frequency to detect a difference in pitch than do individuals with normal hearing.

Preminger and Wiley (1985) compared consonant intelligibility with psychoacoustic acoustic tuning curve data and found that sensorineural hearing loss subjects with nearly normal psychoacoustic tuning curves yielded better consonant intelligibility test results.

The upward spread of masking phenomena has been found to influence persons with high-frequency sensorineural hearing loss (Danaher & Pickett, 1975;). This potential interference with consonant recognition is exacerbated if hearing aids deliver excessive low-frequency amplification. Not all studies confirm the importance of spread of masking with sensorineural subjects. Danaher and Pickett (1975) cautioned that upward spread of masking may not be as much a trait of sensorineural hearing loss as the higher SPL of the stimuli used in testing subjects with sensorineural hearing loss.

Patients with sensorineural hearing loss have much greater difficulty hearing in noise than do normal listeners or persons with conductive or mixed hearing losses (Hodgson, 1995; Olsen & Tillman, 1968). Part of the difficulty may relate to the broader filtering activity of the cochlear loss, and some may be related to the upward spread of masking.

Cochlear Damage, Loudness Perception, and Intensity Resolution

Interestingly, the point at which sounds become uncomfortably loud, or the loudness discomfort level (LDL), is about the same SPL for persons with sensorineural hearing loss as it is for others. This creates a phenomenon known as recruitment (Hodgson, 1995). Loudness recruitment and its relationship to losses of cochlear origin are well known (Fowler, 1936; Steinberg & Gardner, 1937). This abnormally rapid loudness growth is related to the fact that that absolute threshold is elevated, but the level at which sounds become uncomfortably loud is still normal. The net result is a much narrower range of loudness between what is barely heard and what is too loud. This narrowed dynamic range obviously presents a challenge when considering the use of a hearing aid. Because of recruitment, one might expect people with cochlear hearing losses to have intensity discrimination that is better than normal. People with cochlear hearing loss perform as well or better than normal if one compares them at equal sensation levels (SL); however, at equal SPL, the person with impaired hearing may be worse than normal for intensity discrimination (Moore, 1996). Moore further stated that, "in everyday life, hearing impaired people often listen at lower SL's than normally hearing people, so their intensity discrimination can be worse than normal. However, this does not appear to lead to marked problems, because it is rare in everyday life for critical information to be carried by small changes in intensity."

Cochlear Damage and Temporal Resolution

There are several measures of temporal resolution, and subjects with hearing impairment perform poorly on some but not all. For example, the detection of gaps in bands of noise is more difficult for the persons with hearing impairment, as are some forms of recovery from forward masking. Again, individuals with impaired hearing are markedly worse if comparisons with normal function are made at the same SPL; they are only slightly worse if made at the same SL (Glasberg, Moore, & Bacon, 1987). For the detection of gaps in sinusoids or a series of clicks, individuals with cochlear hearing loss may actually perform a little better than normal subjects (Jesteadt, Bilger, Green, & Patterson, 1976; Moore & Glasberg, 1988).

Measures of temporal modulation transfer function (TMTF) show the amount of amplitude modulation required for the detection of the modulation, plotted as a function of the modulation rate. It has been assumed that listeners who are hearing impaired are less able to perceive high rates of modulation than are normal listeners. This means that the signal needs to be changed and modified drastically for the impaired listener just to detect this change. This may be true for individuals who have high-frequency sensorineural hearing losses (Bacon & Viemeister, 1985).

When high-frequency hearing loss is simulated through low-pass filtering in people who have normal hearing, they decline in the ability to detect high rates of modulation. Furthermore, when Bacon and Gleitman (1992) measured TMTFs in individuals with relatively flat hearing losses, they found that, at equal SPLs, they performed similarly to individuals with normal hearing, but were better able to detect high modulation rates when they were presented at equal but low sensation levels to both groups. Recall again, that a high-frequency hearing loss has a different AI index from a flat loss, and so this explains this difference in ability to detect high modulation rates.

Thresholds of speech sounds are also affected differentially as a function of the duration of the sound in individuals with normal hearing and those with losses of cochlear origin. Sounds of longer duration need a larger increase in amplitude than do shorter duration sounds.

Moore (1996) stated that, even though persons with cochlear hearing loss do not suffer decline in performance on some measures of temporal resolution with controlled artificial laboratory stimuli, they do in general have more difficulty than listeners with normal hearing in the unpredictable fluctuations of sounds in everyday life. Again, this is because listeners detecting a controlled artificial sound is a different task than detecting a complex speech stimuli that must be stored, integrated, and processed in a myriad of ways by the auditory cortex to yield a behavioral conversational response. All this is beyond the "detection" tasks, which are the only abilities tested in the controlled laboratory.

Presbyacusis and Cognitive Dysfunction

The proportion of elderly people in the United States has increased substantially. The U.S. Census Bureau predicts that the number of elderly will increase from 35 million in the year 2000 to 71 million in 2030. Thus the audiologist is fitting hearing aids to more elderly hearing impaired patients than ever before.

The term presbyacusis is used to describe hearing loss caused by the aging process. Elderly hearing aid patients, however, will most likely come to one's office with hearing difficulties resulting from a variety of factors including presbyacusis.

Although part of their hearing difficulties may be sensory in origin and relate to the pure-tone audiogram, aging can also cause metabolic changes affecting the endocochlear potential (Schmiedt, 2010) and neural changes affecting the auditory pathways (Humes, 2007; Stach, 2000), as well as cognitive problems that may not be specifically related to the auditory system but can significantly reduce the benefit derived from amplification.

NOISE AND SPEECH PERCEPTION IN PERSONS WITH HEARING IMPAIRMENT

As mentioned earlier, it is well known that individuals with hearing losses of cochlear origin have much greater difficulty in perceiving speech in a background of noise than do listeners with normal hearing or persons with conductive or mixed losses. This increased disability in noise may be due, in part, to the spread of masking described by Martin and Pickett (1970) and the abnormal widening of critical bands in pathological ears (Preves, 1995).

Plomp (1994) described a variety of research that measured the speech reception threshold for sentences (s SRT) in a background of noise. The results are expressed in signal-to-noise ratios (SNR) necessary to yield 50% understanding of the sentence material. Invariably, persons with cochlear hearing loss needed an increase in the signal relative to the noise for understanding. The necessary increase ranged from 2.5 dB for mild hearing losses to 7 dB for moderate to severe losses. An even larger increase in SNR is needed when the noise fluctuates, as with a single competing speaker. The increase in speech intensity necessary to achieve threshold in this type of competing noise can range from 9 dB to as much as 25 dB (Baer & Moore, 1994; Eisenberg, Dirks, & Bell, 1995). Figure 2–4 from Killion (1997) illustrates the increase in signal-to-noise ratio required to maintain 50% intelligibility as a function of hearing loss. As is evident in the figure, persons with a 30 dB hearing loss would require a 4 dB increase in SNR, whereas people with an 80 dB hearing loss may need as much as a

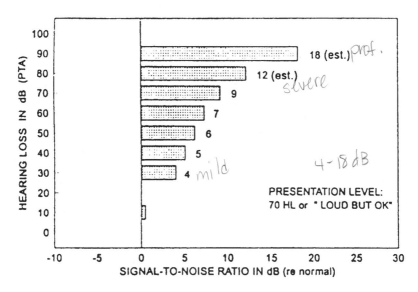

Figure 2–4. Smoothed-average SNR versus HL data. (From Killion, M. (1997). Hearing aids past, present, and future: Moving toward normal conversations in noise. *British Journal of Audiology, 31,* 141–148. Copyright 1997 by Academic Press. Reprinted with permission.)

12 dB increase in SNR to maintain the same 50% level of comprehension.

Signal Processing and Speech Perception

A wide variety of signal processing strategies have been incorporated in hearing aids over the past several years. These include adaptive compression, directional microphones, multichannel compression, digital feedback suppression, high-frequency expansion, directional microphone polar plot manipulation, wide dynamic range compression, compression by bands, and syllabic compression. These have been incorporated in programmable and now digital hearing aids. Multimemory hearing aids allow the user access to different combinations of these processing variables designed to suit different listening situations. Although many of these features have enhanced speech understanding in quiet, they have fallen short of the mark in noise (Killion, 1997).

Compression in its various forms can limit the output of a hearing aid to a level that is safe and comfortable to the listener. With adjustments to compression threshold (CT) and compression ratio (CR), compression can also allow the listener to maintain higher gain for faint and mid-level sounds than he or she would be able to do with a linear instrument. Compression also reduces the need for repeated volume adjustments by the listener. Adaptive compression in selected channels also controls for varying and manipulating the output of hearing aids, thus yielding perhaps the best prediction results and the best SNR for each channel.

The question of whether speech perception is better through compression or linear aids is less clear. Compression applied to low-frequency amplification, as in so-called automatic signal processing (ASP) aids has produced mixed results (Moore, 1996). Studies that seem to suggest benefits may be partly due to the reduction in distortion that such aids provide for sounds at high input levels (Van Tassel & Crain, 1992).

Multiband compression has been found to provide improvement in the comprehension of speech when a wide range of levels was used (Laurence, Moore, & Glasberg, 1983; Moore, Glasberg, & Stone, 1991; Villchur, 1973). When high-level speech input is presented, as is needed with severe to profound hearing losses, compression does not show an improvement over linear amplification. In some studies, fast-acting compression has been found to improve speech understanding in noise as long as the number of bands was kept small (Laurence, Moore, & Glasberg, 1983; Moore, Glasberg, & Stone 1991). This view remains controversial as most hearing aid manufacturers consider having more bands and channels as being more beneficial and these instruments are sold as more expensive circuitries.

Moore (1991) stated that, in part, the lack of advantage for compression instruments in some studies may be related to unrealistically high gain settings chosen for the comparison linear instruments, settings that make sense theoretically for research but would not be maintained by the patient in real-life due to difficulty in tolerating loud sounds.

Multiband compression systems are intended to perform better in noise than single band systems and linear aids by allowing more gain in the high frequencies in the presence of predominately low-frequency noise. Separate CT and CR for each band should allow the audiologist to enhance speech for each person with impaired hearing. When noise exceeds the compression thresholds in the more important high-frequency bands, however, the speech signal will be reduced along with the noise, and the result may be a reduction in comprehension.

The number of bands of compression that are optimal for improved speech understanding in noise is unclear, although it seems that large numbers may not be better than smaller numbers. Yund and Buckles (1995) described improvement in speech understanding in noise with increasing bands until the number of bands reached eight. Moore (1991) suggested that too many bands may reduce the spectral contrasts in speech, thus compromising understanding. Hickson and Byrne (1997) expressed concern that with single-band compression, audiologists may unwittingly alter the consonant-vowel ratio and thus degrade intelligibility.

Wide dynamic range compression instruments are often sold as self-adjusting instruments. It is advantageous to have at least two bands of compression to differentially compensate for recruitment, which is usually worse in the high frequencies. Moore (1991) stated that there is little evidence that these instruments restore loudness perception to normal, and although many elderly patients appreciate the elimination of a need for a volume adjustment, a significant number of patients prefer to modify the overall gain in specific situations.

The use of directional microphones still provides the greatest improvement in speech comprehension in noise. Improvements in directional microphone design now routinely offer a 5 to 6 dB improvement in SNR (Killion et al., 1998). For some hearing-impaired listeners, this can translate to as much as a 60% increase in speech discrimination performance. Directional microphones may create additional problems in some situations. Take, for example, a business executive who may hear better at a conference when the person across the table speaks, but hears much worse when persons on either side make their comments.

Assistive listening devices such as frequency modulation (FM) systems with remote microphones can provide even greater improvement in SNR than directional microphones. They are seldom accepted, however, because of cosmetic considerations or because they impose additional constraints that the user may not be willing to accept.

Perhaps in the future, artificial modification of speech sounds may make them more audible in a background of noise and thus improve speech understanding. Baer, Moore, and Gatehouse (1993) demonstrated that spectral enhancement of consonant sounds does lead to the improvement of consonant recognition in noise.

CURRENT DIGITAL HEARING AIDS

Digital hearing aids first became commercially available in 1987. Two different companies provided instruments that were eventually withdrawn from the market due to high battery drain, large size, and questionable benefit relative to analog hearing aids.

Approximately a decade later, digital aids were reintroduced in sizes and styles comparable with existing analog aids and with improved power consumption. Today almost all commercially available hearing aids are digital.

Digitization of the acoustic signal has allowed the development of new processing strategies, some of which have improved speech perception with digital hearing aids. We review some, but not all, of these digital circuits as they relate to improved speech perception. It should be noted that a more thorough discussion of digital signal processing is found in other chapters of this text.

Compression

Fast acting wide dynamic range compression appears to be more comfortable than more linear amplification, but studies are mixed in its ability to improve speech intelligibility (Costa & Lorio, 2006; Killion et al., 1997; Shi & Doherty, 2008). Interestingly, Gatehouse, Naylor, and Elberling (2006) suggested that WDRC works better with high-frequency sloping loss, and more linear amplification works better with flat losses. After so many years in amplification, there seems to be a permanent tug-of-war between the implementation of fast-acting compression versus slow acting compression. Schum and Sockalingam

(2010) state that advocates of slower acting compression systems argue that information is embedded in the natural intensity differences between one phoneme and the next. Unvoiced fricatives and stops are supposed to be considerably less intense than stressed vowels. Faster acting systems will alter the natural intensity structure of the speech signal. A slower acting WDRC system will preserve these natural phoneme-to-phoneme intensity differences, whereas a faster acting system will destroy this information.

Digital Noise Reduction (DNR)

DNR circuits are designed to reduce gain when nonmodulating noise is detected. There is no strong evidence that these circuits improve speech understanding in noise, especially when the noise is at least partially composed of competing speakers. There is evidence that the DNR circuit improves tolerance or acceptance of noise, however (Bentler, Wuy, Kettel, & Hurtig, 2008; Hornsby, Ricketts, & Johnson, 2006; Mueller, Weber, & Hornsby, 2006; Peters, Kuk, Lau, & Keenan, 2009; Sarampalis, Kallauri, Edwards, & Hafter, 2009).

Directional Microphones

Directional microphones have long been recognized for providing a significant improvement in speech understanding in background noise, especially when the speech and noise come from different directions. Directional microphones can improve the SNR for all types of noises. More recently developed adaptive directional microphones have been found to be effective as well. A limitation of directional microphones is that, at times, important or meaningful sounds or speech that exists in the null areas of the directional microphones will be suppressed more than they would be with omnidirectional microphones. Some studies suggest no difference between directional microphones-only and those with hearing aids with directional microphones plus noise-reduction circuitry in tandem. It seems that directional microphones are the "active" ingredient within most noise-reduction-algorithms. This is surprising, as most hearing aid manufacturers will charge more for hearing aids that include their proprietary noise-reduction circuitry (Bentler, 2005; Magnusson, Claesson, Person, & Tengstrand, 2013).

Frequency Transposition

Frequency transposition has been around since the late 1960s. Transposition is a strategy in which sounds from an unaidable area or dead region (typically in the high frequencies) are transposed to a lower frequency, aidable area with the hope that speech recognition will be improved. Moore and Malicka (2013) have defined a dead region as an "off-frequency listening" or "off-place listening" where a "region in the cochlea where the inner hair cells and/or neurons are functioning so poorly that a tone producing peak vibration in that region is detected by another portion of the cochlea duct." This is termed off-place hearing or listening. Using new assessments such as the Threshold-Equalizing Noise (TEN) test, "a masked threshold that is 10 dB higher than normal is usually taken as indicating a dead region"(Moore & Malicka, 2013). These authors conclude that subjects with dead regions have poorer understanding of speech in noise than those without dead regions. Using amplification, their research indicated that listeners with moderate to severe hearing loss, without dead regions, showed a benefit from amplification for frequencies up to 4 kHz; however, for those listeners with extensive dead regions, there was little benefit, or even a degradation, when amplification was provided for frequencies up to 2 kfe (frequency edge). Kuk, Keenan, Korhonen, and Lau (2009) states that early attempts with frequency transposition were not practical enough to be implemented into hearing aids. While lowering speech frequencies, these methods also altered other aspects of speech that were important for recognition. Recent research has focused on such questions as whether frequency compression (where the bandwidth of transposed frequencies are compressed) is better than linear frequency transposition for speech sound perception. Kuk et al. (2009) states that linear frequency transposition is preferable to frequency compression for the improved fricative recognition.

Auditory training is usually recommended to improve the perception of unnatural transposed speech. Evidence that frequency transposition improves speech understanding in people with unusable high-frequency hearing is mixed (Robinson, Stainsby, Baer, & Moore, 2009). Clearly, the benefit is small if it exists and auditory training continues to be recommended.

CONCLUSION

Moderate, severe, and profound hearing losses of cochlear origin often have accompanying residual hearing that is markedly poorer in its ability to discriminate the frequency, intensity, and timing cues in sound —factors that are more important to the understanding of speech than the residual hearing associated with milder losses. Furthermore, the degree of residual impairment appears to be related to the degree of hearing loss: Individuals with profound hearing losses tend to have less useful residual hearing than persons with severe losses, and so on. The same individuals have significantly greater difficulty understanding speech in a background of noise than persons with normal hearing or milder hearing losses.

This reduced ability to understand speech in noise is most likely related to the poorer suprathreshold discrimination abilities of these individuals, as well as the spread-of-masking phenomenon.

It should be remembered that these deficits have been identified utilizing laboratory equipment that offers much a greater ability to reach residual hearing across the frequen-

cies for an individual with hearing impairment than do personal hearing aids. Practical clinical realities often further reduce important sounds of speech needed for optimal understanding. Examples of these clinical realities are: (1) feedback and the unfortunate need to reduce important high-frequency gain to control it; and (2) the patient's personal demand to use only the smallest cosmetically appealing hearing aid, such as a CIC (for completely in the canal) hearing aid. (These small aids may not have enough gain for the hearing loss being treated, or automatic gain reductions imposed by a hearing aid either through its compression circuit or its noise reduction circuit.) Although these automatic reductions in gain may improve user comfort or reduce background noise, they typically also reduce some useful speech information.

New technology, especially digital technology, has improved our ability to address these limitations; however, the question remains open as to whether the purchase of these more expensive devices with their more intricate processing is wasted on individuals who cannot hear or discriminate the nuances they purport to aid. In addition to the new technology and efforts described herein, new objective measures in speech perception have also been recently introduced. In general, these new measures assess listening effort and include "physiologic, recall, and reaction time based paradigms" (Mueller, 2013). Perhaps these will shed new light beyond speech understanding, which includes listener's efforts.

Successful fitting of hearing aids to persons with sensorineural hearing losses of cochlear origin is no small task. These hearing losses present not only losses of hearing sensitivity but also deficits in the frequency, intensity, and temporal processing acuity for sounds that are audible. Advances in hearing aid technology, such as varying types of compression and multiple channels, allow more flexibility in the shaping of the frequency–gain characteristics of the instrument. Nonetheless, improvements in speech comprehension in noise have been modest and remain the primary challenge of the 21st century.

REVIEW QUESTIONS

1. An Articulation Index of _____ indicates that a person should receive about half the speech information necessary for understanding.

2. The Articulation Index addresses amplitude fluctuations over a __30__ dB range.

3. The weakest sound of speech is: _____. *consonants*

4. With sensorineural hearing losses, an increase in the presentation level of speech can result in _poorer discrim_.

5. Hirsch, Reynolds, and Joseph (1954) found that speech intelligibility began to decline when low-pass filters were adjusted below __800__ Hz. *pg 38*

6. Moore (1996) stated that, for hearing losses below __45__ dB, the primary reason a person does not understand is his or her threshold.

7. Persons with sensorineural hearing losses often have psychophysical tuning curves that are _____ than normal. *broader*

8. TMTF stands for _temporal modulation transfer function_.

9. A narrowed dynamic range between threshold and loudness discomfort indicates the presence of _recruitment_.

10. The most significant improvement, at this time, in hearing aid technology to reduce background noise is _directional mics_.

REFERENCES

ANSI. (S3.5-1969). *American national standard methods for the calculation of the articulation index.* New York, NY: American National Standards Institute.

Bacon, S., & Gleitman, R. (1992). Modulation detection in subjects with relatively flat hearing losses. *Journal of Speech and Hearing Research, 35,* 642–653.

Bacon, S., & Viemeister, N. (1985). Temporal modulation transfer functions in normal and hearing-impaired subjects. *Audiology, 24,* 117–134.

Baer, T., & Moore, B. (1994). Effects of spectral smearing on the intelligibility of sentences in the presence of interfering speech. *Journal of the Acoustical Society of America, 95,* 2277–2280.

Baer, T., Moore, B., & Gatehouse, S. (1993). Spectral contrast enhancement of speech in noise for listeners with sensorineural hearing impairment: Effects on intelligibility, quality and response times. *Journal of Rehabilitation Research and Development, 30,* 49–72.

Bentler, R. (2005). Effectiveness of directional microphones and noise reduction schemes in hearing aids: A systematic review of evidence. *Journal of the American Academy of Audiology, 16*(7), 473–484.

Bentler, R., Wuy, Y. H., Kettel, J., & Hurtig, R. (2008). Digital noise reduction: Outcome from laboratory and field studies. *International Journal Audiology, 47*(8), 447–460.

Costa, L. P., & Lorio, M. C. (2006). Hearing aids: Objective and subjective evaluations of linear and nonlinear amplification users. *Pro Fono, 18*(1), 21–30.

Danaher, E., Osberger, N., & Pickett, J. (1973). Discrimination of formant frequency transitions in synthetic vowels. *Journal of Speech and Hearing Research, 16,* 439–451.

Danaher, E., & Pickett, J. (1975). Some masking effects produced by low-frequency vowel formants in persons with sensorineural hearing loss. *Journal of Speech and Hearing Research, 18,* 261–271.

Dubno, J., & Dirks, D. (1989). Auditory filter characteristics and consonant recognition for hearing-impaired listeners. *Journal of the Acoustical Society of America, 85,* 1666–1675.

Eisenberg, L., Dirks, D., & Bell, T. (1995). Speech recognition in amplitude modulated noise of listeners with normal and with impaired hearing. *Journal of Speech and Hearing Research, 38,* 222–233.

Fletcher, H. (1929). *Speech and hearing.* New York, NY: Van Nostrand.

Fletcher, H. (1953). *Speech and hearing in communication.* Princeton, NJ: Van Nostrand.

Fletcher, H., & Galt, R. (1950). The perception of speech and its relation to telephony. *Journal of the Acoustical Society of America, 22,* 89–151.

Fowler, E. (1936). A method for the early detection of otosclerosis. *Archives of Otolaryngology, 24,* 731–741.

Gatehouse, S., Naylor, G., & Elberling, C. (2006). Linear and nonlinear hearing aid fittings—Patterns of candidature. *International Journal of Audiology, 45*(3), 153–171.

Glasberg, B., Moore, B., & Bacon, S. (1987). Gap detection and masking in hearing-impaired and normal hearing subjects. *Journal of the Acoustical Society of America, 81,* 1546–1556.

Hickson, L., & Byrne, D. (1997). Consonant perception in quiet: Effect of increasing the consonant-vowel ratio with compression amplification. *Journal of the American Academy of Audiology, 8*, 322–332.

Hirsh, I., Reynolds, E., & Joseph, M. (1954). Intelligibility of different speech materials. *Journal of the Acoustical Society of America, 26*, 530–538.

Hodgson, W. R. (1995). Discrimination of acoustic signals. In R. Sandlin (Ed.), *Handbook of hearing aid amplification. Volume 1: Theoretical and technical considerations* (pp. 281–297). San Diego, CA: Singular.

Hodgson, W. R. (1997). Speech acoustics and intelligibility. In W. Hodgson & P. Skinner (Eds.), *Hearing aid assessment and use in audiologic habilitation.* Baltimore, MD: Williams & Wilkins.

Hornsby, B. W., Ricketts, T. A., & Johnson, E. E. (2006). The effects of speech and speech like maskers on aided and unaided speech recognition in persons with hearing loss. *Journal of the Academy of Audiology, 17*(6), 432–447.

Humes, L. (2007). The contributions of audibility and cognitive factors to the benefit provided by amplified speech to older adults. *Journal of the American Academy of Audiology, 18*(7), 590–603.

Jesteadt, W., Bilger, R., Green, D., & Patterson, J. (1976). Temporal acuity in listeners with sensorineural hearing loss. *Journal of Speech and Hearing Research, 19*, 357–370.

Killion, M. (1997). Hearing aids: Past, present and future. Moving toward normal conversation in noise. *British Journal of Audiology, 31*, 141–148.

Killion, M. C., Schulein, R., Christensen, L. A., Fabry, D., Revit, L. J., Niquette, P., & Chung, K. (1998). Real-world performance of an ITE directional microphone. *The Hearing Journal, 51*(4), 24–38.

Kochkin, S. (2007). Increased hearing aid adoption through multiple environmental listening utility. *The Hearing Journal, 60*(11), 28–29.

Kryter, K. (1962a). Methods for the calculation and use of the articulation index. *Journal of the Acoustical Society of America, 34*, 1689–1697.

Kryter, K. (1962b). Validity of the articulation index. *Journal of the Acoustical Society of America, 34*, 1680–1702.

Kuk, F., Keenan, D., Korhonen, P., & Lau, C. C. (2009). Efficacy of linear frequency transposition on consonant identification in quiet and in noise. *Journal of American Academy of Audiology, 20*(8), 465–479.

Laurence, R., Moore, B., & Glasberg, B. (1983). A comparison of behind-the-ear high fidelity linear aids and two channel compression hearing aids in the laboratory and in everyday life. *British Journal of Audiology, 17*, 31–48.

Leek, M., & Summers, V. (1993). Auditory filter shapes of normal-hearing and hearing-impaired listeners in continuous broad band noise. *Journal of the Acoustical Society of America, 94*, 3127–3137.

Magnusson, L., Claesson, A., Person, M., Tengstrand, T. (2013). Speech recognition in noise using bilateral open-fit hearing aids: The limited benefit of directional microphones and noise reduction. *International Journal of Audiology, 52*, 29–36.

Martin, E., & Pickett, J. (1970). Sensorineural hearing loss and the upward spread of masking. *Journal of Speech and Hearing Research, 13*, 426–437.

Martin, E., Pickett, J., & Coltin, S. (1972). Discrimination in vowel formant transitions by listeners with severe sensorineural hearing loss. In G. Fant (Ed.), *Speech communication ability and profound deafness* (Paper 9). Washington, DC: A. G. Bell Association for the Deaf.

Minifie, F. (1973). Speech acoustics. In F. Minifie, T. Hixon, & F. Williams (Eds.), *Normal aspects of speech, hearing and language.* Englewood Cliffs, NJ: Prentice-Hall.

Moore, B. (1991). Characterization and simulation of impaired hearing: Implications for hearing aid design. *Ear and Hearing, 12*, 154S–161S.

Moore, B. (1996). Perceptual consequences of cochlear hearing loss and their implications for the design of hearing aids. *Ear and Hearing, 17*, 133–161.

Moore, B., & Glasberg, B. (1988). Gap detection with sinusoids and noise in normal, impaired and electrically stimulated ears. *Journal of the Acoustical Society of America, 83*, 1093–1101.

Moore, B., Glasberg, B., & Stone, M. (1991). Optimization of a slow-acting automatic gain control system for use in hearing aids. *British Journal of Audiology, 25*, 171–182.

Moore, B., & Malicka, A. (2013). Cochlear dead regions in adults and children: Diagnosis and clinical implications. *Seminars in Hearing, 34*(1), 37–50.

Mueller, G. (2013). *20Q: Listening effort—We know it's a problem but how do you measure it?* Retrieved from http://www. Audiologyonline.com

Mueller, H. G., Weber, J., & Hornsby, B. W. (2006). The effects of digital noise reduction on the acceptance of background noise. *Trends Amplify, 10*(2), 83–93.

Olsen, W., & Tillman, T. (1968). Hearing aids and sensorineural hearing loss. *Annals of Otology, Rhinology, and Laryngology, 7*, 717–726.

Peters, H., Kuk, F., Lau, C. C., & Keenan, D. (2009). Subjective and objective evaluation of noise management algorithms. *Journal of the American Academy of Audiology, 20*(2), 89–98.

Plomp, R. (1994). Noise, amplification and compression: Considerations of three issues in hearing aid design. *Ear and Hearing, 15*, 2–12.

Popelka, G., & Mason, D. (1987). Factors which affect measures of speech audibility with hearing aids. *Ear and Hearing, 8*(Suppl.), 109S–118S.

Preminger, J., & Wiley, T. (1985). Frequency selectivity and consonant intelligibility in sensorineural hearing loss. *Journal of Speech and Hearing Research, 28*, 197–206.

Preves, D. (1995). Principles of signal processing. In R. Sandlin (Ed.), *Handbook of hearing aid amplification. Volume 1: Theoretical and technical considerations* (pp. 81–120). San Diego, CA: Singular.

Robinson, J. D., Stainsby, T. H., Baer, T., & Moore, B. C. (2009). Evaluation of a frequency transposition algorithm using wearable hearing aids. *International Journal of Audiology, 48*(6), 384–393.

Sarampalis, A., Kallauri, S., Edwards, B., & Hafter, E. (2009). Objective measures of listening effort: Effects of background noise and noise reduction. *Journal of Speech, Language, and Hearing Research, 52*(5), 1230–1240.

Schmiedt, R. (2010). Aging and the auditory periphery. *Audiology Today.*

Schum, D., & Sockalingam, R. (2010). A new approach to nonlinear signal processing. *The Hearing Review, 17*(7), 24–32.

Shi, L. F., & Doherty, K. A. (2008). Subjective and objective effects of fast and slow compression on the perception of reverberant speech in listeners with hearing loss. *Journal of Speech, Language, and Hearing Research, 51*(5), 1328–1340.

Stach, B. (1995). Hearing aid amplification and central processing disorders. In R. Sandlin (Ed.), *Handbook of hearing aid amplification. Volume 2: Clinical considerations and fitting practices* (pp. 87–112). San Diego, CA: Singular.

Stach, B. (2000). Hearing aid amplification and cen-tral auditory disorders in R. Sandlin (Ed.), *Textbook of hearing aid amplification. Technical and clinical considerations* (2nd ed.). San Diego, CA: Singular.

Steinberg, J., & Gardner, M. (1937). The dependency of hearing impairment on sound intensity. *Journal of the Acoustical Society of America, 77,* 621–627.

Stone, M., Glasberg, B., & Moore, B. (1992). Simplified measurement of impaired auditory filter shapes using the notched-noise method. *British Journal of Audiology, 26,* 329–334.

Van Tassel, D., & Crain, T. (1992). Noise reduction hearing aids: Release from masking and release from distortion. *Ear and Hearing, 13,* 114–121.

Villchur, E. (1973). Signal processing to improve speech intelligibility in perceptive deafness. *Journal of the Acoustical Society of America, 53,* 1646–1657.

Yund, E., & Buckles, K. (1995). Enhanced speech perception at low signal-to-noise ratios with multi-channel compression hearing aids. *Journal of the Acoustical Society of America, 97*(20), 1224–1240.

CHAPTER 3

Custom Hearing Aid Earshells and Earmolds

CHESTER Z. PIRZANSKI

INTRODUCTION

Digital technology has made a large impact on hearing instrument design and fitting. Digital signal processing contributed to better frequency equalization and the use of multiple-band compression with variable parameters. It has been used to improve feedback cancellation, noise reduction, and adaptive directional-microphone arrays. Now digital acoustics are moving in directions that were not possible with analog hearing aids: neural networks, binaural processing, and adaptive beamforming networks. Today's digital hearing aids communicate with each other wirelessly to keep the sound picture real in both ears. They also connect through Bluetooth devices with cell phones, mp3 players, laptops, TVs, and video games to create a private link for communication.

The hearing health care industry has embraced in recent years another challenge —the widespread application of digital imaging and computer-aided design and manufacturing (CAD/CAM) technology in manufacturing custom ear-level hearing aids and earmolds. The main advantage of this new process is the precision with which it captures and reproduces the shape of the ear impression, so that the earmold is accurately rendered and effectively manufactured. Additionally, the turnaround time is reduced for clinics that are equipped with three-dimensional scanners. Electronic transmitting the three-dimensional model of the impression eliminates the time for the impression to be shipped to the manufacturer.

Digital technology is providing the technical platform to eliminate the ear impression and replace it with a digital scan of the external ear. Scanning the ear has always been a dream in the hearing care profession, and we are now moving closer to the day when it may be a reality.

This chapter discusses a variety of topics related to the physical and acoustic aspect of hearing aid shell and earmold fittings.

THE HUMAN EAR

The ear is the organ that detects sound. Sound is a form of energy that moves through air, water, and other matter, in waves of pressure. Sound is the means of auditory communication, including frog calls, bird songs, and spoken language. Although the ear is a sense organ that recognizes sound, it is the brain and central nervous system that *hears*. The ear changes sound pressure waves from the outside world into a signal of nerve impulses sent to the brain. Human beings localize sound within the central nervous system, by comparing arrival-time differences and loudness from each ear, in brain circuits that are connected to both ears.

When describing parts of the body, we use terms to define position and direction. The body may be sectioned in one of three planes relative to a three-dimensional coordinate system (X-Y-Z). Human body planes and anatomical directions and positions are provided in Figure 3–1.

The word *ear* may be used correctly to describe the entire organ or just the visible external portion. The external ear is shown in the sagittal, frontal, and transverse views in Figure 3–2. The outer ear that collects sound is the most external portion of the ear. It includes the pinna (called auricle), the ear canal (called external acoustic meatus), and the very most superficial layer of the eardrum (called the tympanic membrane). The pinna projects from the side of the head and serves to collect the vibrations of the air by which sound is produced; the ear canal leads inward from the bottom of the auricula and conducts the vibrations to the tympanic cavity. The pinna is of an ovoid form with its larger end directed upward. Its lateral surface is irregularly concave, directed slightly forward, and presents numerous eminences and depressions. The prominent rim of the auricula is called the helix. Another curved prominence, parallel with and in front of the helix, is called the antihelix. The antihelix describes a curve

BODY PLANES
MEDIAN (A)
The median plane divides the body into left/right halves.
SAGITTAL (B)
The plane dividing the body into unequal left and right parts and parallel to the median plane. The terms median and lateral relate to this plane.
CORONAL, FRONTAL (C)
The plane dividing the body into equal/unequal front and back parts. The terms anterior/posterior relate to this plane.
TRANSVERSE, CROSS HORIZONTAL (D) The horizontal plane divides the body into upper (cranial) and lower (caudal) parts. Cross/transverse sections are perpendicular to the long axis of the body or other structures and may not be horizontal.

ANATOMICAL DIRECTIONS/POSITIONS
CRANIAL, SUPERIOR (E)
These terms refer to a structure being closer to the head or higher than another structure in the body.
CAUDIAL, INFERIOR (F)
These terms refer to a structure being closer to the feet or lower than another structure in the body.
ANTERIOR, VENTRAL (G)
These terms refer to a structure being more in back than another structure in the body.
POSTERIOR, DORSAL (H)
These terms refer to a structure being more in back than another structure in the body.
MEDIAL (I)
This term refers to a structure being closer to the median plane than another structure in the body.
LATERAL (J)
This term refers to a structure being further away from the median plane than another structure in the body.

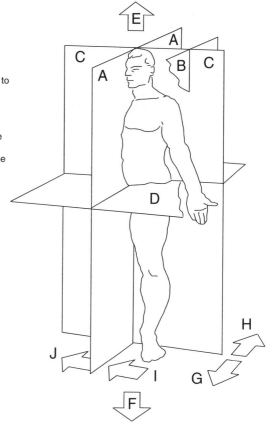

Figure 3–1. Human body planes, anatomical directions, and positions.

around a deep, capacious cavity, the concha, which is partially divided into two parts by the crus; the upper part is termed the cymba concha, the lower part the cavum concha. In front of the concha, and projecting backward over the ear canal, is a small pointed eminence, the tragus, so called from being generally covered on its under surface with a tuft of hair, resembling a goat's beard (from Greek *tragos*). Opposite the tragus, and separated from it by the intertragic notch, is the antitragus. Below this is the lobule (Gray's Anatomy, 2010).

The ear canal has two bends, with the eardrum located beyond the second bend, except in cases such as surgical patients and those with developmental anomalies or mal-

formations (i.e., atresia, stenosis, etc.). These bends, observed in the transverse view of the ear, give the canal a unique but consistent pattern of parallel lines: The tragus line tends to be parallel to the line of the canal medial end. These two bends have approximately the same angle.

The skin at the canal aperture is thick and contains glands as well as hair follicles. The glands make cerumen (also called ear wax). The canal skin is applied to cartilage. This cartilage is soft and forgiving, and can be stretched by an earmold and still remain within comfort limits. The cartilage is also subject to shifting resulting from jaw movements. The jaw's downward movement commonly stretches the anterior ear wall and

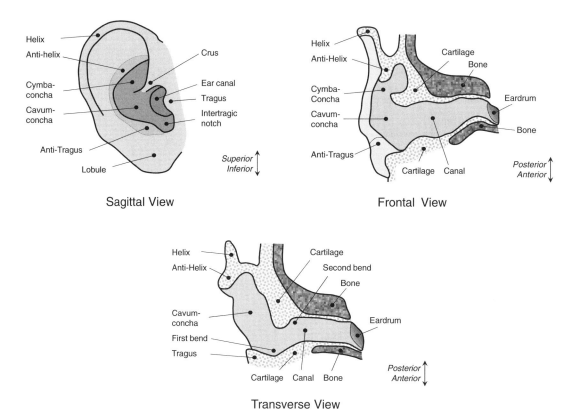

Figure 3–2. Side view and cross-sections of the external human ear: **A.** Sagittal view (or Lateral), **B.** Frontal view (or Coronal), and **C.** Axial view (or Transverse).

increases the volume of the ear canal. Beyond the canal second bend, the cartilage thins and eventually disappears, and the ear wall becomes more rigid. The underlying tissue has no subcutaneous layer, is thin, and highly vascular. The skin of the bony canal is the most delicate skin in the human body and is tightly applied to the underlying bone.

THE EAR IMPRESSION

A custom hearing aid requires an earpiece to couple the device with the ear canal, both acoustically and physically. For a BTE (behind-the-ear) hearing aid, the coupler is an earmold, for an in-the-ear hearing aid it is an earshell. To make a custom earmold or earshell, a model of the ear is required. The model, called an ear impression, is obtained by filling the external ear with soft putty plastic, commonly silicone. The silicone polymerizes and sets in the ear within minutes, becoming a true negative replica of the ear. There is a direct relationship between the technique with which the ear impression is made, the skill level of the technician who crafts the earmold, and the patient's satisfaction with the hearing instrument.

Research data indicates that hearing aid shells and earmolds have a greater chance of being feedback free and comfortable if ear impressions:

1. Have no underfilled areas such as gaps, weld marks, or air pockets;
2. Illustrate the two bends of the auditory passage in full;
3. Have high after-cure dimensional stability;

4. Adequately reflect the softness of the cartilaginous tissue of the ear; and

5. Demonstrate the increase in the ear canal diameter resulting from the jaw's downward movement.

Figure 3–3 shows a transverse view of the ear with an ear impression made past the canal second bend, and an earmold crafted from that impression. Note the location of the ear canal's first and second bends and the canal parallel structure.

Otoscopic Examination

Preparation for taking an ear impression must include hygienic procedures that are strictly followed as a matter of routine: Wash your hands thoroughly with soap and warm water before and after making the impression, unless gloves or a pistol injector is used. Clean the specula of the otoscope, ear-light tip, syringe, and so on, with an antiseptic solution. Some equipment used in otoscopy is not meant for reuse, and therefore the cleaning of these pieces is inappropriate.

During otoscopic examination:

1. Check the ear canal for foreign objects, excessive wax, abnormal growths, or any condition that is out of the ordinary. Determine whether or not wax removal is appropriate. If removal is contradicted or beyond your scope or comfort level, a referral to an otologist or otolaryngologist is recommended.

2. Check the ear canal for size to determine how large an oto-block needs to be used. Blocks that are too small may get pushed down the canal by the impression material and allow the material to flow past the block. Blocks that are too large may not go far enough into the ear canal. If you are dealing with a postsurgical ear, use a larger oto-block than normal, or several oto-blocks.

3. Check which way the canal twists and bends. Look for the second anatomical bend. This will give you an idea of which direction to push the block for insertion in the proper position.

4. Encourage the patient to open and close their mouth to determine the effects of

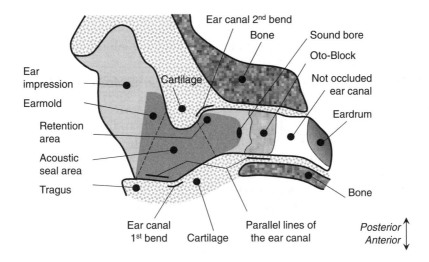

Transverse view

Figure 3–3. The transverse view of the human ear shown with an ear impression taken past the canal second bend and an earmold crafted from the impression.

mandibular movements on the ear canal wall. Look at the anterior ear wall at the canal aperture. If any movement is apparent, taking an open-mouth impression is recommended.

5. Check for landmarks in the canal. Look for any bumps, hollows, or ridges and circle them later on the finished impression. This ensures that the earmold lab technician will not fill the voids assuming they were air pockets or other imperfections.

Tools and Accessories

Depending on the impression-taking technique and material, the selection of tools and accessories employed for impression making will vary. This includes the selection of oto-blocks, syringes, pistol injectors, mouth props, and other items.

Oto-Block

The function of an oto-block is to prevent impression material from reaching the eardrum. All ear impressions should be taken with an oto-block. Oto-blocks are made of cotton or foam and come in a variety of sizes. Foam oto-blocks can come standard with a thread, or pressure relief with a ventilation tube. A vented block consists of a dam made from a slow recovery foam and a ventilation tube. The purpose of the tube is to equalize air pressure, make impression removal easier, and reduce the risk of vascular irritation.

Flattening the cotton ball out helps to seal the canal so the impression material does not flow around it. Cotton tends to be more comfortable for deeper canal impressions. However, in a draining ear or a post-surgical ear canal, cotton fibers may adhere to the canal wall and provide a host for bacterial infection.

Mouth Prop

A mouth prop is a white styrofoam block (see Figure 3–7). It is used to take ear impressions with the client's mouth wide open. The prop must be inserted into the patient's mouth prior to syringing the impression material and must remain there until the impression has cured.

Marking Card

When an impression for a hearing aid with a directional microphone is taken, use a marking card to imprint the horizontal plane of the ear in the hardening silicone. The mark in the impression will allow the earmold lab technician to properly align the microphones on the hearing aid faceplate.

Impression Syringe

Syringes are most commonly used for impression taking. They are loaded from the back. The impression material is deposited in the barrel and moved forward with the insertion of the plunger. Loading is commonly a one-step operation. However, in some syringes, two-step loading is required. First, the impression material is deposited in the larger chamber. Then, with the insertion of the plunger, the material is pushed into the smaller chamber. There are over 10 different models of syringes on the market. The most commonly recommended are syringes that are easy to load, self-cleaning, offer a good grip, and require minimum pressure to operate.

Manual and Motorized Injectors

There are four different pistol injectors available in audiology: (1) manual injector, (2) manual injector S50, (3) motorized Injector Control, and (4) motorized cordless Ez-mix HI injector. Images of the injectors are provided in Figure 3–4.

There are two types of cartridges for the injectors: 48 mL and S50. The manual injector is designed for the 48-mL cartridge, and the S50 injector is suitable for the S50 cartridge. Both motorized injectors can be used with either type of cartridge.

Injectors offer a "mess-free" work environment. The injector can be assembled within

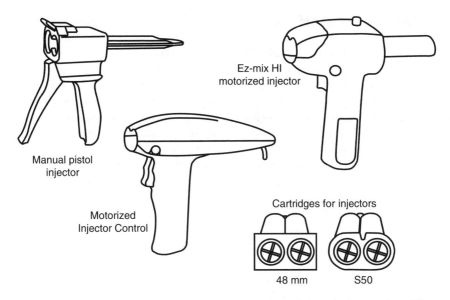

Figure 3–4. Pistol injectors and cartridges used in audiology for impression taking.

a couple of minutes and does not require any advanced maintenance. The impression material is provided in a dual-barrel cartridge. With a push on the trigger, a two-part silicone is automatically mixed in the mixing canula and dispensed directly into the ear. There is little material wasted because only the necessary amount of silicone is mixed.

Manual pistol injectors present unique difficulties in the process of making the impression. The amount of material delivered from one pull on the hand-crank lever is not adequate to take one impression. This necessitates a mid-process recocking of the injector (releasing the lever so the ratchet can reset itself), which in turn interrupts the flow of impression material. The injector has to be recocked three to four times to fill the average ear. Typically, the recocking is evidenced by voids and air pockets in the finished impression.

The motorized electric Injector Control from Dreve operates on a 12V battery pack or an AC adapter. Either is attached to the pistol's handle through a coiled wire. The adapter also doubles as the battery-recharging device. By depressing the trigger, the electric motor is engaged, and the silicone is automat-

ically mixed and dosed. This eliminates the repetitive hand action and prevents shaking movements that are common with manual injectors. The speed of injection is controlled with the push on the trigger and is up to 1 ml/sec. This allows for filling the ear within 5 to 10 seconds.

The Ez-mix injector runs on an AC adapter or a rechargeable battery pack. The battery is housed in the pistol's handle, which makes the pistol truly portable. The type of cartridge must be specified while ordering the injector because each type of cartridge (48-ml or S50) requires a different retainer and push pads. The speed of injection and drip-free feature are similar to Injector Control.

Mixing Canulas

Mixing canulas for cartridges come in different sizes to best match the size of the ear canal. Canulas are disposable and cannot be reused. Each new impression requires a new canula, unless two impressions are taken subsequently as for a binaural fitting. After the impression is taken, the canula is to be left attached to the cartridge until next impression is made.

Impression Materials

Consideration is to be given to the selection of the impression material. The right choice will increase the chance of a successful fitting.

The most commonly used impression materials are addition-cure vinylpolysiloxanes, called silicones. The material is mixed by blending two putties (A and B) at 1:1 ratio. Other impression materials include condensation-cure silicones (25:1 mixing ratio) and powder-and-liquid (e.g., acrylic).

The components for all silicones are supplied in contrasting colors to provide means of indicating when a uniform, streak-free mix is achieved. Impression materials differ not only in the type of cure, mixing procedures, and color, but also in after-mix viscosity, contraction ratio and stress relaxation, as well as in setting time, after-cure hardness, and effectiveness of the release agent.

Viscosity

Viscosity of an impression material is defined as a measure of the material consistency before polymerization. Viscous means having a thick or sticky consistency. A silicone can be of low, medium, or higher viscosity. A low-viscosity silicone has a soft consistency, a higher viscosity silicone is denser. Although the consistency of currently available impression materials significantly varies from one material to another, manufacturers generally do not provide a description of viscosity.

Assessing impression material viscosity by its color or brand name can be misleading. Manufacturers of impression materials sell their product in a variety of shades to various distributors. This means that a yellow silicone being sold under one brand name may be a different viscosity than another yellow silicone offered under another brand name. On the other hand, a green silicone provided by different distributors, often under a different price, may have identical viscosity.

Silicones offered in a rectangular-flange 48-mL cartridge are all low viscosity. Silicones in the rounded-flange S50 cartridge are either low or medium viscosity. Hand-mixed silicones are medium or higher viscosity.

There are no higher viscosity silicones available in cartridges. Still, the clinician may come across "high" (or firm) viscosity silicones in S50 cartridges offered by some suppliers. In this author's classification scheme, these silicones are not as dense as higher viscosity hand-mixed silicones for syringes. It is unlikely that true higher viscosity silicones will be available in cartridges. The concern is that injectors used in audiology are not strong enough to extrude a higher viscosity silicone though a mixing canula. This suggests that a clinician who wants to employ a higher viscosity silicone will have to choose one from the hand-mixed variety that is available only for syringes.

Figure 3–5 shows the viscosity of silicone impression materials distributed by Egger. Note that materials offered in both 48-ml and S50 cartridges are low viscosity. The medium viscosity A/II silicone in the S50 cartridge is as viscous as A/II for syringe. Higher viscosity silicones are available only for syringes. Clinicians may use trade shows and convention exhibits to get familiar with the variety of impression materials available from local suppliers, discuss the impression materials they use, and inquire about better alternatives.

Cartridge silicones are regarded by some audiologists as superior to syringed silicones as they supposedly flow more freely into the ear canal and fill all crevices and undercuts. This opinion is incorrect. All currently available cartridge silicones are formulated as thixotropic materials, which means that their ability to flow freely is eliminated. With either type of silicone, the ear impression is molded by injection, not by free flow.

A medium or higher viscosity silicone is better to use on patients having hair in their ears. When syringed into the ear, a denser silicone will press down the hair. In contrast, a light silicone will flow through the hair making the impression painful to remove and leaving substantial voids and flaws on its surface.

Shore Value

The shore value of an impression material refers to the finished impression hardness 1 hour after the impression was made. The

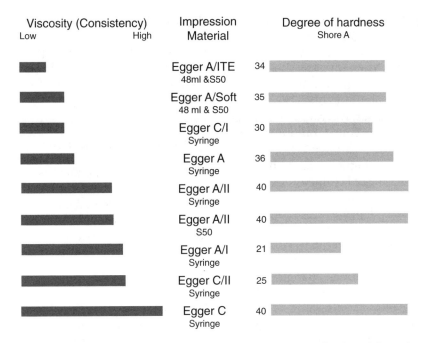

Figure 3–5. Egger Otoplastic impression material selection. Adapted from egger Otoplastik + Labortechnik GmbH, http://www.egger-labor.de with permission.

lower the shore value, the softer the finished impression. Clinicians often relay on the shore value as the guideline for the silicone consistency. There is an opinion that silicones with a higher shore value are more viscous. That is not necessarily correct. As provided in Figure 3–5, there is no apparent relationship between the viscosity of a silicone and its shore value. In fact, in this group of silicones, the lower viscosity silicones are as hard after curing as the more viscous silicones. Therefore, the shore value must not be used as a guideline for the consistency of a silicone. From the practical point of view, the shore value of an impression material is irrelevant to the clinician.

Contraction Ratio

This parameter relates to the material shrinkage with time. Silicone impression materials typically shrink 0.1% to 0.7% in 7 days. Shrinkage of less than 1% is negligible in terms of the resulting dimensional accuracy and earmold fitting.

Stress Relaxation

Stress relaxation describes the viscoelastic nature of the cured material. A finished ear impression must not change shape as a result of its removal from the patient's ear, during shipping or in-lab processing. Impressions made from silicone will recover from stress such as removal from the ear in 99%, which is quite satisfactory.

Impression Material Shelf-Life

The shelf-life of most silicones is 1 year. Expired silicones should not be used because they may not cure.

Impression Techniques

The ear canal is a dynamic environment. During mastication, smiling, yawning, and head movements, the cartilage in the ear canal expands and compresses. The reader can appreciate ear canal dynamics if they examine their ears in the following fashion: Place your little finger deep into the ear and press its soft part against the front ear wall. While moving your jaw, feel the ear wall movement as you are opening your mouth and then when you are closing your mouth to bite. This demonstration, in most cases, will reveal that the ear canal widens when your mouth opens and narrows when you bite down.

As shown in Figure 3–6, with mouth opening, the cartilage is pulled forward and the canal expands. The amplitude to which the canal widens depends on the subject. In contrast, with biting, the condyle of the jaw moves closer to the ear canal, compresses the cartilage, and reduces the canal diameter. These anatomically driven changes in canal dimensions are the cause for poorly fitting earmolds or shells.

Although the changes in the ear canal size and shape are real and obvious, the manner in which ear impressions should be taken is debated. Commonly one of three techniques is used: closed/relaxed mouth impression, chewing impression, or open mouth impression.

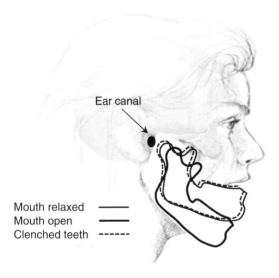

Figure 3–6. The lateral view of a human head illustrating the movement of the condyle of the jaw in the proximity of the ear canal. Image adapted from *TMJ Disorders* (http://www.nidcr.nih.gov/Oral-Health/Topics/TMJ/TMJDisorders.htm). Jaw drawings and positions based on x-ray images of the author's head.

Closed/Relaxed Mouth Impression

In this technique during impression syringing and curing, the patient behaves naturally. They may talk or just relax for the time the material cures in the ear.

Chewing Impression

In this method, the patient is encouraged to smile, talk, and chew vigorously as soon as the silicone is syringed into the ear. All these actions are supposed to produce a more natural impression that notes these changes.

Open Mouth Impression

This technique captures the magnitude of the canal widening with the mouth opening. In order to take an open mouth impression, the patient must open his or her mouth wide before the impression material is injected, hold the mouth open during the injection, and do not let their mouth close until the material is fully cured. Because holding the mouth wide open can be uncomfortable, the use of a mouth prop is recommended. The mouth prop should remain in the mouth as long as the impression cures.

A mouth prop can be used in two ways, as illustrated in Figure 3–7. First, it can be inserted upright between the front teeth (A). This will allow for making two impressions simultaneously, and this method is satisfactory in most cases. Still, some feedback may occur when the patient chews food predominantly on one side.

The other method is to insert the prop lengthwise in the corner of the mouth at the side the impression is taken (B). This will permit taking only one impression at a time. If an impression from the other ear is needed, another mouth prop must be used in the same manner. This second method will produce impressions that are anatomically more accurate and will ensure that the resulting hearing aid be less susceptible to acoustic feedback, particularly when the client is eating or chewing.

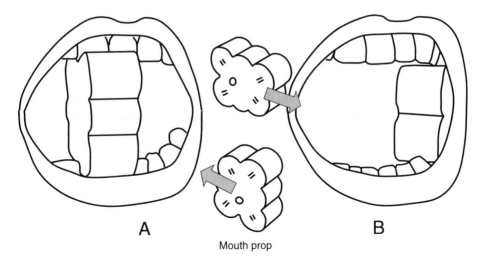

A   B

Mouth prop

Figure 3–7. Options in placing a mouth prop for taking an open-mouth impression.

Impression Taking

All ear impressions can and should be taken with an oto-block inserted past the ear canal second bend. The use of the oto-block not only prevents impression material from reaching the eardrum by providing a resistance, but also helps to replicate the shape of the ear canal and, most importantly, the flexibility of the canal cartilage. When impression material is injected, the material flows up against the oto-block, spreads, and stretches the cartilaginous canal tissue out toward the ear aperture. The canal opens up, and its increased diameter is captured on the impression. This process is critical in order to build a comfortable and feedback-free earmold. In contrast, with a shallow oto-block position, the impression material will not stretch the cartilage within the seal area, and the resulting earmold may fit loosely, have retention problems, and be susceptible to acoustic feedback.

To insert an oto-block, place the block in the opening of the ear canal with your fingers or a pair of tweezers. Gently pull up the back of the ear, as you would for otoscopic examination. Then, using the ear-light, slide the block into the ear canal and past the second bend. Brace your little finger against the side of the head to prevent ear injury, should the patient make a sudden movement. Use the earlight to see the penetration, the blockage of the canal, and the block's position. Do not push the oto-block straight in, but rather gently ease it in by pushing the top and bottom on the sides of the block, so that you are walking the oto-block slowly into place. Make sure you have inserted the block past the canal second bend and verify its proper position with an otoscope. When inserting vented oto-blocks, use an earlight with a slotted tip.

When the oto-block is properly situated in the ear canal, insert a mouth prop into the patient's mouth as discussed above and offer paper tissue (Kleenex) in case the patient drools.

Mix impression material according to the manufacturers guidelines. If you wear gloves, use a mixing pad and a spatula. Products containing sulfur—often found in latex gloves and hand lotions—can react with impression material preventing proper setting. Mixing must be thorough but fast.

While taking ear impressions for large ears, prepare more than one dose of silicone for each ear. Measuring syringes can be more convenient for this than measuring spoons or premeasured packets. To maintain proper proportions of mixing, opt for a one-to-one silicone and measure out 7 mL or 8 mL of each putty.

Impression materials provided in cartridges are mixed automatically when the silicone is dispensed into the ear. After attaching a cartridge with a mixing canula to the injector, repeatedly squeeze the trigger until the silicone appears at the end of the mixing canula. Bleed a small amount of the mixed silicone and check that both components mix thoroughly. If a syringe is used, depress the plunger until the material starts to flow out of the tip.

Pull the pinna up and back and insert the tip of the canula or syringe far into the ear canal. Do not seal the ear canal with the tip when you start filling the ear. If you use a syringe, you have to see the moment the impression material comes out from the canal and covers the tip to a depth of about 3 mm. Continue filling the ear and simultaneously withdraw the syringe keeping the tip imbedded in the silicone. If you use a pistol injector, start withdrawing the mixing tip from the canal just before the material touches the canula. This is called the leading technique. If the silicone covers the tip, the finished impression may have voids and air pockets.

After the ear canal is filled, dispense the material into the concha. First, fill the undercut at the antitragus, then move up and fill in the helix area. You need to see the material coming back from the undercuts before you proceed to the next area. Finish the impression by filling the rest of the concha. If the impression material is syringed into the center of the concha, air may be trapped in the undercuts, and the impression will have voids. The whole operation of filling the ear should be one complete motion.

Let the material cure in the ear undisturbed. Do not touch it, and do not apply any pressure to its surface. Kieper et al., 1991 found that making a "tighter" impression by pressing the material further into the ear created a worse, not a better seal for the resulting earmold. Four to ten minutes after filling the ear (depending on the silicone used), test the outer surface of the impression by indenting or scratching the surface. If the impression does not retain the indentation, it is ready to be removed. To facilitate impression removal, ask the patient to open and close their mouth several times. This will break the seal between the impression and ear wall. Next, gently press the pinna away from the impression, turn the impression's helix portion forward, or lift the lower portion of the impression up. Bring impression straight out from the ear while holding the oto-block thread. Examine the ear for tissue soreness, slight bleeding, or other potential problems. Gently wipe each ear with tissue to remove any residue.

Before an impression is mailed to the lab, carefully check that it is suitable for the earmold to be made: If a long canal is requested, the canal portion on the impression should be adequately long. If a full helix or helix lock is needed, the helix portion on the impression must be fully imprinted. If a large vent is necessary, the diameter of the canal area on the impression is to be at least 1 mm larger than the diameter of the vent prescribed.

For a monaural fitting, sending one satisfactory impression to the earmold lab is enough. However, if two impressions taken from the same patient's ear are sent, explain the reason on the order form and mark the impressions clearly for easy identification. If the two impressions are open-mouth and closed-mouth impressions, code the open-mouth impression with the letter "O" and the closed-mouth impression with the letter "C."

Ear Canal Dynamics

The dynamics of the ear canal and the wide diversity that exists among the population often pose challenges in the fitting of custom earmolds and hearing aids. These challenges commonly include acoustic feedback, discomfort, inadequate retention, and the sound going on and off.

For years, earmold labs have been unable to agree on which technique and material result in the best impression: some labs recommend soft low-viscosity silicones, some prefer medium viscosity, while others advise the use of a firmer higher viscosity silicone. Recommendations relative to mandibular movements also vary. Certain labs insist on having the patient chew, others prefer impressions taken while the patient's mouth is relaxed or open. A considerable number of labs claim that the technique and material are irrelevant as long as the impression is complete.

This inconsistency in advice should be of concern to clinicians; keeping track of who-wants-what relative to the various labs is a challenge for offices that order earmolds from numerous sources. With all this contradictory advice, clinicians wonder if it really matters how the impression is taken, who is right, and what makes the best impression for their patients. The appreciation of what is appropriate in impression taking comes from understanding the dynamics of the ear canal.

Axial Magnetic Resonance images provided in Figure 3–8 visualize the longitudinal axis and size of the condyle and show the effect of jaw position on its location relative to the ear canal (Oliveira & Hoeker, 2003). The condyle of the mandible has been outlined to facilitate its identification and the border between the cartilaginous and osseous regions has been clearly outlined by a solid white line. Note the substantial width of the condyle and its close proximity to the anterior

aspect of the ear canal with at least two thirds of it being in front of the cartilaginous region of the canal. This clearly visualizes the opportunity for its significant influence on canal activity. With the opening of the mouth, the condyle moves forward, pulls the cartilage in front of the ear canal, and expands the canal.

Comparing digital images of open mouth impressions and closed mouth impressions, Oliveira found that open mouth impressions commonly resulted in wider canals. In one quarter of the ears, the increase in the canal volume was equal to or greater than 8 mm^3/mm, which is an equivalent of a 1.5-mm vent. The insert in Figure 3–9 shows an impression taken with a subject's mouth closed, inserted into bisected investment cast from an open mouth impression taken from the same subject. An anterior gap can be seen. This is the articulation area where the ear canal is most frequently affected by mandibular movements.

Data in another Oliveira study (Oliveira, Babcock, & Venem, 2005) showed that 60% of the subjects had asymmetrical changes in the ear canal volume: with the opening of their mouth, one ear canal exhibited an increase in the canal volume that was an equivalent of a 1-mm vent. Sound leakage that occurs

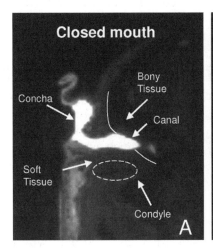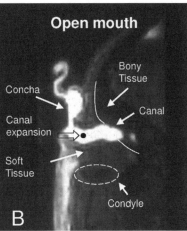

Figure 3–8. Axial MR images visualize the longitudinal axis and size of the condyle and show the effect of jaw position on its location relative to the ear canal. Adapted from Oliveira and Hoeker, 2003, p. 273, with permission.

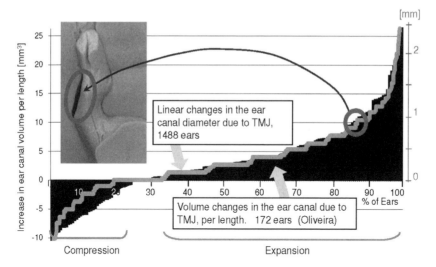

Figure 3–9. Comparison of research data. Data regarding ear canal TMJ activity obtained by Pirzanski and Berge is consistent with Oliveira's research. Adapted from Oliveira and Hoeker, 2003, p. 274, with permission.

through this uncontrolled and undesirable "venting" can be—and often is—a nightmare in hearing instrument fittings.

Research reported by Garcia and Staab (1995) pointed out that ear canals in some clients were remarkably soft and readily stretched when filled with a more viscous (heavier) silicone, often more than 20%.

Pirzanski and Berge (2005) compared ear impressions taken with various techniques and materials from both ears of 744 subjects to further investigate the nature and extent of ear canal dynamics. The impressions were taken by the audiologists enrolled in the distance education doctor-of-audiology (AuD) degree program at the Salus University, School of Audiology.

The research method compared the diameter of the ear canal in the anterior-posterior direction on four ear impressions taken from the right and four impressions from the left ear of each subject. The first two sets of impressions from each ear were made with a low-viscosity silicone and a higher viscosity silicone, with the subject's mouth closed. The two other impressions were taken with the subject's mouth closed and mouth open, using a higher viscosity silicone.

To find if there were any parallels between this and previous research, the data obtained on ear canal expansion/compression with jaw actions were compared with the data from Oliveira (Oliveira & Hoeker, 2003). The charted function (gray line) in Figure 3–9 is the linear increase in the ear canal diameter in the anterior-posterior direction with mouth opening. Although there were some differences in the compression area, in the expansion area the similarity of both studies was striking.

Figure 3–10 illustrates ear canal expansion/compression measured with three different impression techniques. The data for each curve were sorted from the smallest to the largest value. It was a surprise to find that the population of these subjects had their ear canals expanded with the mouth opening almost as much as with a more viscous silicone. The curve for the open-mouth higher viscosity (OM HV) condition showed greater canal widening compared with the other two conditions.

Further analysis of the OM HV impressions demonstrated that (with the data still sorted from the smallest to the largest value) the right ears of the subjects were as dynamic as the left ears, see Figure 3–11. In fact, these

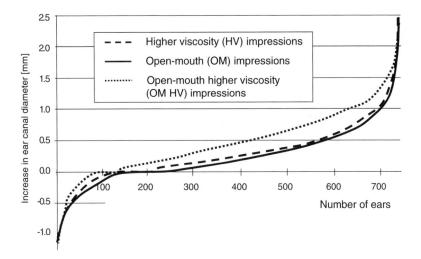

Figure 3–10. Ear canal compression/expansion at the seal area measured with three different impression techniques. Impressions taken with a higher viscosity silicone and the subjects' mouth opened stretched the ear canal at the seal area most.

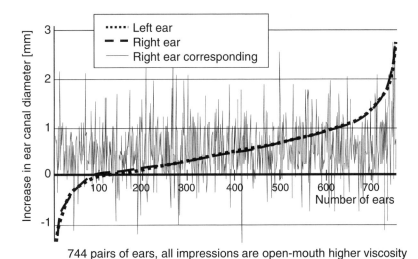

744 pairs of ears, all impressions are open-mouth higher viscosity

Figure 3–11. Asymmetry in ear canal dynamics. Although the subjects' left and right ears exhibited similar dynamics, the two ears belonging to the same individual were in most cases asymmetrical.

two curves look almost identical. This does not mean that the two ears of each of the 744 subjects had similar dynamics. In fact, they often did not. The rugged third curve illustrates the actual expansion in the right ear canal with the corresponding left ear of the same subject. Obviously, there were asymmetries in those dynamics.

The impact of asymmetry in ear canal dynamics is evident in the structure of hearing aid remakes. In a study Pirzanski and Berge (2010) investigated a total of 337 cases of patients fitted binaurally where one or both instruments required a remake. In all cases, the patients had similar hearing loss in both ears. The aids were built with consecutive serial numbers, thus it was assumed that one technician made both shells and assembled both instruments. The results showed that binaural remakes were the least common and accounted only for 32%. Hearing aid remakes for the left ears were at 35%, and for the right ears at 33%. This number of more than 60% remakes occurring only for one hearing aid in a binaural fitting corresponds surprisingly well with the fact that over 60% of human ears exhibit asymmetry in ear canal dynamics significant enough to lead to a fitting problem (Oliveira et al., 2005; Pirzanski & Berge, 2005).

Figure 3–12 illustrates ear canal dynamics from yet another perspective. Employing the digital imaging technology, an image of a closed-mouth low-viscosity (CM LV) impression and an OM HV impression were combined. When the canal area was cross-cut at various levels, an interesting pattern in the canal expansion appeared. First, the OM HV impression was larger in most areas. Second, the canal did not expand evenly in all ana-

tomical directions like a balloon would. It expanded only in certain areas and to a varying degree, all the way between the canal second bend to the canal aperture, reaching a maximum of 0.8 mm. The area of maximum stretching is shifting from the anterior area in section 1 to inferior area in section 3 and then partially returning to the anterior area in section 5. It is clear that expansion of an ear canal is unique, and often different between both ears of the same person.

It is known that ear canal dynamics not only adversely affect the aid's acoustic seal and cause retention problems but may also render the earmold uncomfortable. Ear soreness is reported with earmolds that are loose and as such require frequent pushing back into the ear. The friction between the earmold and canal irritates the ear.

Open mouth impressions made with viscous silicones will not eliminate all earmold and hearing aid problems but will reduce their number. A comparison of the number of remakes experienced by two clinicians working in the same office and using the same impression material found that the clinician who used the open mouth technique had 50%

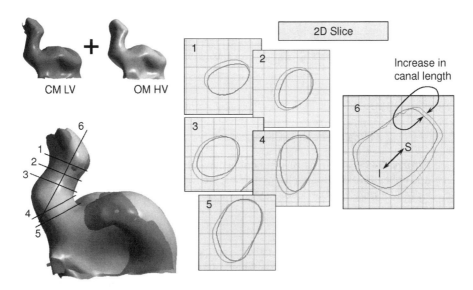

Figure 3–12. Cross-section through combined images of a closed-mouth low-viscosity impression and an open-mouth higher viscosity impression show the unique pattern of the ear canal expansion. Images created with 3Shape A/S software. http://3shape.com

less remakes compared with the other who routinely took closed mouth impressions. A review of 1,900 earmold fittings completed in a hospital setting found that a switch from a lower-viscosity to a higher viscosity silicone reduced the percentage of remakes from 10 to 14% to 5%. In these studies (Pirzanski & Berge, 2010)—prior to the change—the clinicians involved considered their hearing instrument remakes low.

Evaluation of Ear Canal Dynamics

It sounds reasonable that if the extent of the ear canal softness and the magnitude of the canal widening with jaw movements could be correctly quantified during patient examination, the clinician would be able to select an impression material of appropriate viscosity and decide whether or not taking an open mouth impression is justified.

To find if examining the ear provides reliable information about the ear dynamics, Pirzanski and Berge (2005) asked the audiologists to evaluate each ear of their subjects and classify it as having the canal cartilage soft, medium soft, or firm. Mandibular activity in the ear canal was classified as none, moderate, or severe. These perceptions were then compared with impression measurements. Stretching in the ear canal below 0.5 mm was considered minor, widening from 0.5 mm to 1 mm moderate, and expansion over 1 mm significant. This study covered 744 subjects.

The results showed that predictive value of observations relative to the magnitude of TMJ movements was 81% accurate for inactive ear canals and 17% and 10% accurate for ear canals with moderate and severe TMJ movement, respectively. The total number of accurate observations concerning TMJ movements was below 50%. These findings were consistent with Oliveira's study (Oliveira et al., 2005).

For canals classified as soft, medium soft, and firm, the number of predictions consistent with the measurements were 8%, 16%, and 83%, respectively. Accurate predictions regarding ear canal softness were made for only 34% of the ears.

The high number of accurate predictions for inactive and firm ear canals should not surprise the reader; as shown in Figure 3–10, most human ears are relatively firm and affected by mandibular movements only to a minor extent. The low number of accurate observations for soft and dynamic ear canals is a concern because these ears are the most difficult to fit with earshells and earmolds. Because the dynamics of the ear canal cannot be predicted in most cases, as a precaution, all ear impressions should be taken as open-mouth higher viscosity impressions, from all subjects and for all fittings that require an accurate acoustic seal and secure fit, including hearing protectors and swim plugs.

If the ear canal is firm and not affected by mandibular movements, the open-mouth higher-viscosity impression will not differ from an impression taken with any other technique. However, if the ear canal is soft and/or active, the open-mouth higher viscosity impression will most precisely capture the canal dynamics. This will offer the greatest probability that the earmold will have a satisfactory seal as well as fit securely and comfortably.

Pediatric Impressions

The pediatric population of patients wearing hearing aids is different from the adult population. Because children's ears grow fast, they are commonly fitted with BTE hearing instruments instead of custom ear-level hearing aids. When the earmold becomes loose after several weeks or months of service, the cost of ordering a new earmold is considerably less than the cost of manufacturing a new hearing aid.

Choosing the appropriate impression material and technique for a child is often considered a challenge because there is little information published on this topic.

Research data obtained from comparing dimensions of impressions taken from children ages 3 to 12 and adults 20 to 60 showed that ear canals in children were less dynamic and firmer than in adults, as provided in Figure 3–13. The firmness of the pediatric ears

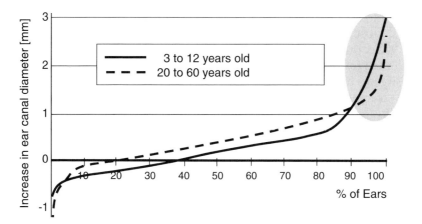

Figure 3–13. Age-related magnitude of ear canal dynamics.

may come as a surprise because it is commonly believed that ear canals in children are soft. Still, note that in each group, there were individuals with remarkably soft and dynamic ears. These ears are circled in the upper right corner.

Because of the fact that the dynamics of the ear canal tissue cannot be accurately assessed prior to impression taking, it is recommended to take pediatric impressions with the same technique as adult ears: using a higher viscosity silicone and the open mouth technique.

Infants

Schedule the appointment around nap time or feeding time. Advise mom or dad to bring the baby in hungry and sleepy. Ask them to feed them in the waiting room and by the time you see the child, they are content and asleep. Leave the child in their car seat if they are sleeping or buckle the child in their stroller and have the parent hold down their head with one ear up.

Small children are usually calmer with the parent holding them.

Toddlers

Toddlers and younger children can be challenging because they are afraid of the unfa-

miliar. The tough age is between 2 and 5, especially if the child had a lot of ear infections and medical treatment; they appear worried that there will be pain associated with the process. Try not to use the sound booth or the office where hearing aid programming is done, so they don't place a connection with the impression to the room where they will need to be often. If appropriate, take impressions in the classroom. Even the 3-year-olds don't want to look like they are afraid in front of their peers. The same child, who would cry and arch their back trying to get off their parent's lap, will sit like a little soldier in front of their classmates. Give lots of praise and compliments to the child.

Equipment seems to be what scares children. Make it child friendly. Place a cardboard animal or cartoon cutout on the otoscope. Use syringes with smiley faces on them (like Westone's kid's syringe). If the child has a stuffed animal or doll with them, pretend to examine its ears and let the child look in the toy's ear with the otoscope.

Describe the oto-block as an "ear pillow." Tickle the child's ear with the cotton block and tell them it will tickle again when you will be inserting it. When you do, ask them if it tickles . . . most children will laugh.

If you intend to take an open mouth impression, and a mouth prop cannot be used, the "alligator game" may be more appropriate.

To play the game, face the child with your face in theirs as you will be playing along with them. Tell the child to open their mouth a little bit and make it wider and wider like an alligator, each time repeating the words "wider . . . wider." Once you reach the point where the mouth is sufficiently open wide, perform the impression taking procedure. Remind the child that they cannot close their mouth until the impression is taken out.

For active children, instruct the parent to use a "big bear hug" so the child moves less. Use the term "big bear hug" because you don't want the parent to be too rough and make it a traumatic experience for everyone. For a right ear, have the child sit on the parent's right thigh with their legs between the parent's legs. The child's left arm gets tucked behind the parent's back. This way the child only has one appendage with which to fight. The right ear faces out and the left cheek goes toward the parent's chest. Consider when an insect is buzzing around one's ear, the first reaction would be to swipe it away, cover the ear, or shove the shoulder to the ear in defense —it's automatic. To prevent the child from acting upon such instincts have the parent hold their right shoulder down away from the child's head by using their left hand. The parent then uses their right hand to gently hold the head into their chest. The child is now restrained by the parent while at the same time held as if in embrace, hence "the big bear hug." This method gives little room for squirming and flailing about, certainly making the job quicker and easier.

Some children may have to be restrained by another person or with a papoose (straight jacket), and you may end up taking the impression on a crying child. At times, such situations can be avoided if you take the impression under sedation for ABR or for PE tubes, if the medical clearance is obtained.

Use treats or a sticker as a reward for good behavior. It is best to ease children with nonfoods. Be cautious about offering a lollipop or candy, as the child may have food and dye allergies. Ask the parent first. If food treats work for you, keep a supply of candies that are not manufactured in the same place as nuts and are Kosher; this is important for many.

Children

Most children age 5 and up are usually straightforward. Involve the child in the whole process because in most cases, this is just the beginning of a lifetime of earmold impressions. Show the child your equipment and tell (sign to) them about what you are doing. Keep your voice low but excited, like this is the best thing that has ever happened to them. Make a big deal about how cool it is to see how the inside of the ear is shaped. Practice with the child plugging their ears, so they can have some idea of what to expect. If you use TV to entertain the child, turn the sound off. This way the child will not notice the moment the ear is filled with the impression material and everything becomes quiet for a while.

If not everything went well, relax and take comfort in the thought that during the next visit, the child will be more at ease and your subsequent impressions will go smoother.

Handling Ear Impressions

Ear impressions can be shared with the earmold lab in two ways. The first is the traditional way in which the impression is put into a box and mailed to the lab along with the paperwork. The other is to scan the impression in the office and submit the electronic file via an electronic ordering system or the manufacturer's website.

The device used for in-office impression scanning is called iScan and was introduced by Siemens. The device is about the size of a printer (Figure 3–14) and uses three-dimensional technology with color-coded triangulation. The impression is affixed to a rotating platform where a projector illuminates it with colored light stripes from different angles. While a camera is capturing the pattern of the impression surface, the iScan software processes the data with high precision

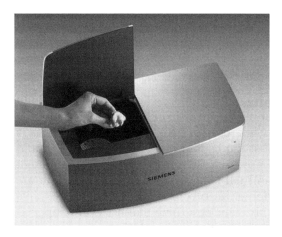

Figure 3–14. The iScan—the portable office impression scanner. Courtesy of Siemens Hearing Instruments.

into a virtual three-dimensional model. Using iScan and the e-order form makes the ordering of custom hearing aids and earmolds faster, eliminates most mistakes in ordering, and provides the clinician with 365-day, 24/7 interaction with the company. With the electronic ordering, the clinician may order a replacement of the hearing aid or earmold by using the iScan file without having to take a new impression.

Direct Ear Scanning

At this time, there are no commercially available devices for direct ear scanning that would eliminate the process of taking the physical impression. The most promising, still in the experimental stage, is a system developed at the Massachusetts Institute of Technology where a stretchy, balloon-like membrane is inserted into the ear canal and inflated to take shape of the canal. The membrane is filled with a fluorescent dye that can be imaged with a tiny fiber-optic camera inside the balloon. Scanning the canal takes only a few seconds, and the entire procedure takes only a few minutes. Because the camera captures three-dimensional images quickly, it can measure how much the shape of the canal shape alters when the pressure changes, or when the subject eats or talks.

EARSHELL AND EARMOLD MANUFACTURING

Earshells and earmolds are manufactured in the traditional manual fashion and with the CAD/CAM method. The method employed depends on the equipment available at the manufacturing site and the earmold material. Today, almost all earshells and a significant number of hard and soft earmolds are manufactured with digital technologies. Further in this chapter, earmolds and earshells are called earmolds to avoid repetition of the two terms together. When a distinction between the two products is needed, each term will be used separately.

Figure 3–15 illustrates the basic flow of the digital manufacturing process and its traditional manual counterpart.

Rapid manufacturing of custom earpieces has three sources of input: (1) silicone impressions, (2) scans of impressions obtained from office scanners (like iScan), and (3) ready to print files. Silicone impressions are the most common. A growing number of impressions are sent via e-mail, particularly for Siemens customers. The ready to print files are usually shared between manufacturing facilities to shorten the manufacturing time.

Digital Manufacturing

The digital method of earshell and earmold manufacturing includes: impression scanning, virtual modeling, and shell printing. The three stages are linked to a computer server that integrates the data and creates the final hearing aid shell. Any changes can be made at any stage without affecting the integrity of the data stored during previous stages.

Scanning

During scanning, the ear impression is photographed by several digital cameras. As a laser beam scans across the impression, a "point cloud" (or a "wire-frame") of the impression is generated. The computer interpolates

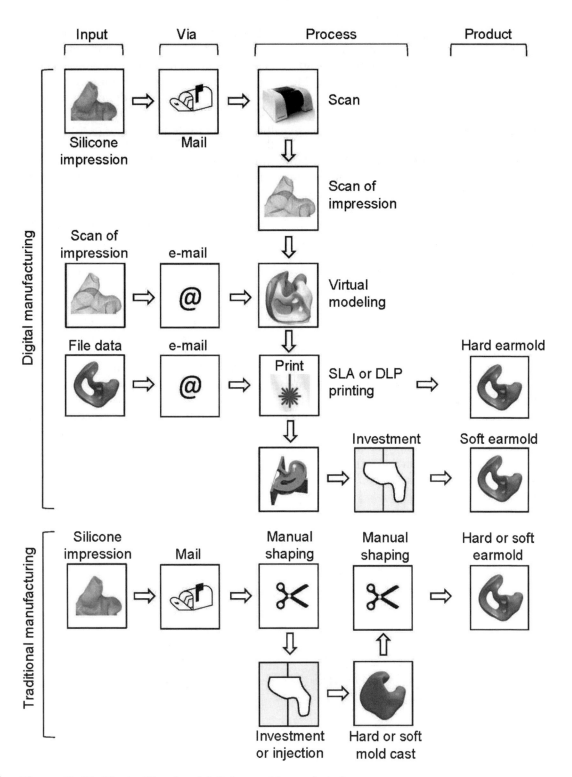

Figure 3–15. The traditional and digital earmold manufacturing processes.

the data and creates a virtual model of the impression. Impression scanning can be performed at the earmold lab or in the clinician's office. Scanning of one impression takes 2 to 4 minutes.

Modeling

Modeling is the process where the technician (or modeler) modifies the virtual impression with three-dimensional modeling software and creates a virtual hearing aid shell. An accurate ear impression is necessary to make a properly fitting earpiece. There are a number of operations that the modeler performs with the virtual impression to model the virtual shell. Parts of the impression that are not necessary are removed. In a procedure called surface offset, the whole impression or only certain parts of it are enlarged. This is similar to waxing in the conventional approach. The amount of the material added or removed is shown in colors to visualize the changing fitting exactitude of the shell.

Afterward, the technician experiments with the size of the shell and different placements of the virtual components (to include IC chip, receiver, microphone, faceplate, vent, receiver tubing, wax guard, etc.) in the virtual shell until the best possible placement is achieved. Most of these operations are aided by the software to make the modeling process easier and time effective.

The image of the virtual impression is used throughout the modeling as a virtual control mold. This allows the modeler to see the extent of the modifications performed and the anticipated fit of the finished hearing aid in the patient's ear. The main advantage of virtual modeling is that the modeler can try out different modifications or layouts of the electronics before settling on the final plan. That is, all changes are reversible until the modeler approves their design. In addition, all impression shaping—including the exact amount of material added or removed are recorded in the computer. Figure 3–16 shows a virtually modeled hearing aid with the electronic components inside. Modeling a hearing aid takes approximately 5 to 10 minutes.

Virtual modeling of an earmold is faster and takes only 3 to 5 minutes. After selecting the earmold style, sound bore and vent option, the software proposes the earmold configuration that can be accepted or altered by the modeler. Figure 3–17 shows the initial stage in earmold modeling and the finished modeling where the earmold is fitted in the virtual control mold just before the file is saved and sent for printing.

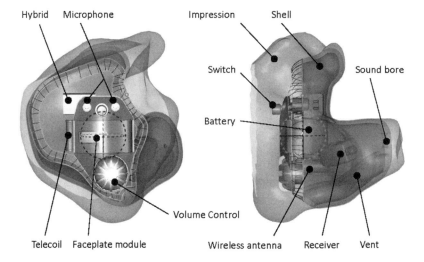

Figure 3–16. Virtual modeling of a custom full-shell hearing aid. Courtesy of Unitron.

Printing

Printing is the term used for the actual production of the shell or earmold. There are two technologies available: Stereo Lithographic Apparatuses (SLA) and Digital Light Processing (DLP). These two technologies are similar. During the printing process, the printer uses a laser or exposure to visible light to harden the photosensitive resin into shells that have been modeled during the modeling stage. The shells are printed in a pool of liquid ultraviolet light sensitive acrylic along with the receiver bore and vent, as well as the support frame (Figure 3–18). Thin layers of the acrylic (1/10 mm thickness) are hardened with the laser beam to form the shell. For example, a canal style shell that is 20 mm in total length will require 200 layers. It takes approximately 2 to 4 hours to complete the printing depending on the number and style of shells being made.

After shell printing, the support frame is removed, the vent and receiver bore cleaned from the remaining uncured liquid acrylic with a vacuum or pressurized air, and the

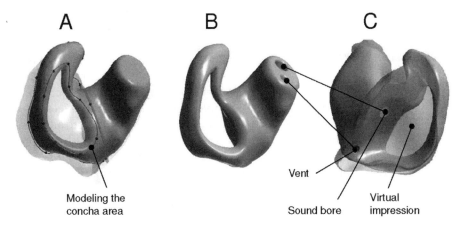

Figure 3–17. Earmold modeling stages: **A.** the initial layout of a skeleton earmold; **B.** the virtual earmold with sound bore and vent; **C.** earmold inside the virtual ear impression. Courtesy of Westone Laboratories and 3Shape A/S.

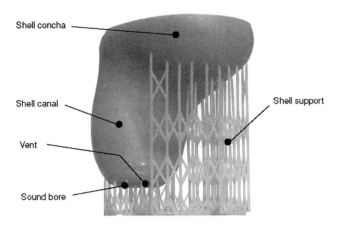

Figure 3–18. A canal style hearing aid shell printed in the SLA technology. Courtesy of Oticon A/S.

shell cured under ultraviolet light. This direct printing is used only for hard earshells and hard earmolds. That is because there are no soft, light curing resins available for digital printing.

To manufacture a soft earmold with the support of rapid manufacturing, the earmold is first modeled virtually and then software creates an injection mold, which is the negative of the soft mold. The injection mold is printed in hard acrylic, complete with the sound bore and vent, and filled with silicone. After the silicone mold hardens and is removed from the injection mold, the soft earmold is ready for final cosmetics and shipping to the customer.

Manual Earmold Manufacturing

Traditional earmold labs find rapid manufacturing technologies expensive. To be cost effective and competitive, they continue the manufacturing of soft and hard earmolds based on manual labor. In this process, hard earmolds and soft earmolds (made from silicone, vinyl, and polyethylene) are cast, shaped, and drilled by earmold laboratory technicians.

The manufacturing of an earmold begins with the removing of the oto-block from the impression, and the lateral process is cut to make a base. The impression is then cut down to an appropriate size for the model ordered. It is detailed so that the finished mold can be easily inserted into the client's ear. The style, hearing loss, impression size, and shape determine how much trimming is done. The shaped impression is dipped into hot wax or lacquered. The number of times it is dipped and the wax temperature determine the thickness of the coating. In general, the severity of the hearing loss or the clinician's request will determine the extent to which the impression is built-up.

The waxed impression is invested. There are two kinds of investing techniques. For earmolds made from thermoplastics such as vinyl and polyethylene, the cast is made from a hard plaster so that it will withstand the pressure and temperature at which the molten plastic is injected into the cast. For other earmold materials, such as acrylic (Lucite) and silicone, the cast is made from hydrocolloid (gel).

The investment is filled or injected with the earmold material and allowed to cure. The mold is then shaped with cutters and burrs. The sound bore and vent are drilled, and the earmold tube is installed. The finished earmold is buffed and shined, or lacquered.

Insta-Mold

The Insta-Mold allows the clinician to make custom silicone earmolds, noise protectors, and floatable swimmolds, at any location and in only minutes. Insta-Mold cures to the shape of the ear. In this method, the impression is the final product. After removing the mold form the ear, the excess material is trimmed off, the sound bore and vent drilled, and the mold is lacquered for improved cosmetics or a snugger fit. Insta-Mold silicones are hypoallergenic. They are formulated with high molecular weight polysiloxanes and reinforcing fillers for strength, durability, and water repellency (Insta-Mold, 2010).

This material is highly regarded in countries that lack well equipped earmold laboratories. The finished earmold is ready to fit and significantly less expensive than a custom earmold made from an ear impression.

Objectives in Earmold Shaping

An ear impression is a model of the patient's ear. During the manufacturing process, the impression is shaped to meet the product specifications provided in the order form and to satisfy the wearer with the quality of the earmold physical fit and cosmetic appearance.

Fulfilling technical specifications is easier than ensuring the earmold satisfactory fit. This relates to the fact that human ears differ in size and shape, softness, and dynamics. An earmold of a given style and material that fits well in one patient's ear may not be appropriate for another wearer. To ensure that earmolds satisfy the greatest populations of customers, earmold labs developed several objectives for impression shaping. These objectives apply to both rapid and manual manufacturing, and soft and hard earmolds, and include:

1. Easy insertion,
2. Adequate retention,
3. Sufficient acoustic seal,
4. Comfort, and
5. Correct sound direction.

For practical reasons, earmold surfaces are divided into fitting and nonfitting (Figure 3–19). A nonfitting surface neither makes contact with the ear nor contributes to the earmold/shell fit. For example, the lateral plane of an earmold is a nonfitting surface. Fitting surfaces meet with the ear and can be critical or semicritical. Critical surfaces include areas at the tragus, antitragus, and helix. The ear canal is also a critical fitting area. Semi-critical surfaces include the medial planes of the concha and helix. These surfaces make contact with the ear but do not affect the fitting of the earmold.

Retention

One of the most critical aspects in impression shaping is to ensure that the resulting earmold will stay securely in the ear, or in other words, have a satisfactory retention (Pirzanski, 2010).

It is a common belief that the closer the shape of an earmold or earshell resembles the impression, the better the fit of the instrument. Although this may be true in some fittings, in general, fewer fitting problems occur if the impression is skillfully shaped by the lab technician. This is related to the fact that the ear canal wall is supported by different anatomical structures such as muscles, cartilage, fat and bone, all possessing different softness and sensitivity. These factors must be accounted for in impression detailing.

Any area on the earmold body that is larger medially than laterally provides retention. Retention areas are critical fitting surfaces. Figure 3–20 shows the most common retention areas and their location in the ear. Retention in the canal is found where the ear canal widens in the superior-inferior or anterior-posterior plane, or both. Retention in the ear concha is provided by the surfaces

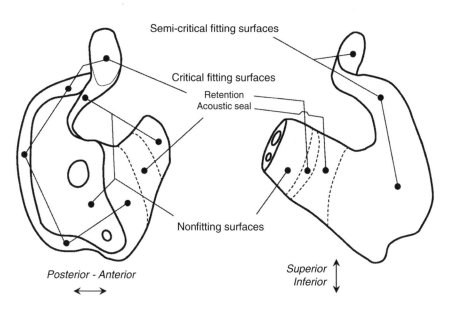

Figure 3–19. Fitting and nonfitting surfaces on an earmold.

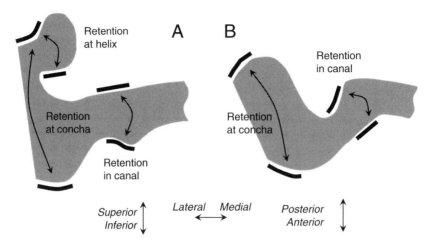

Figure 3–20. Common retention areas on an ear impression.

of tragus, antitragus, and helix. Specifically, it is how much these surfaces limit the mold's movement out from the ear concha.

Insertion

Human ears have complex shapes with prominences, constrictions, and bends. An earmold can be difficult to insert due to:

1. Deep tragus, antitragus, and/or anti-helix area;
2. Helix area extended toward the ear canal;
3. "Bottle neck" at the canal aperture;
4. Sharp upward angle in the ear canal; or
5. Sharp first and second bends in the ear canal.

Constrictions in the ear concha and canal can make insertion of the earmold difficult or simply impossible. It is feasible to streamline the shape of the earmold by removing the difficult to insert areas during impression shaping. However, if this is done, the earmold may lack retention and easily move out from the ear. A balance in impression trimming is necessary. First the earmold must be inserted into the ear, and remain there securely fit. Commonly, surfaces that define earmold easy insertion do not make contact with the ear.

The superior-inferior view of the ear is useful to discuss insertion and retention for concha earmolds. The ear shown in Figure 3–21A has a complex shape of the helix and the ear canal. There are two constrictions in the pinna and one in the ear canal that may impede proper insertion of this earmold. The first constriction is at the helix aperture (x). The wide helix area on the earmold is to pass through it. The second constriction is between the canal and the helix (y). The cartilage of the crus is to pass through it. The third constriction is in the ear canal (z). The wide earmold tip is to move through it.

Each of the three constrictions is shown in a separate insert at the bottom of Figure 3–21 to illustrate the complexity of the problem. The pieces of the *Mold* and the *Ear* in those inserts look like pieces of a puzzle. Readers who have interest in solving puzzles know that joining pieces on a flat surface, without lifting up one of the pieces, cannot be done. In earmold fittings, where the mold is partially inserted into the ear canal, with its helix upward, few maneuvers can be performed by the patient trying to insert the mold. If the earmold is not properly shaped, the presence of only one constriction can make insertion difficult. Two or three constrictions can prove insertion impossible.

The remedy is to trim the earmold in a fashion that reduces the width of the helix area and the width of the canal tip, without affecting the mold acoustic seal. The earmold

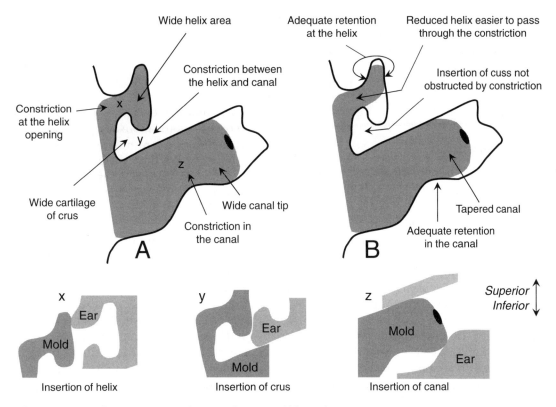

Figure 3-21. Shaping the concha area for earmold insertion.

shown in Figure 3–21B is properly detailed; it is easy to insert and has adequate retention. The area at the canal aperture is not to be trimmed because of risk of a loose fit and feedback.

Acoustic Seal

A whistling sound can be heard at times from an earmold. It is called acoustic feedback and occurs when sound leaking from the ear canal reaches the hearing aid microphone, is amplified by the hearing aid, and causes audible signal oscillation. A leakage can occur through the vent or, in a case of a loosely fitting earmold, through a gap between the ear wall and the earmold, or both. A loose fit can occur for several reasons; it can be that the impression was made with a light silicone, mandibular movements widened the canal, or the patient lost weight. In most earmolds and hearing aid shells, the acoustic seal occurs

between the ear canal first and second bend, and is a critical fitting surface. The ear canal in this area is soft and moderately sensitive. This allows for the earmold snug fit without any sensation of discomfort or tightness. In lab impression shaping and processing are critical in obtaining effective seal. Commonly, enhanced seal is achieved through applying offset or wax on the impression.

Comfort

To be appreciated by the patient, an earmold must be comfortable to wear. If not, the patient will avoid using the earmold and/or the hearing aid. Discomfort often results from earmolds having long canals. When the canal is long enough to reach past the ear canal second bend where the ear wall is thin and tightly applied to the underlying bone, discomfort is likely. To make the earmold comfortable, the canal area must be trimmed or tapered. Earmolds are comfortable if they fit snugly in the canal cartilage and make no contact with the canal bony portion. In other words, earmold comfort is determined by the combination of fitting surfaces at the canal aperture and nonfitting surfaces deeper in the canal.

Sound Direction

Human ears can be straight, or have moderate or acute bends. It is often believed that the sound bore location on the earmold canal tip is critical for the earmold performance. That is not necessarily correct. When we talk to each other, we do not talk directly into the other person's ear. In fact, we often talk facing the other person, or sitting beside them. Still, the sound will travel through the air and ear canal and reach the other person's eardrum with clarity. The same applies to earmolds; when enough space is allowed in front of the sound bore, the sound will travel through the bends of the canal and reach the eardrum.

Challenges in Impression Shaping

The challenge in impression detailing is that all the above objectives, which are insertion, retention, seal, comfort, and sound direction, must be applied to ear impressions having different size and shapes. The more complex the shape of the ear, the more complex the shaping of the impression must be. Figure 3–22 provides examples of shaping the canal area of an ear impression. This ear canal has two acute bends. While shaping this particular impression, the modeler must consider that:

1. The acoustic seal area extends from the canal aperture to the canal second bend,
2. The retention area is at the canal second bend,
3. Comfort is achieved when the earmold makes no contact with the sensitive skin of the ear past the canal second bend,
4. For easy insertion, the earmold tip is to be slimmer, not wider, that the narrowest constriction present in the canal, and

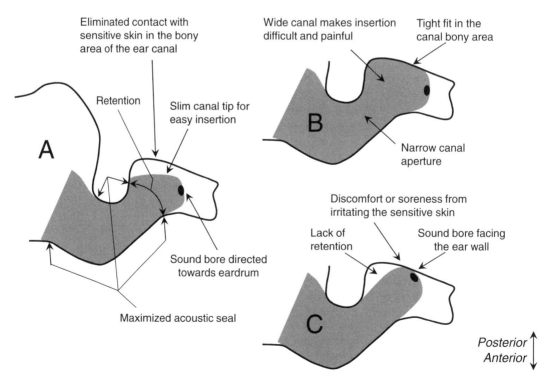

Figure 3–22. Approaches to detailing the earmold canal area for insertion, retention, and comfort.

5. The sound bore is to be directed toward the eardrum, not the canal wall.

Shaping A in Figure 3–22 is the most adequate; the earmold canal tip is not touching the sensitive skin in the bony area. The mold is slim enough to pass through the canal aperture. The sound bore is directed toward the eardrum. The widening on the mold deeper in the canal is the retention area that ensures the earmold secure fit. The seal area is maximized.

The earmold in Figure 3–22B is not as proper. The canal tip is slightly rounded. This mold can be difficult to insert and remove from the ear due to the fact that the wide canal tip is to be forced though the narrow canal aperture. When worn, the earmold will rub the delicate skin deep in the canal causing soreness and discomfort. If this earmold is not completely inserted due to discomfort, it will allow for sound leakage and feedback.

In contrast, earmold C in Figure 3–22C is tapered to the extent that the retention area is entirely removed. Even though this earmold may be easy to insert, it may work out of the ear canal and be susceptible to feedback. In addition, this pointy canal can be uncomfortable and perceived by the wearer as excessively long. Due to the sound bore facing the ear wall, the clarity of the sound can be compromised.

An additional reason to trim the canal tip is that some ears are stretched by the impression material lengthwise, as illustrated in Figure 3–12. If the canal length in the impression is not adjusted, the resulting earmold may have the canal longer than the patient's ear, and fit poorly.

Full-shell hearing aids made for ears with an oversized helix, deep antitragus, and/or a narrow antitragus notch are difficult to fit. Figures 3–23 shows two hearing aids that have different complexity of their concha. Hearing aid A is easy to insert, hearing aid B is not. Its small faceplate and large shell indicate that the concha opening in the pinna is much smaller than the inside of the concha. A half shell or a shell with reduced helix would be proper for this ear.

Figure 3–24A illustrates a case where a CIC hearing aid is difficult to insert due to insufficient tapering of the shell tip. When pushed into the ear, the CIC stretches across the first bend of the canal and creates three contact spots that prevent further insertion: the first at the canal tip, the second at the canal retention area, and the last at the seal area. Unfortunately, the clinician cannot see

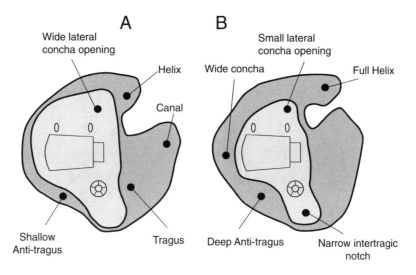

Figure 3–23. Individual differences in the size of the ear concha.

the first two contact spots. They will discern only the third where the CIC pushes on the tragus. If shell modification is carried out at this area, it may help insertion but will likely damage the seal area to the extent that acoustic feedback will occur. Shell modification should start with trimming down the canal tip to make the shell slimmer and straighter. A properly shaped, partially inserted, CIC hearing aid is shown in Figure 3–24B.

Even a properly detailed earmold may be difficult to insert if the patient pushes the earmold in the ear horizontally. In ears where the canal rises sharply upward, the earmold may not go in, or will go in scratching and hurting the ear. In such ears, the earmold should be pushed upward to the ear canal, see Figure 3–25.

Patients with dynamic ear canals not only report that their earmolds have poor retention and feedback issues, but also cut the sound off when they open their mouth. The perception is that mandibular movements are able to rotate the earmold in the ear canal to the extent that the sound bore is partially or totally blocked by an ear wall. This reasoning is incorrect. Two impressions, a closed mouth and open mouth, taken from a patient may

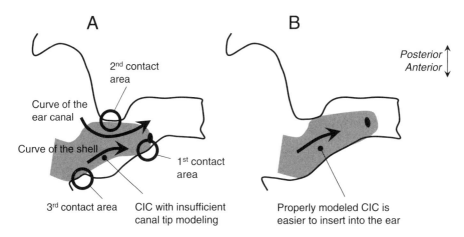

Figure 3–24. Challenges in inserting a deep canal fit earmold.

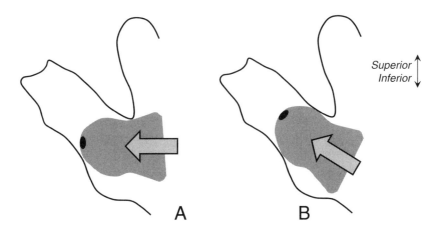

Figure 3–25. Earmold insertion to ear canal with a steep angle upward.

show differences in the canal shape and width, but the open mouth impression will not show a constriction able to block the sound bore on the earmold. The perceived reduction in the instrument loudness in conjunction with mandibular movement actually has another reason; it is that the mouth opening widens the ear canal and reduces the sound pressure, a case illustrated in Figure 3–26. With the subject's mouth closed, the earmold seals the canal well, and there are no sound leaks. When the patient opens their mouth, the volume of the ear canal increases and leaks occur. The receiver has to move now a larger volume of air than previously required. Because the hearing aid amplification level has not changed, the sound pressure in the expanded canal is considerably lower, and the instrument's loudness reduced to the point that the hearing aid is perceived as dead. This effect of the sound going on and off affects mainly low and moderate power hearing aids where the sound leaking from the canal is not strong enough to trigger feedback. In powered hearing aids, the expansion of the ear canal will allow for enough sound radiation back to the microphone to trigger feedback.

If retention is the problem, a micromold or canal style earmold can be made with a canal lock. A canal lock is a small plastic protrusion from the earmold that extends into the ear concha, rests against the antitragus, and secures the fit of the mold in the ear, see Figure 3–27. Before this option is requested, the impression should be evaluated to see that the antitragus will offer retention. Some ears have the antitragus area flat and are not suitable for a canal lock. In addition, consider that canal lock enhances the mold retention, not the acoustic seal. If feedback occurs with mandibular movements, taking a new open mouth impression is more proper than ordering a canal lock.

For ears that have limited retention areas in the ear canal, a concha earmold is recommended. Still, if the mold is to fit securely, the concha ring must rest against the lateral concha wall, see Figure 3–28. If the ring is styled too much to provide retention, the earmold can dislodge, break the seal, and trigger feedback. Full concha and shell style earmolds that are not styled as much as skeleton earmolds offer a more secure fit and, as a result, pose a lower risk of acoustic feedback. That is why earmolds that occupy more of the ear concha are often credited for superior seal (Pirzanski, 2001). Note that for this ear, the canal length is critical. If the canal is extended

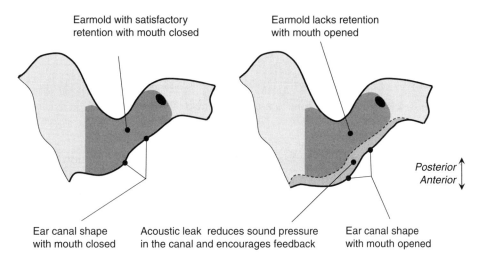

Figure 3–26. Widening in the ear canal resulting from mouth opening and its effect on earmold fitting in the ear.

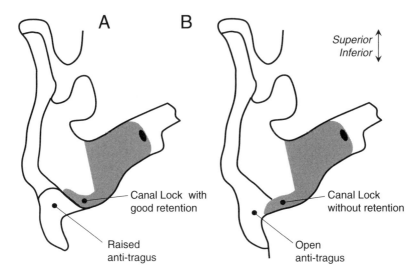

Figure 3–27. Earmolds with a canal lock: **A.** satisfactory retention at the antitragus; **B.** no retention at the antitragus.

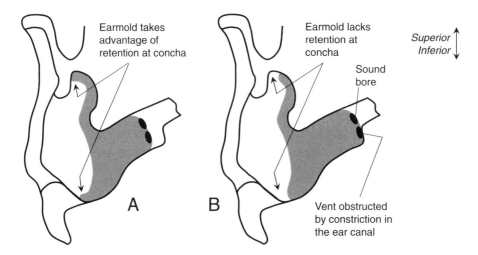

Figure 3–28. Shaping the concha area for earmold effective retention.

to the constriction, the vent may be blocked by the ear wall.

Patients always attempt to insert hearing aids and earmolds into the ear canal as far as possible. They simply have no means of knowing how deeply the mold is inserted and believe that it will stop at the right location. This may not be true. If the cartilage is soft, a CIC or small ITC hearing aid may not stop at the designated location but be inserted deeper, as provided in Figure 3–29. This deep insertion opens several possible scenarios regarding how the patient and the clinician may perceive the poor fitting.

First, if discomfort in the canal is reported, the common conclusion is that the aid is tight. In contrast, if this deeply inserted and poorly sealed hearing aid feeds back, the aid

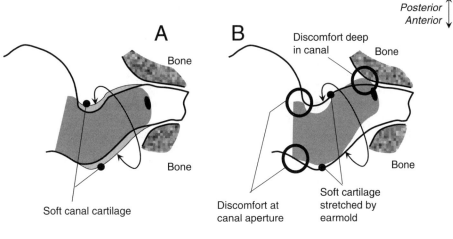

Figure 3–29. An ITC hearing aid inserted deeply into a soft ear canal can cause a variety of fitting problems and confuse the clinician over the cause for the problem.

will be perceived as loose. In addition, this aid may refuse to stay in the ear because the overstretched cartilage will push it out. In such a situation, the clinician may incorrectly conclude that the shell is too short. Another possibility is that with the cartilage stretched by the aid sore spots occur. These symptoms may lead the clinician to believe that the aid is too long, or tight, or that the patient is allergic to the shell material.

These scenarios illustrate how challenging hearing aid troubleshooting can be and that the perception of the problem may be different from the real problem.

Small custom earmolds used with thin-tube BTEs and RIC hearing aids, commonly called micromolds, pose their own challenges in insertion, retention, and acoustic seal. They are known to easily work out of the ear, compared with other earmold styles. This poor retention may have two reasons. The first is that the deep fit and small size reduce the critical fitting areas on the earmold that provide retention. The second is that the tube connecting the mold with the hearing aid is quite rigid and encourages the mold movement and dislodging from the ear.

As far as insertion is concerned, micromolds with a deep fit can be difficult to insert to the designated area for patients with bigger fingers, particularly if their ear canal is long and narrow, as illustrated in Figure 3–30. A partially inserted micromold can be uncomfortable, seal the ear poorly, be susceptible to acoustic feedback, or slip back from the ear. Still, if pushed deep to the bony area, it can be uncomfortable. A longer micromold, which offers the same cosmetics and fits as deeply, is easier to insert. In addition, its extended body allows for the canal tip tapering, which enhances comfort and prevents sore spots.

Earshells for In-The-Ear Hearing Aids

Selecting appropriate custom in-the-ear amplification is a process of integrating shell and circuitry characteristics that satisfy what the patient wants and needs with what is physically and electroacoustically possible. Fitting hearing aids is an inexact science. Options are influenced by many factors, including

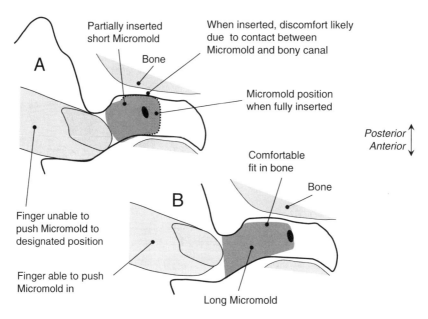

Figure 3–30. Challenges in inserting micromolds deep into the ear canal.

ear anatomy, type and degree of hearing loss, technology, cost, medical conditions, lifestyle, and an individual's capabilities and communication needs.

Earshell Styles and Materials

Custom hearing aids are distinguished by the following nomenclature.

Completely-In-The-Canal (CIC)

CICs are the smallest of all the models that are available today. They fit completely into your ear canal (hence the name!) and are virtually invisible to other people—usually only a small plastic pull-out string protrudes from the canal and maybe visible to people who are looking *very* closely at the ear. The pull out string is necessary to enable the wearer to pull the hearing aid out of the ear. Because of their small size, CIC hearing aids are the least powerful. They are recommended to people with mild to moderate hearing loss. A smaller version of a CIC hearing aid is called IIC (Invisible-In-Canal). It comes with fewer or none custom controls, such as tele-

coil or a programing push button, but offers the best possible cosmetics. Images of custom hearing aids fitted in the ear are illustrated in Figure 3–31.

In-The-Canal (ITC)

ITC fits at the canal aperture and is shadowed by the tragus, which makes it little visible in the ear. ITC hearing aids are the most popular and most flexible—designed to manage a wide range of hearing needs.

Full-Shell (FS)

FS hearing aids fit into the concha portion of the ear and are designed to accommodate a range of hearing conditions, usually more acoustic power, a larger battery, and oversized controls. Custom made according to the shape of an individual's ear, they provide maximum retention and are appreciated by wearers with manual dexterity problems.

Custom hearing aids use three types of batteries; number 13, number 312, and number 10. The 13 battery will power a hearing aid for approximately 15 days for a 16-hour per

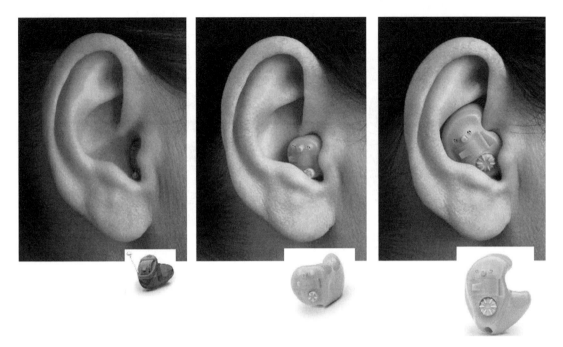

Figure 3–31. Images of custom hearing aids fitted in the ear: completely-in-the canal (CIC), in-the-canal (ITC), and full-shell (FS). Courtesy of Unitron.

day use. The 312 battery will last 10 days and the 10 battery for 5 days, under the same use conditions. For more severe hearing losses, a lager battery is required. This in return may require a larger hearing aid shell.

Shells for custom hearing aids are made hollow to house electronic components such as the microphone, amplifier, receiver, and battery. The lateral opening of the shell is composed of the faceplate with the microphone, battery compartment, optional volume control, as well as additional controls and switches.

The clinician and the patient should be realistic regarding the hearing aid fit in the ear. Some ears are too small to make a true CIC or inconspicuously fitting ITC. When ordering a CIC, check that the canal area captured in the impression is wide enough to accommodate the receiver and the faceplate. If not, consider an ITC hearing aid.

In cases where the FS style is ordered and cosmetics are a priority, opt for the low-profile FS. A low profile FS uses the 312 size battery, which is not as thick as the 13 size

(Figure 3–32). This allows the technician for modeling the battery partially in the canal area. In addition, the volume control wheel on a low profile faceplate is smaller and as such easier to accommodate. As a result, the low profile shell is shallower and the cosmetics of the instrument enhanced.

New hearing aid users may come to their initial evaluation with an idea of the devices they want to wear. This may be based on what they have seen advertised, observed a friend or relative wear, or simply want "the ones that don't show."

Many experienced hearing aid users express a preference for a certain style because they want to: (1) replicate what they are already using, (2) change to something more cosmetically appealing, or (3) obtain features their current hearing aids do not provide. Patient motivation is critical to success with amplification.

Experienced clinicians know that when patients' preferences and expectations are fulfilled, they will be more likely to work cooperatively during the trial period and

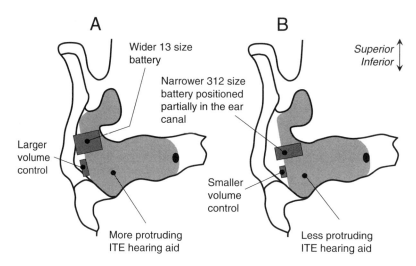

Figure 3–32. Comparison of size between a FS and low profile-FS hearing aid.

beyond. Studies correlating personality traits with prefitting expectations indicate that extroverted patients report more benefit from their hearing aids; persons who feel in control of their lives, and those with less anxiety, also report greater benefit with amplification.

Every electronic hearing aid has a microphone, a loudspeaker (commonly called a receiver), a battery, and electronic circuitry. The electronic circuitry varies among devices, even if they are the same style. The circuitry falls into three categories based on the type of audio processing (analog or digital) and the type of control circuitry (adjustable or programmable).

Microphone

Hearing aids in the 1990s had only an omnidirectional microphone. Today hearing aids have a directional microphone that amplifies sounds from in front more than sounds from other directions. This means that sounds originating from the direction the listener is facing are amplified more than sounds from behind or in other directions. If the speech is in front of the listener and the noise is from a different direction, then compared with an omnidirectional microphone, a directional microphone provides a better SNR. Improving the SNR improves speech understanding in noise. Directional microphones work best when the distance to the talker is small. They are not available on CIC hearing aids.

Digital Audio and Programmable Control

Modern hearing aids have the audio circuit and the additional control circuits fully digital. The clinician programs the hearing aid with an external computer temporarily connected to the device and can adjust all processing characteristics on an individual basis. Digital circuitry allows implementation of many additional features not possible with analog circuitry, can be used in all styles of hearing aids, and is the most flexible. Digital hearing aids can be programmed with multiple programs that can be invoked by the wearer, or that operate automatically and adaptively. These programs reduce acoustic feedback (whistling), reduce background noise, detect and automatically accommodate different listening environments (loud versus soft, speech versus music, quiet versus noisy, etc.), control additional components such as multiple microphones to improve spatial hearing, transpose frequencies (shift high frequencies that a wearer may not hear to lower frequency regions where hearing may be better), and implement many other features.

Digital circuitry also allows control over wireless transmission capability for both the audio and the control circuitry. Control signals in a hearing aid on one ear can be sent wirelessly to the control circuitry in the hearing aid on the opposite ear to ensure that the audio in both ears is either matched directly or that the audio contains intentional differences that mimic the differences in normal binaural hearing to preserve spatial hearing ability.

Streamer

Audio signals from digital hearing aids can be sent wirelessly to and from external devices through a separate module, often a small device worn like a pendant and commonly called a "streamer," which allows wireless connection to yet other external devices. This capability allows optimal use of mobile telephones, personal music players, remote microphones, and other devices. With the addition of speech recognition and internet capability in the mobile phone, the wearer has optimal communication ability in many more situations than with hearing aids alone. This growing list includes voice activated dialing, voice activated software applications either on the phone or on the Internet, receipt of audio signals from databases on the phone or on internet, or audio signals from television sets or from global positioning systems.

Telecoil

Telecoils (T-coils), sometimes referred to as "Telephone Coils," allow audio sources to be directly connected to a hearing aid, which is intended to help the wearer filter out background noise. They can be used with telephones, FM systems (with neck loops), and induction loop systems (also called "hearing loops") that transmit sound to hearing aids from public address systems and TVs.

Hearing loops are used in churches, shops, railway stations, and other public places. In the United States, several states have passed legislation that requires hearing professionals to inform patients about the usefulness of telecoils.

Considerations in Size and Shape of the Ear

Manufacturers' suggested fitting ranges are used as guidelines, but there are many situations in which the style of instrument will be determined by factors other than degree and slope of hearing loss. If a particular shell option appears to be on the borderline of a recommended fitting range, the dimensions of the ear canal, the intended placement of the microphone, and the impedance of the middle ear can help predict if it is realistic to try that style. Adults and children with the same hearing loss will have different gain and output requirements because of the differences in ear canal volume. Ear canal volume is smaller in children than adults resulting in higher ear canal SPL. This will have significant influence on the interpretation of diagnostic tests, real ear measurements, and the response characteristics of the hearing aid. With deep-canal fittings (regardless of shell style), there is an increase in gain, output, and high-frequency emphasis.

Except for obvious physical conditions such as atresia, a malformed pinna or concha, or a surgically modified ear, it is often difficult to predict that a patient will have a good result from a particular type of shell on the basis of physical and otoscopic inspection of the ear. If the hearing loss is well within a fitting range, CICs or ITCs may be the best choice for some patients.

In a surgically modified ear canal with a large volume of 5 to 10 cc, the output speech production level can decrease by 10 to 20 dB SPL. Conversely, a stiff middle ear system secondary to ossicular fixation, tympanosclerosis, or another condition, can increase eardrum SPL (gain and output) by 10 to 20 dB (Gudmundsen, 2003).

Medical Conditions

Patients who have mastoid cavities suffer repeated ear infections medial to the earmold. Although this problem may be solved by venting when it is appropriate, the repeated infections are usually not the fault of the earmold (assuming that there is no allergic reaction to the mold material). They often are related to pockets of residual disease, or moisture from the upper respiratory tract and middle ear that has not been sealed off from the rest of the mastoid cavity. In the majority of cases, if hearing aid use is necessary in patients who are plagued with repeated otitis media, the problem can be solved by revision surgery (Sataloff, 2003).

Hearing aid shell and earmold materials undergo extensive testing to ensure that they can be used for contacting the skin. Tests such cytotoxicity, skin irritation, and dermal sensitization are conducted to validate a material and define it as noncytotoxic, nonsensitizer, and nonirritant. Hearing aids and earmolds are generally assumed to be medical devices that only contact healthy skin. In the case of a medical device contacting breached or compromised surfaces, the use of the materials may not be tested and/or advisable. Simply put, the material testing may not support this type of use, and any reaction may require a medically trained person to evaluate the site to ensure that the skin is not compromised.

Manufacturers use two standards to direct activities related to biological safety of medical devices—ISO 14971 Risk Management and ISO 10993 Biological Evaluation of Medical Devices. They prepare evaluation documents on the biological safety of medical devices that are put on the market. This includes: use considerations of the medical devices (exposure), selection of materials and available information on those materials (chemical composition), any potential hazards or risks, historical information on the safe use of the material, and biological testing required to bridge knowledge gaps. This is called a biological safety evaluation.

The MSDS (material safety data sheet) document gives information of a material in its raw form. MSDS typically is used in industrial settings for safe use of a material or chemical during processing steps and does not necessarily reflect biocompatibility of the finished product.

European manufacturers issue a Declaration of Conformity that declares that the product is meeting the requirements specified in 93/42/EEC Medical Device Directive. MSDS information and Declaration of Conformity are available directly from their website; see an example in Figure 3–33.

Clinicians concerned with the quality or properties of materials used in hearing aid manufacturing may request supporting documents from the earmold lab.

Dexterity

Changing batteries, adjusting rotary controls, switches, or push buttons for volume control, T-coil, direct audio input, or directional microphones could be problematic for persons with limited dexterity. Small hearing aids are not the aids of choice if a person's manual dexterity precludes easy insertion and removal custom shells, particularly CICs. Ease of management may be improved with the addition of removal strings, removal notches, built-up controls, batteries with long pull tabs, or packaging that facilitates easy insertion, automatic T-coil activation, cerumen guards, and wind screens.

It is difficult to predict who will need or want manual controls. Some patients prefer no adjustments, other patients prefer some degree of manual control. Push button switches are available for functions such as T-coil, volume control, or multiple memories. If a clinician thinks a particular style of hearing aid compromises ease of management, it will save time and disappointment if the patient is asked to perform potentially difficult tasks before final decisions are made regarding style and features. Users will usually acknowledge their limitations and opt for the style best suited to their abilities.

When fitting a first-time user, advise them on the proper insertion technique and watch them practice. Some new patients unin-

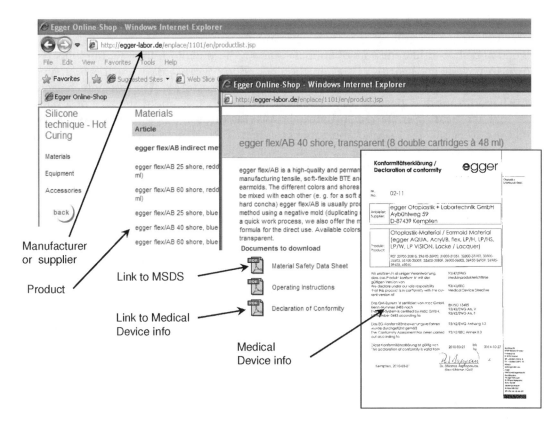

Figure 3–33. Information regarding earshell and earmold materials such as MSDS and Declaration of Conformity can be obtained directly from the Internet. Adapted from egger Otoplastik + Labortechnik GmbH, http://www.egger-labor.de with permission.

tentionally rotate their hand when bringing the hearing aid to ear level. Therefore, they will attempt to insert the earshell with its concha positioned backward across the ear.

A CIC can be inserted more easily if the patient pulls the pinna backward and inserts the aid forward and upward into the ear canal. The pulling of the ear with the other hand from behind the head will stretch the canal and is particularly helpful for patients possessing canals with sharp bends.

Custom Hearing Aids for Children

Clinicians are skeptical about fitting children with custom hearing aids. One consideration is that ear shape changes as children grow and frequent recasing (remake) will be necessary. Other concerns include a higher incidence of outer and middle ear infections in children,

risk of loss, damage, or injury, and reliability of performance compared with BTEs. Self-image, cosmetic concerns, and refusal to wear hearing aids are a reality, particularly with adolescents. Clinicians who work with adolescents indicate that custom hearing aids are not a logical progression for all children. They report that children are uneasy about using custom hearing aids, and that having custom hearing aids, including CICs, does not necessarily ensure that children will wear them more. Other clinicians report that custom hearing aids including CICs are a viable fitting option for children.

Earmolds for Behind-The-Ear Hearing Aids

An earmold is an individually fabricated ear insert that channels the sound reproduced by a hearing aid receiver to the eardrum. In the early days, sound collectors were made of wood and shaped like the ears of animals known to have acute hearing. Later, in the 1800s, hearing coronets and trumpets were horn-shaped sound collectors of various sizes that the hearing-impaired individual would use to help collect sound and funnel it into the ear canal. As is the case today, one of the concerns of the hearing-impaired user was appearance. Listening trumpets were incorporated into ladies' fans, men's walking canes, and pieces of furniture.

By the end of the 19th century, custom earmolds were made with the use of Stents dental modeling wax. The wax was pressed into the concha bowl and canal aperture. After the impression was removed from the ear and the excess was trimmed, the impression was coated with a metallic powder. The impression was then placed in a bath of copper sulfate with an anode. Electric current was applied to create a coat of pure copper to adhere to the metallic powder. Once the copper was thick enough, the wax would be melted away. The resulting copper earmold was then smoothed, polished, and shaped by hand. This earmold would then be attached to the sound collector, and the finished hearing aid would be ready for use.

Around 1922, the first stock earmolds to approximate the adult human ear were introduced. The first commercially available custom earmolds in the United States were made by the S. S. White Dental Manufacturing Company and were sold for a price of $10 each (Cartwright, 2003).

Hearing instruments benefited greatly from research and development in the field of electronics that was undertaken prior to and during the war years 1939–1945. The vacuum tube continued to shrink in size, and the first printed circuits were developed. These smaller tubes and printed circuit designs were quickly incorporated into the manufacturing process by the hearing instrument industry. The early 1950s gave birth to the transistor, and the march toward miniaturization continued. Most people would assume that the transistor radio introduced us to transistor technology; in reality, it was a hearing instrument manufacturer who used this technology as a replacement for the vacuum tube.

Body-worn aids were the first type of modern hearing aid. The case, which contains the amplifier, is about the size of a pack of playing cards and is worn in the pocket or on a belt. The earmold is connected to the case via a cord. Today, body aids have largely been replaced by BTE hearing aids. There are two styles of hearing aids being worn behind the ear. They include the following.

BTE

BTE aids consist of a case, a tube, and an earmold. The case is small and made of plastic. It fits behind the pinna. The case contains the amplification system and the speaker. The tube is used to route the sound from the hearing aid case to the earmold. The color of the BTE components (case, tube, and earmold) range from inconspicuous skin tones to bright colors and optional decorations.

BTEs can be used for mild to profound hearing losses and have several advantages over custom hearing aids. One advantage is that they tend to be more durable. This is because the electrical components are located outside the ear. This reduces the amount of earwax and moisture to which the electrical components are subjected. Another advantage is that BTEs can be connected to assistive listening devices, such as classroom FM systems. FM listening systems have wireless receivers integrated with the hearing aid. A separate wireless microphone can be given to a partner to wear in a restaurant, in the car, during leisure time, in the shopping mall, at lectures, or during religious services. The voice is transmitted wirelessly to the hearing aid eliminating the effects of distance and background noise. FM systems have shown to give the best speech understanding in noise of all available technologies.

Another advantage of a BTE hearing aid is that if the earmold no longer fits the user, the earmold can be replaced for a fraction of the price of a new custom hearing aid. BTE hearing aids are typically prescribed for children. This is because children need a durable hearing aid, often need assistive listening devices, and can quickly outgrow the size of the earmold.

Earmold tubes are made of clear soft plastic. The sound produced by the receiver passes through the earhook and earmold tube into the ear canal. Number 13 earmold tubes are the most common. The number 13 name comes from the standardized wire gauge system for the diameters of round, solid, electrically conducting wire. In this system, #13 tube, with the nominal inside diameter of 0.076 inches fits over #13 copper wire of the nominal outside diameter of 0.071 inches. National Association of Earmold Laboratories standardized the outside diameter of standard, heavy wall, and double wall earmold tubing, keeping the inside diameter the same as insulation tubing, that is 0.076 inches, or 2 mm. Earmold tubes are prebent. Prebending gives the earmold tube a close-to-the-ear fit and makes them less visible. More severe hearing losses require thicker tubes to prevent sound radiation and feedback. Table 3–1 shows earmold tubing selection guidelines.

Special 13 tubes made of a denser material, called Dri tubes, are used for patients that are affected by moisture condensation occurring in the regular earmold tube.

Recent innovations in hearing electronics include BTE hearing aids with thin acoustic tubes that provide an open ear canal fit. A fine clear tube connects the BTE with the ear canal. Inside the ear canal, a small soft silicone dome or a custom highly vented earmold holds the tube in place. This design is intended to reduce the occlusion effect and help users with normal hearing in the lower frequencies. BTE hearing aids with thin tubes are generally used for mild to moderate high frequency losses. Thin tubes come with an internal diameter either 0.9 mm or 1.3 mm and are made in several lengths to match the size of the patient's ear. The larger 1.3 mm thin tube can deliver more acoustic power. They are also prebent with one end pointing toward the ear canal. With such a design, thin tubes are made specifically for the right or left ear. Red or blue markings indicate for which ear the tube is made, and the description of the tube length (0, 1, 2, 3, etc.)

Receiver-In-Canal (RIC)

At a first glance, these hearing devices are similar to the BTE aid. There is, however, one crucial difference: The speaker (receiver) of the hearing aid is placed inside the ear canal and thin electrical wires replace the acoustic tube of the BTE aid. There are some advantages with this approach. The sound of the hearing aid is smoother than that of a traditional BTE hearing aid. In acoustic tubes, the amplified signal generated by the speaker in the BTE creates a peaky frequency response. With a RIC hearing aid, the receiver is right in the ear canal and is therefore free of this distortion. RIC hearing aids are made with a small behind-the-ear case, and the wire connecting the hearing aid and the receiver is extremely inconspicuous.

RIC hearing aids are all digital and can be programmed to accommodate two distinct hearing losses, a sloping high-frequency loss and a more severe hearing loss covering a wider range. This type of hearing aid does not require an occluding earmold, so it leaves the ear canal open, providing a more natural sound quality to the user's own voice.

Table 3–1. Earmold Tube Selection

Earmold Tubing Styles		Suggested Loss	Loss in Decibels
13 Standard Wall	(2 mm × 2.9 mm)	Mild to Moderate	30 to 50
13 Heavy Wall	(2 mm × 3.3 mm)	Moderate to Severe	50 to 70
13 Double Wall	(2 mm × 3.6 mm)	Severe to Profound	70 to 100

For those who have a high-frequency loss, the open ear will hear low frequency sounds naturally, through the ear canal, offering a more natural sound quality than a hearing aid that occludes the ear canal. For individuals who have a wider range of severe hearing loss, meaning that there is a loss in the low frequencies as well as the high frequencies, having the receiver placed down in the ear canal will provide more gain and thus fit a greater hearing loss. Samples of BTE and RIC hearing aids are shown in Figure 3–34.

Earmold Style and Materials

The earmold style and material is selected based on the severity and type of the patient's hearing loss, anatomical properties of the ear, patient's manual dexterity, allergic conditions, personal preferences, and difficulty with any previous hearing instrument fitting. In addition, the style and material selected

for the earmold depends on the style of the hearing aid prescribed.

Earmolds are made in three basic styles: concha, canal, and micromold. Each style has substyles that differ mainly in cosmetics. Common earmold styles are shown in Figure 3–35.

Earmold materials vary in their physical properties, particularly in the degree of softness, extent of shrinkage, and finishing characteristics. The softness of a given material is described as the shore value. Earmolds made from soft materials have 25 to 70 Shore A hardness. The lower the shore value, the softer the material. Most earmold labs offer, often under different names and different prices, the following earmold materials.

Acrylic

It is a crystal clear hard hypoallergenic material that is resistant to breakage. It is the most popular for manufacturing hard earmolds.

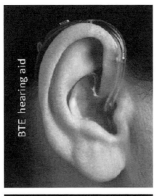

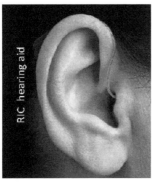

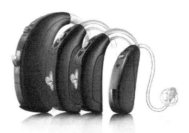

BTE and BTE thin-tube hearing aids

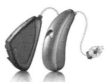

RIC hearing aids

Figure 3–34. BTE and RIC hearing aids. Courtesy of Unitron.

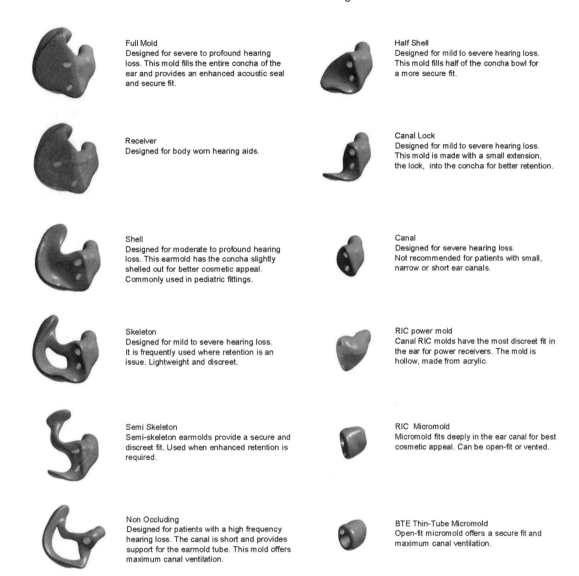

Full Mold
Designed for severe to profound hearing loss. This mold fills the entire concha of the ear and provides an enhanced acoustic seal and secure fit.

Half Shell
Designed for mild to severe hearing loss. This mold fills half of the concha bowl for a more secure fit.

Receiver
Designed for body worn hearing aids.

Canal Lock
Designed for mild to severe hearing loss. This mold is made with a small extension, the lock, into the concha for better retention.

Shell
Designed for moderate to profound hearing loss. This earmold has the concha slightly shelled out for better cosmetic appeal. Commonly used in pediatric fittings.

Canal
Designed for severe hearing loss. Not recommended for patients with small, narrow or short ear canals.

Skeleton
Designed for mild to severe hearing loss. It is frequently used where retention is an issue. Lightweight and discreet.

RIC power mold
Canal RIC molds have the most discreet fit in the ear for power receivers. The mold is hollow, made from acrylic.

Semi Skeleton
Semi-skeleton earmolds provide a secure and discreet fit. Used when enhanced retention is required.

RIC Micromold
Micromold fits deeply in the ear canal for best cosmetic appeal. Can be open-fit or vented.

Non Occluding
Designed for patients with a high frequency hearing loss. The canal is short and provides support for the earmold tube. This mold offers maximum canal ventilation.

BTE Thin-Tube Micromold
Open-fit micromold offers a secure fit and maximum canal ventilation.

Figure 3–35. Custom earmold styles. Three-dimensional scans shown on images were captured using 3Shape A/S 3D-scanner, http://www.3shape.com

Red and blue colors may be available to indicate right and left ear usage. Earmolds in all styles and configurations can be made from acrylic. It is easy to modify, grind, and buff.

Vinyl

Vinyl is a soft, flexible material in which most earmold styles can be fabricated. Available in clear and light pink colors. It is popular for children and seniors. Easy to modify and grind. The shore rating is from 45 to 55. Vinyl earmolds may discolor from the contact with earwax and body oils.

Silicone

This material is a flexible, inert rubber. Silicone earmolds are very durable and do not shrink. Silicone earmolds can be made clear, light pink, or made with solid pastel colors, or with glitter, or color swirls, which makes them attractive for children. Most earmold styles can be fabricated in this material. The exceptions are semiskeletons and nonoccluding styles. Silicone is commonly used for fabrication of soft micromolds. The shore rating is from 25 to 70. This material is difficult to modify. Silicones earmolds are often lacquered for protection from moisture and body oils.

Polyethylene

This material is used in extreme allergy cases. Generally, it is not popular due to its milky white color. Polyethylene earmolds look and feel waxy, and float in water.

Digitally Manufactured Earmolds

Earmolds made with digital modeling and printing technologies are fabricated with hard acrylics or soft silicones, clear or colored. Vinyl and polyethylene earmolds are made manually.

Pediatric Earmolds

Colors are popular with children and are often requested to match the color of the BTE casing. Girls love the rainbow swirl colors and glitter earmolds. For boys, earmolds with a logo of a sport or football team or a cartoon character are great. A number of earmold labs in Europe offer a great selection of such logos. Earmolds for children can be made from different colors for right and left ears to help them easily identify which earmold (and hearing aid) goes on which ear.

The parents of children being fit with hearing aids for the first time may not want bright colored earmolds that attract attention to the child's hearing loss. This can be a possible sign that the parents are still working through some emotional issues with acceptance of their child's hearing loss. The clinician may help to negotiate a compromise—a bright BTE casing and a skin tinted earmold to make the parents more accepting.

Acoustic Seal and Comfort

Acoustic seal and comfort are commonly the key concerns in selecting the earmold material. Proper acoustic seal between the earmold and the ear canal is necessary to prevent the occurrence of acoustic feedback. Traditionally, the effectiveness of the earmold seal is controlled through the thickness of impression coating, commonly made of wax. The problem is that wax adheres in different thicknesses at different points of the impression. This is because the impression is curved and thus retains wax differently at various locations. This may distort the shape of the earmold.

Fifield (2010) wondered whether there was a better method of improving the earmold acoustic seal than waxing. He developed the multilayer impression, a technique in which the impression was taken in several stages to maximize canal cartilage stretching in order to obtain an airtight seal. This technique was time consuming and never gained popularity. However, before it faded out, several interesting studies and observations were made. One of them is of particular interest.

Macrae (1990) compared the effectiveness of the earmold seal relative to various molding conditions. His study was conducted as follows: Two impressions were taken from the same ear of sixteen subjects. The first impression was taken following the traditional technique; the other was a multilayer impression taken with Fifield's method. Four wax coatings of varying thickness were used to make four earmolds from the first impression, one earmold for each coating condition. Earmolds A were made with the thinnest impression coating, whereas earmolds D with the thickest (Figure 3–36). Multilayer impressions were not waxed prior to making earmolds E. All earmolds were made from the same silicone. A pressure seal test was administered to establish the efficiency of each earmold sealing.

Macrae found that the seal varied significantly among earmolds and strongly depended on the thickness of the wax applied to the impression: earmolds A sealed in 15%, whereas earmolds D sealed in 65%. Generally, the thicker the coating, the more effec-

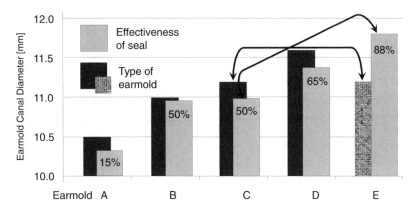

Figure 3–36. Earmold tightness versus effectiveness of sealing. Data adapted from Macrae, J. (1990). Static pressure seal of earmolds. *Journal of Rehabilitation Research and Development, 27*(4).

tive the seal was. Interestingly, earmolds E made from nonwaxed multilayer impressions sealed most effectively, reaching 88%. This better seal was achieved despite the fact that earmolds E had smaller canal diameters than the extra-tight earmolds D. Earmolds C, which had on average the same canal diameter as earmolds E, provided a much less effective seal, just 50%.

These results can be explained as follows: The ear canal tissue is soft, but its softness is not a rubber-like flexibility. Certain areas of the cartilage appear to be more forgiving than others (see Figure 3–12). The extra tight earmolds D did not correspond properly with the anatomical structures of the subjects' ears. They overstretched the cartilage in some areas but did not stretch it enough in other areas allowing for a relatively poor seal and leakage. The most effective seal in earmolds E was achieved by the employment of the multilayer impression. Although the multilayer impression stretched the ear tissue more than the traditional impression, the stretching reflected the natural cartilage forgiveness. Therefore, the fit of the resulting earmold was anatomically most accurate.

Canal cartilage stretching is desirable and beneficial for hearing instrument fittings under the condition that it is carried out through impression taking, not through thick impression waxing.

It is doubtful that soft earmolds can prevent acoustic feedback by "adjusting" to the shape of the ear. A loosely fitting soft earmold is smaller than the actual patient's ear and allows for sound leakage around the earmold. When such an earmold is forced deeper into the ear, the leakage may be reduced and feedback eliminated. This, however, will distort the earmold shape, and in most cases, it will not bring a lasting effect. The earmold will eventually recover from the stress applied and become loose again.

There are some thermoplastic materials that soften under body temperature. However, it should not be assumed that an increase in the earmold softness will improve its seal. A loose-fit earmold will not become tighter just because the material becomes softer.

There were experiments in manufacturing earmolds from thermoplastics that expanded in the patient's ear under body temperature and provided an airtight seal within minutes of insertion. The presumption was that the ear tissue would stretch and conform to the tighter earmold, whereas the softness of the earmold would prevent discomfort. While some patients benefited from these materials, others complained of the excessive tightness after the earmold expanded. As for the general patient population, the idea of manufacturing self-sealing earmolds produced a limited success.

Soft earmolds do not prevent acoustic feedback related to jaw movements. Consider that the increase in the ear canal volume (see Figure 3–12) would require the earmold to expand instantaneously when the mouth is opening, and then compress just as quickly when the mouth was closing. There are no balloon-like soft earmolds that would increase and decrease their volume in a split second. The likelihood of breaking the acoustic seal by jaw movements is similar for both soft and hard earmolds.

Another study tried to determine whether clinicians fit soft or hard earmolds more successfully (Pirzanski & Maye, 1999). A total of over 2,000 earmolds were investigated. Approximately one half of them were made from soft materials such as silicone and vinyl, the rest were hard acrylic earmolds. The parameters of the molding process were monitored throughout the study to ensure consistent manufacturing. The study found that soft earmolds required just as many remakes as the hard earmolds.

These research data suggest that soft materials do not enhance the acoustic seal in earmolds. Rather, feedback and loose fit in earmolds is controlled by the impression-taking technique, the viscosity of the impression material, and the parameters of the in-lab molding process.

While inserting a soft earmold, the patient may have difficulty guiding the canal portion of the earmold into the ear canal. In some ears, the canal on the earmold can bend backward, resulting in improper insertion. The softer the earmold, the more difficult insertion can be. Firmer or hard earmolds are more suitable for these patients.

Contrary to the common belief that the more the ear concha is occupied by the earmold body, the more effective the seal; two separate studies found that all earmold styles are capable of providing an equally effective acoustic seal.

Kuk (1994) found that there was no difference in REIG (real ear insertion gain) among the shell, canal, and skeleton earmolds, while the full concha earmold permitted the least amount of maximum REIG (Figure 3–37). Analyzing REAT (real ear at threshold) data, Pirzanski (2000) noted that

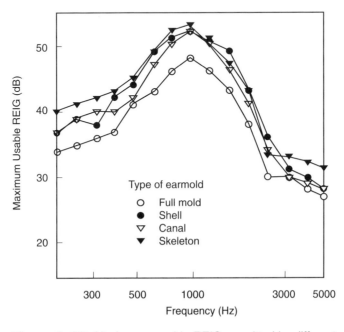

Figure 3–37. Maximum useable REIG permitted by different style earmolds. Reprinted from Kuk, 1994, pp. 44–51. Courtesy of the American Academy of Audiology.

in most subjects, canal molds sealed as effectively as full molds, if not better.

These findings further support the supposition that acoustic seal in earmolds and custom hearing aids occurs in the ear canal. This means that the bulk of the earmold at the concha is irrelevant as a factor contributing to the earmold seal.

The sound escaping from the ear canal radiates to all directions. However, it is the path from the anterior ear canal wall to the microphone that is the shortest. This is the path that triggers feedback. A larger concha or extended helixes do not prevent acoustic feedback because the concha and helix are not in the path of the leaking sound to the microphone. The impression taking technique appears to be far more critical for proper acoustic seal than the earmold style.

Mandibular movements not only widen the ear canal but may also change the angle between the ear canal and concha. As a result, a hard-body full-concha mold can be forced out of the ear. This problem can be remedied in two ways: (1) If the ear provides adequate in-canal retention, order a silicone canal earmold; if it does not (2) order a silicone skeleton earmold. The earmold's flexible concha ring will absorb the tissue movement while the canal area will maintain effective seal.

Intuitively, earmolds made from soft materials should be more comfortable than those made from hard materials. Practically, because the ear canal tissue in human ears is softer than soft mold materials, the softness of the earmold is irrelevant. It is the ear tissue that has to conform to the earmold, not the earmold to the ear. The clinician can experience this first hand by pressing the canal portion of a soft earmold (of average size) against his or her thumb, or open hand. With little pressure applied, it will be the skin that accommodates the earmold.

Venting and the Occlusion Effect

The occlusion effect is commonly described as an unnatural and mostly annoying quality of the voice of a person wearing hearing aids or hearing protectors. As a result, it is often reported by hearing aid users as a deterrent to wearing hearing aids. To experience the occlusion effect, a person has to use their own voice to produce a sustained «eee» sound in a quiet place, and then—after plugging their ears—repeat the same sound. The «eee» will sound louder when the ears are blocked.

Sounds generated within the body (for example from speech, chewing, or running on hard surfaces) reach the hearing mechanism through the vibration of the skull bones into the ear canal. Normally, these sound waves escape from the open ear and are not heard by the person. If the canal is blocked by an earmold, sound pressure is generated in the closed ear canal and transmitted through the conductive mechanism to the inner ear. The effect is like speaking into a barrel.

This phenomenon is caused by the closure effect, called the occlusion effect. The sound is perceived as being hollow or booming in quality and considerably louder. When speaking or chewing, the skull bones vibrate, and the sound waves travel all around the skull creating standing waves. Because the skull is composed of many different bone plates having different densities and different vibration characteristics, the vibratory behavior is quite complicated. Skull shape, size, bone plate strength, and other qualities vary with each individual. Therefore, the occlusion effect will vary greatly from person to person. In addition, the stimulation type, stimulation place, and stimulation intensity determine the strength of perception. The effect will also depend on the natural frequency of the skull, which lies within the speech frequency range (Voogdt, 2010).

Earmolds and hearing aid shells block the ear canal to a greater or lesser extent depending, among other factors, on the depth of the earmold insertion into the canal. A study investigated the relationship between the earmold insertion depth and the magnitude of the occlusion effect. Soft, not vented, earmolds were used. The canal length of those molds varied from 0 mm to 21 mm. The medial end of the molds was not tapered, so they provided a maximum acoustic seal in the ear canal. The marking lines in Figure 3–38 indicate the insertion depth of each earmold. The subject's own voice was used as the stimulus. The difference between the open ear spectrum and the occluded condition was the magnitude of the occlusion effect. The data shows that the initial increase in the earmold canal length elevated the occlusion effect. The maximum sound pressure at the ear drum was measured for earmold M3. Then, as the canal length increased, a progressive reduction was noted. The greatest reduction occurred with the change from mold M5 to M6. This suggests that patients wearing hearing aids can be free from the occlusion effect if the canal on the earmold or earshell extends past the canal second bend and is not tapered. This certainly can be done for straight, tube-like ear canals, which are uncommon. For the great majority of ears, as discussed above, tapering of the earmold canal tip is a must to ensure that the earmold can be inserted into the ear and be comfortable to wear.

A practical alternative to manufacturing deeply sealed earmolds is to make them with properly shaped canals and to vent them. A vent is a channel drilled or cast in the earmold that connects the lateral surface of the mold with the medial end of the canal. To be effective, the vent size should be significantly large. Revit found that a 2-mm vent reduced the occlusion effect by 8.5 dB at 200 Hz. Dillon considers a 2-mm vent a starting point and advises to use a 3-mm vent, if possible (Dillon, 2001; Revit, 1992).

In addition to transmitting sounds out of the ear, a vent also transmits sounds to the ear canal. The vent path is totally nonelectronic. Sounds are transmitted into the ear canal without attenuation up to the Helmholtz resonant frequency of the vent. Above that frequency, the vent attenuates sound, so the hearing aid, when turned off, acts like an earplug.

Helmholtz resonance is the phenomenon of air resonance in a cavity. An example of

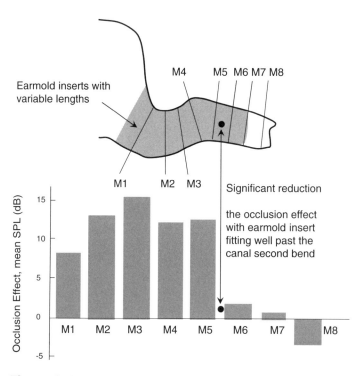

Figure 3–38. Variations in the occlusion effect depending on the insertion depth of an earmold.

Helmholtz resonance is the sound created when one blows across the top of an empty bottle. When air is forced into a cavity, the pressure inside the cavity increases. When the external force pushing the air into the cavity is removed, the higher pressure air inside will flow out. However, this surge of air flowing out will tend to overcompensate, due to the inertia of the air in the neck, and the cavity will be left at a pressure slightly lower than the outside, causing air to be drawn back in. This process repeats with the magnitude of the pressure changes decreasing each time. This effect is akin to that of a mass attached to a spring. In earmolds, air trapped in the vent acts as a *spring*. Changes in the dimensions of the vent adjust the properties of the *spring*: a larger diameter vent makes for a softer *spring*, a small diameter vent makes a harder *spring* that "chokes" the flow of the air.

Figure 3–39 shows a sample of a hearing loss of a person having normal hearing up to 1 kHz. Their hearing deteriorates and becomes severe above 3 kHz. In the area where the person's hearing is normal, it is the vent, not the hearing aid, which transmits the sounds from the environment to the eardrum. In contrast, above 3 kHz, it is the hearing aid that provides the necessary amplification. In the 1 kHz to 3 kHz region, the sound from the vent and the hearing aid combine. In this process, a vent of adequate size is instrumental for obtaining a natural sound. The hearing aid user cannot make a distinction between sounds coming through the vent and sounds coming from the hearing aid receiver. Both sounds blend in the ear canal before they reach the eardrum.

The effectiveness of venting depends not only on the vent diameter but also on the vent length. A vent is a column of air. Air, like any other substance, has mass, and therefore has inertia. The less inertia, the more effective the ventilation. A short vent provides more effective ventilation than a longer vent of the same diameter. This correlation is used in venting micromolds. Because micromolds are worn deeply in the ear where the canal is narrow,

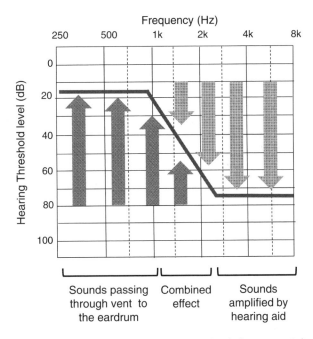

Figure 3–39. A vent of adequate size is instrumental in transmitting sounds into the ear canal for patients with normal hearing in the low frequencies.

a vent larger than 3 mm can rarely be accommodated. However, a 2.5-mm vent that measures only 8 mm in length is as effective as a 4 mm vent that is 20 mm long.

For people with more than 40 dB loss at 250 Hz and 500 Hz, the occlusion effect is rarely a problem. These people need significant low-frequency amplification, so it does not matter if there is an increased sound level when they speak or not.

The presence of a vent in hearing aids and earmolds is often associated with increased risk of acoustic feedback. Feedback occurs if the amplified signal leaking from the ear canal reaches the hearing aid microphone and is amplified again. Modern hearing instruments have advanced feedback managing systems that allow for vents as large as 3 mm without feedback.

Recently, larger vents are also employed for hearing aids with directional microphones. In the past, the concern was that a larger vent allowed low-frequency sound from the rear to pass through the vent without attenuation, thus reducing the directional benefit. Flynn (2004) demonstrated that a directional microphone designed specifically to work with a larger vent provided the same improvement in speech understanding as hearing aids with smaller vents used in previous studies.

With the advanced electronics, selecting the vent size for in-the-ear hearing aids and earmolds has been simplified; manufacturers employ large vents in their hearing devices as a default. In fact, the available vent sizes may not be even listed on the order form. Unless otherwise advised, the hearing aid shell or an earmold is made with the largest possible vent proper for the style, circuitry, and amplification level.

While the occlusion effect is a common problem among hearing aid users, there is a second, similar condition that is sometimes mistaken for occlusion. It is called ampclusion, as related to amplification (Kuk & Ludvigsen, 2002). Ampclusion occurs if the hearing aid excessively amplifies the lower frequencies. This can create a similar auditory booming effect.

If the user complains that their voice sounds unnatural, the underlying cause of the problem has to be established. The easiest way is to turn the hearing aid off, or take the battery out of the instrument, and ask the patient to speak. If the sensation is gone, it is the ampclusion effect, and the problem can be corrected by adjusting the parameters of the hearing aid amplifier. When the problem is still there, it is the occlusion effect. Enlarging or shortening the vent will address the problem. Other solutions include shortening and/or tapering the canal.

Some patients may not benefit from a large vent, or at least the benefit is not obvious. Research conducted by Kampe and Wynne (1996) on 10 adults found that the enlargement of the vent caused an increase in the occlusion effect for one vowel and a reduction for another. In one subject, the introduction of a 2-mm vent into a previously unvented earmold elevated the occlusion effect by 15 dB at 300 Hz for the vowel /ee/, and reduced it by 18 dB for the vowel /oo/ for the same frequency. In another patient, a reversed effect was measured. In addition, real ear measurements were unable to predict how the user would perceive their own voice with a change in the vent diameter.

Increasing the earmold tightness can also reduce the sensation of the occlusion effect because a tighter earmold will reduce vibration of the canal cartilage. Pirzanski (1998) was successful in obtaining several snug-fit, unvented hard CIC size earpieces that eliminated the occlusion effect even though their tapered canal tips lacked an acoustic seal deep in the ear.

Service, Modifications, and Remakes

Earmolds and hearing aid shells require proper maintenance and service. This includes cleaning their surfaces from the dead skin and body oils, and cleaning the sound bore and vent from ear wax. With time, the quality and accuracy of the earmold or hearing aid shell physical fit can deteriorate, and the patient may need a new hearing aid shell or earmold, a procedure called recasing or remake.

Daily Care and Maintenance

Patients may experience acoustic problems with hearing aid performance. Some of the issues can be resolved by the user themselves without visiting the office. Supported with educational materials, the wearer can be trained to:

1. Verify that the hearing instrument is turned on,
2. Verify battery charge, and change the battery if needed,
3. Replace wax filter,
4. Clean the battery contacts with a cotton swab dipped in rubbing alcohol,
5. Verify that the battery is correctly inserted into the hearing instrument,
6. Verify that the microphone and the receiver outlet are free from debris.

Earmold labs and online catalogs offer accessories that help to maintain hearing aids and earmolds in good condition. This, among other items, includes: Dry and Store (for overnight storage, to keep the aid from moisture and allow it to dry), Oto Care kit, earmold blower, wax loops and brushes, Oto ease lubricant, and skin conditioners for ear hygiene and relief of itching ears. Clinicians find the Dry and Store device so effective in conditioning hearing aids that some offer it at no charge to first-time customers to prevent their office visits and save time on moisture related repairs (Pirzanski & Berge, 2010).

Service

Hearing aids and earmolds should be cleaned and serviced every 3 to 6 months. However, people who develop more earwax should have their hearing instruments cleaned on a more frequent basis. Cleaning custom hearing aids (ITE, ITC, CIC) includes:

1. Wipe off the outside of the hearing aid using a soft, dry cloth or tissue to remove any buildup of earwax and body oils.
2. Remove stubborn ear wax buildup with a soft toothbrush.
3. If wax builds up inside the openings of the vent or sound bore, clean the aid under a magnifying glass using a wax loop and a small vacuum, or blower.
4. Replace wax filter.

Cleaning earmolds includes:

1. Wipe off the outside of the BTE hearing aid using a soft, dry cloth or toothbrush.
2. If wax has entered into earmold tube and cannot be cleaned with a wax loop, detach the earmold from the BTE and soak in warm water. Place only the earmold into the water, not the entire hearing aid. Allow the earmold dry before reconnecting it to the hearing aid.
3. If it is an earmold with a thin tube, replace the tube.
4. For micromolds with RIC receivers, detach the receiver, clean the mold, install a new wax filter, and verify that the receiver is not impacted with wax. If it is, replace it.
5. Do not use chemical solvents as they may cause discoloration and harden the earmold itself.

Online catalogs offer a variety of cleaning solutions that are formulated to clean, disinfect, and deodorize earpieces and ITE hearing aids.

Earmold Retubing

If the earmold tube discolors, becomes stiff, or cracks, a trained technician is to replace it. When retubing a hard or vinyl earmold, place the mold in warm water for several minutes, this will weaken the glue holding the tube. Earmold tubes in silicone molds are fixed with a tube lock.

Select a new tubing of the same type that was used originally. Size thirteen tubes have different thicknesses, and a thicker tube than previously used will constrict in the earmold affecting the higher frequencies transmitted into the ear. Some thin tubes may require trimming the length of the end that terminates in the mold. Examine the old tubing to see how the trimming was done; it may be different for tubes used with hard molds from tubes used with soft molds.

Thin tubes have markings that indicate the length of the tube and internal diameter. RIC tubes are also marked with numbers and colors indicating their size. If you cannot establish the length of the tube, use a tool that measures the distance between the canal aperture and the hearing aid.

When removing the RIC receiver from the mold, use the tool provided to release the receiver from the red/blue adapter to which it is snapped. Make sure the user is aware of the fact that if they remove a micromold from the ear by pulling it out by the tube, the thin wires inside can break causing the hearing aid to produce a cracking intermittent sound. A pull-out string is proper for removing the mold from the ear.

In-Office Modifications

Some patients may be unsatisfied with their hearing aids and may opt for returning them. Others, particularly those who see the benefit of improved hearing but are concerned with the aid's poor fit, will appreciate in-office modifications of the hearing aid shell or earmold done by the clinician, or other trained person.

Hearing aid shells made with the rapid manufacturing technology are thin. The shell wall thickness is comparable with the thickness of a credit or banking card. Still, some minor shell sanding or buffing may be enough to relieve a pressure area or make the aid easier to insert. A soft coat can be applied if the shell is loose or works out from the ear canal. A removal handle, or a pull out string, can be installed to help users with poor dexterity.

Earmolds that are solid can be modified to a greater extent. The canal can be shortened, the helix reduced, the vent enlarged. A handheld or bench grinder with a white stone or steel trimmer works well with all hard and vinyl earmolds.

Silicone earmolds are more difficult to modify. Modifications of silicone require a high-speed grinder and the blue stone. Some silicones produce white smoke during grinding, and the burr or stone becomes very hot. Use caution; wear a mask and protective glasses. If a larger area on a silicone mold is to be modified, trim the mold first with a knife or scissors. Then, round the edges with a stone or steel trimmer. Burrs and trimmers with cross-cut edges (serrated) are the most effective for silicone drilling and trimming. Online catalogs offer small tools suitable for use in office.

Remakes

In cases when modifications are ineffective, or not proper, the hearing aid or earmold may have to be returned to the manufacturer to have a new earmold or earshell made. This is called a remake. If a remake is the course of action, the clinician should advise the lab clearly on the problem. Earmold labs appreciate to hear both; the user and the clinician's description of the problem. This gives them better understanding of the issue and more flexibility in finding the proper solution. To provide accurate instructions, the following terms describing the problem should be used; difficult to insert, works out from the ear, loose fit, inadequate retention, uncomfortable, or feedback. Terms such as too big, too tight all over, poor fit, canal too short should be avoided as they may be understood differently by different people. Use simple terminology. Descriptions such as, "The soreness results from tightness of the superior canal eminence, particularly its superior, medial and inferior surfaces" may be difficult to understand for lab technicians and may require help from professional staff, which may delay the processing of the order.

Pictures of poorly fitting hearing aids and earmolds in the ear are helpful and can be included in the box with the paper work, emailed, or attached to the electronic order form. The picture can be compared with the image of the virtual modeling and make troubleshooting accurate, easier, faster, and more objective.

If the digital rapid manufacturing process was used to manufacture the original earmold or earshell, there is no need to provide the earmold lab with a new impression if the reordering or remake occurs within 6 or so months for one of the following reasons:

1. The earmold or earshell is lost or damaged,
2. Change in the style or color,
3. Change in the vent style or size,
4. Remake due to an allergic reaction,
5. The earmold or earshell is difficult to insert into the ear, or
6. New options are to be accommodated on the hearing aid faceplate (like a larger volume control wheel).

In these cases, the reuse of the original file is fully justified. Addressing a nonfit-related issue through the file reprint or modification ensures that the resulting earmold or hearing aid shell will have the same quality of fit and size, an issue important to all.

If a remake due to a fitting problem such as a loose fit, insecure fit, discomfort, sound going on/off, or feedback is needed, taking a new impression is recommended because the problem may be related to the poor quality of the first impression or to changes in the ear canal shape and underlying structures. The new impression will accurately capture the extent of those changes and ensure the proper fit of the new earmold. Remodeling the impression that was inferior in the first place may be a long way to satisfy the patient with the fit of the earmold.

It is a common request to remake hearing aid shells and earmolds with longer canals. Most earshells and earmolds have adequately long canals. The tip of the canal is tapered for the mold insertion and comfort. Because the tip does not make contact with the ear, making it longer will not improve the mold retention; in fact it can make insertion difficult. Loosely fitting earshells and earmolds need, in most cases, a snugger fit, not a longer canal.

Remakes of hearing aids and earmolds are not common. Typically, five to 10 hearing aids in 100 will require a remake within the first 3 months of the aid use, for any reason, including style and color change, and lost and damaged aids. Earmolds for BTEs require fewer remakes, micromolds more.

The first remake usually addresses the fitting issue, and the hearing aid will serve the user well for the next several years. Some hearing aids require more than one remake. In binaural fittings, it is usually one hearing aid in the pair that fits poorly. This causes frustration among clinicians who cannot comprehend why a hearing aid in one ear fits well from the very beginning while the other requires multiple remakes. Manufacturers are often blamed for inadequate manufacturing standards, insufficient quality control, and lack of proper training. Although this may be true in some cases, those poor fittings can be linked to patients with soft and dynamic ear canals. A significant number of ears are asymmetrical in softness and dynamics to the extent that only one hearing aid is at risk of a fitting problem. File modifications are not recommended for such remakes. Certainly, the clinician may insist that the lab modifies the original impression over and over again to get a better fit. A simpler and more effective way is to provide the lab with an open mouth higher viscosity impression, if such was not made for the original earmold. In general, if a second remake fails to address the fitting issue, a change in the impression material or technique, or both, is needed.

Sources of Information

The Internet and websites are a popular and up-to-date source of information. Hearing aid manufacturers, earmold labs, and dispensing offices advise their customers on topics such as symptoms of hearing loss, types and styles of hearing aids, and newest products and models. Educational materials and product catalogs can be viewed and downloaded. Tips for hearing aid maintenance or quick troubleshooting are offered. A local hearing instrument specialist or audiologist can be located. Popular topics about the ear anatomy, health problems, and trends in technology are provided by numerous websites including Wikipedia—a free online encyclopedia (Figure 3–40).

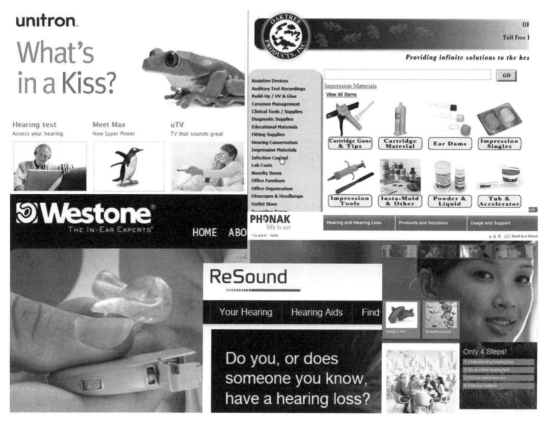

Figure 3–40. The Internet and websites are a popular and up-to-date source of information about hearing health, hearing aids, and earmolds.

More traditionally oriented clinicians looking for advice or a second opinion are always welcome to call directly the manufacturer's Customer Service for help and support.

REVIEW QUESTIONS

1. Human ear canal observed in the transverse view commonly has:
   a. One sharp bend.
   b. The number of bends depends on how old the patient is.
   c. Two bends that give the canal shape similar to the letter "S."
   d. Thick hair close to the eardrum.
   e. B and D.

2. The cartilaginous tissue of the ear canal commonly is:
   a. Quite flexible.
   b. Moderately sensitive.
   c. Lined with earwax.
   d. Changing with jaw movements.
   e. All of the above.

3. The following is/are true:
   a. Any impression is sufficient to make a properly fitting earmold.
   b. The use of a mouth prop is recommended to prevent accidental jaw closing while the material cures in the ear.
   c. A hearing aid has a better acoustic seal if the impression is taken with a low viscosity (runny) impression material.

d. The shorter the canal portion of the impression, the better the instrument's retention.

e. The oto-block should be removed from the impression before the impression is forwarded to the otoplastic lab.

4. Insertion of the oto-block past the ear's second bend is necessary to:
  a. Imprint the first and second canal bend on the impression.
  b. Eliminate voids and air pockets on the impression.
  c. Prevent bleeding while removing the impression from the ear.
  d. A and B.
  e. None of the above.

5. An earmold to be appreciated by the user must have:
  a. Sufficient acoustic seal.
  b. Adequate in-ear retention.
  c. Proper sound direction.
  d. Comfortable fit for extended use.
  e. All of the above.

6. An earmold manufactured from an open-jaw impression commonly:
  a. Has a small vent.
  b. Has better seal, retention, and comfort than an earmold built from a closed jaw or chewing impression.
  c. Is more difficult to modify.
  d. Is rejected by the user.
  e. Has a long crooked canal.

7. An earmold manufactured from an impression taken with a low-viscosity (runny) impression material may:
  a. Be loose.
  b. Feed back.
  c. Be uncomfortable.
  d. Work out of the ear.
  e. All of the above.

8. The shore value of an impression material refers to the material:
  a. After cure hardness.
  b. Color.
  c. Flow characteristics.
  d. Stress relaxation.
  e. None of the above.

9. Acoustic seal area in most earmolds occurs:
  a. At helix.
  b. At the concha.
  c. Between the ear canal anatomical first and second bend.
  d. Past the second bend.
  e. All over the earmold.

10. The following is/are true:
  a. Silicone earmold materials typically have 90 Shore hardness.
  b. Shrinkage in earmold materials typically exceeds 5%.
  c. Earmolds made of vinyl prevent acoustic feedback better than molds made of silicone.
  d. All of the above.
  e. None of the above.

11. Ear inflammation can be caused by:
  a. A loose or tight hearing aid fit.
  b. Allergic reaction to the earmold material.
  c. Difficulty in earmold insertion.
  d. All of the above.
  e. B and C.

12. Retention for a canal style earmold can be found:
  a. At the helix or antitragus.
  b. In the canal.
  c. At the antitragic notch.
  d. All over the earmold.
  e. Is not necessary for the earmold proper fit.

13. The following is true:
  a. RIC hearing aids are analog programmable.
  b. RIC hearing aids have the receiver located in the ear canal.
  c. IIC hearing aids feature a 3-mm volume control.
  d. CIC hearing aids are too small to accommodate a vent.

e. Streamers serve for hearing aid cleaning.

14. Custom micromolds are made
a. Only from soft materials.
b. From hard or soft materials.
c. From stents dental modeling wax.
d. From expandable polyurethane foam.
e. From vulcanized rubber.

15. The occlusion effect results from
a. Eating chips with ketchup.
b. Talking, chewing, or laughing.
c. The closure of the ear canal, for example by an earmold.
d. Incorrect amplification characteristics of the hearing aid.
e. Is inherited.

Answer Key

1. c
2. e
3. b
4. d
5. e
6. b
7. e
8. a
9. c
10. e
11. d
12. b
13. b
14. b
15. c

REFERENCES

Cartwright, K. (2003). Custom earmolds: Art or Science. *Seminars in Hearing, 24*(4), 265–275.

Dillon, H. (2001). *Hearing aids*. New York, NY: Thieme.

Fifield, D. (2010). A new ear impression technique to prevent acoustic feedback with high-powered hearing aids. *Volta Review, 82*(1), 33–39. Reported in Pirzanski, C. (2000). Secrets of the multilayer impression-taking technique. *Hearing Review,* 7(10), 22–27. Retrieved from http://www.hearing review.com/issues/articles/2000-10_01.asp

Flynn, M. (2004). Maintaining the directional advantage in open fittings. *Hearing Review, 12*(11), 32–36. Retrieved from http://www.hearingreview.com/issues/articles/2004-11_04.asp

Garcia, H., & Staab, W. (1995). Solving challenges in deep canal fittings. *Hearing Review, 2*(1), 34–40.

Gray's Anatomy. (2010). *The external ear.* Retrieved from http://www.theodora.com

Gudmundsen, G. (2003). Physical options for custom hearing aids. *Seminars in Hearing, 24*(4), 313–322.

Insta-Mold Products. (2010). Retrieved from http://www.instamold.com

Kampe, S., & Wynne, M. (1996). The influence of venting on the occlusion effect. *Hearing Journal, 49*(4), 59–66.

Kuk, F. (1994). Maximum usable insertion gain with ten earmold designs. *Journal of American Academy of Audiology, 5*, 44–51.

Kuk, F., & Ludvigsen, C. (2010). Ampclusion management 101: Understanding variables. *Hearing Review, 10*(8), 22–32. Retrieved from http://www.hearing review.com/issues/articles/2002-08_02.asp

Macrae, J. (1990). Static pressure seal of earmolds. *Journal of Rehab Ressearch and Development, 27*(4), 397–410.

Oliveira, R., Babcock, M., & Venem, M. (2005). The dynamic ear canal and its implications. *Hearing Review, 12*(2), 18–19. Retrieved from http://www.hearingreview.com/issues/articles/2005-02_01.asp

Oliveira, R., & Hoeker, R. (2003). Ear canal anatomy and activity. *Seminars in Hearing, 24*(4), 265–275.

Pirzanski, C. (1998). Diminishing the occlusion effect: Clinician/manufacturer relative factors. *Hearing Journal, 51*(4), 66–78.

Pirzanski, C. (2001). Factors in earmold style selection: Starting (and finishing) right. *Hearing Review, 8*(4), 20–24. Retrieved from http://www.hearing review.com/issues/articles/2001-04_01.asp

Pirzanski, C. (2010). Earmold retention issues: Why do these earmolds keep falling out? *Hearing Review, 17*(5), 26–34. Retrieved from http://www.hearing review.com/issues/articles/2010-05_02.asp

Pirzanski, C., & Berge, B. (2000–2010). *Earmold acoustics and technology.* Doctoral level course, Salus University School of Audiology. Retrieved from http://audonline.org

Pirzanski, C., & Berge, B. (2003). Earmold impressions: Does it matter how they are taken? *Hearing Review, 10*(4), 18–20. Retrieved from http://www.hearing review.com/issues/articles/2003-04_01.asp

Pirzanski, C., & Berge, B. (2005). Ear canal dynamics: Facts versus perception. *Hearing Journal, 58*(10), 50–58. Retrieved from http://journals.lww.com/thehearingjournal/Fulltext/2005/10000/Ear_canal_dynamics_Facts_versus_perception.8.aspx

Pirzanski, C., Chasin, M., Klenk, M., Purdy, J. (2000). Attenuation variables in earmolds for hearing protection devices. *Hearing Journal, 53*(6), 44–50.

Pirzanski, C., & Maye, V. (1999). *Variances in the remake rate of earmolds made of hard and soft materials.* Starkey Labs Canada. Internal study.

Revit, L. (1992). Two techniques for dealing with the occlusion effect. *Hearing Instruments, 43,* 16–18.

Sataloff, R. (2003). Abnormal anatomy of the external auditory canal. *Seminars in Hearing, 24*(4), 277–280.

Voogdt, U. (2010). *The occlusion effect.* Retrieved from http://www.bernafon-maico.com

Some paragraphs in this book chapter are updated from articles published by this author in The Hearing Review *in April, May, July, August, and September of 2006, and are used with permission. All these five articles are available online at http://www.hearingreview.com*

CHAPTER 4

Principles of High-Fidelity Hearing Aid Amplification

MEAD C. KILLION
PATRICIA A. JOHNSON

INTRODUCTION

The 20th century saw the emergence of many technologies related to amplification of sound for the listener with hearing impairment, ranging from a turn-of-the-century nonelectric ear trumpet to the fully digital hearing aid of the 1990s. The 21st century brings continuing advances including nonoccluding open-fit hearing aids and wireless integration of communication devices (e.g., hearing aids to phone, cell phone, computer, or TV). As technology has advanced, the market lifespan of technology has rapidly decreased. In the 1970s, a new technology might have a lifespan of 6 to 12 years, whereas today, with flexibility in signal processing made possible by digital platforms, a new technology may have a lifespan of 1 to 2 years (D. Smriga, personal communication, 2010). As technology advanced, the retail price to the consumer increased substantially: 77% over the 10-year period of the early 1990s to 2000. One might conclude that the newer technology, with its significantly higher price tag, improved satisfaction with hearing aids. Consumer surveys, however, indicated that over the 10-year period in which the price increased 77%, overall consumer satisfaction remained *unchanged* (Kochkin, 2002). Specific problems—namely, speech intelligibility in noise—have not been solved by hearing aid signal processing. Satisfaction with hearing aids in noisy situations was highest (51%) for single-channel multiple memory hearing aids in 1996 (Kochkin, 1996). By 2005, when digital hearing aids made up 90% of fittings in the United States, satisfaction with hearing aids in noise remained at 51% (Kochkin, 2005). Despite the move to digital signal processing, one half of all hearing aid users remained dissatisfied with hearing aid performance in noisy situations.

All known experimental evidence suggests that speech intelligibility in noise, patient satisfaction, and sound fidelity are highly correlated. That is, the best intelligibility and greatest patient satisfaction is achieved with hearing aids that have the highest fidelity. High fidelity in hearing aids is achieved by first understanding the physics of sound as it relates to sound arriving at the normal ear, and then applying those principles to the amplification of sound so that hearing-impaired listeners obtain a more normal listening experience. It is also necessary to understand the nature of hearing impairment as it relates to gain requirements. Design solutions to the hearing-in-noise problem lie not in hearing aid signal processing, but rather in measuring the degree of the hearing-in-noise deficit and applying signal-to-noise enhancing technologies to remediate the problem.

What Is High Fidelity?

Fidelity is defined as accuracy and exactness. In sound reproduction, fidelity is the degree of accuracy with which sound is reproduced. High-fidelity sound bears very close resemblance to the original sound. High-fidelity hearing aids, then, should be acoustically and subjectively transparent: listeners should receive the same audio quality with high-fidelity hearing aids as they would receive listening directly to the sound. Fidelity can be quantified in terms of frequency response, amplitude, and time. Distortion produced in any of these domains results in reduced fidelity.

High fidelity as a concept applied to the amplification of sound for hearing-impaired listeners is not new; studies defining aspects of high fidelity have been conducted for the past 80 years (e.g., Snow, 1931). Transducers capable of producing high-fidelity sound in hearing aids are also not new: high-fidelity, low distortion microphones have been available since the 1970s, and low distortion receivers since the late 1980s. What appears to be lacking is recognition of the fact that high-fidelity sound reproduction provides the best sound quality and speech intelligibility for all listeners.

Ear Canal Acoustics

High-fidelity design requires that we account for amplitude and frequency response characteristics in the normal, open ear. Nature provides each of us with a hearing aid in the form of external ear resonances and "horn" action, which combine to produce substantially greater eardrum sound pressure levels than those present in the sound field. This canal resonance amounts to approximately 15 to 20 dB of gain around 2.7 kHz (Wiener & Ross, 1946) in a normal ear canal. The sound pressure at the microphone inlet of a hearing aid, on the other hand, will generally be only about 5 dB greater than that in the sound field, depending on the exact location of the microphone (Kuhn & Burnett, 1977; Madaffari, 1974). Thus, the hearing aids must first provide 10 to 15 dB of acoustic gain in the 2.7 kHz frequency region simply to compensate for the gain eliminated by occluding the open ear. In contrast, little compensation is required at low frequencies where the eardrum pressure and the pressure available to the hearing aid microphone are essentially the same.

Coupler Response for Flat Insertion Gain

For engineering purposes, the required hearing aid gain, output, and frequency response are best defined in terms of the coupler response of the hearing aid. The Coupler Response for a Flat Insertion Gain (CORFIG) curve is influenced by the choice of coupler, the selection of reference sound-field conditions, and differences among individuals' external ear resonances, eardrum impedances, and other factors. A great deal of simplification is provided if we ignore individual differences and choose a manikin of average anthropometric dimensions and a coupler ("occluded-ear simulator") that approximates the acoustic impedance of an average ear. The KEMAR manikin (Burkhard & Sachs, 1975) meets the first requirement, while the modified Zwislocki (1970) coupler meets the second requirement up to 7 or 8 kHz (Sachs & Burkhard, 1972). Unpublished experiments comparing eardrum-pressure response on real ears with the response measured in the Zwislocki coupler were conducted at Etymotic Research during the development of the ER-4, 16-kHz bandwidth high-fidelity

earphones. These experiments indicated that the Zwislocki coupler also provides a reasonably good representation of the ear in the 8- to 16-kHz region, despite the fact that the acoustic side branches in the coupler, which simulate the motion of the eardrum, have little effect above 8 kHz. The motion of the eardrum itself is so small above 8 kHz as to have little effect on the pressure developed in front of the eardrum (see the complete analog of the ear given by Goode, Killion, Nakamura, and Nishihara, 1994).

The location of the hearing aid microphone itself naturally affects the real-ear response of the hearing aid. Figure 4–1 shows the Zwislocki-coupler CORFIG curves from Killion and Monser (1980) for three sound-field reference conditions (0°, 90°, and random incidence), based on measurements with a KEMAR manikin. The inset drawings illustrate three locations for the microphone inlet: BTE (a behind-the-ear hearing aid case in which the microphone is located over, and not behind, the ear), ITE (in the ear), and CIC (completely in the canal) hearing aids. The curves for the ITE aid were obtained for a microphone inlet approximately flush with the plane of the pinna, because at the time these data were obtained, most ITE aids filled the entire concha.

Reference Sound-Field Condition

As Figure 4–1 indicates, it is impossible to design a conventional ITE or BTE aid that will have a perfectly flat (matched to average ear canal resonance) frequency response for the user at all angles of incidence. The response-versus-source angle effects of the open ear are not duplicated at either of these microphone locations. Where speech discrimination in face-to-face (near-field condition) listening situations is the only consideration, the appropriate reference condition might be a 0°-incidence sound wave. Where sound quality is the dominant criterion, this is an extremely poor choice of references because a sharp minimum occurs for frontal sound at about 7 kHz. Fortunately, in both home and concert listening, the reflected energy substantially exceeds the energy arriving

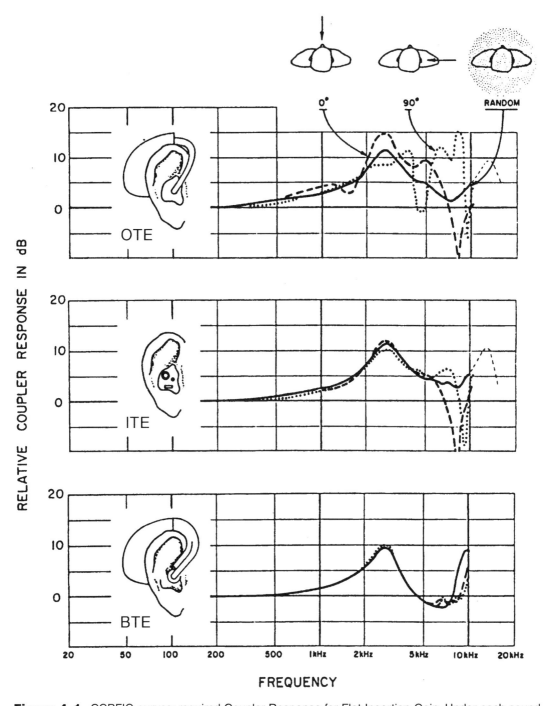

Figure 4–1. CORFIG curves: required Coupler Response for Flat Insertion Gain. Under each sound field condition, these curves represent the difference between the open-ear pressure at the (eardrum-position) Zwislocki-coupler microphone and the pressure measured at the microphone pickup position as noted. From CORFIG: Coupler Response for Flat Insertion Gain (1980) by M. C. Killion and E. L. Monser IV, in G. A. Studebaker & I. Hochberg (Eds.), *Acoustical factors affecting hearing aid performance*. Baltimore, MD: University Park Press. Reprinted with permission.

directly from in front (Olson, 1967) and is free of unusual nulls. Under those circumstances, the appropriate design compromise for a high-fidelity hearing aid would appear to be a flat insertion gain for random-incidence sound. This conclusion is consistent with the results of the psychoacoustic experiments reported by Schulein (1975).

The CIC aid requires no compromise between conflicting frequency response requirements, because the coupler response that provides a flat insertion gain response for 0°-incidence sound also provides a flat insertion gain response for all angles once the microphone inlet is inside the ear canal entrance (Shaw, 1974).

Any of the microphone locations used in binaural hearing aids will preserve basic interaural time and intensity differences so important to binaural localization (Licklider, 1949), and the head-motion-induced changes in interaural phase and intensity that are so important to the externalization of sound (Wallach, 1940). What is not as clear is the relative importance of the pinna and concha cues to everyday localization, auditory spatial perception, and the binaural squelch of noise and reverberation. Informal experiments (such as taping the pinna tightly to the side of the head) have suggested that the pinna and concha provide relatively weak cues to localization compared with those provided by head movement and interaural time and intensity differences. Such a conclusion is consistent with anecdotal evidence indicating that many individuals who need artificial pinnae wear them only on social occasions, that is, primarily for cosmetic reasons.

Frequency Response

Bandwidth

The bandwidth of sound heard by the very young, normal-hearing human ear comprises the range of 20 Hz to 20 kHz. It is logical that preserving as much of this bandwidth as possible should be a goal of high-fidelity sound reproduction. Olson (1957) concluded that

"the reproduction of orchestral music with *perfect* fidelity (emphasis ours) requires a frequency range of 40 to 14,000 cycles and a volume range of 70 dB," whereas Fletcher (1942) concluded that "*substantially complete* fidelity (emphasis ours) in the transmission of orchestral music is obtained by use of a system having a volume range of 65 dB and a frequency range from 60 to 8,000 cycles per second." Both judgments were based on similar data, primarily those of Snow (1931), and the differences between the two conclusions reflected the level of fidelity required and the music to be reproduced. Snow's listeners rated quality close to 100% for a frequency range of 40 Hz to 14 kHz, and slightly above 90% for a frequency range of 60 Hz to 8 kHz. Interestingly enough, later tests reported by Muraoka, Iwahara, and Yamada (1981) on the audio bandwidth requirements for unlimited digital recordings indicated that their listeners could reliably detect the bandwidth restriction only with a 14 kHz cutoff frequency (but not with a 16, 18, or 20 kHz cutoff frequency).

Killion (1979a) concluded that a frequency response extending from 60 Hz to 8 kHz was a reasonable minimum goal for a high-fidelity hearing aid. This was confirmed in fidelity rating experiments in which three panels of listening judges (24 average, untrained listeners; six trained listeners; and five "golden ear" listeners) each rated a pair of experimental BTE hearing aids with 8-kHz bandwidth as comparable in fidelity to a pair of good studio monitor loudspeakers with 20-kHz bandwidth. Figure 4–2 shows their frequency response curves, labeled OTE and MS, respectively. The irregularity in the frequency response of the loudspeakers was apparently judged as important a defect as the 8-kHz bandwidth limitation of the OTE aids.

The 8-kHz-bandwidth hearing aids were rated *much* higher in fidelity than a pair of "PP" headphones popular at the time (Koss PRO-4AA) in which exaggerated bass and treble response were widely noted. The good fidelity ratings for the BTE aids were consistent across four different selections of program material, including a piano trio selection chosen because the drummer's brush-on-cymbal sound provided substantial energy above 10 kHz.

Informal experiments conducted by Gudmundsen and Killion (1998) using a high-fidelity loudspeaker playing a piano trio recording, indicated that 12 out of 14 hearing aid wearers could hear the difference between a 16 kHz bandwidth and the 4 to 5 kHz bandwidth typical of many hearing aids. For these tests, the participants removed their hearing

aids and the presentation level was set to 85 dB SPL, which is typical of nightclubs. Of the 12 participants who could tell the difference, 10 preferred the wider bandwidth.

Bandwidth and Speech Intelligibility

Skinner and Miller (1983) did a series of experiments on the effects of bandwidth on word recognition scores in quiet and noise,

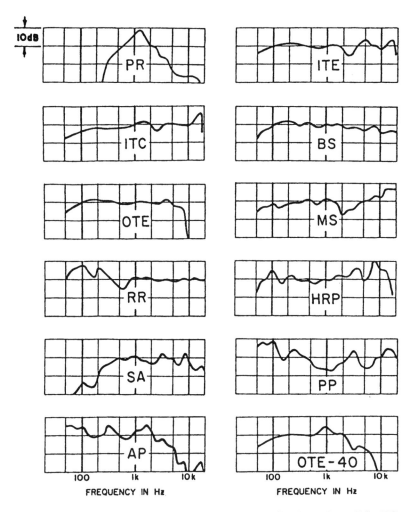

Figure 4–2. Effective relative room response (loudspeakers BS, MS, and RR), relative real-ear field-referenced response (headphones HRP, PP, and AP), pocket radio (PR), speech audiometer (SA), and relative insertion response (binaural hearing aids ITE, ITC, OTE, and OTE-40) of 12 sound systems studied by Killion (1979a). Note: At the time, OTE (over the ear) was becoming a popular substitute for the BTE (behind the ear) label, because the microphones were no longer hidden behind the ear in the better designs. The original BTE term has now become dominant.

for listeners with moderate to severe hearing loss. They found that all listeners scored best with the widest audible bandwidth, which had an upper limit of 7.1 kHz (the upper cutoff of their 6.3 kHz third-octave band). The widest possible audible bandwidth is also desirable when fitting children with hearing aids, because it enhances perception of high-frequency consonants during their learning years. The phoneme /s/, for example, carries significant linguistic importance in the English language, serving multiple linguistic functions (i.e., plural, tense, and possessive case). A bandwidth extending to 10 kHz may be required for adequate perception of /s/ and /z/ by hearing-impaired children, particularly when sounds are spoken by women and children (Stelmachowicz, Lewis, Sangsook, & Hoover, 2007).

Bandwidth can also affect localization ability; Musicant and Butler (1984) reported that front-back errors in their experiments went from about 1% to nearly 10% when their normal-hearing subjects listened to broadband noise through a 4 kHz low-pass filter. Edwards et al. (2010) found similar results (Figure 4–3).

Considering all these data, it is reasonable to conclude that providing a *minimum* upper bandwidth of 8 kHz is important to high-fidelity sound reproduction. Fortunately, even a 16-kHz bandwidth has been practical since 1979, as demonstrated by the experimental ITE aids whose fidelity rating is shown in Figure 4–2.

Smoothness

The smoother the hearing aid frequency response, the higher the fidelity. Perfect smoothness is not required, however. Bucklein (1962) studied the effect of 10- and 20-dB peaks and dips at 3.2 kHz in an otherwise flat-response transmission system. Although

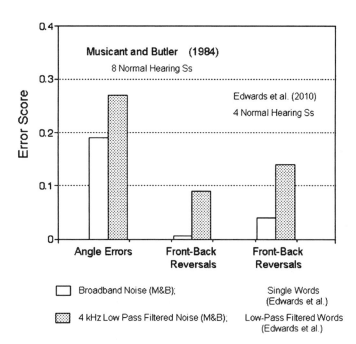

Figure 4–3. Localization errors versus bandwidth. Data (broadband noise and 4 kHz low-pass filtered noise) adapted from Musicant and Butler (1984); data (single words and low-pass filtered words) adapted from Edwards et al., 2010. Both studies showed a significant increase in localization errors from low-pass filtering.

100% of his observers could detect both the 10- and 20-dB peaks, only 10% could recognize the narrowest (less than ⅓ octave) 10-dB dips. Similarly, in a study of the difference limen for formant amplitude, Flanagan (1957) found that a change of 3 dB in the amplitude of the second formant could be detected approximately 50% of the time.

Toole (1981, 1984, 1986) published several findings from 10 years of investigating high-fidelity loudspeakers (and high fidelity in general). He observed (personal communication) that loudspeakers that receive the highest fidelity ratings exhibited frequency responses within a ±1.5 dB tolerance from 100 Hz to 1 kHz, widening to about ±3 dB between 1 and 2 kHz, and then +1.5/−3 dB from 2 kHz to 10 kHz.

From these results, it seems reasonable to infer that a response irregularity in a high-fidelity system of approximately 3 dB can be detected (under appropriate conditions when the source material is speech), but is not likely to be objectionable. Even much larger response irregularities have been found to be minimally objectionable (Dillon & Macrae, 1984) or even preferable (Cox & Gilmore, 1986) under some experimental conditions. However, in addition to sound quality, the issues of feedback and usable gain must be considered. Peaks in the frequency response predispose a hearing aid to feedback, whereas a smooth frequency response reduces the likelihood of feedback. A smooth response can also extend the range of usable gain, because hearing aid volume is often "set to the peaks." When a peak exceeds user discomfort, the natural response is to reduce the gain, which reduces gain throughout the frequency response and can result in decreased audibility for important speech and environmental sounds.

Is there a way to reliably estimate directly from the frequency response curve what the fidelity rating would be if an extensive (and expensive) listening test was performed? With some limitations, the answer is "yes." Consumers Union (CU) adopted a procedure (Consumer Reports, 1977a) based on Stevens Mark VII Loudness calculations (Stevens, 1972) to rate the frequency response

accuracy of high-fidelity loudspeakers using their measured response in 21 ⅓ octave bands with center frequencies of 125 to 12,500 Hz. Killion (1979a) extended the calculations to a 25-band score by including the four ⅓-octave bands between 50 and 100 Hz.

With either procedure, the loudspeakers are driven with a wideband "pink" noise (equal energy in each ⅓-octave band). In the 25-Band Accuracy method, the reference level is a presumed perfect loudspeaker that produces 74 dB SPL in each of the 25 ⅓-octave bands, or 88 dB SPL. Using the Stevens Mark VII loudness calculations, this corresponds to a calculated loudness of 88.6 sones. (Note: The similarity of the two numbers is a coincidence: The Sone and SPL scales intersect near 88.)

The drive voltage to the loudspeaker under test is next adjusted and measured by trial and error until the calculated loudness of its output is also 88.6 sones. A "percentage error" is then calculated from the deviations from a perfect score (100%), averaged over the 25 ⅓-octave bands. To accomplish this: (a) the calculated loudness produced in each band is divided by the ideal loudness for that band, (b) the resulting ratio is subtracted from 1.0, and (c) the absolute value of that result is taken as the relative error for that band. Thus, a measured power equivalent to either 0.5 or 1.5 times the ideal loudness would produce a 50% error for that band. A loudspeaker with a perfectly flat "power response" everywhere except for a 9 dB dropoff in the 1000-Hz band (half loudness by Stevens Mark VII) would have a calculated accuracy of 98% [(50% + 24 × 100%)/25 = 98%].

The original 21-Band Accuracy Score obtained in 1977 by Consumers Union on 16 models of low-priced ($100 to $200 per pair) high-fidelity loudspeakers ranged from 63% to 93%, with a median value of 80%. Listening tests were said to have borne out the utility of the Accuracy Score, although Consumers Union stated that "experience has taught us that a group of listeners won't readily agree on which of two speakers is more accurate when the speakers' scores differ by eight points or less" (Consumer Reports, 1977b). The utility of the newer 25-Band Accuracy Score was confirmed in extensive listening-test experiments reported in the first author's PhD thesis (Killion, 1979a). Systems with different frequency response inadequacies were given subjective ratings by listeners, which showed an excellent correlation between the subjective ratings and the calculated 25-Band Accuracy Score, provided the systems didn't buzz, crackle, or otherwise audibly distort. Figure 4–4 shows the comparison between fidelity rating and calculated 25-band Accuracy Scores for a variety of loudspeakers, earphones, and hearing aids rated on three selections of program material: orchestra, piano trio, and live voice.

A more detailed look at some frequency-response examples is useful. The frequency response of six of the tested sound systems from the first author's PhD thesis (Killion, 1979a) is shown in Figure 4–5.

The important conclusion of these experiments was that it was possible to design hearing aids with a judged fidelity and cal-culated Accuracy Score comparable with the expensive studio monitor loudspeakers popular in Chicago recording studios in the 1970s, and better than that of the Koss PRO4AA stereo headphones, which were the most popular hi-fi headphones available at the time. Following these frequency response design guidelines 10 years later, the K-AMP hearing aids were developed. Their fidelity was verified by their use by professional musicians, including four members of the Chicago Symphony Orchestra.

Amplitude Response

Hearing Aid Gain

Because hearing impairment creates the need for hearing aids in the first place, it must be accommodated, but done in such a way as to give the hearing aid user a "normalized"

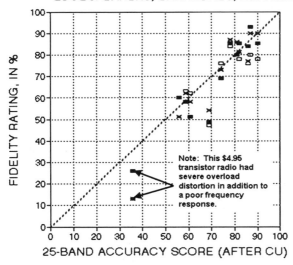

Figure 4–4. Comparison of subjective fidelity rating (100% means no audible difference between the test sound and reference sound), and 25-Band accuracy score averaged over orchestra, jazz trio, and live voice. For purposes of comparison among the subject groups, 7 percentage points were added to each Golden Ears score. Without that addition, the more-critical Golden Ears scores followed the same trend, only 7 points lower.

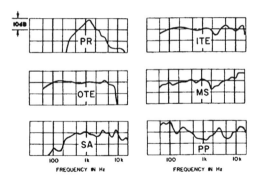

TABLE 1. Overall fidelity ratings for seven sound systems obtained from 24 Untrained Listeners.

	Fidelity ratings		
Sound system	First day	Second day	Average
ITE hearing aids	74.2	77.3	75.7
OTE hearing aids	74.7	76.0	75.4
Monitor speakers	73.1	72.3	72.7
Popular head phones	59.2	59.5	59.3
Speech audiometer	50.0	48.4	49.2
Discount stereo	47.3	46.8	47.1
Pocket radio	12.5	12.8	12.6

Figure 4–5. Frequency response of six of the sound systems used in listening tests shown in Figure 4–2, with details on the ratings inset as Table 1 (Adapted from Killion, 1979a). Note: Hearing aid responses are insertion gains (referred to KEMAR open ear response); all others are relative to the reference loudspeaker system response. The frequency response of the discount stereo is not reported.

loudness experience. There is substantial evidence that many persons with mild or moderate hearing impairment have normal hearing for high-level sounds and thus no amplification is required for high inputs.

As early as 1937, Steinberg and Gardner (1937) reported that many persons with impaired hearing had essentially normal hearing for high-intensity sounds: their hearing loss was obvious as a loss of normal sensitivity for *low*-intensity sounds. This phenomenon is commonly referred to as loudness recruitment. Figure 4–6 (Scharf, 1978) illustrates this phenomenon for a "typical listener with a 40 dB hearing loss due to a cochlear impairment."

The data of Lippman, Braida, and Durlach (1981), Lyregaard (1988), and Hellman and Meiselman (1993) also provide information on how a person with cochlear hearing loss perceives loudness compared with a person with normal hearing. Subjects with 40 dB or less hearing loss had normal loudness for high-intensity sounds. Even for subjects with 60 dB hearing loss, only 8 dB of gain was required to restore normal loudness for high input levels. Pascoe's data on 508 ears (Pascoe, 1988) indicated that with the proper amount of hearing aid gain, limiting should not be required even for high input levels (Figures 4–7A & 4–7B).

Three additional studies indicated that persons with hearing impairment can have essentially normal hearing for moderate or high-level sound. Punch (1978) found no significant difference between hearing aid sound-quality judgments made by 10 subjects with normal hearing and 10 subjects with sensorineural hearing loss listening at the most comfortable level, even though some subjects had moderate-to-severe losses at high frequencies. Lindblad (1982) found that subjects with sensorineural hearing loss were as good at detecting nonlinear distortion in high-level material as subjects with normal hearing. Finally, some of Toole's (1986) listeners had mild-to-moderate high-frequency hearing loss and still exhibited excellent reliability in their fidelity ratings of high-fidelity loudspeakers.

On a more basic level, the following attributes of hearing have been found to be within normal limits at sufficiently high-intensity levels, even in the presence of mild-to-moderate cochlear impairment:

1. Frequency selectivity determined from the "Fletcher Critical Band" can be inferred from tone-in-noise masking experiments (Jerger, Tillman, & Peterson, 1960; Palva, Goodman, & Hirsh, 1953)
2. Frequency selectivity determined from psychophysical tuning curves (McGee, 1978)
3. Frequency discrimination (Gengel, 1973)
4. Loudness summation for complex sounds (with cochlear impairment below 50 dB; Scharf & Hellman, 1966)
5. Loudness discrimination (Scharf, 1978).

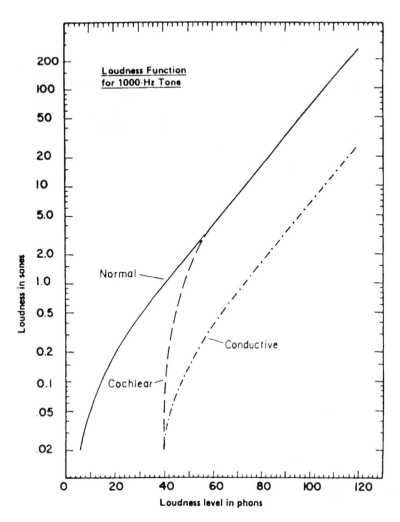

Figure 4-6. Loudness of a 1000 Hz tone as a function of the loudness level for a normal-hearing listener, a typical listener with a cochlear impairment (and recruitment), and a typical listener with a conductive impairment. From Scharf, B. (1978). A model of loudness. A summation applied to impaired ears. *Journal of the Acoustical Society of America, 40,* 71–78. Reprinted with permission.

In addition to the psychophysical data, there is physiological evidence that high-level electrical potentials in the cochlea can be normal in some cases of mild cochlear impairment. The whole-nerve action potential recorded in laboratory animals (Wang & Dallos, 1972) or recorded from the ear canal in humans (Berlin & Gondra, 1976) is often normal. Indeed, both the waveform and latency of the entire auditory brain stem evoked response may appear entirely normal at high levels in some persons.

A discussion of the physiology of hearing impairment is beyond the scope of this chapter, but it appears that outer hair cells function to improve the low-level sensitivity of the ear, while the primary function of audition appears to rest on the inner hair cells. Post-mortem hair-cell counts on patients with hearing impairment who had good speech recognition in noise typically show hair-cell loss restricted to outer hair cells, consistent with normal or near-normal hearing for high-level sounds, even with the loss of outer hair

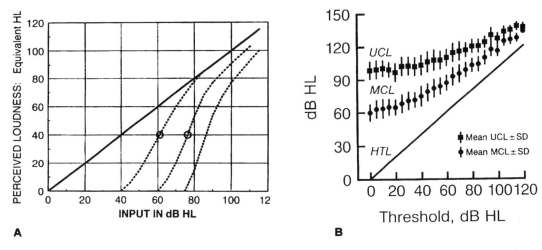

Figures 4–7. A. Loudness data of Lippman et al. (1981) and Lyregaard (1988) combined; **B.** MCL and UCL data of Pascoe (1988). These data provided the logic for the FIG6 fitting formula.

cells, as long as most of the inner hair cells function properly.

The obvious conclusion is that whenever a person has normal or near-normal hearing for high-level sounds, hearing aids should not amplify high-level sounds: the hearing aids should be so acoustically transparent that they subjectively disappear. The term "unity insertion gain" describes the condition in which hearing aids provide neither amplification nor attenuation of the incoming sound.

For soft sounds, hearing aids must provide enough gain to compensate for the loss of sensitivity to low-level sounds (i.e., the loss of sensitivity that is plotted on the threshold audiogram). If hearing loss for low-level sounds is frequency dependent (sloping hearing loss), more amplification for low-level sounds is required at some frequencies than at others. This requirement, in combination with the requirement for unity acoustic gain at some or all frequencies for high-level sounds, implies that both the frequency response of the hearing aids as well as the gain must depend on the input level. The hearing aids should make soft sounds audible, moderate sounds (conversation) clearly audible and comfortable, and loud sounds loud, but not uncomfortably loud. If

these criteria are accomplished, a more natural loudness experience is achieved. Wide Dynamic Range Compression (WDRC) circuitry meets these requirements.

There have been several attempts to specify the proper hearing aid gain response for varied input levels: NAL-NL1; DSL[i/o]; IHAFF; and FIG6, as summarized in Dillon (2001), and CAMEQ2-HF (Moore, Glasberg, & Stone, 2010). To the authors' knowledge, none except FIG6 specify the most obvious property: Provide unity gain in the regions where the wearer has no loudness loss (Killion & Fikret-Pasa, 1993; Figure 4–8).

Peak Output Levels

There is no easy answer to the question of what the maximum undistorted output of a unity-gain, high-fidelity sound reproduction system should be. A reasonable approach is to consider input levels typically encountered by hearing aid users and the peak undistorted output levels the hearing aid receivers are capable of producing.

In everyday conversation, the highest levels at the hearing aid microphone are usually generated by the user's own voice. The data of Dunn and Farnsworth (1939) indicate that the overall speech levels measured at the

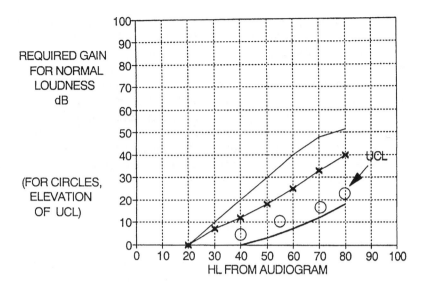

Figure 4–8. Figure 6 from Killion and Fikret-Pasa (1993) was subsequently called the "FIG6" gain prescription. It was derived from the data of Figure 4–7A and 4-7B. It shows the estimated gain required to restore loudness for various level signals, independent of frequency. The upper curve is for 45 dB SPL signals, the middle curve is for 65 dB SPL signals, and the lower curve is for 95 dB SPL signals. The UCL data suggest that the required high-level gain is safe (UCL and MCL data adapted from Pascoe, 1988).

talker's ear were about equal to levels 30 cm in front of the speaker's mouth. Thus, the Dunn and White (1940) data on instantaneous peak levels in speech measured at 30 cm may be used directly: In normal conversational speech, instantaneous speech peaks of 90 to 95 dB SPL occur with some regularity (in 1% to 5% of ⅛-second intervals). Because of the head-shadow, high frequencies will be attenuated somewhat, but since the majority of the peak energy lies below 1 kHz, this will have little effect on the overall peak levels. Unless the conversational level increases, therefore, the instantaneous peak levels at the microphone will be 90 to 95 dB SPL, a range that has often been used as the goal for the level of minimum undistorted input in hearing aid design. Higher inputs are not uncommon; a shout can easily produce 100 to 105 dB instantaneous peak SPL at the microphone of the speaker's own hearing aid. The first author, a choir director, can still easily produce a 112 dB instantaneous (oscilloscope) peak SPL singing a high "F." Years ago, his then two-year-old daughter consistently produced 114 dB peaks saying "Hi Dad" three feet from the hearing aid microphone. Other commonly encountered sounds such as a finger snap at arm's length can produce a 100 to 110 dB instantaneous peak SPL, while keys jangling or a spoon dropped onto a plate can produce a 110 to 115 dB instantaneous peak SPL. Even in 2011, such sounds can still be a common source of complaints about hearing aid distortion.

Live Music

In live performances of classical music, Marsh (1975) reported that "a fully scored orchestral passage in a Mendelssohn symphony reaches approximately 95 dB on a decibel meter" for someone sitting in a main-floor seat at Chicago's Orchestra Hall. Marsh reported that approximately the same levels are reached during a similar passage in the front seats at outdoor amphitheaters such as Chicago's Grant Park, or at the edge of Highland Park's

Ravinia Festival stage. The typical instantaneous peak factor for an orchestral passage of this sort is 5 to 10 dB, indicating instantaneous peaks of 100 to 105 dB SPL at these three Chicago-area locations. Similarly, for a typical listening position in a large music hall, Olson (1967) reported the instantaneous peak sound pressure level as 100 dB SPL. During the last 20 years, one of the authors has carried a sound level meter (SLM) to concerts. The Chicago Symphony Orchestra has produced a peak SLM reading of 104 dBA during a Mahler symphony, measured in a seventh-row, center balcony seat. At the other extreme, the quietest piano passage in Strauss's Burlesque for Piano and Orchestra in D Minor was 35 dBA. The same level was measured on a solo viola during a performance of the Elgar/Payne Symphony No. 3.

Performers have more stringent requirements, as discussed by Killion (2009) and illustrated in Figure 4–9.

Surprisingly high decibel levels are even encountered at audiology convention events where bands are playing. At an opening night party of one audiology convention, the levels in the dance area at the beach ranged from 108 to 112 dB on a sound level meter (A-Fast). All things considered, an undistorted *input* capability of 115 dB instantaneous peak SPL—referred to the sound field—appears to be a minimum requirement for a high-fidelity hearing aid.

Distortion

Undistorted Output Requirements Versus Frequency

In a high-fidelity sound reproduction system, the peak undistorted output levels need to be determined. The frequency distribution of the maximum instantaneous peak levels for

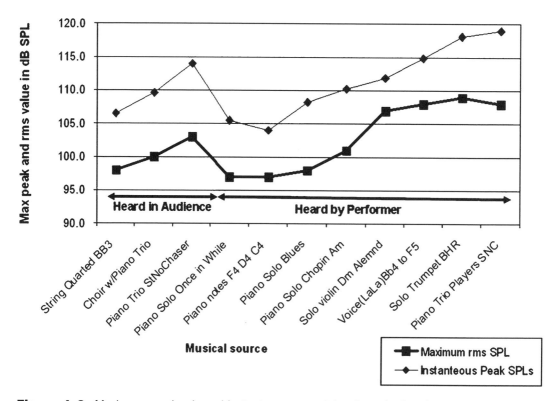

Figure 4–9. Maximum rms levels and instantaneous peak levels at the hearing aid microphone as heard in the audience and by the performing musicians. Reprinted from Killion, 2009, with permission from Allied Media, LLC.

a 75-piece orchestra was given by Fletcher (1931) and is shown in Figure 4–10.

The undistorted output requirements fall off with frequency with typical speech and music inputs. This fact has been used since the 1940s to allow "hiss reduction" in recordings by preemphasizing the signals with a high-frequency boost. The effect of the preemphasis, which is corrected in playback, is to improve the SNR of recorded material at the expense of a reduced high-frequency overload capability. For example, adding a 75 μs, high-frequency pre-emphasis (6 dB per octave upward slope above a 2.1 kHz corner frequency) remains the standard in FM broadcasting. Similarly, Audio Engineering Society (AES) standards for prerecorded tape and phonograph records call for a preemphasis ranging from 75 to 150 μs (Roys, 1968).

Because of the amplification of the external ear, a hearing aid receiver must produce some 15 dB greater output near 2.8 kHz than would be indicated by the spectrum of peaks in speech and music in the sound field. From this and other considerations (discussed in detail in Killion, 1979a), it is possible to arrive at the dotted curve in Figure 4–10, which shows the estimated instantaneous peak (sine-wave) output requirements for a high-fidelity hearing aid operating at unity insertion gain for high-level signals. A 10-dB safety factor is desirable; fortunately, even a 127-dB eardrum pressure peak corresponds to only 112 dB SPL in a 2cc coupler at 3 kHz because of the normal 15 dB real-ear coupler difference (RECD) at 3 kHz. This output is easily reached with Class B or Class D receivers.

Input Noise Level

Ideally, the input noise level of a hearing aid should be less than that of ambient noise levels likely to be encountered by the user, in which case it will seldom be heard. It is important to distinguish input noise from amplified ambient noise, which is often ascribed to the hearing aid until the wearer learns to localize and recognize quiet high-frequency sounds.

The A-weighted noise level during a quiet period in a theater or auditorium may drop to 32 dB (Fletcher, 1942; Olson, 1967). The first author has observed the sound level meter drop to its minimum reading, 30 dBA, on several occasions in Chicago's Symphony Center. Residential noise levels are generally higher. Seacord (1940) measured noise levels in a large number of residential rooms and

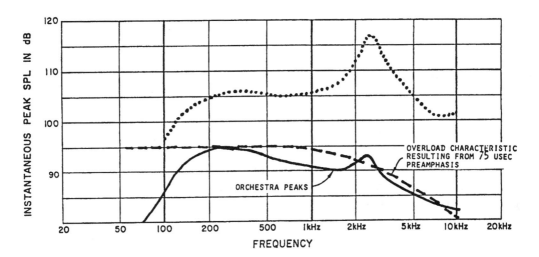

Figure 4–10. Maximum peaks produced in half-octave bands by a large orchestra, referred to audience area (*solid line*). Instantaneous sine wave peak eardrum pressure required of a hearing aid to reproduce a large orchestra (*dotted line*). From Killion (1979a). Note: Orchestra peaks correspond to instantaneous wideband peaks of 105 dB SPL or peak readings of 95 dB SPL on a sound level meter set to "C, Fast."

found an average level of 43 dBA; 90% of the levels fell between 33 and 52 dBA. Seacord's data (1940) have found common acceptance, although it is generally believed that greater use of forced-air heating and air-conditioning systems has increased average levels since his data were obtained.

Macrae and Dillon (1986) reported a more lenient target after they determined the maximum hearing aid equivalent input noise levels *acceptable* to their subjects. A hearing aid in which input noise *just met* their ⅓-octave limits at each frequency would have an overall A-weighted equivalent input noise of 38 dB SPL.

The input noise level in today's hearing aids is determined almost entirely by the microphone noise level. Because the predecessor of this chapter appeared in 2000, a slow but steady improvement in the noise level of subminiature microphones has resulted in typical A-weighted noise levels equivalent to a 23 dBA SPL ambient noise level in some models. Even in a quiet auditorium, the microphone noise level would add less than 1 dB to the apparent A-weighted ambient level. The aided threshold determined by typical microphone noise levels is within a few dB of normal threshold and can be better than normal with special design (Killion, 1979a). The internal noise of the modern hearing aid should thus not degrade a high-fidelity design.

Nonlinear Distortion

The terms "distortion" and "nonlinear distortion" in this chapter refer to distortion that results in the generation of new frequencies in the output that were not present in the input. An example of nonlinear distortion is clipping that occurs from an overloaded amplifier. Total harmonic distortion and intermodulation distortion both measure the relative strength of new frequencies created by nonlinearity when sine-wave signals of one or more frequencies are present at the input.

In a study of the amount of distortion tolerable in a high-fidelity system, Olson (1957) found that total harmonic distortion

levels of approximately 1% were just detectable and that total harmonic distortion levels below 3% were not considered objectionable in a system with an 8-kHz upper cutoff frequency. Intermodulation distortion levels below 2% are generally inaudible on musical material, and even gross distortion levels (6% to 12%) are sometimes inaudible. In general, the barely audible distortion levels of any kind for musical material are at least 10 times greater than the barely audible distortion for a pure-tone signal (Milner, 1977).

The levels above are measured in the sound field. The traditional 2cc coupler measurement of a hearing aid produces relative distortion numbers that are roughly equivalent. If a more accurate comparison is desired, the hearing aid output can be measured using a "diffuse field inverse" filter following the ear simulator, as described by Killion (1979a).

A complicating factor when determining allowable distortion for a sound reproduction system is the fact that the ear's sensitivity to distortion is level dependent. At low sound pressure levels, the level of any harmonic or intermodulation distortion products may lie below the normal threshold of hearing. At high sound pressure levels, the increased upward spread of masking (Wegel & Lane, 1924) and the distortion of the ear itself may mask externally generated distortion products. Thus, no single-number distortion specification applies at all listening levels.

The tests reported by Olson (1957) were carried out in a small listening room at a level of "about 70 dB." Assuming that this level was close to the 75 dB levels reported by Olson for similar listening tests, it corresponds to instantaneous peak levels of approximately 85 dB SPL. This is only slightly greater than the 70 to 80 dB SPL that the masking literature indicates is the region in which the ear should be most sensitive to distortion. Thus, values for detectable and tolerable distortion obtained by Olson and others should be considered a requirement for high-fidelity hearing aids at output levels between about 50 and 90 dB SPL, measured at the eardrum or in an ear simulator. Below 50 dB and above 90 dB, less stringent criteria are required, so relaxing specifications to 10% at 30 dB and 110 dB eardrum SPL appears reasonable. Killion (1979a) describes a variety of psychoacoustic measures of the ear's own distortion that support this choice.

The last issue in determining reasonable distortion criteria is probably the most important one. Unless the precise distortion mechanism (peak clipping, center clipping, curved transfer characteristic) is understood, no single distortion measurement can provide reliable information as to how sound quality will be judged by a listener. For example, 1% of "soft peak clipping" distortion may be inaudible, but 1% of center clipping distortion may be intolerable. Similarly, Peters and Burkhard (1968) found that the 40% total harmonic distortion produced by one system with half-wave rectification had a negligible effect on speech discrimination, while another system with 20% total harmonic distortion from extreme crossover distortion (center clipping) resulted in a loss of 40 percentage points in word recognition.

In light of the available information, a reasonable initial goal for distortion limits for a high-fidelity hearing aid with an 8 kHz bandwidth is shown in Figure 4–11. Listening tests should always be used as a final check.

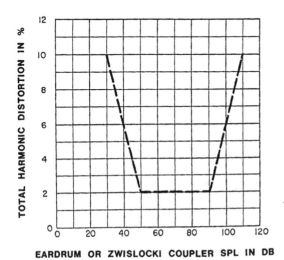

Figure 4–11. Estimated maximum hearing-aid distortion that will be inaudible for speech or music inputs, as a function of level. From Killion (1979a).

Automatic Gain Control Characteristics

To provide a normalized loudness experience, sufficient gain is needed to make soft sounds audible and conversation comfortable. In contrast, unity gain is often required for high-level sounds.

The low-level gain required in a high-fidelity hearing aid can be readily estimated. Although gain numerically equal to the user's hearing loss would be required to restore threshold to audiometric zero, such a large amount of gain is unacceptable (Lybarger, 1944; Martin, 1973).

Under most circumstances, the masking produced by background noise levels commonly encountered in homes, offices, and other locations make it impossible to detect sounds less than 15 to 30 dB above audiometric zero. Based on the average room noise and spectral data of Seacord (1940) and Hoth (1941), Killion and Studebaker (1978) estimated that the masking effect of typical residential room noise produces a nearly uniform 23-dB "hearing loss" across the 250 to 4 kHz speech frequencies. Olson (1957) calculated a 20 to 22 dB loss using slightly different assumptions. More gain than the amount required to make background noise audible will be "empty gain" that makes everything louder but does not improve the detection of soft sounds. These considerations suggest that the gain required to improve aided sound-field thresholds to 20 to 25 dB HL is probably sufficient for most wearers.

The input level at which the gain should be reduced to unity can be estimated. Examination of clinical data and the literature on recruitment indicates that recruitment is typically complete (loudness sensation is essentially normal) for sounds corresponding to 80 dB HL or greater. Some time ago, Barfod (1978) reported that in some cases a nearly linear relationship exists between the degree of hearing loss and the hearing level at which recruitment is complete. Barfod's subjects all had steeply sloping high-frequency loss with nearly normal low-frequency hearing. All his hearing losses below 50 dB HL were characterized by complete recruitment above 75 dB HL. By way of illustration, Figure 4–12 shows two hypothetical hearing losses with their corresponding areas of presumably normal hearing, based on Barfod's loudness data.

As a practical example, assume a user has a 45 dB HL cochlear impairment with complete recruitment for sounds above 80 dB HL. By our assumptions, he requires a maximum gain of 25 dB (45 minus 20) for sounds at 20 dB HL, and unity (0 dB) gain for sounds at 80 dB HL and above. (For speech, 80 dB HL corresponds to 95 dB SPL in a 0°-incidence sound field.)

Optimum Amplitude Input-Output Characteristics

To avoid constant adjustments of the volume control, an Automatic Gain Control (AGC) system is required. To introduce the minimum degradation in perceived sound quality, the operation of the AGC system must be unobtrusive. Compression is universally used in the broadcast and recording industry (Blesser & Ives, 1972). As originally defined at Bell Telephone Laboratories (Mathes & Wright, 1934), compression amplification meant what is now sometimes called logarithmic compression (to distinguish it from some of the misuses of the term; i.e., a con-

stant ratio between the logarithms of the input and output signal amplitudes). When input and output levels are expressed in dB, for example, a compression ratio of 2:1 corresponds to a 5 dB increase in output level for each 10 dB increase in input level.

The idea of applying compression amplification to hearing aids is not new, dating back at least to Steinberg and Gardner (1937). Wide dynamic range compression amplification was apparently first reduced to commercial practice in hearing-aid designs by Goldberg (1960, 1966). It was commonly believed that because compression brought up the audible level of background noise, it would degrade speech intelligibility in noise. Villchur (1973, 1996) was the first to demonstrate that the opposite could be true: By increasing the audibility of both the speech and the noise, the net result was better intelligibility in noise with compression than in quiet without compression.

Figure 4–13 illustrates input-output characteristics (Killion, 1979b) for a hearing aid intended to meet the requirements of the example discussed above. There are four stages of amplification illustrated in Figure 4–13: a low-level, constant-gain stage; a mid-level, constant-compression ratio (2:1) stage; a high-level, unity-gain stage; and a very high-level, compression-limiting stage. In

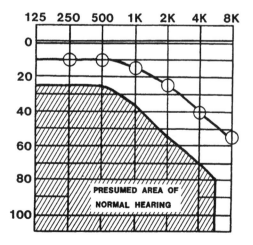

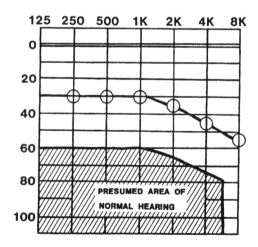

Figure 4–12. Threshold audiograms for two hypothetical subjects, with areas of presumed normal hearing. Data adapted from Barfod, 1978.

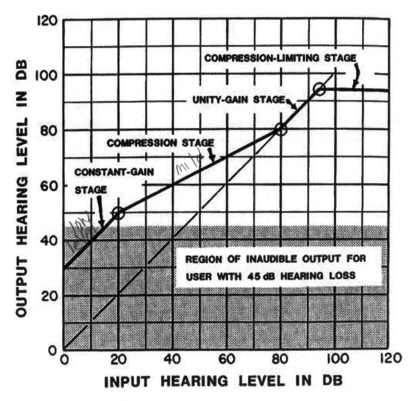

Figure 4–13. Presumed ideal hearing aid input-output characteristics for a listener with 45 dB hearing loss and complete recruitment above 80 dB HL.

the K-AMP design, the compression-limiting stage was not invoked, and loudness discomfort was virtually never a complaint.

The input-output characteristics illustrated in Figure 4–13 are quite different from any of the three other types that were commonly employed in hearing aids at the time the first edition of this chapter was written (shown for comparison in Figure 4–14): Output limiting (peak clipping or low-distortion compression limiting), AVC (automatic volume control), and wide dynamic range compression. Properly adjusted, output limiting can prevent amplified sounds from ever becoming too loud, but linear amplification combined with output limiting often makes a large proportion of sounds too loud. An automatic volume control can ensure that all sounds are amplified to the most comfortable listening level, but the resulting restriction of the dynamic range lends a highly unnatural

sameness to all sounds. Wide dynamic range compression comes closest to the "ideal" characteristic of Figure 4–13 but continues to perform signal processing even for loud sounds, when the hearing aid should simply reproduce sound as it naturally occurs.

Level-Dependent Frequency Response

Few threshold audiograms are flat; a greater loss at the higher frequencies is common. For low-level sounds, high-frequency emphasis in the hearing aid frequency response is required to make the entire range of soft speech sounds audible without over-amplifying low frequency sounds. For high-level sounds, on the other hand, unity gain (and thus a flat frequency response) is required.

The need for a level-dependent frequency response was discussed by Barfod (1976),

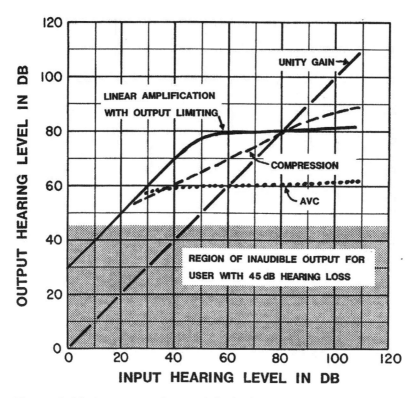

Figure 4–14. Input-output characteristics for three conventional approaches to dynamic range reduction in hearing aids.

Goldberg (1960, 1972), Skinner (1976, 1980), and Villchur (1973, 1978). Level-dependent frequency response can be achieved in several ways. The technique most often described in the literature is the use of multichannel compression amplification, with the compression ratio in each channel chosen to compensate for the degree of hearing loss in that frequency band (Villchur, 1973). An alternate method that provides equivalent performance for persons with mild-to-moderate hearing impairment is a single-channel compression amplifier with level-dependent frequency response. Figure 4–15 shows the level-dependent frequency response characteristic (Killion, 1979b) used in the K-AMP.

AGC Time Constants

The attack and release time constants of the AGC system used to obtain the desired input-output characteristics throughout the operating range are an important consideration in any sound processing system. As discussed by Lippman (1978), the proper choice of time constants depends on the goal of the AGC system of the hearing aid. Early experiments of Ahren et al. (1977) and Schweitzer and Causey (1977) indicated the attack time should be as short as possible, and the release time between 30 and 100 ms, to maximize speech intelligibility. When the goal is to maximize sound quality, on the other hand, the ideal compression attack and release times are not as clear, as discussed by Blesser and Ives (1972). They reported that values of 10 ms and 150 ms for attack and release times, respectively, were accepted for use in the broadcast industry.

However, even under ideal conditions, such as those found in professional recording studios, the optimum choice of attack and release times for minimum perceived distortion is highly dependent on the program material. Thus, any choice of fixed attack and release times will be "wrong" at least part

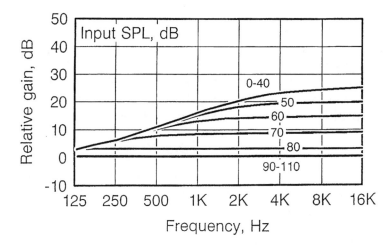

Figure 4–15. Level-dependent frequency response (compression ratio set for 2:1) of the first author's experimental amplifier. Note the high-frequency emphasis for low-level inputs and the flat frequency response for high-level inputs.

of the time. A solution to this dilemma that has been used for some time in the broadcast industry is "Adaptive Compression" or "Variable Recovery Time." This technique automatically varies the release time dependent on the duration of the high-level signal that activated the compression action.

Fikret-Pasa (1993) found an interesting result when comparing peak clipping and two low-distortion compressors (each set to 8:1 compression ratio), with one utilizing a fixed 50 ms recovery time and the other utilizing variable-recovery-time compression. Eight subjects having moderate to severe hearing loss repeated IEEE sentences (IEEE, 1969) spoken by a female talker in four-talker babble. The SNR for 50% correct was calculated for each condition. All subjects obtained the worst SNR (poorest performance) with peak clipping, and the best SNR with variable-recovery-time compression. The industry-typical 50 ms recovery time compression scores were in between. The average SNRs required for 50% correct words in noise were:

Peak clipping	20 dB SNR
50 ms compression	14 dB SNR
Variable recovery time compression	9 dB SNR

The presumed explanation (Teder, 1991) is that a 50-ms recovery time quickly brings the background noise up to the level of the desired speech, making it more difficult for the listener with hearing impairment to use speech envelope cues to help separate the two.

In the case of wide dynamic range compression circuits using relatively low compression ratios (and increasing gain for quiet sounds rather than limiting gain for loud sounds), the principal benefit of variable recovery time is better subjective fidelity. This allows a long-sound recovery time to 500 ms or more, substantially reducing the "pumping" sound that accompanies typical 50 ms recovery, while simultaneously reducing the recovery time after short transients (hand clap, finger snap, etc.) to only 20 ms.

IMPLEMENTATION OF THE GUIDELINES IN HEARING AIDS

A Brief History of High-Fidelity Hearing Aids

The quest for this type of high-fidelity hearing aid began in the late 1970s with the design of hearing-aid-size microphones used in recording and broadcast studios. In 1979, Killion (1979a) demonstrated that available transducers could provide hearing aids with objective frequency response accuracy and subjective fidelity ratings comparable with those of highly regarded stereo loudspeaker systems.

K-AMP

By the end of the 1980s, only two things were missing from hearing aids: a broadcast-quality input amplifier that could handle loud inputs without distortion, and a low-distortion output amplifier with a low enough battery drain to be practical for use in small hearing aids. Both amplifiers became a reality in tiny integrated circuit chips introduced in 1989.

The input amplifier, developed by Etymotic Research with the help of a $500,000 grant from the National Institute on Aging, was labeled the K-AMP amplifier. Consuming less than 0.25 mA, it provided low-distortion, wide-dynamic-range compression with TILL (Treble Increase at Low Levels) level-dependent frequency response, and the ability to handle 115 dB SPL input peaks without audible distortion (Killion, 1993).

The output amplifier was the Class D chip, developed by Etymotic Research for Knowles Electronics. The Class D amplifier produced 110 to 115 dB maximum undistorted output, yet required only a small fraction of the power required by typical hearing aid power amplifiers, making it practical for use in small hearing aids.

Two additional developments made high-fidelity hearing aids more practical: soft-tip, deeply sealed earmolds and CIC (for completely-in-the-canal) hearing aids. Zwislocki (1953) first observed the elimination of the occlusion effect with a deep seal; Killion, Wilber, and Gudmundsen (1988) demonstrated its effectiveness and practicality. By sealing in or near the bony portion of the ear canal, the canal-wall vibration caused by speaking, chewing, or blowing on a horn can be isolated from the eardrum. Thus, an earmold or hear-

ing aid that seals deeply in the ear canal (past the second bend) can eliminate the annoying "hollow voice" occlusion effect discussed in Killion et al. (1988). They also reduce the likelihood of feedback by improving the seal and reducing the sound-producing vibration of the earmold.

Digi-K

The Digi-K (Etymotic Research, 2002) retained the basic virtues of the K-AMP design, with the addition of four programmable memories and a patented method of obtaining a nearly perfectly smooth frequency response from unit to unit. A series of tunable filters are used to flatten the response peaks, after which the appropriate CORFIG equalization is applied (BTE, ITE, CIC, etc.). As of this writing, the K-AMP and Digi-K are still available in the United States from General Hearing Instruments, and they continue to be the hearing aids of choice for performing musicians (M. Chasin, personal communication, 2011).

Who Are the Beneficiaries?

Persons with mild-to-moderate sensorineural hearing loss are the primary beneficiaries of high-fidelity hearing aids, although many persons with moderate and moderate to severe sensorineural loss are also successful users of high-fidelity hearing aids. Individuals with no useful high-frequency hearing will derive little benefit from an extended high-frequency bandwidth (Hogan & Turner, 1998; Rankovic, 1991; Skinner, 1980). However, even individuals with severe high frequency losses often prefer the sound quality provided by high-fidelity hearing aids in the regions where they have useful residual hearing (R. Juneau, personal communication, 2003).

Two critical factors in any successful hearing aid fitting are appropriate counseling and an established trust between the professional and the person with hearing impairment. Because of this, any hearing aid that makes previously unheard sounds audible can be the basis of a successful fitting. However, when fitting musicians and trained listeners, no amount of counseling or trust can overcome the auditory distortions produced by non-high-fidelity hearing aids, regardless of their level of signal processing or cost.

Success of High-Fidelity Hearing Aids

The high-fidelity hearing aids described in this chapter have been available for over 20 years. In the first article on the K-AMP amplifier, the final sentence read "The ultimate test of this amplifier design will be the degree of its acceptance by hearing-impaired wearers" (Killion, 1988). The subsequent acceptance was beyond expectations: a large percentage of all circuits sold for over a decade had K-AMP amplifiers, and wide dynamic range compression processing is now found in nearly all hearing aids. Although subsequently introduced digital circuits provide more signal-processing features, no analog or digital signal processing amplifier introduced in the last 22 years equals the judged fidelity and 16 kHz bandwidth of the K-AMP design, with the exception of its successor, the Digi-K (Etymotic Research, 2002).

Musicians as Judges

One of the most challenging tests of a hearing aid is whether or not a musician can wear it while performing, because the circuit must be capable of handling peak SPLs created by the musicians themselves. In the case of virtuoso violinists, this amounts to 115 dB at the left ear (closest to the violin body). As an amateur violinist, it has been gratifying to the first author that several now- retired violinists in the Chicago Symphony Orchestra wore K-AMP hearing aids during rehearsal and performance. It is now understood that a loss of sensitivity for soft sounds does not have to interfere with a musician's ability to play.

In contrast, this same author has tried a wide variety of popular all-digital hearing aids with disappointing results while directing a choir. Most of the hearing aids overload (distort) so badly with the live choir and piano levels that it is impossible to listen for choral balance and intonation. The errors introduced by the hearing aids overwhelm those of the choir!

The problem of handling performance-level SPLs without distortion may explain the comment made by Chasin (personal communication, June 7, 1999): "Out of the last 200 hearing aid fittings on musicians, 180 of them were K-AMPs. Musicians seem to like the low distortion levels of the K-AMP in high-volume environments—perhaps it has to do with the high input limiting level of the K-AMP that distinguishes it from other hearing aids, including digital products." (Chasin's comments were reaffirmed in more recent trials as this chapter was being prepared.) The issue of overload distortion was discussed recently by Killion (2009). Since that time, at least one company has introduced a widely available digital hearing aid that does not overload on live music, and has excellent AGC characteristics. Unfortunately, it has only a 7 kHz bandwidth.

Fidelity: The Listening Tests

As digital signal processing hearing aids became widely available in the 1990s, advertising claims of "CD sound quality" were frequently seen. To evaluate the fidelity of various digital hearing aids, Killion (2004a) created A-B-A listening comparisons processed through seven manufacturers' digital hearing aids, as well as the K-AMP analog hearing aid, the Digi-K digital hearing aid, and the unaided open ear. All hearing aids were programmed for a 40 dB flat hearing loss using the manufacturer's autofit software. Recordings were made through the nine hearing aids and "open ear" on a KEMAR manikin, utilizing a live string quartet (made up of Chicago Symphony Orchestra players) and a jazz trio as the input signal. Sixty five normal-hearing listeners were asked to rate the fidelity of the hearing-aid-processed music passages using the unaided open ear recordings as the "perfect reference" condition. Results for the string quartet fidelity ratings are shown in Figure 4–16.

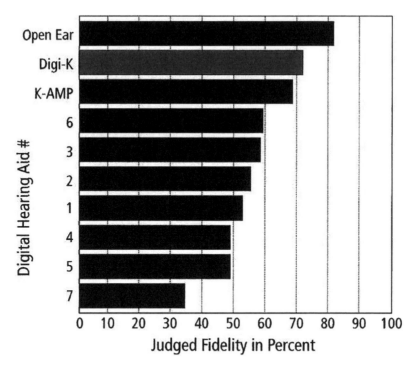

Figure 4–16. Judged fidelity of seven popular digital hearing aids, K-AMP and Digi-K. Recordings of a live string quartet were made through each hearing aid, placed on a KEMAR manikin.

Can the fidelity ratings of normal-hearing listeners be relevant to listeners with hearing loss? Killion (2004a) conducted the same listening comparisons detailed above on 16 subjects with mild-to-moderately-severe sloping sensorineural hearing loss. These subjects gave the same average fidelity ratings as the 65 normal-hearing listeners, suggesting that fidelity is fidelity: That is, when sound is audible, persons with hearing loss judge fidelity the same as persons with normal hearing. A similar result was obtained with a smaller group of subjects listening to a jazz piano trio (Figure 4–17).

In a separate listening test, subjects were also asked to place a dollar value on the quality of the sound when each comparison was played. The dollar ratings obtained from the smaller group of subjects (see Figure 4–17) are shown in Figure 4–18. The results were similar to those obtained from the larger group as reported in Killion (2004a). The hearing-impaired listeners were less willing to pay for low fidelity sound than the normal-hearing listeners, presumably because the normal-hearing listeners don't have to purchase and *wear* the hearing aids.

Within the last couple of years, informal recordings of recent premium digital hearing aids have produced similar results (with one exception) for live piano, trumpet, violin, and voice. The exception was one hearing aid that passed all informal listening tests for sound quality. Its only deficit was a restricted (7 kHz) bandwidth. *which brand*

Performance in Noise

SNR Loss

Nearly any hearing aid can help listeners understand speech in noise when both speech and noise are inaudible with the open ear.

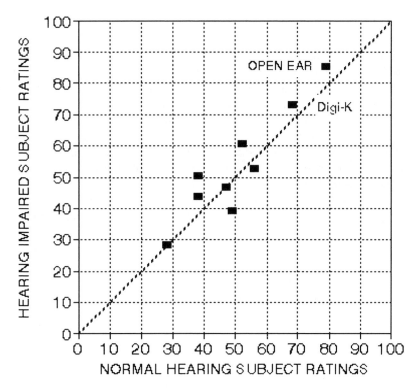

Figure 4–17. Comparison of fidelity judgments from 9 hearing aid wearers and 19 normal-hearing subjects. Recordings of a live jazz piano trio were made through 7 popular digital hearing aids, the Digi-K the "open ear" on a KEMAR manikin.

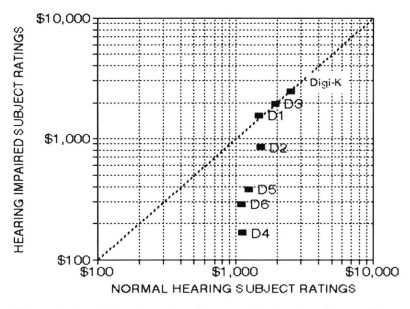

Figure 4–18. Dollar value ratings for seven digital hearing aids (see Figure 4–17 for details).

Unfortunately, many digital hearing aids *degrade* the listener's ability to hear in noise compared with the open ear when the noise levels are at 83 dBA (70 dB HL) and above, typical of cocktail parties and noisy restaurants. At those levels, most sounds are audible *unaided* for someone with moderate hearing loss. Truly high-fidelity hearing aids can avoid such degradation, but do not improve the listener's ability to hear in noise (Bentler & Duve, 2000).

Tests that quantify a listener's ability to hear in noise have become an important part of evaluating a patient for amplification (Etymotic Research, 2001, 2005; Killion, Niquette, Gudmundsen, Revit, & Banerjee, 2004; Nilsson, Soli, & Sullivan, 1994; Soli & Nilsson, 1997; Taylor, 2003). These tests estimate the SNR at which a listener correctly identifies 50% of key items (e.g., words-in-sentences or sentences). Understanding 50% of words-in-sentences translates to almost 90% intelligibility for conversation, as knowledge of the language, awareness of the conversational topic, and visual cues contribute to speech understanding (e.g., Figure 4–19). In contrast, only 8% of speech cues (i.e., an AI of 8%) are needed for repeating digits from zero through nine. These results are similar to those of Miller, Heise, and Lichten (1951), who found a 20 dB lower SNR was required for a "list" of two words compared with that required for an open set of monosyllables.

When testing performance in noise, results are compared with average performance of a group of normal-hearing listen-

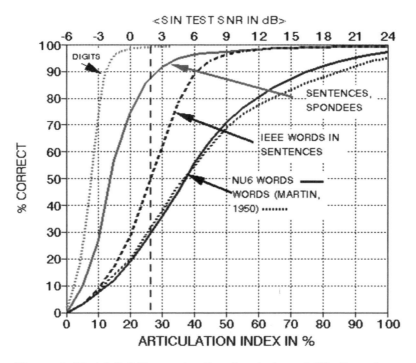

Figure 4–19. Intelligibility as a function of context, word difficulty, and proportion of speech cues audible (Articulation Index). When audibility is controlled by masking noise, each 3 dB increase in masking noise causes a 10 percentage-point decrease in AI. Normal performance on the QuickSIN test (IEEE words in sentences) is 50% words correct at 2 dB SNR, or an AI of 26%. At that SNR, nearly 90% of sentences will be understood. From Killion, M. C., and Mueller, H. G. (2010). Twenty years later: A NEW Count-The-Dots method. *The Hearing Journal, 63*(1), 10, 12–14, 16–17. Reprinted with permission.

ers on the same materials. SNR loss is the dB increase in SNR required by a person to understand speech in noise, compared with the average score of the normal-hearing group (test norm). For example, if normal-hearing listeners require a +2 dB SNR to understand 50% of key words in noise, and a hearing-impaired listener requires a +8 dB SNR on the same material, the hearing-impaired listener has a 6 dB SNR loss (8 − 2 = 6). Knowing the SNR loss aids in decision-making for amplification (e.g., a listener with a 6 dB SNR loss would generally do well with directional microphone hearing aids). However, for a listener with a 12 dB SNR loss, the 4 dB SNR improvement provided by typical dual-microphone digital directional hearing aids (Killion, 2004b) leaves an 8 dB SNR loss, which will result in virtually zero intelligibility in the typical cocktail party or high-noise restaurant. This is illustrated in Figure 4–20. (Note: With a typical open-canal fitting, the 4 dB directional microphone improvement is cut in half.)

A wired or radio-frequency remote-microphone system, which can provide 15–20 dB improvement in SNR, can restore intelligibility for persons needing more SNR improvement than directional microphones can provide. If the listener chooses not to use such a system, the professional can at least help prevent disappointment with the "performance of the hearing aids" by counseling the listener on what to expect given their SNR loss and technology choice.

At one time, many of us assumed we could estimate the degree of SNR loss from the audiogram. Unfortunately, this is not true. Figure 4–21 shows a plot of SNR loss versus pure-tone-average (PTA) hearing loss. Each asterisk represents an individual listener with hearing impairment. Note the range in performance: an 8 dB SNR loss was found for listeners having pure-tone averages

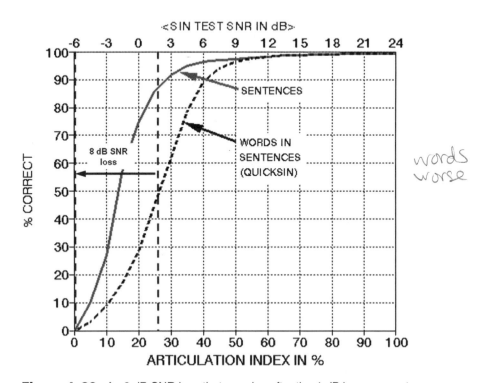

Figure 4–20. An 8 dB SNR loss that remains after the 4-dB improvement of a directional microphone will leave the wearer unable to understand anything at all in a typical cocktail party or noisy restaurant.

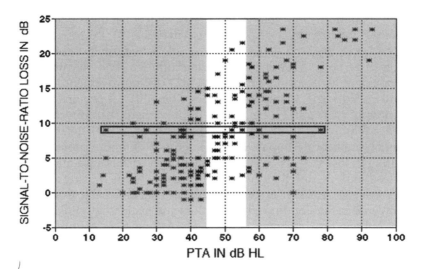

Figure 4–21. SNR Loss versus Hearing Loss (3F PTA) in 100 patients. SNR loss cannot be predicted from the pure-tone audiogram: Patients with 8 dB SNR loss had PTAs ranging from 14 to 78 dB HL, and patients with PTAs of 45 to 55 dB HL had SNR losses of 2 to 22 dB.

ranging from 14 to 78 dB HL. Likewise, those with PTA hearing thresholds of 45 to 55 dB HL had SNR losses ranging from 2 to 22 dB. SNR loss cannot be predicted from the pure-tone audiogram (Killion & Niquette, 2000).

The Quick Speech-in-Noise (QuickSIN) test (Etymotic Research, 2001; Killion et al., 2004) was developed to: (1) provide a quick way to estimate SNR loss; (2) assist professionals in choosing appropriate amplification and other assistive technologies; and (3) provide information useful in counseling patients regarding realistic expectations. The QuickSIN consists of IEEE (1969) sentences in four-talker babble (Auditec of St. Louis, 1971). Each list takes approximately one minute to administer and score. The QuickSIN is appropriate for adults since its sentences are at a high school language level.

The BKB-SIN Test (Etymotic Research, 2005) was developed for use with children and adults for whom the QuickSIN is too difficult (some elderly and cochlear implant users). The BKB-SIN uses the Bamford-Kowal-Bench (BKB) sentences (Bench et al., 1979) in four-talker babble (Auditec of St. Louis, 1971). East list pair takes approximately three minutes to

administer and score. The BKB sentences are at approximately a first-grade reading level, and the test has normative data for adults and children down to age five.

Directional Microphones

Hearing aid circuitry cannot solve the hearing-in-noise deficit experienced by listeners with significant SNR loss (Christensen, 2000; Killion, 1997a, 1997b), and engineers have looked for other solutions to improve the SNR for these listeners.

Directional microphones improve the SNR for sounds coming from in front of a listener by attenuating sounds arriving from the sides and the rear. Directional microphones in hearing aids are not a new development, although today's directional microphones provide substantially more benefit than the pre-1990s directional microphones (Killion et al., 1998).

Contemporary directional microphones are designed in two ways: (1) using two omni microphones and electrically subtracting the outputs (called a dual-omni approach); and (2) using a single directional microphone with two ports and acoustically subtracting the outputs following a delay (called a single-cartridge approach). Both methods provide good directivity if designed and implemented correctly.

Killion et al. (1998) evaluated the performance of a single-cartridge directional microphone (D-MIC) in real-world environments. In this study, recordings were made from hearing aids equipped to record from the outputs of both the omnidirectional and the directional microphones simultaneously. Recordings in a variety of environments were accomplished, and results indicated SNR improvements in the directional condition ranging from 4 dB in reverberant environments (e.g., restaurants and cocktail parties) to 11 dB in outdoor (nonreverberant) environments. These improvements in SNR translated to significant improvements in speech recognition scores in noise, ranging from 30% to 60%.

Coupling a well-designed directional microphone with a high-fidelity hearing aid amplifier will provide listeners with mild-to-moderate hearing loss substantial benefit when listening in both quiet and noisy environments. Listeners with moderate and severe SNR losses require greater improvements in SNR to function in noisy places, and can be helped with wireless assistive devices such as personal FM systems and the Companion Mics Multi-Talker Noise Reduction System (Etymotic Research, 2006). The Companion Mics system is unique in that it is the only system that provides a 15 to 20 dB improvement in SNR for up to three talkers.

SUMMARY AND CONCLUSIONS

In this chapter, we have presented the design characteristics required for high-fidelity amplification. An understanding of these characteristics is essential for making decisions about amplification for listeners with hearing impairment. Current hearing aids have eliminated many of the major problems with older technologies including distortion, narrow bandwidth, and peaks in the response. However, high-fidelity hearing aids have not solved the speech understanding problems experienced by hearing-impaired listeners in noisy environments. Fortunately, SNRs can be improved by the use of good directional microphones and other SNR-enhancing technologies. Professionals who measure their patients' SNR loss are in the best position to prescribe the appropriate technology and counsel their patients regarding realistic expectations from hearing aids and SNR-enhancing options.

REVIEW QUESTIONS

Principles of High-Fidelity Hearing Aid Amplification

1. What deficits in older hearing aid technology have been overcome by modern hearing aid technology?
   a. Distortion
   b. Narrow bandwidth
   c. Peaks in the frequency response
   d. All the above

2. A WDRC circuit is one in which:
   a. Amplification is only provided in the frequency regions where hearing loss is present.
   b. Compression is applied at high input levels so that the signal doesn't get clipped.
   c. Gain is dependent on the input level to the hearing aid.
   d. All input levels receive the same amount of gain.

3. Who are the primary beneficiaries of high-fidelity hearing aids?
   a. Musicians
   b. Persons with loss of sensitivity for soft sounds and normal hearing for loud sounds
   c. A & B
   d. Persons with profound hearing loss

4. What should the minimum upper bandwidth be for a high-fidelity hearing aid?
   a. 8kHz
   b. 7kHz
   c. 6kHz
   d. 4kHz

5. High-fidelity hearing aids are not widely available because:
   a. Research is lacking on what constitutes high fidelity in hearing aids.
   b. Normal-hearing listeners cannot judge the fidelity of hearing aids because they don't have hearing loss.
   c. High-fidelity transducers (microphones, amplifiers, receivers) are not available.
   d. None of the above.

6. What should be the maximum total harmonic distortion of a high-fidelity hearing aid for output levels of 50 to 90 dB SPL?
   a. 2%
   b. 3%
   c. 5%
   d. 10%

7. Listening tests (A-B-A comparisons) completed by normal-hearing and hearing-impaired listeners have shown:
   a. Hearing-impaired listeners cannot accurately judge fidelity.
   b. Normal-hearing listeners cannot accurately judge fidelity.
   c. Normal-hearing and hearing-impaired listeners give the same fidelity judgments.
   d. None of the above.

8. Which technology can improve SNR?
   a. High-fidelity hearing aids
   b. Directional microphones
   c. Digital hearing aids
   d. WDRC hearing aids

9. Measuring the SNR loss is important because:
   a. It cannot be predicted from the puretone audiogram.

b. It provides information useful in selecting amplification.
c. It provides information useful in counseling regarding realistic expectations.
d. All of the above.

10. Which technology received the highest fidelity rating by normal-hearing and hearing-impaired listeners?
    a. Digi-K
    b. Digital aid #1
    c. K-AMP
    d. Digital aid #4

Answer Key

1. D
2. C
3. C
4. A
5. D
6. B
7. C
8. B
9. D
10. A

REFERENCES

Ahren, T., Arlinger, S., Holmgren, C., Jerlvall, L., Johansson, B., Lindblad, A. C., . . . Sjogrem, G. (1977). *Automatic gain control and hearing aids* (Report TA No. 84). Stockholm: Karolinska Institutet, Technical Audiology.

Auditec of St. Louis. (1971). Four-talker babble. 2515 S. Big Bend Boulevard, St. Louis, MO, 63143–2105.

Barfod, J. (1976). *Multichannel compression hearing aids* (Report No. 11). Technical University of Denmark, Acoustics Laboratory.

Barfod, J. (1978). Multichannel compression hearing aids: Experiments and consideration on clinical applicability. *Scandinavian Audiology*, Suppl. 6, 315–340.

Bench, J., Kowal, A., & Bamford, J. (1979). The BKB (Bamford-Kowal-Bench) sentence lists for partially-hearing children. *British Journal of Audiology, 13*, 108–112.

Bentler, R. A., & Duve, M. R. (2000). Comparison of hearing aids over the 20th century. *Ear and Hearing, 21*(6), 625–639.

Berlin, C. I., & Gondra, M. I. (1976). Extratympanic clinical cochleography with clicks. In R. P. Rubin, C. Eberling, & I. Salomon (Eds.), *Electrocochleography*. Baltimore, MD: University Park Press.

Blesser, B. A., & Ives, F. (1972). A reexamination of the S/N question for systems with time-varying gain or frequency response. *Journal of the Audio Engineering Society, 20*, 638–641.

Bucklein, R. (1962). Horbarkeit von Unregel-makigkeiten in Frequenzgangen bei akustischer Ubertragung. *Frequenz, 16*, 103–108.

Burkhard, M. D. & Sachs, R. M. (1975). Anthropometric manikin for acoustic research. *Journal of the Acoustical Society of America, 58*, 214–222.

Christensen, L. A. (2000). Signal-to-noise ratio loss and directional-microphone hearing aids. *Seminars in Hearing, 21*(2), 179–200.

Consumer Reports. (1977a). How CU's auditory lab tests loudspeaker accuracy. *Consumer Reports TNG-3*. Mount Vernon, NY.

Consumer Reports. (1977b). Low-priced loudspeakers. *Consumer Reports, 42*, 406–409.

Cox, R. M., & Gilmore, C. (1986). Damping the hearing aid frequency response: Effects on speech clarity and preferred listening level. *Journal of Speech and Hearing Research, 29*(3), 357–365.

Dillon, H. (2001). Prescribing hearing aid performance. In *Hearing aids*. New York, NY: Thieme.

Dillon, H., & Macrae, J. (1984). *Derivation of design specifications for hearing aids* (NAL Report No. 102). Australia: National Acoustical Laboratories.

Dunn, H. K., & Farnsworth, D. W. (1939). Exploration of pressure field around the human head during speech. *Journal of the Acoustical Society of America, 10*, 184–199.

Dunn, H. K., & White, S. D. (1940). Statistical measurements on conversational speech. *Journal of the Acoustical Society of America, 11*, 278–288.

Edwards, B., Kalluri, S., Valentine, S. Carlile, S., Best, V., & Wolfe, J. (2010). *The effect of hearing aid microphone location on spatial perception*. Podium presentation at the American Auditory Society meeting, Scottsdale, Arizona.

Etymotic Research. (2001). *QuickSIN Speech-in-Noise Test, Version 1.3* [CD]. 61 Martin Lane, Elk Grove Village, IL, 60007.

Etymotic Research. (2002). Digi-K digital hearing aid amplifier.

Etymotic Research. (2005). *BKB-SIN Speech-in-Noise Test, Version 1.03* [CD]. 61 Martin Lane, Elk Grove Village, IL, 60007.

Etymotic Research. (2006). *Companion mics multitalker noise reduction system, user guide*. 61 Martin Lane, Elk Grove Village, IL, 60007.

Fikret-Pasa, S. (1993). *The effects of compression ratio on speech intelligibility and quality* (Doctoral dissertation, Northwestern University, 1990). University Microfilms, Ann Arbor, MI.

Flanagan, J. (1957). Difference limen for formant amplitude. *Journal of Speech and Hearing Disorders, 22*, 205–212.

Fletcher, H. (1931). Some physical characteristics of speech and music. *Bell Systems Technology Journal, 10*, 349–373.

Fletcher, H. (1942). Hearing, the determining factor for high-fidelity transmission. *Proceedings of the Institute of Radio Engineering, 30*, 266–277.

Gengel, R. W. (1973). Temporal effects in frequency discrimination by hearing impaired listeners. *Journal of the Acoustical Society of America, 54*, 11–15.

Goldberg, H. (1960). *A new concept in hearing aids*. Flushing, NY: Dynaura.

Goldberg, H. (1966). *Hearing aid*. U.S. Patent No. 3229049. Filed August 4, 1960.

Goldberg, H. (1972). The utopian hearing aid: Current state of the art. *Journal of Auditory Research, 12*, 331–335.

Goode, R. L., Killion, M. C., Nakamura, K., & Nishihara, S. (1994). New knowledge about the function of the human middle ear: Development of an improved analog model. *Otolaryngology-Head and Neck Surgery, 109*(5), 899–910.

Gudmundsen, G. I., & Killion, M. C. (1998). High-frequency bandwidth changes: Recognition and subjective preference (Unpublished data).

Hellman, R. P., & Meiselman, C. H. (1993). Rate of loudness growth for pure tones in normal and impaired hearing. *Journal of the Acoustical Society of America, 93*(2), 966–975.

Hogan, C. A., & Turner, C. W. (1998). High-frequency audibility: Benefits for hearing-impaired listeners. *Journal of the Acoustical Society of America, 104*, 432–441.

Hoth, D. F. (1941). Room noise spectra at subscriber's telephone locations. *Journal of the Acoustical Society of America, 12*, 499–504.

IEEE. (1969). *Recommended practice for speech quality measurements, Appendix C*. Institute of Electrical and Electronics Engineers. Global Engineering Documents, Boulder, CO.

Jerger, J. F., Tillman, T. W., & Peterson, J. L. (1960). Masking by octave bands of noise in normal and impaired ears. *Journal of the Acoustical Society of America, 32*, 385–390.

Killion, M. C. (1979a). *Design and evaluation of high-fidelity hearing aids* (Doctoral dissertation, Northwestern University, 1990). University Microfilms, Ann Arbor. MI.

Killion, M. C. (1979b). *AGC circuit particularly for a hearing aid*. U.S. Patent No. 4,170,720.

Killion, M. C. (1988). An "acoustically invisible" hearing aid. *Hearing Instruments, 39*(10), 39–44.

Killion, M. C. (1993). The K-AMP hearing aid. *American Journal of Audiology, 2*, 52–74.

Killion, M. C. (1997a). SNR loss: "I can hear what people say, but I can't understand them." *Hearing Review, 4*(12), 8–14.

Killion, M. C. (1997b). Hearing aids: Past, present, future: Moving toward normal conversations in noise. *British Journal of Audiology, 31*, 141–148.

Killion, M. C. (2004a). Myths that discourage improvements in hearing aid design. *Hearing Review, 11*(1), 32–40, 70.

Killion, M. C. (2004b). Myths about hearing in noise and directional microphones. *Hearing Review, 11*(2), 14, 16, 18, 19, 72, 73.

Killion, M. C. (2009). What special hearing aid properties do performing musicians require? *Hearing Review, 16*(2), 20–31.

Killion, M. C., & Fikret-Pasa, S. (1993). The 3 types of sensorineural hearing loss: Loudness and intelligibility considerations. *The Hearing Journal, 46*(11), 31–36.

Killion, M. C., & Monser, E. L. (1980). CORFIG: Coupler response for flat insertion gain. In G. A. Studebaker & I. Hockberg (Eds.), *Acoustical factors affecting hearing and performance.* Baltimore, MD: Park Press.

Killion, M. C., & Mueller, H. G. (2010). Twenty years later: A NEW count-the-dots method. *The Hearing Review Journal, 63*(1), 10, 12–14, 16–17.

Killion, M. C., & Niquette, P. A. (2000). What can the pure tone audiogram tell us about a patient's SNR loss? *The Hearing Journal, 53*(3), 46–53.

Killion, M. C., Niquette, P. A., Gudmundsen, G. I., Revit, L. J., & Banerjee, S. (2004). Development of a quick speech-in-noise test for measuring signal-to-noise ratio loss in normal-hearing and hearing-impaired listeners. *Journal of the Acoustical Society of America, 116*(4), 2395–2405.

Killion, M., Schulein, R., Christensen, L., Fabry, D., Revit, L., Niquette, P., & Chung, K. (1998). Real-world performance of an ITE directional microphone. *The Hearing Journal, 51*, 24–38.

Killion, M. C., & Studebaker, G. A. (1978). A-weighted equivalents of permissible ambient noise during audiometric testing. *Journal of the Acoustical Society of America, 63*, 1633–1635.

Killion, M. C., Wilber, L. A., & Gudmundsen, G. I. (1988). Zwislocki was right . . . a potential solution to the "hollow voice" problem. *Hearing Instruments, 39*(1), 14–17.

Kochkin, S. (1996). Customer satisfaction and subjective benefit with high performance hearing aids. *Hearing Review, 3*(12), 16–26.

Kochkin, S. (2002). 10-year customer satisfaction trends in the US hearing instrument market. *Hearing Review, 9*(10), 14–46.

Kochkin, S. (2005). Customer satisfaction with hearing instruments in the digital age. *The Hearing Journal, 58*(9), 30–43.

Kuhn, G. F., & Burnett, E. D. (1977). Acoustic pressure field alongside a manikin's head with a view towards in situ hearing-aid tests. *Journal of the Acoustical Society of America, 62*, 416–423.

Licklider, J. C. R. (1949). Basic correlates of the auditory stimulus. In S. S. Stevens (Ed.), *Handbook of experimental psychology.* New York, NY: Wiley.

Lindblad, A. C. (1982). *Detection of nonlinear distortion on speech signals by hearing impaired listeners* (Report TA105). Stockholm: Karolinska Institutet Technical Audiology.

Lippman, R. P. (1978). *The effect of amplitude compression on the intelligibility of speech for persons with sensorineural hearing loss.* (Doctoral dissertation, Massachusetts Institute of Technology, 1978.) University Microfilms, Ann Arbor, MI.

Lippman, R. P., Braida, L. D., & Durlach, N. I. (1981). Study of multichannel amplitude compression and linear amplification for persons with sensorineural hearing loss. *Journal of the Acoustical Society of America, 69*(2), 524–534.

Lybarger, S. F. (1944). U.S. Patent Applications S.N. 543,278. Filed July 3, 1944.

Lyregaard, P. E. (1988). POGO and the theory behind. In J. Jensen (Ed.), *Hearing aid fitting: Theoretical and practical views.* Proceedings of the 13th Danavox Symposium, Copenhagen, 81–94.

Macrae, J., & Dillon, H. (1986). *Updated performance requirements for hearing aids* (NAL Report No. 109). Australia: National Acoustical Laboratories.

Madaffari, P. L. (1974). Pressure variation about the ear. *Journal of the Acoustical Society of America, 56*, S3(A).

Marsh, R. C. (1975). Tweeters in the grass, alas. *Chicago,* 76–78.

Martin, M. C. (1973). Hearing aid gain requirements in sensorineural hearing loss. *British Journal of Audiology, 7*, 21–24.

Mathes, R. C., & Wright, S. B. (1934). The compandor—An aid against static in radio telephony. *Bell Systems Technology Journal, 13*, 315–322.

McGee, T. (1978). *Psychophysical tuning curves from hearing impaired listeners.* (Doctoral dissertation, Northwestern University). University Microfilms, Ann Arbor, MI.

Miller, G. A., Heise, G. A., & Lichten, W. (1951). The intelligibility of speech as a function of the context of the test materials. *Journal of Experimental Psychology, 41*(5), 329–335.

Milner, P. (1977, June). How much distortion can you hear? *Stereo Review,* pp. 64–68.

Moore, B. C. J., Glasberg, B. R., & Stone, M. A. (2010). Development of a new method for deriving initial fittings for hearing aids with multi-channel compression: CAMEQ2-HF. *International Journal of Audiology, 49*, 216–227.

Muraoka, T., Iwahara, M., & Yamada, Y. (1981). Examination of audio-bandwidth requirements for optimum sound signal transmission. *Journal of Audio Engineering Society, 29*, 2–9.

Musicant, A. D., & Butler, R. A. (1984). The influence of pinnae-based spectral cues on sound localization . *Journal of the Acoustical Society of America,* 75(4), 1195–1200.

Nilsson, M. J., Soli, S. D., & Sullivan, J. A. (1994). Development of the hearing in noise test for the measurement of speech reception thresholds in quiet and in noise. *Journal of the Acoustical Society of America,* 95(2), 1085–1099.

Olson, H. F. (1957). *Acoustic engineering.* New York, NY: Van Nostrand.

Olson, H. F. (1967). *Music, physics, and engineering.* New York, NY: Dover.

Palva, T., Goodman, A., & Hirsh, I. J. (1953). Critical evaluation of noise audiometry. *Laryngoscope, 63,* 842–860.

Pascoe, D. P. (1988). Clinical measurements of the auditory dynamic range and the relation to formulas for hearing aid gain. In J. Jensen (Ed.), *Hearing aid fitting: Theoretical and practical views* (pp. 129–152). Proceedings of the 13th Danavox Symposium, Copenhagen.

Peters, R. W., & Burkhard, M. D. (1968). *On noise distortion and harmonic distortion measurements* (Industrial Res. Prod. Report No. 10350–1). Franklin Park, IL: Knowles Electronics.

Punch, J. D. (1978). Quality judgments of hearing aid-processed speech and music by normal and otopathologic listeners. *Journal of the American Audiology Society, 3,* 179–188.

Rankovic, C. M. (1991). An application of the articulation index to hearing aid fitting. *Journal of Speech and Hearing Research, 34,* 391–402.

Roys, H. E. (1968). Record industry association of America Standards for prerecorded tape & phonograph records. *Journal of the Audio Engineering Society,* 16(1), 18–20.

Sachs, R. M., & Burkhard, M. D. (1972). Earphone pressure response in ears and couplers. *Journal of the Acoustical Society of America,* 51, 140(A). (Available as Industrial Research Products Report No. 20021–2 to Knowles Electronics.)

Scharf, B. (1978). Comparison of normal and impaired hearing. I. Loudness, localization: II. Frequency analysis, speech perception. *Scandinavian Audiology,* Suppl. 6, 4–106.

Scharf, B., & Hellman, R. P. (1966). A model of loudness summation applied to impaired ears. *Journal of the Acoustical Society of America, 40,* 71–78.

Schulein, R. B. (1975). In situ measurement and equalization of sound reproduction systems. *Journal of Audio Engineering Society, 23,* 178–186.

Schweitzer, H. D., & Causey, G. D. (1977). The relative importance of recovery time in compression hearing aids. *Audiology, 16,* 61–72.

Seacord, D. F. (1940). Room noise at subscriber's telephone locations. *Journal of the Acoustical Society of America, 12,* 183–187.

Shaw, E. A. G. (1974). Transformation of sound pressure level from the free field to the eardrum in the horizontal plane. *Journal of Acoustical Society of America,* 56(6), 1848–1861.

Skinner, M. W. (1976). *Speech intelligibility in noise-induced hearing loss: Effects of high-frequency compensation* (Doctoral dissertation, Washington University). University Microfilms, Ann-Arbor, MI.

Skinner, M. W. (1980). Speech intelligibility in noise-induced hearing loss: Effects of high-frequency compensation. *Journal of the Acoustical Society of America, 67,* 306–317.

Skinner, M. W., & Miller, J. D. (1983). Amplification bandwidth and intelligibility of speech in quiet and noise for listeners with sensorineural hearing loss. *Audiology, 22,* 253–279.

Snow, W. B. (1931). Audible frequency ranges of music, speech, and noise. *Bell Systems Technology Journal, 10,* 616–627.

Soli, S. D., & Nilsson, M. J. (1997). Predicting speech intelligibility in noise: The role of factors other than pure-tone sensitivity. *Journal of the Acoustical Society of America, 101,* 3201–3201(A).

Steinberg, J. C., & Gardner, M. B. (1937). The dependence of hearing impairment on sound intensity. *Journal of the Acoustical Society of America, 9,* 11–23.

Stelmachowicz, P. G., Lewis, D. E., Sangsook, C., & Hoover, B. (2007). Effect of stimulus bandwidth on auditory skills in normal-hearing and hearing-impaired children. *Ear and Hearing,* 28(4), 483–494.

Stevens, S. S. (1972). Perceived level of noise by Mark VII and decibels (E). *Journal of the Acoustical Society of America, 51,* 575–601.

Taylor, B. (2003). Speech-in-noise tests: How and why to include them in your basic test battery. *The Hearing Journal,* 56(1), 40–46.

Teder, H. (1991). Hearing instruments in noise and the syllabic speech-to-noise ratio. *Hearing Instruments, 42,* 15–18.

Toole, F. E. (1981). Listening tests—Turning opinion into fact. *Journal of the Audio Engineering Society, 30,* 431–445.

Toole, F. E. (1984). Subjective measurements of loudspeaker sound quality and listener performance. *Journal of the Audio Engineering Society, 33,* 2–32.

Toole, F. E. (1986). Loudspeaker measurements and their relationship to listener preferences: Part 2. *Journal of the Audio Engineering Society, 34,* 323–348.

Villchur, E. (1973). Signal processing to improve speech intelligibility in perceptual deafness. *Journal of the Acoustical Society of America, 53,* 1646–1657.

Villchur, E. (1978). A critical survey of research on amplitude compression. *Scandinavian Audiology,* Suppl. 6, 305–314.

Villchur, E. (1996). Multichannel compression in hearing aids. In C. Berlin (Ed.), *Hair cells and hearing aids.* San Diego, CA: Singular.

Wallach, H. (1940). The role of head movements and vestibular and visual cues in sound localization. *Journal of Experimental Psychology, 27,* 339–368.

Wang, C. Y., & Dallos, P. (1972). Latency of whole nerve action potentials: Influence of hair cell normalcy. *Journal of the Acoustical Society of America, 52*, 1678–1686.

Wegel, R. L., & Lane, C. E. (1924). The auditory masking of one pure tone by another and its probable relation to the dynamics of the inner ear. *The Hearing Review, 23*, 266–285.

Wiener, F. M., & Ross, D. A. (1946). The pressure distribution in the auditory canal in a progressive sound field. *Journal of the Acoustical Society of America, 18*, 401–408.

Zwislocki, J. J. (1953). Acoustic attenuation between the ears. *Journal of the Acoustical Society of America, 25*, 752–759.

Zwislocki, J. J. (1970). *An acoustic coupler for earphone calibration* (Report LSC-S-7). Syracuse, NY: Syracuse University, Laboratory of Sensory Communication.

CHAPTER 5

The Many Faces of Compression

THEODORE H. VENEMA

INTRODUCTION

Compression often is referred to as automatic gain control (AGC) because it changes the gain of the hearing aid as the input intensity SPL changes. In this chapter, the use of the word "compression" is maintained. Compression is a big word in the realm of hearing aids. Toward the end of the decade of the 1990s, hearing aid specifications all hailed the advent and eminence of compression, and all kinds of compression hearing aids began to be sold by almost every hearing aid manufacturer. Here at this point, it must be emphasized that the decade of the 1990s witnessed the flourishing of compression advances, and this was at the tail end of the reign of analog hearing aids. Today's digital hearing aids utilize the same types of compression; however, they do so with digital software algorithms, rather than by means of the exclusive use of resistors, capacitors, and other hard-wired, physical electrical components.

Almost all digital hearing aids are adjusted or digitally programmed by the fitting software provided by their specific manufacturers. With the initial "quick-fit" adjustments or even with subsequent "fine tuning," however, the compression characteristics of the digital hearing aid are usually buried under the surface, nowhere to be seen on the screen. The specific compression characteristics of the digital hearing aids are more often seen when more specific fitting options are selected. In many instances, even the paper hearing aid specification sheets, published by the hearing aid manufacturers, usually omit many of the compression specifics of today's digital hearing aids. What's more, even when similar types of compression are found in the vast plethora of hearing aid products, the manufacturers tend to call or label them by completely different marketing terms or monikers.

This is why the decade of the 1990s was the "golden" age of compression. Almost all hearing aids then were analog, and each model was composed of one specific type of compression or another. Wide dynamic range compression (WDRC) was beginning to emerge, and seasoned clinicians were put into the position of having to learn it as a new type of compression. Manufacturers regularly held seminars where compression types were outlined, explained, and compared.

At that time, clinicians could manually adjust the compression by the screwdriver potentiometer control or trimmer (sometimes called "trimpots) of the hearing aid; however, changing to another *type* of compression meant choosing another hearing aid. Although today's digital hearing aids still include the same types of compression, the compression characteristics are typically sculpted under the surface by the fitting software itself. The ease of adjusting today's digital hearing aids by means of programming software has thus actually served to cloud clinicians' understanding of compression itself.

In the early 1990s, many graduate programs in audiology were guilty of not teaching compression very well, often because there was but one course in hearing aids. In addition, the teacher of that class often did not really understand compression very well. Those were the days when the manufacturers possessed most knowledge of compression. As a result, the universities generally relied on these manufacturers to educate their students. Today that has all changed; most audiology and hearing instrument specialist programs offer at least two hearing aids classes, where compression is covered quite well. Still, with today's fitting software, many clinicians lose their sound grasp on the many types of compression and clinical applications as to when to fit what type.

Compression in hearing aids would ideally seek to address compression in the cochlea, a magnificent nonlinear sensory organ. Our attempts to restore "normal" hearing with our best signal processing technology and a myriad of fitting methods, however, have met with limited success. Even the most advanced hearing aid technology does not restore normal hearing. The human cochlea, with the differential roles played by the outer and inner hair cells, has a majesty not easily imitated by even the most sophisticated digital algorithms.

It should be noted at the start of our discussion that there are *two essential goals* in the fitting of hearing aids: (1) provide gain to compensate for the hearing loss, and (2) increase the SNR, so that the client can better separate speech from background noise. The first goal is accomplished by means of gain and compression. To that end, compression *per se* is a gain issue. The second goal is accomplished by means of Directional Microphones (Dmics) and to a lesser extent, by digital noise reduction (DNR). This chapter does not get into the topics of Dmics and DNR, as that is a separate topic; the focus here is to specifically explore the technical areas of compression in hearing aids.

To understand *why* and *how* certain types of compression are clinically utilized, we must understand the various types of compression. Anything less makes the clinician a blind follower of manufacturer fitting software. To appreciate compression types as they are combined in today's digital hearing aids, it behooves the clinician to understand compression types as they once stood alone in yesterday's analog hearing aids. We, therefore, begin to explain and describe each type of compression separately, as they used to be offered in yesterday's analog hearing aids. It is hoped that this type of discussion will help clinicians understand the rationale behind the same types of compression found in today's digital hearing aids.

This chapter starts with a preliminary discussion of input/output graphs, reflecting the performance of linear hearing aids. We begin here because basic concepts must be understood before discussing nonlinear (compression) hearing aids. Compression has many "faces"; that is, there is no one simple dimension by which to describe it. To appreciate the topic of compression, we can liken it to a piece of sculpture. We need to walk around and view it from several different angles to appreciate the entire piece. Accordingly, compression in hearing aids will be reviewed along two separate dimensions: (1) output limiting compression, which was the first type of compression used in hearing aids, versus wide dynamic range compression (WDRC), which emerged in the early 1990s, and (2) the maximum power output (MPO) compression control that adjusted the output limiting compression adjustment versus the threshold knee-point (TK) control, which was used to adjust WDRC. In the mid 1990s, the concepts of bass and treble increases at low level input (BILL and TILL) became popular. These are discussed as two subsets or types of WDRC.

Common clinical applications of compression are still used today. In general, those with mild-to-moderate sensorineural hearing loss (SNHL) often are fit with WDRC hearing aids, which utilize a TK type of adjustment. Those with severe-to-profound hearing loss often are fit with output limiting compression, and these hearing aids use MPO type of adjustment. Expansion (as opposed to compression) is also reviewed in this chapter because it is also commonly employed in today's digital hearing aids (it was not used in analog hearing aids). Expansion presents a unique solution to microphone and internal amplification noise associated with WDRC hearing aids. This is especially true in quiet listening environments, and the noise is most often audible to those with mild-to-moderate

SNHL, where the hearing in the low frequencies is good enough to hear the low-frequency internal noise of the hearing aid in question.

Last, dynamic, as opposed to static, compression characteristics are reviewed. The concepts underlying attack/release times often are poorly understood by clinicians. Some of the more popular applications of attack/release times in hearing aids are discussed, including adaptive compression, syllabic compression, and automatic volume control. There is some detrimental interaction between attack/release times and actual compression ratios, and these are briefly described. Today's digital hearing aids tend to default to the use of relatively fast attack/release times in the low-frequency channels and variable attack/release times for the higher frequency channels.

The purpose of this chapter is to explain the concepts of compression as they are relevant to students, and also to clinicians who fit hearing aids for a daily living. Readers will not find citations of other literature throughout this chapter, along with a corresponding list of References at the end. This is for two reasons: (1) The author did not utilize other sources to put together the chapter, and (2) the explanations of compression are generic. Any specific observations regarding compression throughout arise from clinical experience of the writer, and not from any "cutting edge" research. Consider this chapter also as a history of compression development, as it began with analog hearing aids and continues in today's digital hearing aids.

INPUT/OUTPUT GRAPHS AND LINEAR HEARING AIDS

Input/output (I/O) functions are the most common way to explain compression, and they can appear on any specs found on any software from any hearing aid manufacturer. It may thus be a good idea to make them your friends. Ideally, clinicians should be able to ignore the written content on the specs sheets from any hearing aid manufacturer, look only at the I/O functions, and be able to tell what type of compression is being shown.

On any I/O function, the x-axis shows input sound pressure level (SPLs) and the y-axis shows output SPLs. The diagonal lines within the axes are the "functions," and they represent the working of the hearing aid. The functions on each graph show the *difference* between corresponding input and output levels; in other words, the functions show the *gain* of a hearing aid for different input SPLs.

Notice that on input/output functions, the values of input and output are always expressed as "dB SPL." This is because they are each referenced to some absolute value, representing 0 dB SPL (e.g., this could be 0.0002 dynes/cm^2). Whenever gain is the value of interest, the reader might notice it expressed simply as "dB." This is because gain is a *relative* decibel value that is not referenced to any specific sound pressure representing 0 dB SPL. The reader might recall being specifically taught that one cannot simply arithmetically add decibel values together; this is true for adding two decibel values that are each separately referenced to some *absolute* pressure representing 0 dB SPL. One *can* simply add dB values together (or subtract dB from one another, for that matter) if simply adding a *relative* dB value to an absolute dB value that is referenced to .0002 dynes/cm^2. For example, an input of 50 dB SPL plus a gain of 50 dB equals a total output of 100 dB SPL. This is an often overlooked fact when discovering the decibel. In our field, we often *do indeed* simply add decibel values together.

The most important formula for understanding hearing aid function is: input + gain = output. For most input/output functions, linear gain is represented by 45° diagonal lines. The point where any gain line suddenly takes a bend is called the compression "threshold," or "knee-point," and it is at this point that "compression" begins. The "knee-point" of compression above the input axis shows the input SPL where compression begins. From now on, the term "knee-point" is used to describe the input when compression begins.

The gain shown in many input/output functions is linear to the left of (or below) the knee-point, which means that for any increase of input SPL, there is a correspondingly equal increase of output SPL. For example, if the hearing aid has a gain of 60 dB, then a 10 dB SPL input will result in a 70 dB SPL output, a 20 dB SPL input results in a 80 dB SPL output, and so on (Figure 5–1). This is a compression ratio of 1:1, because for every 10 dB of input increase, there is a corresponding 10 dB of output increase. The difference between input and output is of course, the gain.

Figure 5–1 actually shows an old "linear" hearing aid of yesteryear. Linear gain is seen to the left of the knee-point, but to the

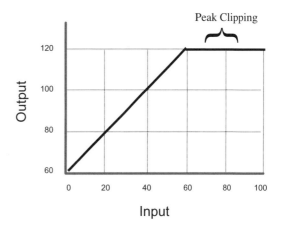

Figure 5–1. Linear amplification. With linear amplification, the output increases at the same rate as the input increases. In this example, the gain of the linear hearing aid is 60 dB. For 20 dB inputs, the output is 80 dB; for 60 dB inputs, the output is 120 dB; for 100 dB inputs, the output would be 160 dB (if not for output limiting). People with sensorineural hearing loss usually cannot stand much more than about 120 dB SPL, and so linear circuits introduce "peak clipping." This means that any output more than 120 dB SPL gets clipped, or "cut off." Peak clipping means that the diaphragm inside the receiver is actually "slapping" against the sides of the receiver walls, which in turn, produces a very distorted sound quality for the listener.

right of the knee-point, the line is completely horizontal. This demarcates the MPO of that linear hearing aid. For this linear hearing aid then, the gain is 60 dB, and the MPO is 120 dB SPL. Note that for input levels of 60 dB SPL or more, the output begins to no longer increase along with the input. Here, the linear hearing aid goes into "peak clipping," where the sinusoid back and forth movement of the receiver diaphragm is literally "slapping" the metal sidewalls of that same receiver. In this case, the peaks are truly "clipped," and the output result might be a complex square wave rather than a simple sine wave. When new harmonics are added to the input in

this manner, the result is distortion. This is why linear hearing aids with peak clipping were known to distort at high input levels, especially when the gain or VC was set to a high position.

Now take a look at Figure 5–2, which shows "compression" instead of linear gain. At input levels beyond 60 dB SPL, something different happens; it is not peak clipping but rather, *compression* that occurs. Note how the MPO does *not* take a straight horizontal direction to the right; instead, it rises at a shallower slope. In this example, the MPO is limited with a bit of "give." Instead of hitting one's head against a cement ceiling, it's

Compression Amplification

Output = input + gain

- •Compression circuits: different gain for different inputs

- •Knee point: at 60 dB inputs

- •Line at rising angle:
  - •compression
  - •outputs increase < inputs

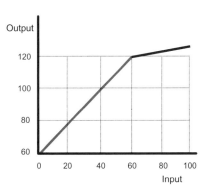

For inputs > 60 dB SPL compression limits MPO

Figure 5–2. Compression amplification. With compression, the output increases in a linear fashion, entirely along with the input, up until the knee-point. The knee-point is the bend in the line function on the input/output graph. Beyond (to the right of) the knee-point, the output still increases with input increases, but this increase is no longer at a corresponding 1:1 rate. It is at this point, that compression begins. In this example, the compression ratio is 4:1, which means that 4dB input increases are accompanied with only 1 dB output increases. Contrast this situation to that of linear peak clipping, as shown in Figure 5–3. With peak clipping, the output increases stop abruptly. That is, further input increases do not result in any further output increases. In this example, the gain of the compression hearing aid is 60 dB. For 20 dB inputs, the output is 80 dB; for 60 dB inputs, the output is 120 dB; this is still linear gain. For 80 dB inputs, however, the output is 125 dB, because with a 4:1 compression ratio, a 20 dB input increase results in a 5 dB output increase. Similarly, for a 100 dB input, the output is 130 dB SPL.

as if some sponge was attached to the cement ceiling, thus softening the thud. In fact, that is how the first compression came to be; it was a method of limiting the MPO *without* the distortion caused by peak clipping. More is discussed on output limiting compression later on in this chapter.

With compression, the gain is "nonlinear" because the gain *changes* as a function of input SPL. The hearing aid provides linear gain (where the gain function is at a 45° angle) until input levels seen below the knee-point are reached; above that intensity level, compression begins. When there is compression, an increase in input SPL does *not* correspond to an equal increase in the output SPL. On the contrary, the gain for input SPLs "above" or to the right of the knee-point is *less* than the gain for input SPLs "below" the knee-point. The slope of any line to the right of a compression knee-point shows the effect of compression on the gain of the hearing aid (see Figure 5–2). A compression knee-point, for example, at an input of 60 dB SPL means that the hearing aid provides linear gain for input levels up to 60 dB SPL. For inputs above that intensity level, compression begins. When there is compression, an increase in input SPL does not result in an equal (linear) increase in output SPL. The gain for input SPLs "above" or to the right of the knee-point is less than the gain for input SPLs "below" the knee-point.

For input sound pressure levels to the right of or above the knee-point, compression thus determines the MPO of the hearing aid. The MPO is shown by the general "height" of any line that is to the right of the knee-point. Always remember that compression is really a gain-related issue. Only with regard to input, does compression affect the sum total MPO. Thus, on input/output functions showing compression, for input sound pressure levels to the right of (or above) the knee-point, compression determines the MPO of the hearing aid.

Compression ratios are the *amount* of compression provided by the hearing aid once compression begins. Compression ratios can be visualized on an input/output graph by the slant of the line after the knee-point.

A 10:1 compression ratio means that for every 10 dB increase of input SPL, there is only a 1 dB corresponding increase to the output SPL. A 2:1 compression ratio means that for every 10 dB increase of input SPL, there is a corresponding 5 dB increase to the output SPL of the hearing aid. Higher compression ratios indicate *more* compression, that is, *less* gain than linear gain.

In summary, for the subsequent input/output graphs you encounter, it is helpful to see the 45° angle lines as representing linear gain; the shallower lines that continue on to the right of the knee-point can be seen as representing the MPO as controlled by compression. Think of the knee-point as the "when" of compression, and the ratio as the "how much" of compression. Compression is often referred to as AGC because the gain of the hearing aid changes as the input intensity SPL changes.

OUPUT COMPRESSION VERSUS INPUT COMPRESSION

In the "old days" of the 1990s, much was made of the difference between output and input compression. In today's digital hearing aid, however, digital algorithms can mathematically imitate the actual effects of output versus input compression. Readers can skip over this portion if in a hurry. Otherwise, for the interest of learning how these elements were found and utilized in analog hearing aids, as well as for the sake of practicing how to read and interpret input/output functions, readers can indulge in this topic now.

An oft-mentioned concept used to separate output from input compression in *analog* hearing aids is that output compression hearing aids had a compressor located between the amplifier and the receiver, while input compression hearing aids had a compressor located between the microphone and the amplifier. Whether this was true or not is one thing; but it was of precious little value to the clinician fitting a patient who had presbycusis.

For the clinician (and the client), however, the major difference between output and input compression was where the *VC* sat in the circuit (see bottom of Figure 5–3). In analog hearing aids, the manipulation of the VC had very different effects on the performance of the hearing aid, thus giving it either output or input compression. If the VC was left in one position, however, there would be no difference between input and output compression at all.

For analog output compression hearing aids, the VC was literally hard-wired or situated "early on" in the circuit; it was located between the microphone and the amplifier (Figure 5–3, bottom left). For input compression hearing aids, the VC was situated almost dead last in the circuit, just in front of the receiver that sends sound into the ear (Figure 5–3, bottom right). Different VC locations lead to dramatic differences in what they do. The two functions in Figure 5–3 show the different effects of the VCs with output compression hearing aids (top left) and input compression hearing aids (top right).

As said earlier, in today's digital hearing aids, digital algorithms can mathematically mimic the effects of different physical VC locations in analog circuits. In this way, a digital hearing aid does not have to be locked into being either input or output compression. The programming software of the digital hearing aid can simply create the effects of input or output compression.

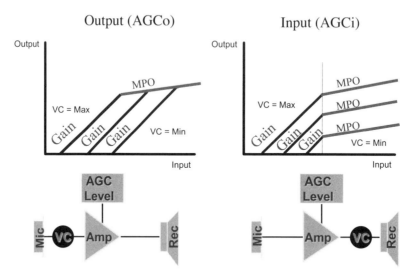

Input Versus Output Compression: Volume Control Effects

Figure 5–3. Input versus output compression: Volume control effects. Input/output graphs and simple circuit schematics showing relative VC positions for output compression (*left*) and input compression (*right*). For each graph, the parallel diagonal lines rising from the *x*-axis represent linear gain, the corners represent the threshold knee-point of compression, the line(s) to the right of the knee-points represent the maximum power output (MPO). The position of the VC in the circuits determines its effect. For output compression (*left*), the VC affects gain and knee-point, but not MPO. For input compression (*right*), the VC affects gain and MPO, but not knee-point.

Output Compression

For output compression hearing aids (Figure 5–3, top left), the VC affects the *gain* but not the MPO. The three 45° diagonal gain lines in each graph show the effects of three different VC positions upon the gain of the hearing aid. The right-most line actually shows minimum gain, with the VC position *lowered* to a minimum position. The left-most line shows maximum gain, with the volume control *raised* to a maximum position.

To make this clear, it may help to draw some more lines here. From the right-most knee-point on the output compression graph, draw a vertical line down to the input axis. From the same knee-point, draw a horizontal line to the output axis. This shows that at the minimum VC setting, some X amount of input is needed to give some Y amount of output. If similar vertical and horizontal lines are drawn from the left-most knee-point, it may become clear that for the maximum VC position, less input is needed to give about the same amount of output. At low VC positions, lots of input is needed to result in some amount of output. At high VC positions, less input is needed to give about the same amount of output. This means that the gain is increased as the VC position is raised.

The input/output function also shows that once "past" or to the right of the knee-point, in the region of compression, there is only one MPO line that is common to all three diagonal lines. This shows that, for output compression hearing aids, the VC does not affect the MPO. Output compression was touted as being suitable for *high-power* hearing aids, because for these hearing aids, clinicians should be very concerned about providing excessive output, as this can potentially damage hearing even further.

Note that the VC also changes the compression knee-point. In analog hearing aids, this is because the compression knee-point was adjusted "later on" in the circuit after the VC; the compressor was always set to wait for some steady amount of voltage that will tell it to compress (Figure 5–3, bottom left). The VC affects the amount of input signal that will arrive at the compressor of the hearing aid. If this amount of input voltage is not enough to tell the compressor to compress, then it will not act. Only when the VC sends the required input signal voltage that the compressor is "waiting for," will the compressor then "do its thing." Again, in today's digital hearing aids, these actions are mimicked mathematically in the digital software algorithms.

Input Compression

For input compression hearing aids, the effects of the VC are completely different (see Figure 5–3, top right). For input compression, the volume control affects both the gain *and* the MPO. Again, three diagonal gain lines for three different volume control positions are shown. Once again, the right-most 45° diagonal gain line shows the lowest VC setting, and the left-most gain line shows the highest or maximum VC setting. It is obvious that the MPO is also affected by the VC because once "past" or to the right of the knee-point, the height of all three gain lines also changes.

There is no specific, intended design feature or clinical fitting advantage to have the VC affect the MPO on input compression hearing aids. Rather, on analog hearing aids, this feature was simply a by-product of the VC placement in the circuit. In addition, the VC placed early on in the circuit simply allowed for another control—the TK control—to be placed near the end of the circuit (more on this control will be described later on in the next section). At any rate, those with mild-to-moderate SNHL have a larger dynamic range than those with severe SNHL and can more easily accommodate an MPO that rides up and down with VC adjustments. Input compression hearing aids are, therefore, often moderate-power hearing aids, intended for mild-moderate SNHL.

Note also for input compression hearing aids, that the VC does not affect the knee-point of compression. As Figure 5–3 (bottom right) shows, the compressor is situated before the VC. This means that the VC does nothing to the knee-point because the compression knee-point is already determined.

Input/output graphs are not the only way to look at the differences in the VC effects. The clinician is apt to be familiar with the frequency responses (gain as a function of frequency) seen on a hearing aid test box screen or printout, as shown in Figure 5–4. Here, the effects of the VC on gain and MPO are readily apparent for output compression (left graph) in comparison with input compression (right graph). For output compression, the VC increases and decreases the gain; for input compression, both the gain and the MPO are affected by the VC.

Clinical Uses of Input and Output Compression

Input and output compressions were never described as being "better" or "worse" than each other; they were always explained as simply being different, having different clini-

cal applications. Output compression was seen as being good for severe-to-profound SNHL where the dynamic range is very small. For these clients, the clinician might worry that an excessively high VC position could cause damage to remaining hair cells or residual hearing. On the other hand, an output compression circuit would ensure that the VC affects only the gain and not the MPO. For the same reason, on older analog hearing aids, which were either output or input compression, output compression was also often selected for use on children. The parent, teacher, or caregiver did not need to worry about excessive MPO causing further hearing loss, when the little person ran into the house with the VC on a full-on position.

Input compression in analog hearing aids was generally recommended for mild-to-moderate SNHL where the dynamic range is larger, and there is consequently more room for "play" on MPO. Again, input compression in analog hearing aids also allowed for the use of the TK compression control, which was of special use for those with mild to mod-

Input Versus Output Compression:
Volume Control Effects on Frequency Response

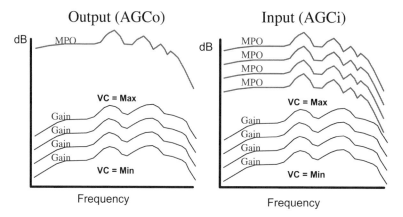

Figure 5–4. Input versus output compression as seen on frequency responses. Frequency responses showing relative volume control positions for output compression (*left*) and input compression (*right*). The VC for output compression adjusts the gain, but not the MPO; for input compression, the VC adjusts the gain along with the MPO.

erate SNHL. Mild-to-moderate presbycusis is the most common type of hearing loss. Input compression hearing aids thus had a large potential fitting application. Today, most digital hearing aids incorporate the use of input compression for soft inputs, along with output compression for louder inputs.

In addition to testing each type of compression on a hearing aid test box, one could also *hear* the effects of output versus input compression (the cochlea is an excellent acoustic analyzer). To hear the differences between output and input compression, one would talk softly into each hearing aid while adjusting the VC; with both output and input compression, the volume would go up and down, because the VC adjusted the gain on both. When talking loudly into each while adjusting the VC, the volume would change mostly when listening to the input compression hearing aid, because only on these hearing aids was the VC adjusting the MPO.

COMPRESSION CONTROLS: MPO CONTROL VERSUS "TK"

Here we turn to view another face of compression: the effect of manipulating the compression knee-point control. For this topic of compression, turn away from input versus output compression and think of the VC as frozen in a constant position; we are simply manipulating another variable here.

There are two types of compression knee-point adjustments: (1) the earlier or original type of compression adjustment of the MPO, and (2) a relatively newer type of adjustment of the threshold knee-point (TK) that appeared in the early 1990s. On analog hearing aids, both potentiometer controls actually adjusted the knee-point of compression; however, the effect of the MPO control was most pronounced on the actual MPO, while that of the TK control was mostly upon the gain for *soft* input sounds; for some reason, the TK control got the privilege of the name "TK." The effect of each of these is presented in Figure 5–5. Both I/O functions in

the figure represent input/output functions similar to those shown in Figures 5–1, 5–2, and 5–3. Again, on today's digital hearing aids, these adjustments are made mostly automatically on the fitting software.

MPO Compression Control

The left graph in Figure 5–5 shows the effects of the MPO compression control. It was typically found in conjunction with output compression. When hearing aids were all analog, there were *some* input compression hearing aids that also utilized the MPO compression control. Again, it should be appreciated that in the decade of the 1980s, when compression first appeared in hearing aids, this type of control was used as a way to limit the MPO without the distortion caused by peak clipping. Therefore, all hearing aids with compression—either output or input—utilized this type of compression control. Toward the middle of the 1990s, the analog *input* compression hearing aids began to utilize a different kind of compression control—the "TK" control. More is discussed on this control later in this section.

The MPO compression control affects the knee-point and the MPO. It does so by adjusting the voltage level that the compressor of the circuit needs to begin compressing. As the control is turned to a maximum position, the compression knee-point is raised, along with the MPO. At a maximum knee-point setting, the compression hearing aid is actually in a linear (1:1) gain mode for a wide range of soft to average input SPLs; compression will not occur until input sounds that are higher than the intensity level specified by the knee-point are reached. At this maximum knee-point setting, the MPO is also increased. Note from Figure 5–5 (left-most graph), that the MPO compression control does *not* affect the gain; the 45° diagonal, linear gain line does not change in position with changes to the compression control settings.

If you had (or have) an analog hearing aid with this control, the effects of this adjustment can be heard in addition to being tested

Different Ways of Adjusting AGC

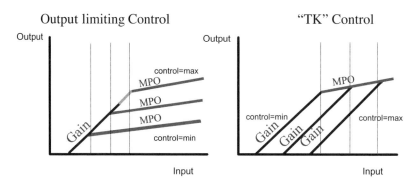

Output limiting control: Affects Kneepoint & Output

"TK" control: Affects Kneepoint & Gain

Figure 5–5. Different ways of adjusting AGC. Input/output graphs showing effects of two different types of compression controls (VC is assumed to be held constant at some position). For both graphs, the diagonal line(s) rising from the *x*-axis represent the linear gain; the corners represent the threshold knee-point of compression; the line(s) to the right of the knee-points represent the maximum power output (MPO). Both controls adjust the knee-point of compression, but that is where the similarity ends. The MPO compression control affects MPO, and the TK control affects gain for soft input sound pressure levels only.

on a hearing aid test box (the cochlea is an excellent acoustic analyzer). To hear the effect of this compression control, you must speak *loudly* into the hearing aid, because only then will the input sound plus the gain reach the MPO (a low-intensity input sound, such as a soft voice, plus the gain of the hearing aid may not result in an output that reaches the MPO). As the MPO compression control is turned from a maximum position to a minimum position, the knee-point of compression as well as the MPO are reduced; one should notice that the amplified loud voice becomes softer. This is because the compression control affects the MPO, not the gain.

TK Control

The TK control is completely different. On analog hearing aids, it emerged as a type of compression control much later than the original MPO type of compression control. Many clinicians during the 1990s were initially confused by the TK control because it works so very differently from the MPO compression control. On digital hearing aids today, the TK control works the same way, but it may not always be called a "TK" control. It may be seen on digital software as the left-most, or lower, knee-point on a rather complex looking input/output function (which we look at later on in this chapter).

The right-most graph in Figure 5–5 shows the effect of the TK control. Technically, any compression control affects the knee-point of compression, but electrical engineers probably will be quick to note that the term "threshold knee-point" is an input-related term, and rarely encountered with output compression hearing aid circuitry. At any rate, on analog hearing aids, the TK control was always found in conjunction with input compression, more specifically, with a certain subset of input compression known as "wide dynamic range compression" (WDRC), which we discuss in the next section. In older analog hearing aids, the TK control was first associated with hearing aids using the KAmp circuit that first appeared in the very late 1980s. Along with that circuit, the TK control began to be known as a separate entity from the relatively earlier MPO type of compression control.

The TK control affects the threshold knee-point of compression and also the gain for *soft* input SPLs, especially those below 60 dB SPL. This is because the TK control adjusts the knee-point of compression over a range of relatively low input levels, from around 40 to 60 dB SPL. Like all compression hearing aids, those with the TK control provide greater linear gain below the threshold knee-point of compression. However, because this knee-point is found at relatively soft inputs, the TK control can be seen as a gain booster for soft sounds. Unlike the MPO compression control, the TK control does not affect the MPO.

The input/output graph for the TK control (Figure 5–5, top right) looks similar to the graph showing the VC effects for output compression (Figure 5–3, top left). This is because the TK control operates in a similar manner to the VC for output compression hearing aids. On analog hearing aids with WDRC, the TK potentiometer was located at the input stage of the hearing aid (recall that in analog hearing aids the VC for output compression was positioned before the compressor and amplifier). It thus affected the amount of input signal that arrives at the compressor of the circuit, just like the VC did for output compression hearing aids.

It is very important to note that the leftmost gain line, where there is greatest gain, shows the TK set to the *lowest* knee-point position. The right-most gain line, where there is the least amount of gain, shows the TK set to the *highest* knee-point position. As the compression knee-point with the TK control is lowered, the gain for low-intensity input sounds is *increased*. Similarly, as the

compression knee-point with the TK control is raised, the gain for low-intensity input sounds is decreased.

Again, if you had (or have) an analog hearing aid with a TK control, you could hear its effects. Then *listening* to a hearing aid with a TK control, it is important to let just the ambient noise of the room into the microphone in order to hear the effect of turning the control. With any input greater than the compression knee-point (set by the TK control), the effect of adjusting the TK will not be audible. This is very different from the MPO compression control where loud input sound becomes louder to the listener as the knee-point is raised, and the MPO is increased.

Clinical Uses of MPO and TK Compression Controls

Because the MPO compression control affects the MPO and not the gain, it can be used to limit the MPO to protect the client who wears the hearing aid from further hair cell damage and hearing loss. This type of compression control is especially useful for those clients who have a severe or profound hearing loss and a limited dynamic range. The output limiting type of compression control can be adjusted, so that it limits the MPO of the hearing aid to a level that corresponds to the client's loudness tolerance levels. Some clinicians opt to set the MPO (measured in dB SPL) to be about 15 dB higher than the client's reported loudness tolerance levels (measured in dB HL). The rationale here is that the difference in dB HL versus dB SPL is close to an average of about 15 dB for the speech frequencies. As mentioned earlier, the MPO compression control was most often found on *output* compression hearing aids, which were also more suited for severe-to-profound hearing loss.

As mentioned before, the TK control was initially associated with the KAmp, which was a specific type of input compression hearing aid; namely, WDRC. This is discussed in further detail in the next section. The purpose behind the TK control is an attempt to imitate the function of the outer hair cells of the cochlea. It should be noted that in the cochlea, outer hair cells amplify soft sounds (approximately less than 40 to 50 dB SPL), so that the inner hair cells can sense them. Use of the TK control is, therefore, most appropriate for mild-to-moderate SNHL. There is no real rule for adjusting the TK control; after all, what rule would one use to determine whether to adjust the TK control to say, 40 dB SPL versus 60 dB SPL inputs? The main reason the TK is adjustable in the first place, is to reduce the gain for quiet incoming sounds. A TK setting for maximum gain in quiet (e.g., the knee-point set at 40 dB SPL) environments could result in the client being able to hear the internal amplifier and microphone noise of the hearing aid itself. The audible hiss can be annoying, especially for the cli-

ent who has excellent low-frequency hearing. In general, raising the knee-point setting of TK control so as to reduce the gain for very soft input sounds is not an issue for the client who presents with a flat, moderate SNHL. In today's digital hearing aids, "expansion" is commonly used along with the TK control, in order to reduce the audibility of the "hissing" sounds in quiet.

Let's summarize where we have come so far. Four input/output functions are shown in Figure 5–6. The top and bottom functions on the left side fit together well; they both describe the two aspects of compression we have discussed so far, which are often combined on high-power hearing aids. The top-left function shows the VC effects found on output compression; the client can adjust the gain by means of the VC, without any wor-

Putting It All Together:
Output/Input Compression & Compression Control Types

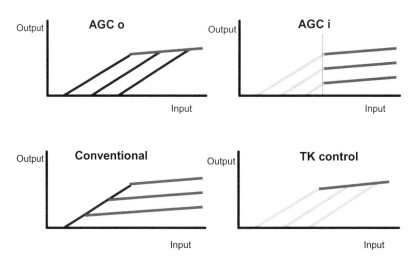

Figure 5–6. Putting it all together: Output/input Compression and compression control types. A summary of: (1) Input versus output compression and (2) MPO compression control versus TK control is shown here. The VC effects for input versus output compression can be seen on the top two graphs, while the effects of the different compression controls are displayed on the bottom two graphs. Most often, for severe-to-profound hearing loss, output compression was associated with the MPO compression control (*left hand graphs*). For mild-to-moderate SNHL, input compression is often associated with the TK control (*right-hand graphs*).

ries about affecting the MPO. The bottom-left function shows the MPO adjustments that can be made by the hearing health care professional, based on the client's loudness discomfort levels. Together, on high-power hearing aids, these gain and MPO adjustments can be seen to work well as a team.

The two functions on the right show a combination of two compression characteristics that are commonly found together on moderate-power hearing aids. The top-right function shows that with the VC, the client adjusts both the gain and MPO simultaneously. This is a satisfactory characteristic for moderate-power hearing aids because these cannot normally produce sufficient MPO that could further damage one's hearing. The bottom-right function shows the effects of the TK adjustment control, which, like the MPO compression control, is set by the hearing health care professional. As mentioned earlier, many clinicians were initially confused by the TK control and how it worked. Again, it is very important to note that the left-most gain line, where there is greatest gain, shows the TK set to the *lowest* knee-point position. The right-most gain line, where there is the least amount of gain, shows the TK set to the *highest* knee-point position. As the compression knee-point is lowered, the gain for low-intensity input sounds is increased. Similarly, as the knee-point is raised, the gain for low-intensity input sounds is decreased. The general rule for setting the TK control was to set it as low as possible, in order to provide as much gain for soft incoming sounds as possible. Theoretically, the hearing aid would thus imitate the role of the outer hair cells.

Last, note that the bottom-right function for the TK control looks similar to the top-left graph showing the VC effects for output compression. On the older analog hearing aids, the TK control, like the VC on output compression hearing aids, was positioned before the compressor and amplifier. It thus operated in a similar manner to the VC for output compression hearing aids, by changing the amount of input signal that arrives at the compressor of the circuit. This is exactly what the VC did in the older analog hearing aids with output compression. With digital hearing aids, of course, all of these characteristics are achieved by means of mathematical software algorithms.

OUTPUT LIMITING COMPRESSION VERSUS WDRC

Two faces of compression have been discussed: (1) Input versus output compression, and (2) MPO compression control versus the TK control. Again, the topic of input versus output compression has become quite outdated, with the advent of digital hearing aids. The topic of types of compression adjustment, however, is indeed quite relevant, as is evident in the fitting software of most digital hearing aids. We now encounter the third and final "face" of compression, and this concerns "output limiting" compression versus WDRC. These are really, two different compression schemes—they do not concern specific controls or adjustments. Each of these compression schemes refers to specific ranges of compression threshold knee-points and compression ratios. The effects of output limiting compression and WDRC can be seen in Figure 5–7. Once again, both functions in the figure are input/output functions, similar to those previously shown in this chapter.

Output Limiting Compression

Output limiting compression was typically associated with *output* compression hearing aids that used an MPO type of compression control. As such, these three properties together were associated with high-power hearing aids for severe-to-profound SNHL. Today, two of these properties are most relevant for severe-to-profound hearing loss; namely, type of compression control and type of compression scheme. Let's look at output limiting compression and see how it differs from WDRC.

The salient features of output limiting compression are shown in the left-most function of Figure 5–7. Output limiting compression is associated with "high" compression knee-points and high compression ratios. A high knee-point means that the hearing aid begins to compress at relatively high input SPLs (i.e., 60 dB SPL or more). Below the knee-point, the hearing aid provides linear or its most maximum gain.

We have already mentioned that compression ratios are the *amount* of compression provided by the hearing aid once compression begins. Recall that compression ratios can be visualized on an input/output function by the slant of the line after (to the right of) the knee-point. A 10:1 compression ratio is almost horizontal compared with that of a 2:1 ratio. Always remember that compression implies less gain than linear gain. A high compression ratio is roughly defined by most practitioners as being greater than 3:1 or 4:1. Higher compression ratios indicate *more* compression.

It should also be noted here that there is a law of diminishing returns with compression ratios. There is a big difference in gain between a linear 1:1 ratio versus a 2:1 compression ratio. There is, however, not much difference between compression ratios of

Output Limiting
Versus
Wide Dynamic Range Compression

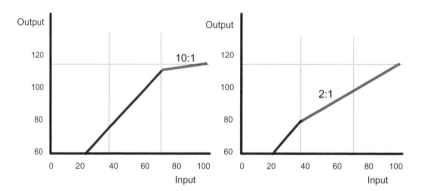

Figure 5–7. Output limiting versus wide dynamic range compression. Input/output graphs also show effects of output limiting compression (*left*) and wide dynamic range compression (*right*). For both graphs, the diagonal lines rising from the x-axis represent the gain; the corners represent the threshold knee-point of compression; the lines to the right of the knee-point represent the MPO. The hearing aid gain is the same (60 dB) for each type of compression. The gain function, however, is very different for each type of compression. Output limiting compression has a high knee-point and a high compression ratio; linear (maximum) gain is provided for soft to medium input levels, and a high degree of compression suddenly limits the MPO. The focus of this compression combination is to "limit the ceiling" of loudness tolerance. WDRC has a low knee-point and a low compression ratio; linear (maximum) gain takes place only for very soft inputs, while a weak degree of compression occurs for medium to intense input levels. The focus of this compression combination is to "lift the floor" of hearing sensitivity.

10:1 versus 20:1. Think of standing in a room facing a wall 10 meters away; if you cut the distance to 5 meters, you have moved much closer to the wall. If you continue to apply the same rule of halving the distance, you will continue to get closer to the wall but at a slower rate. It is indeed true too, that in fact, you will never actually reach the wall.

Output limiting compression hearing aids have a high knee-point and a high ratio of compression. They provide a strong degree of compression over a narrow range of inputs (Figure 5–7, left graph). Below the threshold knee-point, the output limiting compression hearing aid provides linear gain for a wide range of input SPLs. In other words, it "waits" for a fairly high input SPL to go into compression, but once it goes into compression, it *really* goes into compression.

Output limiting compression hearing aids have some similarities to linear hearing aids. They both give a fixed amount of gain over a wide range of different input SPLs, and then they both "suddenly" limit the output SPL. As mentioned earlier, the main difference between them is that linear hearing aids use peak clipping to limit the output, and output limiting compression hearing aids use a high ratio of compression to limit the output. The advantage of limiting the MPO with compression is that it introduces less distortion than peak clipping.

WDRC

WDRC hearing aids became extremely popular on analog hearing aids during the 1990s. It is important to categorize where WDRC properly fits in the overall spectrum of the many faces of compression, because then, it can be appreciated for what it is, and what it is not.

WDRC is shown in Figure 5–7 (right graph). The TK control was used to adjust WDRC and like the TK control, WDRC was always associated with *Input* compression hearing aids. Recall, however, that not all input compression was WDRC; some analog input compression hearing aids used output limiting compression, which was adjusted by an MPO type of compression control. When teaching classes in hearing aid compression, the writer often referred to these as the "odd ball" hearing aids, because they offered two ways to change the MPO; namely, the VC as well as the MPO compression control. Today, of course, these analog hearing aids have long since left the stage.

WDRC is associated with *low* threshold knee-points (below 60 dB SPL) and *low* compression ratios (less than 4:1). As the right-most function of Figure 5–7 shows, the WDRC hearing aid is almost always in compression, because all kinds of inputs, from very soft speech to a scream, will cause it to go into compression. Perhaps it was called "wide dynamic range compression" because of its low knee-point, which allows compression to take place over a wide range of input intensity levels.

Once the WDRC hearing aid goes into compression, however, it does not provide a great ratio or degree of compression (Figure 5–7). Basically, WDRC provides a weak degree of compression over a wide range of inputs. The effect of WDRC is very different from output limiting compression or the old linear hearing aids, for that matter. Unlike those hearing aids that suddenly reduce the gain once the input SPL exceeds a certain amount, WDRC gradually reduces the gain for a wide range of input SPLs.

Clinical Applications of Output Limiting Compression and WDRC

When comparing output limiting compression with WDRC, it may be most useful and helpful to look closely at their names. The main clinical difference between the two is that output limiting compression does its work above its knee-point; it reduces or limits the output for high input SPLs. On the other hand, WDRC does its work *below* its knee-point; it increases its gain for sounds below the knee-point by providing most gain for soft input sounds.

Why would clinicians desire a choice between these two types of compression? To answer this question, it may be a good idea to take another look at loudness growth, shown as the dotted lines and solid gray lines on the graphs of Figure 5–8. Both graphs show the loudness growth functions of someone with normal hearing compared with that of someone with mild-to-moderate SNHL. The client who has outer hair cell damage usually has mild-to-moderate SNHL. For this person, the "floor" of hearing sensitivity is elevated compared with normal, although the "ceiling" of loudness tolerance is similar to normal. The appropriate goal of amplification is to restore normal loudness growth, and to accomplish this goal, we need to amplify soft sounds by a lot and loud sounds by little or nothing at all.

Here is some food for thought: It is no coincidence that, on the one hand, the KAmp,

WDRC, and on the other, oto-acoustic emissions and the knowledge of the role of the outer hair cells, became clinically popular at around the same time—the late 1980s and early 1990s.

Figure 5–8 shows output limiting compression (left) and WDRC (right) superimposed on two identical loudness growth graphs. Both output limiting compression and WDRC may do the same thing for inputs of 80 dB; they may both reach the point where output sounds are perceived as being "too loud," but the *way* that each type of compression arrives at this common point is completely different. The author once attended an American Academy of Audiology conference seminar on compression given by F. Kuk back in 1996, who provided a very illustrative analogy. Output limiting compression was compared with a teenager speeding down

Loudness Growth
&
Types of Compression

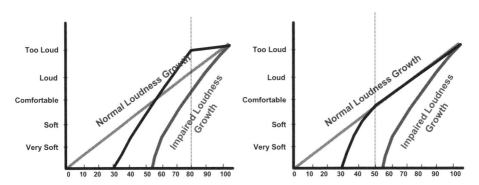

Figure 5–8. Loudness growth and types of compression. For mild-to-moderate SNHL, which is most common, re-establishing normal loudness growth is more easily achieved with WDRC than with output limiting compression. In both graphs, the x-axis represents the physical dimension of input sound intensity to the hearing aid; the y-axis represents the psychoacoustic dimension of loudness perception (similar to Figure 5–1). In this example, both output limiting compression and wide dynamic range compression make 90 dB inputs sound "too loud." But the high knee-point and high compression ratio for output limiting compression, make inputs of 70, 80, and 90 dB all sound "too loud" as well. This does not occur for WDRC, because it has a low knee-point and a low compression ratio.

the road in a relative's car who sees a stop sign at the end of the road and slams on the brakes and screeches to a stop. WDRC was compared with an elderly person who starts out at a normal speed, but on seeing the stop sign far ahead, ever so cautiously applies a foot gently to the brakes and slows to a stop over a long distance.

In the above analogy, normal loudness growth is the road. Some problems occur when trying to restore normal loudness growth with output limiting compression (Figure 5–8, left-most graph). First, there is an "overshoot" of normal loudness growth. The worst problem, however, is that amplified 70, 80, and 90 dB inputs all sound the same and are perceived as being "too loud." This does not restore normal loudness growth. The right-most graph shows WDRC applied to the same goal of restoring normal loudness growth. If restoring loudness growth is the goal, then the lower knee-point and lower compression ratio that are provided by WDRC are clearly a much better fit, because soft sounds are perceived as louder, while loud sounds do not exceed the listener's comfort levels.

Maybe another reason for the term "WDRC" is that the low knee-point and low compression ratio reduce a normally large dynamic range into the smaller one associated with mild-to-moderate SNHL. For example, a low compression ratio of 2:1 will compress a dynamic range of 100 dB into one of 50 dB.

Does this mean that all those with mild–moderate SNHL should "drive like the elderly person?" Not really. A listener with mild–moderate SNHL may have become accustomed to wearing linear hearing aids with peak clipping, or those that provide linear gain and limit the MPO with output limiting compression. For this listener, a sudden switch to WDRC might be too big a jump, and WDRC might be rejected because it is not "loud" enough. Although WDRC will amplify soft input SPLs by a lot, it will not amplify average intensity input SPLs by the same amount, and it is *this* difference that the listener accustomed to linear amplifica-

tion may find frustrating. Output limiting compression may result in the "overshoot" of normal loudness growth as seen in the left graph of Figure 5–8, but the listener may have become accustomed to the sound. In this case, WDRC must be introduced gradually and with considerable counseling about what to expect from the hearing aids. Many such patients/clients can adjust to WDRC, but others cannot seem to let go of their need for more power and refuse to make the change. It is significant to note that even for today's digital hearing aids, the fitting software of some manufacturers still asks if the client prefers Linear or WDRC!

For the client with severe-to-profound hearing loss, output limiting compression might be a better choice than WDRC. These clients might prefer a strong, linear gain over a wide range of input SPLs, at least until the output SPL becomes close to their loudness tolerance or uncomfortable loudness levels. Furthermore, these clients often have worn this kind of hearing aid in the past. High-power output limiting compression hearing aids will give lots of gain for soft sounds and the same "lots of gain" for average input sounds, such as speech, making it quite audible.

It should be appreciated that output limiting compression hearing aids had similar gain characteristics as linear hearing aids; they both provided linear gain over a wide range of soft to moderately intense input levels. More is discussed about this similarity near the end of this chapter. In general, these two types of hearing aids did differ in one significant way: Instead of using peak clipping to limit the MPO, as the old linear hearing aids did, output limiting compression hearing aids offered a high degree of compression to accomplish the same thing. This introduced a lot less distortion than peak clipping.

It must be said here that linear gain can sound very "clean" and clear. This is because there is no compression taking place, which *can* audibly distort the sound quality. Linear gain can sound quite pleasing, as long as the input plus the gain does not *saturate* the hearing aid or, in other words, add up to equal the MPO. In short, output limiting compression may definitely be preferred by clients with severe-to-profound hearing loss. Recall too, the WDRC amplifies soft input sounds by a lot, and loud input sounds by less. This would imply that for the waveform of input speech, the more intense peaks would be given less gain than the less intense valleys. The net effect here is that important contrasts in speech are decreased, thus making the input speech less intelligible. This has often been touted as a problem with WDRC.

WDRC can also be described in terms of its affect on the frequency response (Figure 5–9), much like we did with output versus input compression (see Figure 5–4). Here it becomes quite evident that the gain of a WDRC hearing aid is highly dependent upon the input SPL, over a wide variety of input levels. In contrast with output limiting compression, where the gain reduces abruptly once a higher input sound level reaches the hearing aid, WDRC acts like a "trampoline";

its gain fluctuates with any input sound levels above its low knee-point. Because of this phenomenon, WDRC is sometimes called "input level dependent compression."

For the purpose of sticking to clear definitions, a hearing aid with plain WDRC would tend to offer a fairly similar degree of compression across the frequencies. This is shown in Figure 5–9, where the difference in gain for each of the various input levels is consistent across the frequency response of the hearing aid. In the 1990s, some analog hearing aids with WDRC did exactly that. On those hearing aids, the low- or high-frequency gain could be adjusted, and such adjustments would result in an *equal* gain reduction for all input levels, For example, to fit someone with a sloping high-frequency hearing loss, the clinician would cut some of the low-frequency gain. In Figure 5–9, this would be seen as an equal drop in all three lines on the graph across the low frequen-

WDRC: Displayed as a Frequency Response

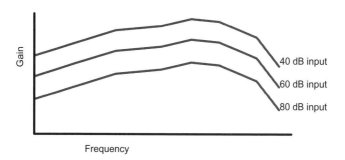

Figure 5–9. WDRC displayed as frequency response. The effects of WDRC can also be seen on a frequency response, with varying input intensities. While the volume control is set to a typical preferred level, WDRC provides very different amounts of gain for widely ranging input intensities. These differences in gain would not be apparent with output limiting compression; very similar amounts of gain would be provided for the 40 and 60 dB SPL inputs. In other words, the bottom two functions would be much closer together.

cies. The reason the point of an equal amount of WDRC applied across the frequencies is highlighted here is to point out how WDRC can also be specifically applied more at some frequencies than at others. This is explained further in the next section.

BILL AND TILL: TWO TYPES OF WDRC

Bass increase at low levels (BILL) and treble increases at low levels (TILL) are two types or subsets of WDRC. There are other names that pertain to these categories, such as LDFR (level-dependent frequency response), FDC (frequency-dependent compression), and ASP (automatic signal processing). Basically, these terms all boil down to at least one similar thing; namely, compression occurs more in some frequencies than in other frequencies. Where compression occurs, it will be WDRC, with a low knee-point and a low compression ratio. The simplest classification of these types of compression is that of BILL and TILL.

The advent of BILL took place in the mid 1980s; TILL came along with the analog KAmp circuit, around 1989. So BILL is a bit older than TILL. BILL first appeared in a circuit known as the "Manhattan" circuit, created by the now swallowed up company called "Argosy." It was called the Manhattan circuit because in a long-ago naming contest at the American Speech-Hearing Association, someone said its circuit board looked like the skyline of Manhattan. In subsequent circuits using BILL, it was also sometimes referred to as "automatic signal processing" (ASP).

Basically, BILL was WDRC confined to the bass frequencies, and TILL was WDRC confined to the treble frequencies. In any compression hearing aid, the compression knee-point is often set at somewhat different input SPLs for different frequencies. Hearing aid specs in North America don't show this; rather, they show the compression knee-point on input/output graphs at 2000 Hz only. The reason is because 2000 Hz is a very impor-

tant frequency required for the recognition of audible speech.

BILL and TILL were unique hearing aids, designed to make compression occur at *very* different input SPLs for different frequencies. BILL hearing aids had a low knee-point for the low frequencies and a higher knee-point for the high frequencies. Low-frequency input would not have to be very intense to set the BILL hearing aid into compression, but high-frequency input would have to be much more intense to cause compression. This meant that the BILL circuit would go into compression very often with low-frequency inputs, and not as often with high-frequency inputs (Figure 5–10). BILL is basically WDRC confined to the low frequencies.

Figure 5–10 shows a simple set of gain and frequency graphs for BILL (left graph) and TILL (right graph) circuits. BILL (left graph) has a very broad or flat frequency response with soft inputs (e.g., 40 dB SPL). If input sound is produced so that it is at 40 dB SPL all across the frequency range, then the gain and frequency response of the BILL hearing aid would look something like the top flat line on the graph. As the input across frequencies is increased in intensity to 60 dB SPL, the gain and frequency response will reveal a decrease in gain for the low frequencies. As the input intensity is increased to 80 dB SPL, the gain for the low frequencies will drop even more.

The main idea behind the BILL circuit was to enable better listening for speech while in background noise. That is, the "hubbub" of low-frequency background noise will be suppressed by compression, with the high-frequency sounds that render clarity for speech still receiving a full measure of gain. As mentioned earlier, BILL first appeared in the "Manhattan" circuit; in the mid 1990s, Oticon took the concept of BILL and utilized it in the analog two-channel Multi-Focus hearing aid in 1995. Later on, in 1997, Oticon again championed BILL in its first digital product, the DigiFocus. Oticon's stated purpose was to reduce the upward spread of masking. Cochlear physiology and, in particular, the

BILL vs. TILL
Two Types of WDRC

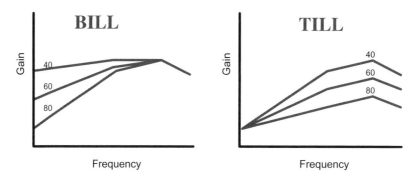

Figure 5–10. BILL versus TILL: Two types of WDRC. For each graph, the gain (*y*-axis) across a frequency range (*x*-axis) is shown for three different input levels. The left graph shows BILL. As inputs decrease in intensity, low-frequency gain increases. Note that WDRC takes place only at the low frequencies, where the line functions are furthest apart. The right graph shows TILL. As inputs decrease in intensity, high-frequency gain increases. Again, WDRC here only takes place at the higher frequencies. This is evident because the lines are furthest apart at the high frequencies. Early examples of BILL were the Manhattan circuit and the Oticon Multifocus. The right graph shows treble increase at low levels (TILL). As inputs decrease in intensity, high-frequency gain increases. The KAmp was an early example of a TILL circuit.

asymmetrical shape of the traveling wave envelope dictate that low frequencies mask high frequencies better than high mask lows (known as the "upward spread of masking"). BILL was seen as a way to fight the upward spread of masking, so as to increase speech intelligibility in background noise.

TILL (right graph) is completely different. The original analog TILL hearing aids were those that utilized the K Amp circuit. These hearing aids first appeared around 1989 and quickly became extremely popular. The knee-point was set at a low knee-point for the high frequencies. With TILL, high-frequency input will not have to be very intense to cause compression. This means the TILL circuit would go into compression very often with high-frequency inputs, and not as often with low-frequency inputs. TILL is basically WDRC confined to the high frequencies.

Figure 5–10 (right graph) shows a TILL response. For the TILL hearing aid, low-intensity input SPLs of 40 dB across the frequency range would result in a gain and frequency response that has more of a high-frequency emphasis. As the input is increased to 60 dB SPL, the high-frequency emphasis will decrease relative to the gain for the low frequencies. With inputs of 80 dB SPL, the gain for the high frequencies will decrease even more. In some TILL in-the-ear hearing aids, the 80 plus dB SPL response was intended to resemble the resonance of the open, unaided ear, thus providing an acoustic "transparency" for intense inputs when amplification is not needed.

The main idea behind TILL was to emphasize the high-frequency sounds of speech for the listener who most typically has high-frequency hearing loss. This client will have a reduced dynamic range for the high frequencies. Compared with that for normal hearing, the "floor" of hearing sensitivity will be elevated, although the "ceiling" of loudness tolerance will not.

COMMON CLINICAL COMBINATIONS OF COMPRESSION

Let's summarize where we have come so far. Leaving the dimension of input versus output compression behind, two dimensions of compression have been woven together so far: (1) MPO compression controls versus the TK control, and (2) output limiting compression versus WDRC. These static aspects of compression are still often found together in two common compression combinations, and each combination can serve a different clinical population (Figure 5–11). Although

there are no absolute maxims for endorsing one type of compression over another, there are, however, some trends, as described here. It is important to reinforce here, yet again, that an appreciation of these historic types of compression, as they first appeared in analog hearing aids is essential in order to understand today's digital hearing aid technology.

A Compression Combination for Severe-to-Profound Hearing Loss

Output limiting compression, along with the use of an MPO compression control, work well together in the same circuit. This combination has several features for clients with severe-to-profound hearing loss, which usually results in a small dynamic range (i.e., about 20 dB). With high-power hearing aids, protection of residual hearing is critical for

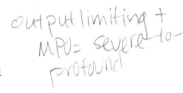

Summary: Applying Compression

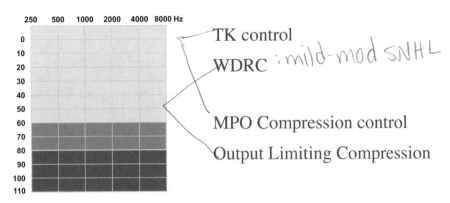

Figure 5–11. Loudness growth and types of compression. WDRC, originally a type of input compression that utilized the TK control, was found to be well suited for fitting mild-to-moderate SNHL. Output limiting, which was almost always used with output compression circuits, and which is adjusted with an MPO control, was similarly found to be well-suited for fitting severe-to-profound hearing losses. Today, both are commonly used in digital hearing aids. The diagonal lines in the range from 60 to 80 dB hearing losses, represents a "gray" area of intersection for the fitting of either type of hearing aid.

MPO + kneepoint = directly proportional

these clients. Independent from the VC, an MPO compression control in the hearing aid also changes the compression knee-point, and this adjusts the MPO (see also Figure 5–6). Specifically, as the knee-point is raised, the MPO is also raised. The output limiting compression in the hearing aid means that the compression knee-point occurs at a relatively high input level, along with a high ratio or degree of compression. If the hearing aid has a high-power circuit, the client receives lots of linear gain for soft to at least conversational speech input levels, but once the output comes close to the individual's loudness tolerance levels, the hearing aid suddenly provides a high degree of compression, so as to limit the output. Although normal loudness growth has not been achieved for these clients, they do get a strong degree of amplification along with a limited maximum output.

WDRC + TK = mild-mod SNHL

A Compression Combination for Mild-to-Moderate Hearing Loss

WDRC, along with the use of a TK control also work well together in the same circuit (see Figure 5–11). This combination has several features that address the needs of clients with mild-to-moderate SNHL, which usually results in a dynamic range of at least 40 dB to 60 dB. With input compression, the VC does not affect the knee-point of compression, but it does affect the gain and the MPO together. A TK control changes the knee-point of compression, and it also specifically affects the gain for soft incoming sounds (see also Figure 5–6). Recall that the TK control adjusts the gain for soft input sounds. Specifically, as the knee-point is *lowered*, the gain for soft inputs is *increased*. The WDRC in the hearing aid means that the knee-point of compression occurs at a relatively low input level, along with a low ratio or degree of compression. WDRC hearing aids usually had a medium-power circuit, which means the client received linear gain for only very soft input levels. The hearing aid was otherwise

in a low degree of compression over a wide range of medium to intense input levels. With these features, WDRC offers a greater degree of amplification for soft input sounds and less amplification for sounds that are well within a client's dynamic range.

Recall that for clients with mild-to-moderate SNHL, the cochlear damage most often concerns the outer hair cells. As a result, the "floor" of hearing sensitivity is raised, while the "ceiling" of loudness tolerance may be quite similar to that of normal hearing. WDRC is applicable to the largest clinical population (i.e., those persons with mild-to-moderate SNHL).

As the philosopher John Quine once said, "Categorization is the essence of intelligence." BILL and TILL are two types of WDRC, but not all WDRC is specifically BILL or TILL. The analog KAmp hearing aid circuit of the 1990s was TILL, a type of WDRC. The analog Oticon Multifocus hearing aid, also of the 1990s, was BILL, another type of WDRC. Recall that BILL hearing aids offer most compression for the low frequencies, and TILL offers most compression for the high frequencies. A straight WDRC hearing aid that is neither BILL nor TILL offers a more similar degree of compression across the frequencies. Today's digital hearing aids readily and commonly utilize all types of compression mentioned so far.

Now let's place all the hearing aids we have discussed together, next to each other, on a clinical "spectrum" (Figure 5–12): the old linear gain hearing aid with peak clipping, the newer hearing aids that began to offer output limiting compression (which first appeared in the late 1970s), and the newer still hearing aids that offered WDRC (which first appeared in the 1980s). Linear gain hearing aids with peak clipping were more similar or closer in relationship to output limiting compression hearing aids than to WDRC hearing aids. Thus, output limiting compression is like a bridge between linear gain and WDRC. At the risk of repetition, it is worth repeating a point earlier: Output limiting "does its work" above its threshold knee-point to limit the output, whereas WDRC "does its

Summary
A Clinical "Spectrum" of Hearing Aids

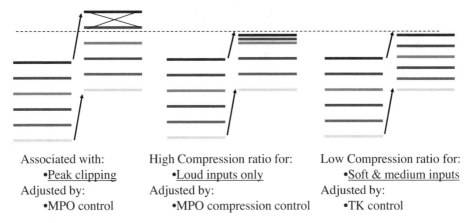

Associated with:	High Compression ratio for:	Low Compression ratio for:
•Peak clipping	•Loud inputs only	•Soft & medium inputs
Adjusted by:	Adjusted by:	Adjusted by:
•MPO control	•MPO compression control	•TK control

Figure 5–12. A clinical "spectrum" of hearing aids. For each of three types of hearing aids shown here, two sets of horizontal lines and arrows are shown. The left lines represent the input, the arrows represent the gain, and the right lines represent the output. The dotted line represents the loudness tolerance level for some particular client. For linear hearing aids, the gain is the same for all input levels. When the output reaches the "ceiling" of loudness tolerance, the output is clipped, resulting in distortion of sound quality. For output limiting hearing aids, only the top "output" lines are squeezed together, because the gain is linear for soft and average input sound, and is dramatically reduced for high-intensity input sounds. For wide dynamic range compression hearing aids, both the input and output lines are evenly spread apart because the gain is gradually reduced as the input intensity increases. A large dynamic range is "evenly" shrunk into a smaller one, which restores normal loudness growth. Figure courtesy of Huup Van den Heuvel, personal communication.

work" below its knee-point to increase the gain for soft sounds.

Linear hearing aids once enjoyed a wide but diminishing range of fitting applicability; they were routinely fit on the majority of clients up until as recently as the late 1980s. Linear circuitry can provide a lot of gain for severe-to-profound hearing losses or less gain for mild-to-moderate hearing losses. The most salient feature of linear gain is that it offers the same gain for all input levels, until saturation or peak clipping occurs. Note on the left-most graphic of Figure 5–12, that soft, average, and loud inputs are all "elevated" by the same amount. The worst thing about

linear hearing aids was that the MPO was limited with peak clipping. Sound limited in this manner was often distorted and had poor quality for the listener.

The output limiting compression hearing aid (usually found together with output compression) once represented compression in general. It was most often associated with high-power circuitry, however, which provides a lot of gain for the client with severe-to-profound hearing loss. As such, it serviced the needs of clients for whom loudness tolerance was a major concern. The middle graphic on Figure 5–12 shows that with its high knee-point of compression and

Digital Hearing Aids Commonly Use Many Channels

Increases Accurate Hz Shaping / Fitting Flexibility

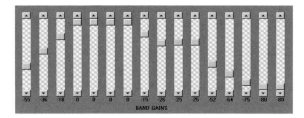

Change gain in each band…
Until desired frequency
response is achieved

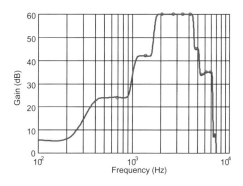

Figure 5–13. Digital hearing aids commonly use many channels. A fictitious frequency band equalizer is shown in the left panel. Each button represents a particular frequency channel. Selective adjustment of adjacent buttons would allow an exquisite sculpting of the frequency response, as shown in the right panel. Digital hearing aids are all multichannel. Their dB/octave slopes can be almost infinite, meaning that adjacent frequency bands can be very independent from each other. Turning the gain up on one band may thus not affect the gain in adjacent bands.

high compression ratio, the output limiting compression hearing aid "elevates" soft and average input levels by the same amount. In this way, it was like the linear hearing aid on the left. Unlike the linear hearing aid, however, the output limiting compression hearing aid had an MPO compression control that enabled compression (instead of peak clipping) to limit the output. This is accomplished without the degree of distortion often associated with linear peak clipping.

In the world of compression in analog hearing aids, WDRC was the "new kid on the block," becoming popular already in the early 1990s. Originally appearing as a type of input compression, WDRC hearing aids often provided less gain than the output limiting

hearing aid. The right-most graph on Figure 5–12 shows that with its low threshold knee-point and low compression ratio, the WDRC hearing aid gave progressively less and less gain as the inputs increase. Recall that the focus of WDRC is to restore normal loudness growth by shrinking a large dynamic range into a smaller one. The gain, however, does *not* decrease to the same degree as the input SPLs increase; otherwise the output would remain the same for all input levels. The gain must go down more slowly than the input SPLs go up.

When WDRC first appeared, experienced clinicians were fond of pointing out the difficulties of fitting WDRC hearing aids on clients who are accustomed to wearing linear hearing aids; these clients initially found that the WDRC hearing aids were "not loud enough." For soft input sounds, the WDRC hearing aids were satisfactory because it is for these sounds that they provided the most gain; however, with their low compression knee-point and low ratio of compression, the WDRC circuit did not provide as much gain as the older linear hearing aids did for average-to-intense input sounds. A common clinical report was that clients who were accustomed to linear peak clipping, therefore, initially rejected WDRC. As a transition to WDRC from linear gain, it was suggested to fit them with output limiting compression, because this type of compression is closer to linear gain. On the other hand, for new clients with mild-to-moderate SNHL who have never worn hearing aids before, WDRC may provide a very good initial fit.

COMPRESSION IN DIGITAL HEARING AIDS

So far, the reader no doubt wonders why it has taken up until this point to finally and specifically address digital hearing aids. True, we have consistently referred to digital hearing aids as something to be discussed later on. But it is the author's strong opinion that digital hearing aids cannot be truly appreciated unless the characteristics of their analog forebears are understood. As mentioned earlier, compression in analog hearing aids had to be understood because those hearing aids typically provided either one type or another type of compression. Successful client fittings relied on such knowledge. That is why the decade of the 1990s was truly the golden age of compression.

These advances in amplification are now "de rigour" in today's digital hearing aids. Digital hearing aids are almost all adjusted by the manufacturer's fitting software. The gain, MPO, compression, and much more, are adjusted and implemented by means of soft-ware, on to the hardware of the digital chip, or the digital signal processing (DSP) core. Compression characteristics and all kinds of other features are automatically combined and separately adjusted on each frequency band or channel of the digital hearing aid, at the flick of the software's "quick-fit" option.

As mentioned at the outset of this chapter, the one drawback of this (in the writer's opinion) is that so much seems buried this way. Clinicians who do not take the time to understand the rationales behind the software's settings are in peril of becoming mere technicians who just push buttons and who don't understand "why." Here, it is important for clinicians to determine which digital hearing aids they most often recommend, and then to actually *listen* to these hearing aids in various environments. Compare the sound quality of different digital hearing aids when they are set up to meet the fitting requirements of some specific hearing loss. Do not completely rely on the marketing claims made by the manufacturers; take the time to check them out with your own ears. Always remember; the cochlea is an excellent acoustic analyzer.

All hearing aids that do not have a digital circuit, or a DSP core, are analog hearing aids. For hearing aids, the term "analog" means that the patterns of electrical current or voltages in the circuit are analogous (similar) to those of the acoustic (sound) input. It is also important to remember the electrical patterns are continuous (not discrete pieces), just like the incoming and outgoing sound waves. When thinking of analog, think about sound being played from old-time record albums on a stereo turntable. The needle wiggles in the grooves on the record, and these wiggle patterns are converted into *analogous* patterns of electricity, which are then amplified. These amplified patterns of electricity are then turned back into sound waves by the speakers (which are like microphones in reverse).

Both analog and digital hearing aids share the fact that they all have microphones and receivers, known as *transducers*. Transducers simply change energy from one form into another (microphones change sound into electricity and the receiver changes electricity back into sound). At the amplifier stage, gain is added to the input, and the sum total electrical current or voltage is sent on to the receiver, where it is converted back into sound. The microphone changes incoming sound into electricity. Transducers like these, for the most part, are all analog.

Digital hearing aids simply have an *additional* transduction process; after the sound is transduced into electricity by the microphone, an analog-to-digital (A/D) converter changes the electrical current into binary sequences of numbers (or digits). These digits can be manipulated in almost any way possible to provide the gain or other digital processing instructions that are needed for someone's hearing requirements. Once the DSP algorithms have been executed (i.e., once the binary digits have been manipulated), the numbers are then changed back into electrical current by a digital-to-analog (D/A) converter. This current is then transduced back into sound by the receiver.

When reading about digital hearing aids, one may encounter the term "algorithm," which is simply a series of mathematical instructions. Numbers lend themselves easily to manipulation, and this ability is what makes digital hearing aids very attractive. Digital circuitry allows the frequency response of the hearing aid to be even more flexible than that of the analog, multichannel WDRC hearing aids. With DSP, the frequency response can be literally "sculpted" to meet the target(s) of gain as closely as possible. Additional digital algorithms provide other, unparalleled flexibility and adaptability not easily accomplished with analog circuitry.

The basic thing to remember about a digital hearing aid is that sound is represented and manipulated by separate or discrete (not continuous) numbers or digits. When reading about digital hearing aids, various terms are encountered: two of these are "sampling rate" and "quantization." These refer to the way a digital circuit converts a continuous analog signal into a sequence of discrete numbers.

In more simple terms, these terms refer to the way in which the frequency and the intensity of sound become represented by numbers.

Digital Architecture: Channels and Bands

Just as the terms "digital" and "programmable" represent essentially different concepts, so do the terms programmable and multichannel. When programmable and multichannel hearing aids are understood as distinct from each other, it can be appreciated how the properties of multichannel and programmability often intersect or are combined.

Programmable hearing aids can be single-channel or multichannel. Similarly, single-channel and multichannel hearing aids can be programmable or nonprogrammable. Features like multiple channels and programmability can be combined, however, and investigation of the offerings by manufacturers will quickly verify that combinations of programmable, multichannel hearing aids abound.

Programmable hearing aids, whether single-channel or multichannel, also can have more than one memory or program. A programmable hearing aid with two or more programs enables the listener to manually choose (by a switch on the hearing aid or by remote control) among the different programs. For the simplest example, a two-program, single-channel hearing aid could be set to meet the needs of a client who wants to choose between two different types of sound qualities. One program will provide optimal gain for listening in quiet or listening to music and here, the widest frequency response may be desired. This program might be set to provide the necessary gain to meet target gain dictated by a fitting method. A second program will provide an appropriate frequency response for difficult listening situations, such as discriminating speech in a noisy background. This second program might be set to provide less low-frequency gain to reduce background noise, and more *diff. band channel*

high-frequency gain to increase audibility for the normally less intense, high-frequency consonants of speech.

To provide different frequency responses for the client, programmable hearing aids with more than one memory (multimemory) typically provide different clusters of trimmer settings for different listening situations. In the example above, settings for Program 1 would be programmed optimally to meet some fitting method target(s). For Program 2, the trimmers could be set to provide more overall gain along with less low-frequency gain (more low-cut). This would create the "teeter-totter" effect in the frequency response: Program 1 would provide more lows and less highs, whereas Program 2 would provide less lows and more highs.

Multimemory hearing aids are not limited to providing different clusters of gain settings for different frequency responses. Different programmed memories can provide also alternate compression characteristics, or permit the client a choice between using directional versus omnidirectional microphone characteristics. One program could provide omnidirectional sound, while another program provides directional sound. Directional microphones are not a new development in the hearing aid industry, but they did experience a revival in the late 1990s, and they continue to receive a lot of attention.

Whereas high-end analog hearing aids are almost always restricted to two frequency bands or channels, digital hearing aids are known to have in excess of 10 bands or channels (see Figure 5–13). Here is a good point to distinguish between "bands" and "channels." In analog hearing aids, the term "frequency band" was used interchangeably with the term "channel." These bands or channels were often separated by filtering, from other frequency regions. This filtering was referred to as "band splitting." In each band, only the gain—and consequently, the output—was adjusted. For today's digital hearing aids, much more than gain can be adjusted independently in each frequency band. It has become industry convention to posit that if only the gain is adjusted, each frequency region is called a "band." This is just convention; there is no official definition of "bands" and "channels." So, if the whole point is shaping the frequency response, then one might call such a hearing aid a "multiband" system.

On the other hand, if more than just the gain is adjusted within a band, then the band would be referred to as a "channel." Lots more than just gain can be adjusted within a band, for example, specific types of compression, such as BILL or TILL, or noise reduction, or feedback reduction. In today's digital hearing aids, therefore, channels are groups of frequency bands that share a digital algorithm. For example, if a group of low-frequency bands has a digital algorithm that instructs it to provide BILL, this group would comprise a low-frequency BILL channel. In the final analysis, it is possible to have more bands than channels, but not the other way around. From now on, let's just use the term channel.

The dB/octave slope of the individual channels in digital hearing aids can be much steeper than in analog hearing aids, and this further increases fitting flexibility. A fairly steep analog slope found in hearing aids was 24 dB/octave. Although a 24 dB/octave slope permits a relatively high degree of independence between channels, it does not allow complete independence. With DSP, the slope between adjacent channels can be almost infinitely steep compared with those of analog multichannel hearing aids. A very steep slope between channels permits an even higher degree of fitting flexibility for various shapes or configurations of hearing loss than that already obtained with analog multichannel WDRC hearing aids. By adjusting the gain and output of each channel, much like the buttons on a stereo equalizer, the frequency response can be literally "sculpted" to meet the target (or targets) of gain as closely as possible.

In summary, there are always tradeoffs to be considered when engineering new digital hearing aids. It behooves of clinicians to listen to digital products with their own ears, and compare sound quality among digital hearing aids before automatically adhering to the claims of the manufacturers who build them. The high-end digital hearing aid from any one specific manufacturer may not necessarily offer the best sound quality. Sometimes, the simpler products, with fewer frequency bands and fewer "bells and whistles," can in fact sound the best.

Digital Combinations of Compression

Digital hearing aids are almost always software-driven. Because of this fact, digital hearing aids simply combine all sorts of compression types. Always remember those building blocks of compression discussed earlier in this chapter; they are fundamental to understanding compression in both analog and digital hearing aids. Readers may recall the functions shown in Figure 5–5; they show the way compression is often adjusted, and it is the way that many clinicians understand compression. The compression ratios hinge from a knee-point that is situated to the left, and over a relatively low-input SPL. Higher compression ratios here result in decreased gain. Compression, however, can also be adjusted from a right-most knee-point (Figure 5–14). Notice on the right-hand function of Figure 5–14, however, that the compression ratios hinge from a knee-point that is situated

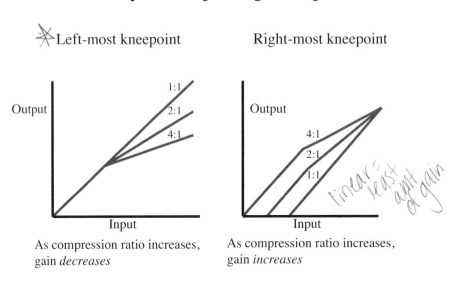

Different Ways of Adjusting Compression

Left-most kneepoint

Right-most kneepoint

As compression ratio increases, gain *decreases*

As compression ratio increases, gain *increases*

Figure 5–14. Different ways of adjusting compression. The left panel shows compression adjustments in the way that most clinicians conceive of them. When hinging from a left-most knee-point, linear (1:1) gain implies greatest gain. Increased compression ratios imply progressively less gain. The right panel shows compression as it originally became available with high-end multichannel analog hearing aids of the mid to late 1990s. This type of compression adjustment was based on the model of normal loudness growth. With compression hinging from the right-most knee-point, linear gain is actually the least amount of gain offered, while increased compression ratios imply increased gain. The objective here was to approximate normal loudness growth with increased compression ratios. Today's digital hearing aids commonly utilize both of these ways of adjusting compression.

to the right, and over a relatively high-input SPL. Here, a higher compression ratio results in *increased* gain.

Digital hearing aids often combine both of these types of knee-points and compression ratio adjustments, so that the input/output graph now has two knee-points (Figure 5–15). Here, maximum gain occurs below the left-most knee-point, and the gain is linear.

Even greater than linear gain can also occur; this is called "expansion," and it will be covered next in this chapter. For now, concentrate on the linear gain shown here, and the WDRC, as well as the output limiting compression. Linear gain occurs below or to the left of the left-most knee-point. WDRC, with its low compression ratio, occurs between the two knee-points. Above the right-most knee-point, output limiting compression occurs with its high knee-point and high compres-

Two Knee-points, with Linear, WDRC, and Output Limiting

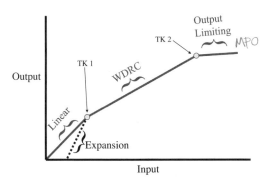

Figure 5–15. Two knee-points, with linear, WDRC, and output limiting. Digital hearing aid fitting software commonly enables clinicians to visualize input/output graphs showing two (or more) knee-points. Each knee-point can be adjusted both vertically and horizontally, to best meet the needs of the client. Linear gain takes place below the left-most knee-point; WDRC occurs between the two knee points, while output limiting compression occurs to the right of the right-most knee-point. In many digital hearing aids, expansion is also offered. Expansion provides greater than linear gain, and it occurs below the left-most knee-point.

sion ratio. The purpose here is to limit the MPO for high input sound levels.

In today's fitting software, input/output graphs sometimes comprise a section, and the results of knee-point and compression ratio adjustments can be seen. On digital hearing aids, two (and sometimes more) knee-points can often be separately and independently adjusted, which in turn, adjusts the compression ratios. Once again, you will not normally encounter compression I/O functions on the surface of the fitting software. On the contrary, you would have to dig around to find them and hence, most clinicians do not look at these functions anymore. The following, however, describes what would happen if you did adjust the knee-points and ratios in the fitting software.

Raising the left-most knee-point vertically increases the compression ratio for soft-moderate level input sounds, which increases the gain for these sounds (Figure 5–16). This accomplishes the same thing as increasing the compression ratio as shown in Figure 5–14. Moving the left-most knee-point to the left does nothing to the compression ratio itself, but it does have the effect of increasing the gain for very soft input sound levels.

Raising the right-most knee-point vertically has the effect of decreasing the compression ratio (Figure 5–17). This increases the gain, but only for the more intense sound inputs of the MPO hearing aid; the most obvious effect is to increase the MPO. Moving the right-most knee-point to the right, again has no effect on the compression ratio, but it does increase the gain for the most intense input sounds. These two adjustments of the right-most knee-point (raising it vertically or moving it horizontally) together accomplish the same thing as adjusting the MPO with the output limiting compression control, as discussed earlier. The digital difference here is the routine and easily accomplished adjustments of knee-points and compression ratios.

In some digital hearing aids, even more knee-points can be specified (Figure 5–18). Some digital hearing aids utilize multi knee-point input/output functions, and their stated

Left Knee-Point Adjustment

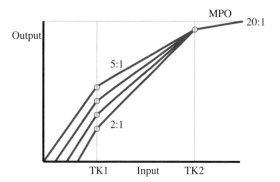

•*Increases compression ratio*
•*Increases gain for soft/mid-level inputs*

Figure 5–16. Left knee-point adjustment. The left-most knee-point can be adjusted vertically and/or horizontally. An increased WDRC ratio results from raising this knee-point (as the compression here hinges from the right-most knee-point). This serves to increase the gain for soft-to-mid-level input intensity sounds. If the same knee-point were to be moved horizontally to the left, this would do nothing to the compression ratio itself, but it would have the effect of increasing the gain for very soft input sound levels.

Right Knee-Point Adjustment

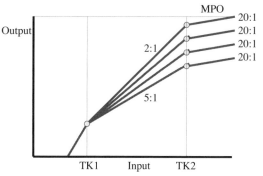

•*Compression ratio decreases*
•*Gain increases for intense input levels*

Figure 5–17. Right knee-point adjustment. The right-most knee-point can also be adjusted vertically and/or horizontally. An increased MPO results from raising this knee-point (as the compression here hinges from the left-most knee-point). This serves to increase the gain for mid to intense input intensity sounds. If the same knee-point were to be moved horizontally to the right, this would again, do nothing to the compression ratio itself, but it would have the effect of increasing the gain for intense levels.

purposes proposed by the manufacturers of these hearing aids are quite interesting. The literature for many of today's' digital hearing aids states the reasoning for their input/output function as follows. Expansion (to be described in the next section), for example, is called "soft squelch," and it appears below the first- or left-most knee-point at around 25 dB SPL. The purpose is to reduce annoying audible internal hearing aid noise that is below the intensity of typical speech. WDRC appears between the first and second knee-points (25 dB to 45 dB SPL), and its purpose is to increase audibility of soft speech, and also, to hear softer sounds that are a further distance away. The compression ratio is increased between the second and third knee-points (45 dB and 65 dB SPL), thus providing less gain for these inputs. The reason is because listening conditions are stated to be quite good between these levels. From 65 dB to about 80 dB SPL, the gain is again linear! At

A Multi-Knee-Point Input/Output Graph

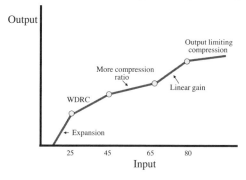

Figure 5–18. A multi knee-point input/output graph. The software for fitting many digital hearing aids often shows input/output graphs that have more than two knee-points. Each can be adjusted by the software, or they can be automatically set to a "best-fit" as determined by the fitting software. Below the left-most knee-point, either linear gain or expansion (commonly called "soft noise squelch") can be selected. Only expansion is shown on this figure. Linear gain, of course, would be a 45° angle.

these levels, speech and noise are commonly mixed together, and people generally prefer increased gain in these situations, so as to hear speech better in these more difficult listening situations. Past 80 dB SPL inputs, the compression ratio is dramatically increased in order to limit the MPO. The point here is that clinicians should make it their business to become good consumers of the products manufacturers provide.

EXPANSION (AS OPPOSED TO COMPRESSION)

Expansion is the opposite of compression. On the basis of everything discussed so far, one might wonder when this would ever be of use. Basically, expansion is a way to reduce internal microphone and amplifier noise that sometimes becomes audible to the listener in quiet, especially those who have good low-frequency hearing. Expansion actually serves to reduce the gain for very soft input sounds (e.g., below 40 dB SPL), and then rapidly increases the gain as inputs increase, up until the first knee-point of compression. Expansion was actually offered on an analog circuit produced by Gennum, the DynamEQIII, but the advent of digital technology precluded its use in hearing aids. Today, most digital hearing aids offer expansion.

Many manufacturers and clinicians are content to think of expansion as an internal noise squelch, but to truly understand what it is doing, here is a description of how and why it works: Figure 5–19 shows expansion on an input/output function, as it is superimposed on typical WDRC, offered by some fictitious hearing aid. The vertical output line is extended downward on this figure,

Expansion

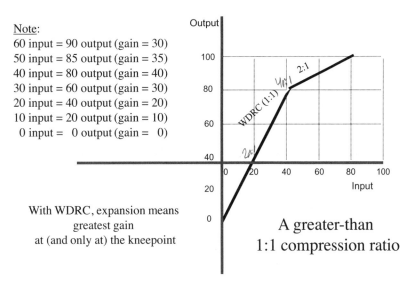

Note:
60 input = 90 output (gain = 30)
50 input = 85 output (gain = 35)
40 input = 80 output (gain = 40)
30 input = 60 output (gain = 30)
20 input = 40 output (gain = 20)
10 input = 20 output (gain = 10)
  0 input =   0 output (gain =   0)

With WDRC, expansion means greatest gain at (and only at) the kneepoint

A greater-than 1:1 compression ratio

Figure 5–19. Expansion. Expansion is the opposite of compression. Unlike WDRC, it provides greater than linear gain for inputs that are below the knee-point of compression. Note in this example, how the gain increases as the inputs increase from 0 dB SPL to 40 dB SPL; for increasing inputs beyond the knee-point, the gain once again decreases. When WDRC is used along with expansion, the greatest gain is delivered at (and only at) the left-most knee-point of compression.

further than usual, in order to show where the function of expansion would terminate. Note that the gain for 0 dB SPL input would be nothing, so the output would also be 0 dB SPL. Note also, how the gain dramatically increases, however, as the inputs increase, up until the knee-point shown here. With greater than 1:1 linear gain, expansion thus provides maximum gain at (and only at) the left-most knee-point seen in most input/output graphs. Hopefully, this left-most, lower knee-point is set at an input level typical to soft conversational speech, because soft speech is then what gets the greatest amount of gain for the listener. Expansion in digital hearing aids commonly offers expansion ratios of 1:5, 1:75, or 1:2. With a 1:2 compression ratio, for example, for each added decibel of input, there would be two decibels of added output.

As mentioned earlier, expansion is mainly used to reduce the gain for soft, internal microphone and amplifier noise. The left graph of Figure 5–20 shows an input/output graph for a typical WDRC hearing aid. This is essentially the same graph for the same fictitious WDRC hearing aid as that shown on Figure 5–19; however, the vertical output line is no longer extended below the horizontal input line. On the left graph, straight WDRC without the use of expansion would provide 40 dB of linear gain below the knee-point. The WDRC here provides a 2:1 compression ratio. Again, the solid line extending downward to the left of the knee-point shows expansion when used with this WDRC hearing aid. The expansion in this example gives a 1:2 input/output ratio. It is important to note that expansion is always offered only below

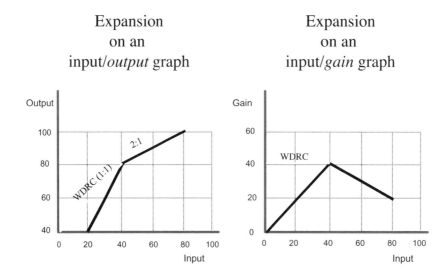

Figure 5–20. Expansion plotted as input/output versus input/gain. The left panel shows expansion on an input/output graph. The example here is the same as that shown in Figure 5–10. The gain of the WDRC hearing aid here in this example is 40 dB. WDRC (*line*) provides linear gain for soft inputs below the knee-point. Expansion is shown as the solid line below the knee-point. Note that its function is steeper than the typical 45° angle function of linear gain. The right panel shows the same expansion and WDRC, only this time, they are displayed on an input/gain graph. WDRC provide a constant (linear) amount of gain for all inputs below the knee-point; once past (to the right of) the knee-point, the gain again drops off due to compression. In comparison, expansion, provides increased gain with increased input levels, up until the knee-point. Again, with expansion, the greatest gain is only at the first knee-point of compression. Hopefully, this maximal gain is provided for soft speech inputs.

the left-most knee-point. Its purpose is to give more than linear gain, but only for very soft inputs.

Here's the rub with expansion; for *really* soft inputs, like 10 dB to 20 dB SPL, there is very little gain. In the example shown in Figure 5–20, there is a dramatic, greater-than-linear increase of gain, however, as the input intensities increase up to the knee-point set at 40 dB SPL. Past the knee-point, the hearing aid goes into compression. The right graph on Figure 5–20 shows the very same hearing aid, but this time the vertical axis shows gain and not output. Note that the WDRC hearing aid in this example is providing a steady amount (40 dB) of gain for all inputs below the knee-point. When the same hearing aid uses expansion, however, there is less gain for the really soft input sounds of 0 dB to 20 dB SPL. Again, with expansion, the maximum gain is seen at, and only at, the knee-point of compression. The gain increases as input sound levels increase up to the knee-point, and then as compression kicks in, the gain is once again reduced. WDRC hearing aids that use expansion and have a knee-point of around 40 dB provide maximum gain for soft sounds of speech.

People who complain that their WDRC hearing aids make a "hissing" sound in quiet are apt to appreciate the benefits of expansion. These people also most likely have good low-frequency hearing. Recall that the focus of WDRC hearing aids is to "lift the floor" of hearing sensitivity, to imitate the outer hair cells, and to amplify soft sounds by a lot and loud sounds by little or nothing at all. Clinicians can counsel their users that the hearing aid is meant to imitate the outer hair cells, and so on. But if he or she has good hearing in the low frequencies, the user may still say, "I hate my hearing aid in quiet because it makes a hissing sound." This is because WDRC by itself is "trying too hard" to imitate outer hair cells. In really quiet surroundings, it will provide maximum gain, and her good low-frequency hearing will pick up unwanted internal microphone and amplifier noise. Expansion thus acts like an internal noise squelch feature. In fact, some hearing aid manufacturer promotional literature calls expansion a "soft squelch" feature. It is useful mostly for those who have mild-moderate SNHL, and would otherwise benefit from WDRC.

DYNAMIC ASPECTS OF COMPRESSION

Until now, compression has been discussed in terms of threshold knee-point and compression ratio. These are sometimes known as the "static" aspects of compression, because they involve the input SPL when compression begins and the degree of compression once it occurs. Sound in the environment, however, is constantly changing in intensity over time, and a compression hearing aid has to respond to these changes in intensity over time. The "dynamic" aspects of compression are known as the "attack" and the "release" times.

The attack and release times are the lengths of time it takes for a compression circuit to respond to changes in the intensity of an input SPL (Figure 5–21). When the input SPL exceeds the knee-point of compression, the hearing aid "attacks" the sound by reducing the gain. Once the input sound falls below the knee-point of compression, the hearing aid "releases" from compression and restores the gain. The attack time is the length of time it takes for a hearing aid to go into compression and reduce the gain; the release time is the length of time it takes for it to come out of compression and restore the gain.

An electrical (and especially a digital) circuit cannot instantly mirror the changes that take place in the environment, because it requires time to respond to these changes. For example, if a compression circuit is to respond to a sudden input SPL increase, it has to wait for at least one cycle of the sound wave to "know" if the increased SPL will remain. A change in gain that occurs faster than the longest cycle or period of incoming sound can in turn, change the fine details of the sound waves, and distortion will result.

Hearing aids are not the only electrical devices that use compression and have

Dynamic Compression Characteristics

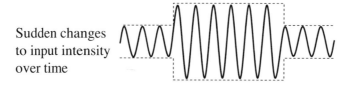

Sudden changes
to input intensity
over time

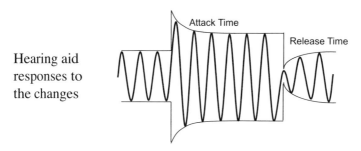

Attack Time

Release Time

Hearing aid
responses to
the changes

Figure 5–21. Dynamic compression characteristics. The top shows a simple description of input sound changing in intensity (vertical dimension) over time (horizontal dimension). The sound has suddenly increased in intensity, and after a while, the sound suddenly decreases in intensity. The bottom shows the output response of a compression hearing aid to the changes in sound input intensity over time. Note that gain has been applied to even the soft input, before the sudden intensity increase. The compression circuitry takes some amount of time to respond or compress the incoming signal that has suddenly increased in intensity. This is the "attack" time. Once the input sound has decreased in intensity, the circuit takes some time to stop compressing. This is the "release" time.

attack/release times. Audiovisual equipment has used input and output compression for many years, and we have heard its effects before. Recall, for example, the television broadcasts in which the sports announcer is talking and the background noise is changing in intensity over time. When a score is made and the audience suddenly increases their cheers, the background noise increases in intensity. It may take a short time for the compression of the audiovisual equipment to attack and reduce the gain of the noise; but this also temporarily reduces the gain for the announcer's voice. When the cheering stops, it may again take some time for the system to release from compression, and the announcer's voice will accordingly take some time to return back to a normal, audible level.

Most attack and release times are set to achieve a best compromise between two undesirable extremes. Times that are too fast will cause the gain to fluctuate rapidly, and this may cause a jarring, "pumping" perception by the listener. Times that are too slow may make the compression act too slowly and cause a real lagging perception on the part of the listener. Quick attack times (i.e., 10 ms or less) might prevent sudden, transient sounds from becoming too loud for the listener. In general, release times need to be longer than attack times to prevent a "fluttering" perception on the part of the listener. Longer release times (i.e., up to 150 ms) tend to prevent severe distortions that occur with fast release times. Inordinately fast release times can cause the hearing aid to track the amplitude of individual cycles of sound waves. Such a rapid modulation of sound can cause a "breathing" or "pumping" perception on the part of the listener.

Just as we have seen with the static aspects of compression, there are lots of "buzz" words that float around when the dynamic aspects of compression are discussed. Different attack and release times are sometimes used to categorize different types of dynamic compression. Various types of dynamic compression methods are discussed briefly below.

Peak Detection

Most early analog compression hearing aids used a technique called peak detection to "track" the peak amplitude of incoming sound waves. If the peak was greater than the compression threshold knee-point, the circuit attacked and began to compress the signal, which reduced the gain. Once the peak was below the knee-point, the compression releases and the gain increases again. Peak detection allowed for a wide variety of times that could separately be specified and assigned as attack and release times; however, these times were constant and fixed for any incoming sound intensity patterns. Most peak detection systems in hearing aids were adjusted to provide quick attack times and longer, slower release times. A typical default attack/release time set were an attack time of 50 ms and a release time of about three times that length, namely, 150 ms.

An advantage of peak detection is that it reacted very quickly to increases in environmental sound levels. Unfortunately, however, it could react inappropriately to very short intense sounds, because the longer release times would keep the gain down after the short intense sound has stopped. This unnecessarily reduced the gain of sounds the listener might have wanted to hear.

With fixed attack/release times, the hearing aid cannot respond differently to different patterns of sound input intensities when needed. Speech is an example of sound that is constantly changing over time. The dynamic acoustic sounds of speech within the world of ever-changing background noise (e.g., the sudden slamming of a door or the constant roar of traffic) posed real problems for the peak detection method and the listener.

"Syllabic compression" and "automatic volume control" (AVC) are two specific sets of attack/release times commonly encountered on today's digital hearing aids. In the past, some high-end analog hearing aids employed the use of either syllabic or AVC. Today, these attack/release time schemes, as well as those of average detection (described later on), can often be selected alternately on fitting software for digital hearing aids. The most high-profile usage of syllabic compression occurred with the advent of the one of the earliest digital hearing aids, the Oticon DigiFocus, in 1997.

Automatic Volume Control

A type of compression known as AVC has often been used during broadcasts with audiovisual equipment. In a comparison with peak detection, AVC has a relatively long attack and long release times; its release times are usually more than 150 ms and can be as long as several seconds. Because of this, it does not respond to rapid fluctuations of sound input. On the contrary, it responds mainly to general, overall changes in sound intensity, which reduces the need for the listener to adjust the volume control manually. The long attack/release times with AVC are intended to imitate the length of time it physically takes for a listener to react to sudden noise increases by raising a hand and manually adjusting the VC on a hearing aid, hence, its name. The most high-profile usage of AVC occurred with the Widex Senso digital hearing aid in 1997. The Senso was the very first digital product to appear in BTE and ITE formats.

Syllabic Compression

"Syllabic compression" refers to the exact opposite of AVC; namely, relatively short attack and release times; its release times vary from less than 50 ms up to 150 ms. The attack/release times are specifically intended to be shorter than the duration of the typical speech syllable, which is about 200 to 300 ms. Short attack/release times allow the hearing aid to compress or reduce the gain for the peaks of more intense speech (usually the vowel sounds), and this provides more uniformity in the intensity of ongoing speech syllables. In other words, syllabic compression reduces the differences between the normally more intense vowels and the softer unvoiced consonants such as /s/. The main premise of syllabic compression is to allow a hearing aid to make the softer sounds of speech more audible without simultaneously making the normally louder parts of speech from becoming too loud.

Syllabic compression is somewhat controversial and not everyone agrees with its use, especially along with WDRC. As mentioned earlier, one criticism of WDRC is that it serves to reduce the peaks in the speech waveform and increases the valleys. In addition, a hearing aid might amplify the noise that is situated between the peaks of speech, and this only further degrades speech intelligibility. Much clinical experience has shown that the use of fast attack/release times (less than 10 ms) and short release times (less than 100 ms) along with WDRC is especially detrimental to speech intelligibility. This is because fast attack/release times enable the WDRC to follow the rapidly changing speech waveform with good precision, reducing it's peak-to-valley contrasts in real time. Syllabic compression along with WDRC can thus compromise the intensity differences between the various phonetic elements of speech and distort the spectral content of speech cues. It is interesting to note that the opposites of AVC and syllabic compression were used in the very first two digital hearing aids (Widex Senso and Oticon DigiFocus). Widex promoted the use of AVC on its Senso digital hearing aid; the reason was because field trial subjects who first tried the Senso liked it best. Recall also that syllabic compression was utilized for the low frequencies on Oticon's Digi-

Focus. There you have it; opposite attack/release time schemes for the first two small-sized digital hearing aids out in the marketplace. The jury was obviously out regarding the best attack/release times. As mentioned earlier, in the mid to late 1990s, Oticon promoted the use of syllabic compression along with BILL, in its analog Multi-Focus hearing aid and digital DigiFocus hearing aids. Here, the intent was to improve aided speech recognition by reducing the upward spread of masking. Thus, not only was WDRC present especially for the low frequencies, but the WDRC was made to act quickly. If the normally loud, low-frequency background noise can be thought of as the bull, and relatively soft, high-frequency consonants as fragile china teacups, then syllabic compression used in conjunction with BILL could be a way to control the raging bull in the china shop.

Adaptive Compression

This type of compression has fixed, quick attack times, but has release times that vary with the length or duration of the intense, incoming sound. For short (transient) intense sound inputs, the release time is short. For sound inputs that are longer in rise time and duration, the release times are longer. The desired result is a reduction of compression "pumping" heard by the listener. Adaptive Compression was originally patented by Telex and then became most commonly associated with the KAmp circuits.

Average Detection

Average detection was first associated with the analog DynamEQII circuit by Gennum. This circuit was one of the original analog two-channel WDRC hearing aid circuits that emerged during the mid-1990s (following the early analog two-channel circuit produced by ReSound). These multichannel hearing aids commonly emerged with BILL being used in the low-frequency channel, and TILL being used in the high-frequency channel. Unlike the peak detection method that tracks the peak amplitude of incoming sound waves, the average detection method looks at the average of incoming signal over a given length of time. When the average SPL exceeds the knee-point of compression, then the gain is reduced. For the purpose of explaining the average detection, its historical implementation in the analog, two-channel DynamEQII will be explained here. It should, again, be recalled that digital hearing aids utilize mathematical algorithms to accomplish similar results.

The analog DynamEQII had "twin" average compression detectors; one was a fast detector and the other was a slow detector (Figure 5–22). The slow average detector averaged sound inputs over a 220-ms time interval (i.e., about $1/5$ of a second) and was in control of the compression system most of the time. When the slow average of incoming sounds exceeded the threshold knee-point of compression, the gain was slowly reduced and was hardly noticeable. With the slow detector alone, however, a short spike of intense sound could be averaged into the overall body of sound taking place over 220 ms. This slow average would not be enough to "tell" the hearing aid to go into compression and reduce the gain. This is where the fast average detector came into the picture. The fast average detector averages sound inputs over time intervals of about 10 ms (i.e., $1/100$ of a second), and it acted when intense transients were not "caught" by the slow detector.

Average Detection for Variable Attack/Release Times

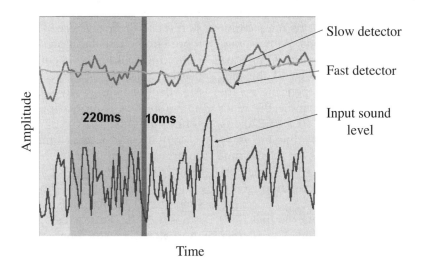

Figure 5–22. Average detection for variable attack/release times. The figure shows the actions of an slow average detector, which in this case averages sound over time intervals of about 220 ms, and a fast average detector, which averages sound over time intervals of about 10 ms. The bottom line represents sound intensity as it occurs over time. The top smooth line represents the input signal when averaged by the slow average detector. Note that the slow average is very flat over time. The top bumpy line represents the input signal when averaged by the fast detector. Note the fast average changes a lot more over time than the slow average. Variable attack/release times between 220 and 10 ms can be provided, depending on how quickly the input sound intensity changes.

When the "fast" average was 6 dB greater than the "slow" average, the fast average detector took over and reduced the gain for the spike of intense sound.

The main result of average detection is that both the attack and release times vary with the length of the incoming intense sounds. This is in direct contrast with the peak detection systems that give constant, fixed quick attack and slow release times for all incoming stimuli. As long as the incoming sounds are below the compression threshold, both types of circuits provide uncompressed gain. With sudden transient loud sounds, however, such as a door slam, the average detection system will provide quick attack and quick release times. On the other hand, the peak detector will provide its usual quick attack and slow release times. Because of the reduction of gain and the long recovery of the peak detection circuit, soft speech spoken right after the door slam may be temporarily inaudible to the listener. The average detection circuit enables a quick recovery of gain after the door slam, because its release time will be quick for short sounds. With average detection, the attack/release times can vary anywhere between the short and the long average detection times, depending on the input sound. In the above example, the attack time could vary between 10 and 220 ms, depending on how quickly the incoming input sound became intense; the release time could also vary between these time constants, depending on how quickly the input sound became quiet again.

The benefit to the listener is that there is less "pumping" perception. The average detection system is a compromise between compression that reacts to every short intense sound and compression that may react too slowly for some sounds that should be compressed. Audible byproducts of compression should not become a nuisance to listeners. Dynamic aspects should be considered when trying to make hearing aids acoustically "transparent."

The various dynamic compression characteristics described above can be selected for most of today's digital hearing aids on the fitting software. For the most part, on most manufacturers' fitting software, the choice is largely between syllabic compression and average detection. Most often, syllabic compression is selected for the low-frequency channels of the digital hearing aid, and average detection is selected for the higher frequency channels.

INTERACTION BETWEEN STATIC AND DYNAMIC ASPECTS OF COMPRESSION

Compression consists of static aspects in one dimension and dynamic aspects in a purely separate dimension. With incoming sounds, the attack/release times of a hearing aid interact with the ratio of compression. The input/output graphs on hearing aid spec sheets show compression ratios that are obtained with constant pure tones, not the stops and starts of sounds like speech. Static compression ratios on spec sheets do not accurately represent the actual compression ratios experienced in real life by clients who wear the hearing aids. Fast attack/release times have the effect of temporarily reducing the ratio or amount of compression for any given sound stimulus.

Attack and release times interact with compression ratios, and these interactions affect the sound quality for the listener. In general, a combination of short attack/release times (e.g., 10 ms) and high compression ratios (e.g., 10:1) cause distortion. If the same short attack/release times are used with low compression ratios (e.g., 2:1), then the sound quality is not as distorted. On the other hand, long attack/release times can be combined with either high or low compression ratios.

Dynamic aspects and static aspects of compression are often found in predictable combinations today. Syllabic compression, with its relatively short attack and release times, is most often associated with WDRC hearing aids that have a low-compression knee-point and a low-compression ratio of less than 5:1. It is less common with output limiting compression hearing aids where the knee-points and ratios of compression are "high." AVC, with its relatively long attack/release times, is most often seen in hearing aids that offer a low-threshold knee-point of compression and high-compression ratio.

DYNAMIC COMPRESSION CHARACTERISTICS IN DIGITAL HEARING AIDS

Digital hearing aids also uniquely implement various types of *dynamic* compression characteristics. It is highly recommended by most manufacturers for clinicians not to meddle with or make large customized changes to suggested software default attack/release time parameters; doing so often causes very poor sound quality to the listener. Today, most digital hearing aid fitting software tends to offer two types for clinicians to choose from: syllabic compression and average detection. Recall that syllabic compression is most successfully used along with low-frequency WDRC or BILL; average detection provides adaptive attack and adaptive release times and has no specified frequency of usage. Many quick-fit options of digital hearing aids default to the use of syllabic compression for the low-frequency channels and average detection for the high-frequency channels.

As can be seen, many manipulations are possible with digital hearing aids. Clinicians can take comfort from fears of too much freedom; the same fitting software that offers these functions and parameters for adjustment also hides them during "quick fit" options. Furthermore, many manufacturers do indeed provide advice, guidance, and fitting solutions on their fitting software.

SUMMARY

■ The 1990s were the "golden" age of compression, because compression types flourished and differentiated, and yet, all hearing aids were still analog. This meant that each hearing aid was confined to providing one type of compression or another. In order to choose the appropriate hearing aid products for their clients, clinicians thus needed to understand each type of compression well, and categorize these among all available types of compression.

■ In this chapter, we reviewed some of the fundamental concepts that are necessary to comprehend before any discussion of compression: input/output graphs and linear hearing aids. Compression was explored along two dimensions:

Assuming that the VC is held at a constant position, the MPO compression and TK adjustments were compared. The MPO compression control affects the threshold knee-point of compression and also the MPO. By raising the knee-point, the MPO is correspondingly increased. The TK control affects the knee-point of compression and the gain for soft inputs only. By raising the knee-point here, the gain for soft input sounds is decreased.

Output limiting compression was compared with WDRC regarding compression knee-points and compression ratios. Output limiting compression has a high knee-point, which means that compression is activated only for relatively intense sound input levels; it also has a high compression ratio. WDRC has a low knee-point and a low compression ratio. These differences separate their respective clinical purposes.

Output limiting compression acts above its knee-point to limit the MPO. WDRC acts below its knee-point to provide most gain for soft input sounds. Output limiting compression is adjusted by an MPO compression control. It can be very appropriate for severe-to-profound hearing loss that usually exhibits a narrow dynamic range. WDRC is adjusted with a TK control, and can be appropriate for mild-to-moderate SNHL. It can be very appropriate for mild-to-moderate SNHL, which usually exhibits a wider dynamic range. This most commonly prevalent degree of SNHL is mostly due to outer hair cell damage, and thus can benefit from the express amplification of soft inputs.

As mild-to-moderate SNHL is very common, and WDRC is correspondingly by far the most popular type of compression used today. Two types of WDRC are BILL and TILL.

■ Dynamic aspects of compression were discussed separately from the static compression aspects of compression threshold knee-point and compression ratio. Different types of attack/release time parameters were discussed. The usual compromise has been to provide fast attack times with longer release times.

AVC and syllabic compression were described as being opposites. AVC has long attack/release times, and syllabic compression offers relatively short attack/release times. AVC is chosen for client comfort; the attack/release times are intended to mimic the length of time it takes for someone to physically adjust the VC. Syllabic detection is chosen to reduce the upward spread of masking. Adaptive compression offers fixed attack times and variable release times, while average detection offers variable attack and release times. Both adaptive compression and average detection are designed to reduce the adverse perception of audible hearing aid amplifier "pumping."

■ The above types of compression were all discussed as they are utilized in today's digital hearing aids. Input/output functions with more than one knee-point were discussed. Output limiting compression and WDRC were also discussed as they pertain to these multiple knee-point input/output functions. Last, dynamic aspects of compression were revisited as they are most commonly found on digital hearing aids.

REVIEW QUESTIONS

1. On input/output graphs, input is always on the vertical axis.　　　　T　F

2. On an input/output graph, the left-most diagonal line indicates the most gain.
   T　F

3. The MPO compression control is the older of the two control types discussed.
   T　F

4. The TK control affects:
   a. MPO.
   b. gain for any input intensity level.
   c. gain for soft inputs only.
   d. none of the above.

5. WDRC is associated with:
   a. high knee-point and high compression ratio.
   b. low knee-point and high compression ratio.
   c. high knee-point and low compression ratio.
   d. low knee-point and low compression ratio.

6. WDRC provides most gain for:
   a. soft input sounds .
   b. medium input sounds.
   c. loud input sounds.
   d. all of the above.

7. As you lower the knee-point with an MPO compression control, you:
   a. increase the MPO.
   b. decrease the MPO.
   c. decrease gain for soft inputs.
   d. increase gain for soft inputs.

8. For mild-moderate SNHL, the following two compression features are often found together:
   a. high knee-point and ratio, TK control.
   b. high knee-point and ratio, MPO compression control.
   c. low knee-point and ratio, TK control.
   d. low knee-point and ratio, MPO compression control.

9. For severe-to-profound hearing loss, the following two compression features are often found together:
   a. high knee-point and ratio, TK control.

b. high knee-point and ratio, MPO compression control.
c. low knee-point and ratio, TK control.
d. low knee-point and ratio, MPO compression control.

10. On input/output graphs, the right-most diagonal line represents the:
a. least gain.
b. least compression.
c. most gain.
d. highest knee-point.

11. A compression hearing aid provides 90 dB output with 40 dB input; what's the gain here?

12. Same hearing aid: knee-point at 50 dB SPL, compression ratio of 2:1; the output for a 60 dB input is:

13. Same hearing aid: knee-point at 50 dB SPL, compression ratio of 2:1; the gain for a 60 dB input is:

14. A compression hearing aid provides 120 dB output with 50 dB input; what's the gain here?

15. Same hearing aid: knee-point at 70 dB SPL, compression ratio of 10:1; the output for an 80 dB input is:

16. Same hearing aid: knee-point at 70 dB SPL, compression ratio of 10:1; the output for a 90 dB input is:

17. Relatively short or quick attack/release times are associated with:
a. Average detection.
b. Adaptive compression.
c. AVC.
d. Syllabic compression.

18. Variable attack and release times are found with the following type of dynamic compression:

a. average detection.
b. adaptive compression.
c. AVC.
d. Syllabic compression.

19. A typical compression ratio for expansion might be:
a. 1:1.
b. 2:1.
c. 10:1.
d. 1:2.

20. You are fitting a hearing aid; the knee-point is 40 dB SPL, and the compression ratio is 2:1. Your real-ear system does not work well for inputs below 50 dB SPL. From the output for a 50 dB SPL input, the calculated gain is 30 dB. What would the gain be if you ran a curve using a 40 dB SPL input? Hint: an I/O graph can really help to figure it out.

Answer Key

1. False
2. True
3. True
4. c
5. d
6. a
7. b
8. c
9. b
10. a
11. 50 dB
12. 105 dB SPL
13. 45 dB
14. 70 dB
15. 141 dB SPL
16. 142 dB SPL
17. Syllabic compression
18. Average detection
19. d
20. 35

CHAPTER 6

Use of Directional Microphone Technologies to Improve User Performance in Noise

YU-HSIANG WU
RUTH A. BENTLER

PERCEPTUAL DISADVANTAGES OF DIRECTIONAL MICROPHONE SYSTEMS
  Lower Output Level
  Higher Internal Noise Level
  Higher Wind Noise Level
  Poorer Sound Localization Performance
CHAPTER SUMMARY
REFERENCES

INTRODUCTION

One of the most common complaints of listeners with hearing loss is difficulty understanding speech in background noise (e.g., Takahashi et al., 2007). Early studies comparing speech recognition performance of listeners with normal hearing to that of listeners with hearing loss have indicated that those with hearing loss require a better SNR than those with normal hearing (e.g., Dirks, Morgan, & Dubno, 1982; Dubno, Dirks, & Morgan, 1984; Duquesnoy & Plomp, 1983; Plomp, 1978; Schum, Matthews, & Lee, 1991). Evidence also has suggested that the detrimental impact of noise on speech recognition performance worsens as hearing deteriorates (Nabelek, 1982; Nabelek & Mason, 1981).

Considerable research and development efforts have been devoted to hearing aid technologies to reduce the detrimental impact of noise, both in processing-based and microphone-based applications. Processing-based techniques (i.e., single-microphone digital noise reduction algorithms) analyze the incoming signal and then alter the gain/output characteristics to enhance speech and/or attenuate noise. Microphone-based techniques (i.e., directional (DIR) microphone technologies) utilize the outputs from multiple microphones to achieve spatially dependent sound sensitivity, thereby improving SNR. Compared with processing-based techniques, DIR technologies seem to hold the most potential for enhancing speech intelligi-

bility by improving the SNR in at least some listening situations. Specifically, DIR microphone hearing aids are designed to be more sensitive to sounds arriving from certain directions (usually in front of the listener) and less sensitive to sounds from other directions (e.g., from behind the listener). If hearing aid users can place the talker of interest in the front and position the noises to the back, DIR technologies can improve SNR, thereby enhancing speech intelligibility.

For many years, DIR technologies were considered a special feature and were only available in high-end hearing aid models. Today, manufacturers offer DIR technologies in most of their hearing instruments, including entry-level devices. Although DIR technologies have also been implemented on other hearing devices such as cochlear implants (e.g., Chung, Zeng, & Acker, 2006) and bone-anchored hearing aids (e.g., Oeding, Valente, & Kerckhoff, 2010), this chapter focuses on traditional ear-worn DIR microphone hearing aids.

HOW DIRECTIONAL TECHNOLOGIES WORK

Omnidirectional Microphone System

To understand how a DIR microphone system works, it is first necessary to understand an omnidirectional (OMNI) microphone system. A typical hearing aid OMNI microphone system is a closed box that is divided into two small chambers by a thin diaphragm (Figure 6–1). Sounds enter the small microphone port and travel into the chamber. The changes in sound pressure cause the diaphragm to vibrate. The vibration of the diaphragm creates a small electrical signal, which is then processed by the electronic circuit of the hearing aid. OMNI microphone systems are equally sensitive to sound pressure arriving from all directions.

Directional Microphone System: First-Order

The sensitivity of the DIR microphone system depends on the origin angle of sounds. This spatial difference in sensitivity is termed

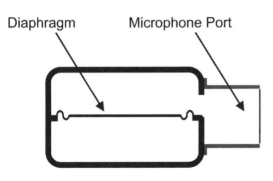

Diaphragm   **Microphone Port**

Figure 6–1. The schematic of an OMNI microphone system. Courtesy of Knowles Electronics.

"directivity." There are several ways to achieve directivity. Two designs are commonly used in hearing aids: the single-cartridge design and the dual-microphone design.

Figure 6–2 shows the schematic illustration of the single-cartridge design. The microphone has one diaphragm housed in a cartridge with two ports allowing sounds to enter on both sides of the diaphragm. The two ports are typically arranged anteriorly-posteriorly on the horizontal plane of the hearing aid as it is placed on the listener's ear. Along the line passing the two microphone ports, the direction in front of the listener is typically defined as 0° and is referred to as the *on-axis* direction. All other directions are considered *off-axis*. Note that there is a mechanical screen, which serves as an acoustic resistor, covering the pathway of the real microphone port.

Now assume a sound source is behind the hearing aid (i.e., 180°). The sound enters the rear port first and then, with a traveling time delay, the front port. This time delay is called *external delay.* The sound entering the rear port is further delayed by the mechanical screen before it enters the chamber. This delay is termed *internal delay.* When the internal delay is set to be equal to the external delay (by choosing an appropriate acoustic resistor), the sound entering the rear port and the sound entering the front port will hit the two sides of the diaphragm simultaneously, cancelling out any movement of the diaphragm. As a result, the microphone will generate no

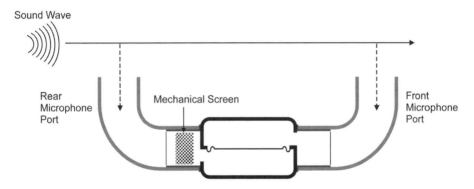

Sound Wave

Rear Microphone Port   Mechanical Screen   Front Microphone Port

Figure 6–2. The schematic of the single-cartridge design of a DIR microphone system.

output because the sound entering one port is subtracted from the sound entering another port. For sounds arriving at the hearing aid from the on-axis direction (0°), the external delay time will be different from the internal delay. As a result, the sounds entering the two ports will not hit the diaphragm simultaneously, resulting in diaphragm vibration and microphone output.

Compared with the single-cartridge design, the dual-microphone design is more commonly used in today's hearing aids. In the simplest dual-microphone system, the spatial sensitivity is achieved by combining two OMNI microphones (Figure 6–3). The acoustic signal is first converted to an electrical or digital signal by each microphone, and then the output signal of one microphone is subtracted from that of the other. Before subtraction takes place, a delay (i.e., internal delay) is applied to the signal from the rear microphone, but now the delay is achieved electronically or digitally. If the internal delay is set equal to the external delay and the

sound is arriving from 180°, output signals from the two microphones will then be identical before subtraction. After signal subtraction, there will be no output from the DIR microphone system.

Although the single-cartridge design differs from the dual-microphone design in structure, these two designs are conceptually equivalent: both rely on the appropriate time difference of the sounds entering the microphone ports and signal subtraction to achieve directivity. This approach is often referred to as *delay-and-subtraction processing*. Because the output of the system is obtained after *one step* of signal subtraction between the sound pressures at the two sides of the diaphragm or between the electronic/digital signals of the two microphones, these systems are classified as first-order DIR systems.

The biggest advantage of the dual-microphone design over the single-cartridge design is the flexibility. Specifically, because the signal delay and subtraction can be achieved digitally, the directivity of the dual-

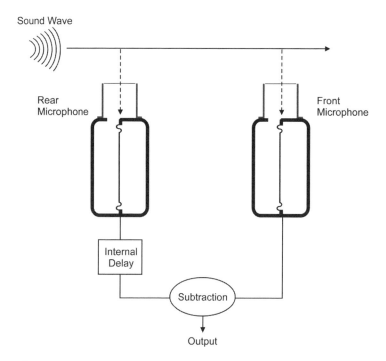

Figure 6–3. The schematic of the dual-microphone design of a DIR microphone system.

microphone design can be easily manipulated. For example, setting the internal delay to be equal to the external delay will, as mentioned previously, attenuate the sound arriving from 180° the most. If the internal delay is programmed to be zero, the microphone system will be less sensitive to sounds arriving from the side of the hearing aid (90° or 270°). This flexibility is the basis of the adaptive DIR system (see the section *Adaptive and Automatic Features*). On the other hand, even though the single-cartridge design can only achieve one directivity pattern (the internal delay is fixed by the acoustic resistor chosen by the manufacturer), this design is free from the potential problem of directivity degradation caused by microphone aging. Specifically, the two OMNI microphones in the dual-microphone design need to be precisely matched in their intensity and phase characteristics in order to achieve and maintain directivity. The dual-microphone system could lose its microphone match over time, thus degrading the directivity. This issue is addressed in the section directivity degradation.

Directional Microphone System: Higher-Order

Directivity can be achieved by combining three microphones. For example, a second-order DIR system has three matched OMNI microphones and uses two steps of signal subtraction between the microphones to achieve directivity (Figure 6–4). The second-order system has been implemented on a commercial hearing aid (Powers & Hamacher, 2002) and is shown to have better SNR improvement than the first-order system (Bentler, Palmer, & Dittberner, 2004; Bentler, Palmer, & Mueller, 2006).

Microphone arrays that consist of multiple microphones have been under development for several years. The microphones in an array can be arranged in any configuration. The simplest configuration is the *broadside array*, in which microphones are placed along the axis perpendicular to the direction of the sound source of interest (e.g., along the listener's forehead using an eyeglass or headband), and the *end-fire array*, in which

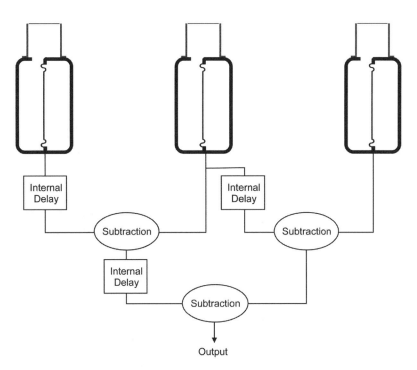

Figure 6–4. The schematic of a second-order DIR microphone system.

microphones are arranged along the axis parallel to the direction of sound source (e.g., on the eyeglass temple). Because of the reasons of cost and cosmetics (Kates, 2008), microphone arrays are rarely used in traditional ear level hearing aids. Recently, higher order DIR systems have been implemented on commercial hearing aids by utilizing binaural wireless transmission technologies to combine the four microphones of two hearing aids (Latzel, 2012).

QUANTIFYING DIRECTIVITY

For clinicians, researchers, and manufacturers, it is important to know if one DIR system has better directivity than the other. The electroacoustic measurement procedures that assess the "goodness" of the DIR microphone system are referred to as *directivity quantification.* Many directivity quantification measures have been suggested. Some of these procedures need special measure-

ment location and equipment and can only be conducted in laboratories; others can be performed at the clinical level.

Directivity Index

Directivity index (DI) is a frequency-dependent numerical index that describes a device's directivity. Strictly defined, the DI, in decibels, is the ratio of the sound pressure of the microphone on-axis response to a sound source in a free sound field to the sound pressure of the microphone off-axis response in a diffuse sound field of the same sound level (Beranek, 1949). This hard-to-understand definition can be illustrated by the following measurement procedures: First let us place a DIR hearing aid in a free sound field (Figure 6–5A). A free sound field is a space without sound diffraction and reflection (Ghent, 2005). (The reader may think of a free sound field as the sound field contained within an anechoic chamber, although the anechoic chamber is designed only to simulate a free sound field.) A loud-

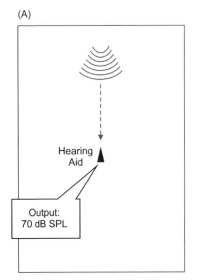

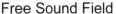

Free Sound Field

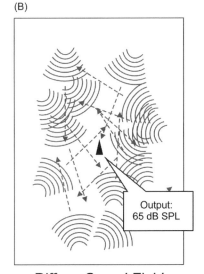

Diffuse Sound Field

Figure 6–5. The illustrations of the DI measurement. Plot A shows a free sound field. A sound of 70 dB SPL arrives at a DIR microphone hearing aid, which has a unity gain, from 0°. The output of the aid is 70 dB SPL. Plot B shows the same hearing aid in a diffuse sound field. Sounds with an overall level of 70 dB SPL propagate in all directions. If the hearing aid output is 65 dB SPL, the DI of this hearing aid would be 5 dB.

speaker is placed at 0° in both vertical and horizontal planes of the hearing aid (i.e., the on-axis position). The loudspeaker generates a sound with a level of, say 70 dB SPL, measured at the microphone port of the hearing aid. If the hearing aid has unity gain, the level of the hearing aid output responding to this on-axis signal will be 70 dB SPL.

Next, let us move the hearing aid to a diffuse sound field (Figure 6–5B). A diffuse field is a space in which the sound energy is uniformly distributed and the sound propagates in all directions with equal probability (Ghent, 2005). (The sound field created by multiple loudspeakers aimed at different directions in an enclosure may simulate a diffuse sound field.) Let's assume that sounds are generated in the diffuse field and the sound level measured at the microphone port is, again, 70 dB SPL. Note that the sounds are now arriving at the hearing aid from all directions (off-axis directions). If in this diffuse sound field the output of the hearing aid is found to be 65 dB SPL, then the DI of this hearing aid will be 5 dB (i.e., 70 minus 65). In other words, this DIR hearing aid can attenuate sound level by

5 dB if the sounds are arriving from all directions, relative to the sound with the same level arriving only from the on-axis direction. Therefore, the DI represents a device's ability to improve the SNR in a diffuse noisy environment in which speech is arriving from 0°. For an OMNI system, the on-axis response in a free field would be equal to the off-axis response in a diffuse sound field, resulting in a DI of 0 dB.

Although the DI represents a device's performance in a diffuse sound field, a sufficiently diffuse field that allows accurate directivity measurements is difficult to create. Therefore, the DI is typically obtained in an anechoic chamber. To obtain a three-dimensional DI, a stimulus signal is sequentially and systematically presented to the hearing aid from different azimuth angles of the horizontal plane and elevation angles in the anechoic chamber (Figure 6–6A). The aid's response to the signal arriving from each angle is recorded. The DI is then be derived mathematically (American National Standards Institute, 2010).

The DI can be measured in various conditions. For example, the DI can be measured

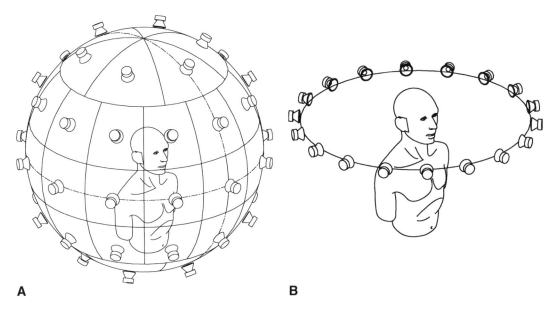

A   **B**

Figure 6–6. The illustrations of three-dimensional (**A**) and two-dimensional (**B**) DI measurements. The stimulus signal is sequentially presented from each location. (Reprinted from ANSI/ASA S3.35-2010 *American National Standard Method of Measurement of Performance Characteristics of Hearing Aids under Simulated Real-Ear Working Conditions*, 2010, with the permission of the Acoustical Society of America, 35 Pinelawn Road, Suite 114E, Melville, NY 11747.)

with the hearing aid hanging freely in space (i.e., free-field DI), or with the hearing aid placed on a manikin's ear (i.e., simulated real-ear aided DI or in situ DI). The latter is also called KEMAR DI because the measure is often performed with a Knowles Electronics Manikin for Acoustic Research (KEMAR). In addition to the three-dimensional DI, the DI can also be measured by presenting the stimulus signal on the horizontal plane only with a 0-degree elevation around the device (i.e., planar DI or two-dimensional DI; Figure 6–6B). Although the three-dimensional in situ DI measure needs a manikin, a larger space, and special equipment to move the signal source around the manikin, this DI measure has been shown to more accurately reflect the benefit that a DIR hearing aid would provide because it takes into account the asymmetric acoustic effect generated by the head and ear (Dittberner & Bentler, 2007a, 2007b). On the other hand, because of the simplicity of the planar DI measurement and because the DI data are frequently used to predict speech recognition tests in which competing noise sources are placed on the

horizontal plane relative to the listener, the planar DI is still widely used (e.g., Ricketts, 2000a; Ricketts, Henry, & Hornsby, 2005; Wu & Bentler, 2007, 2009, 2012a).

A DIR system may have different DI values across frequencies (Figure 6–7). To present the device's directivity and to predict perceptual benefit provided from the DIR system more efficiently, frequency-specific DIs are often obtained and averaged. In order to make the DI more relevant to speech perception, applying frequency-specific importance weightings to the DI values before averaging across frequencies has been suggested (Killion et al., 1998). The weightings most often used are based on the band importance function, which is used in calculating the speech intelligibility index (SII; American National Standards Institute, 1997). This weighted average DI is called the *speech-intelligibility weighted directivity index (SII-DI)* or *articulation index weighted DI (AI-DI)*. The rationale for applying weightings is that when a larger DI value (and therefore greater SNR improvement) occurs in the frequency bands that are more important for speech perception, the DIR sys-

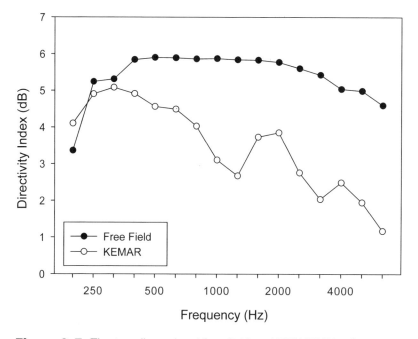

Figure 6–7. The two-dimensional free-field and KEMAR DI values as a function of frequency, obtained from a DIR system that has a hypercardioid directivity pattern (also see Figure 6–8).

tem would provide a greater improvement in speech intelligibility. Although it seems logical to apply the weighting function, Ricketts and his colleagues (Ricketts et al., 2005) found that the differences between unweighted linearly averaged DI and SII-DI were very small and that the SII-DI did not predict the score for speech recognition in noise tests more accurately than the unweighted DI. Therefore, the use of a simple average DI without weighting is suggested (American National Standards Institute, 2010): the average DI is the arithmetic mean of the DIs measured for one-third octave bands with center frequencies from 500 to 5000 Hz.

Polar Plot

To visually demonstrate the directivity pattern, a polar plot is often used. A polar plot is a graph that records the attenuation pattern of a DIR system as a function of angle of incidence. Although the plot does not give the numerical value of the directivity, it qualitatively illustrates how a DIR system responds to sounds arriving from different directions. Figure 6–8 shows several polar plots. The 0°, 90°, 180°, and 270° correspond to the hearing aid's front, right, back, and left, respectively. The center of the circle corresponds to −25 dB, and the radius of the

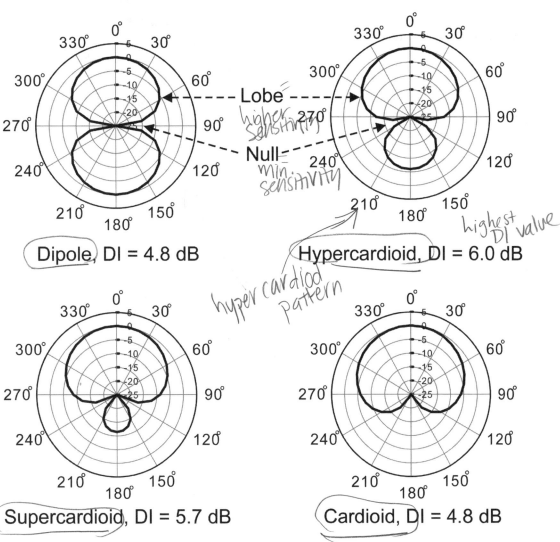

Figure 6–8. Four commonly seen two-dimensional free-field directivity patterns and their DI values.

outermost circle corresponds to +5 dB. The curve shown in the polar plot is the level of hearing aid's response to a sound arriving from a given angle referenced to that to a sound from 0°. For example, the polar plot shown in the right upper corner of Figure 6–8 (the hypercardioid pattern) indicates that the DIR system is 6 dB less sensitive for sound arriving from 180°, relative to sound arriving from 0°. In a polar plot, the area where the microphone system has higher sensitivity is often called a *lobe*, and the area with minimal sensitivity is called a *null*. The polar pattern of the OMNI system that has equal sensitivity to sounds from all directions is a circle at 0 dB.

Figure 6–8 shows four basic directivity patterns of the first-order DIR system measured with the hearing aid hanging freely in space (i.e., free-field polar patterns) and their free-field planar DI values: dipole (with null at 90° and 270°), hypercardioid (with null at 110° and 250°), supercardioid (with null at 125° and 235°), and cardioid (with null at 180°). Note that the hypercardioid pattern has the highest DI value among the directivity patterns.

Figure 6–9 shows the polar patterns of a hypercardioid and a cardioid pattern measured with the hearing aid placed on the manikin's right ear (i.e., in situ patterns). Because

of sound diffraction and reflection effect generated by the head and ear, these in situ directivity patterns are very different from the free-field patterns shown in Figure 6–8. Note that the maximum sensitivity of the DIR system is shifted from 0° in the free-field pattern to approximately 45° in the in situ pattern. Because the DI value is obtained by comparing the off-axis response to the 0° on-axis response, the fact that the on-axis angle is not the one with the highest sound sensitivity results in smaller DI values in the in situ pattern than in the free-field pattern (see the DI values in Figures 6–8 and 6–9).

Clinical Measures of Directivity

For quality control purpose, clinicians need to measure the directivity of DIR hearing aids to ensure that hearing aids meet reasonable and expected quality standards. The quality control procedures need to be completed before hearing aid fitting because newly issued DIR hearing aids may be defective upon receipt (Howell & Saunders, 2008). This process is typically known as *verification*. These quality control measures must be repeated at cer-

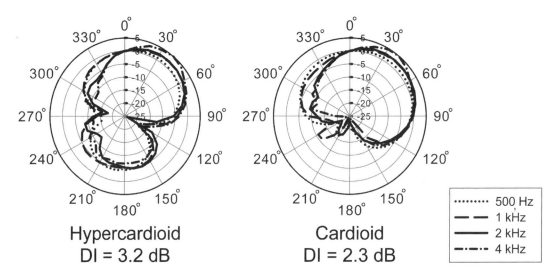

Figure 6–9. The two-dimensional KEMAR polar plots of hearing aids with a hypercardioid pattern and with a cardioid pattern. The hearing aids are placed on the right ear of the manikin.

tain points in the future since hearing aids' directivity could decline over time (American Academy of Audiology, 2006; American Speech-Language-Hearing Association, 1998).

Directivity Degradation

As mentioned previously, the directivity of the dual-microphone system is achieved by subtracting the output of one microphone from the output of another microphone. Therefore, the two microphones of the system must be matched in order to create maximum directivity. That is, the DIR system's two OMNI microphones have to be identical in amplitude and phase characteristics at all times (Csermak, 2000; Edwards, 2000; Kuk, Baekgaard, & Ludvigsen, 2000; Tchorz, 2001; Thompson, 2003). A small amplitude or phase mismatch could completely eliminate directivity or even reverse the polar pattern (i.e., the hearing aid has become more sensitive to off-axis sounds than to on-axis sounds; Kuk et al., 2000; Wu & Bentler, 2012a). The mismatch could be due to the change in amplitude or phase of the microphone that is used over time. This mismatch due to microphone aging is termed *drift*. It has been reported that the average drift is around 0.25 dB after one-year of use (Tchorz, 2001). Fortunately, the drift can be compensated by the hearing aid's automatic compensation algorithm (Chung, 2004b; Tchorz, 2001); its effect on directivity is reported to be relatively small (Csermak, 2000; Tchorz, 2001).

The mismatch created by accumulation of dirt and moisture in the acoustic pathway of the microphone system has a more serious effect on directivity. Clogged microphone ports can generate frequency-dependent change in intensity and phase, which are more difficult problems for the algorithm to correct (Chung, 2004b; Tchorz, 2001). Clogged microphone ports have been shown to have a great impact on directivity and listeners' speech recognition performance (Tchorz, 2001; Wu & Bentler, 2012a). They would affect not only the DIR system with the dual-microphone design, but also the single-cartridge design. Therefore, it is critical for clinicians to

measure and monitor the directivity of DIR hearing aids on a routine basis.

Although the DI and the polar directivity pattern are well-accepted electroacoustic measures of directivity, these measurements generally need an anechoic chamber and require special equipment such as a turntable. Therefore, the DI is not usually measured clinically. A hearing aid analyzer equipped with a small anechoic test chamber (Fonix 8000; Figure 6–10) has recently become available. This equipment enables clinicians to use the polar pattern to verify and monitor the functionality of DIR hearing aids. In addition to the polar pattern, a variety of simple directivity measures have been suggested.

Front-To-Back Ratio

The *front-to-back ratio* is the frequency-dependent ratio (in decibels) of the level of a hearing aid's response to a sound arriving at 0° azimuth (on-axis measurement) to the response to the same sound arriving at 180° azimuth (off-axis measurement). Typically the on-axis and off-axis measurements are performed sequentially; that is, the output of the hearing aid is obtained with the front-facing port aimed toward the sound source, and again with the rear-facing port aimed toward the sound source (Figure 6–11). This simple measure can be easily performed using most hearing aid analyzers or probe-microphone equipment. Unlike the DI, the front-to-back

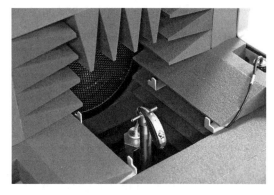

Figure 6–10. The anechoic test chamber of the Fonix 8000. Courtesy of Frye Electronics.

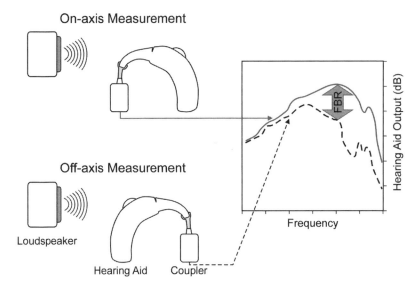

Figure 6–11. The illustrations of the front-to-back ratio (FBR) measurement. The difference in hearing aid's output frequency response curves (*gray solid and black dashed curves in the plot*) between the on-axis and off-axis measurements quantifies the front-to-back ratio (*the double arrow*).

ratio only takes into account sounds coming from two directions. Therefore, the front-to-back ratio is not recommended for comparing directivity across hearing aids (Dittberner & Bentler, 2007a). However, the front-to-back ratio can be used to monitor the directivity within a given hearing aid at periodic hearing aid checks to ensure the DIR system's functionality (Cox, 2009; Ricketts, 2000a, 2001; Ricketts & Dittberner, 2002).

The front-to-back ratio measure has many variants. For example, when evaluating a hearing aid with the polar nulls at angles other than 180°, measurement at the null angle instead of at 180° would demonstrate the maximal signal attenuation provided by the hearing aid (Ricketts, 2001). Wu and Bentler (2012a) further demonstrated that, for the cardioid and hypercardioid patterns, the front-to-back ratio measure that uses 110° in the off-axis measurement correlates to speech recognition performance better than that which uses 180° in the off-axis measurement. The front-to-back ratio measurement could also be conducted in the test chamber of a hearing aid analyzer, in a sound field with the hearing aid hanging freely in space, or on

a manikin/listener's ear using a probe-microphone system (Frye, 2006; Ricketts, 2001).

One factor that affects the front-to-back ratio is the amplitude compression algorithm. Specifically, the design of the DIR system mandates that the microphone output to the off-axis stimulus be reduced. When the on-axis and off-axis stimuli are presented sequentially, the compression algorithm, which takes the microphone output as the input, will provide larger gain in the off-axis measurement than in the on-axis measurement. As a result, the front-to-back ratio value is generally smaller for the hearing aid when in the nonlinear mode than in the linear mode. This compression effect could be problematic in monitoring directivity in a clinical setting because the front-to-back ratio value would be different if the compression ratio has been changed. Therefore, it is preferable to use either the same compression parameters or to set the hearing aid to a linear mode when using the front-to-back ratio at periodic checks (Ricketts, 2001). For the same reason, it is desirable to disable the hearing aid's adaptive features during front-to-back ratio measurement that uses sequential stimuli.

Front-To-Back Ratio Using Simultaneous Stimuli

Although the effect of amplitude compression may impact front-to-back ratio measures using sequential stimuli, certain methods can be used to derive a system's frequency response to each of the simultaneous input signals, thus bypassing the effect of compression (Bell, Creek, & Lutman, 2010; Hagerman & Olofsson, 2004; Puder, 2006; Wu & Bentler, 2007, 2009). For example, two broadband signals consisting of a series of nonoverlapping pure tones could serve as the inputs when presented to the hearing aid simultaneously from on-axis and off-axis angles, respectively. The hearing aid's response to each of the inputs can be filtered out to derive directivity (Bell et al., 2010). Because the on-axis and off-axis signals are processed simultaneously, the compression algorithm will provide the same gain to both signals and will not affect the derived directivity.

The directivity measure using simultaneous input signals has been implemented in a clinical hearing aid analyzer (Audioscan Verifit; Figure 6–12). In this hearing aid analyzer, two input signals consisting of 500 nonoverlapping pure tones, each separated by 16 Hz, are presented from the left and right loudspeakers, respectively. The difference between the two loudspeaker output response curves quantifies the front-to-back ratio.

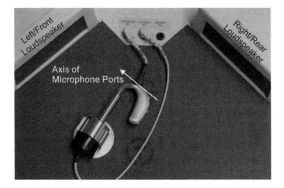

Figure 6–12. The orientation of the hearing aid relative to the left/front and right/rear loudspeakers of the Verifit that uses the simultaneous stimuli to measure microphone directivity.

PERCEPTUAL ADVANTAGES OF DIRECTIONAL MICROPHONE SYSTEMS AND RELATED FACTORS

Because DIR microphone systems are more sensitive to on-axis signals than off-axis signals, DIR processing has the potential to improve speech intelligibility in noise relative to OMNI processing when the speech of interest is on-axis and the noise is off-axis. This perceptual benefit afforded by DIR processing is typically referred to as *DIR benefit* or *DIR advantage.*

In the laboratory, DIR benefit can be quantified by comparing the listener's performance in speech recognition amid noise between the DIR mode and OMNI mode of the same hearing aid, expressed in percentage or decibels. Specifically, speech-recognition-in-noise tests are often administered using two procedures: fixed and adaptive SNR procedures. Fixed SNR procedures measure the extent that a listener can correctly recognize speech (in percentage correct point) at a given SNR. The test SNR is selected before testing and remains unchanged throughout. One widely used fixed SNR speech-in-noise test is the Connected Speech Test (CST; Cox, Alexander, & Gilmore, 1987; Cox, Alexander, Gilmore, & Pusakulich, 1988). For adaptive SNR procedures, the SNR of each trial is determined by the preceding stimuli and responses (Levitt, 1971; Plomp & Mimpen, 1979). Following a correct response, the SNR is reduced (becomes more difficult); after an incorrect response, the SNR is increased (becomes easier). This procedure is repeated several times until it is possible to estimate the SNR (in decibels) at which the listener attains a predetermined criterion performance. If a performance of 50% correct is used as the criterion, the SNR result obtained from adaptive procedures is often called SNR50. One widely used adaptive SNR test is the Hearing in Noise Test (HINT; Nilsson, Soli, & Sullivan, 1994). The DIR benefit in decibels measured by the adaptive procedure can be converted to the improvement in the percentage of correct points by multiplying the benefit value by the slope of the performance-intensity function of the speech material. A 1-dB improvement corresponds to approximately 10 percentage points of improvement (Dillon, 2001).

A large body of literature using laboratory testing has consistently shown that DIR processing provides considerable benefit relative to OMNI processing. The benefit is approximately 20 to 25 percentage points (Bentler, Egge, Tubbs, Dittberner, & Flamme, 2004; Kuk, Kollofski, Brown, Melum, & Rosenthal, 1999; Ricketts et al., 2005; Ricketts & Hornsby, 2006; Valente, 2000; Valente, Sweetow, Potts, & Bingea, 1999; Walden, Surr, Cord, Edwards, & Olson, 2000; Wu & Bentler, 2010a) or 3 to 5 dB (Amlani, 2001; Chung, 2004a). Compared with other hearing aid features such as digital noise reduction algorithms, DIR processing provides substantial benefit in speech intelligibility to the user (Boymans & Dreschler, 2000; Valente, Fabry, & Potts, 1995; Walden et al., 2000).

In addition to benefit in speech intelligibility, researchers have demonstrated hearing aid users' strong preference for DIR processing over OMNI processing for better speech clarity, better sound quality, and less noise annoyance (Amlani, Rakerd, & Punch, 2006; Boymans & Dreschler, 2000; Preves, Sammeth, & Wynne, 1999; Walden et al., 2005; Wu & Bentler, 2010a). DIR processing also increases the listener's noise acceptance. Specifically, the Acceptable Noise Level (ANL) test determines the maximum level of background noise that a listener is willing to accept while listening to running speech (Nabelek, Freyaldenhoven, Tampas, Burchfield, & Muenchen, 2006; Nabelek, Tucker, & Letowski, 1991). Research has shown that DIR processing provides approximately 3- to 5-dB benefit in ANL relative to OMNI processing (Freyaldenhoven, Nabelek, Burchfield, & Thelin, 2005; Kim & Bryan, 2011; Wu & Stangl, 2013). That is, compared with the OMNI mode, listeners are willing to accept a 3- to 5-dB lower SNR when listening to speech with the DIR mode.

The benefit afforded by DIR processing is affected by many factors. These factors are divided into three categories in this chapter: environmental factors, fitting factors, and human factors.

Environmental Factors

Speech and Noise Location

Because DIR processing is designed to maintain the on-axis sensitivity while reducing the off-axis sensitivity, DIR benefit is highly dependent on the locations of speech and noise sources. On one hand, DIR processing could improve speech understanding if speech is presented from in front of the listener, and noise is presented from behind the listener. On the other hand, DIR processing could have a detrimental effect on speech understanding in the speech-back/noise-front configuration (Chalupper, Wu, & Weber, 2011; Lee, Lau, & Sullivan, 1998; Ricketts & Picou, 2013; Wu, Stangl, & Bentler, in press). Although it is assumed that listeners will turn their heads toward the talker of interest, there are some situations in which this is not possible, such as when driving a vehicle (Chalupper et al., 2011; Wu, Stangl, Bentler, & Stanziola, 2013) or while taking notes in a classroom (Ricketts & Galster, 2008). In these cases, the listener's DIR-aided performance could be 4 to 5 dB or 20 percentage points worse than the OMNI-aided performance (Chalupper et al., 2011; Lee et al., 1998; Wu et al., in press; Wu et al., 2013).

When the speech is from in front of the listener, the number and directions of the noise sources could affect DIR benefit (Leeuw & Dreschler, 1991; Ricketts, 2000b). In general, DIR processing provides larger benefit in conditions wherein a single noise source is placed behind the listener than in conditions wherein multiple noise sources are located around the listener (e.g., diffuse noise). This is because the speech and noise sources are more spatially separated in the former configuration than in the later. Ricketts (2000b) demonstrated that the DIR benefit changed from 6 to 7 dB in the speech-0°/Noise-180° configuration to 2 to 3 dB in a configuration that consists of five noise sources around the listener. If the noise source is placed at the angle of the polar null, DIR benefit will be further maximized.

If the benefit of DIR processing is highly dependent on the speech/noise configuration, one may ask how often that speech-front/noise-back configuration occurs in the real world. Cord, Walden, and their colleagues (Cord, Walden, Surr, & Dittberner, 2007; Walden, Surr, Cord, & Dyrlund, 2004) asked hearing aid users to describe numerous acoustic characteristics of their everyday listening environments, including the talker-listener distance, the presence of noise, and the locations of the speech and noise sources. Listeners were also asked to record the time they spent in each kind of listening environment and their preference for DIR or OMNI mode in each environment. The data suggested that the environments in which DIR processing is preferred over OMNI processing (i.e., the talker is located in front of and close to the listener, and noise(s) is (are) present and located other than the front) constitute one-third to one-fourth of the total active listening time in everyday lives. These real-world data support the potential of DIR technologies to provide benefit in the real world.

Reverberation and Distance

If the sound source stops emitting sound in an enclosed space, the sound will bounce off the surfaces and persist for a while; this is called *reverberation*. Reverberation, if long and loud enough, can degrade speech intelligibility. The degree of reverberation is usually expressed in terms of reverberation time, which is measured or calculated as the time it takes for a sound pressure level to decay 60 dB from when the sound is interrupted (i.e., the *RT60*).

DIR benefit decreases as reverberation increases. This is because, in reverberant environments, the noises from sources behind a listener would bounce off the wall and arrive from in front of the listener. Similarly, speech sounds from a talker in front of the listener could arrive from behind the listener. These reflections make the speech and noise signals less spatially separated, resulting in reduced DIR benefit. Hawkins and Yacullo (1984) reported a decrease in DIR benefit from 4 dB to 0 dB as the RT60 was increased from 0.6 to 1.2 sec. Wu and Bentler (2012c) found that increasing RT60 from 0.2 to 0.7 sec resulted in a reduction of DIR benefit from 5.2 dB to 2.7 dB. These findings indicate that reverberation has a significantly detrimental effect on DIR benefit.

The effect of reverberation on DIR benefit further depends on the distance between the listener and sound sources. In a sound field, the sound emitted directly from the sound source attenuates over distance according to the inverse square law: each time the distance from the source is doubled, the level decreases by 6 dB. On the other hand, the sound level of the reflected sound (echoes) is fairly consistent over distance (Figure 6–13). The *critical distance* is the distance at which the direct and reflected sound intensity is equal. For distances shorter than the critical distance, direct-path sound dominates the sound field (i.e., the direct field). Beyond the critical distance, the reflected sound dominates the sound field (i.e., the reverberant field). Ricketts and Hornsby (2003) measured DIR benefit at different talker-listener distances and found that reverberation is less likely to reduce DIR benefit if the distance between the talker and listener is shorter than the critical distance.

SNR

DIR benefit is SNR-dependent (Lurquin & Rafhay, 1996; Walden et al., 2005; Wu & Bentler, 2010a). Walden et al. (2005) measured speech recognition performance with the DIR and OMNI modes at numerous SNRs ranging from −15 to +15 dB using a fixed SNR speech recognition test. The data are illustrated in Figure 6–14. They found that the DIR

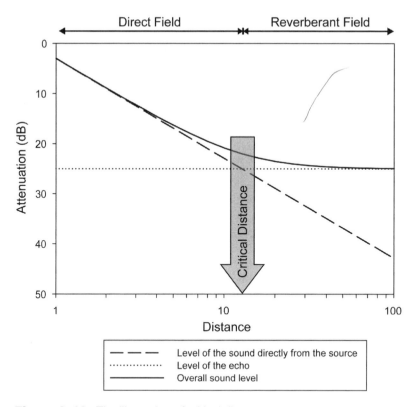

Figure 6–13. The illustration of critical distance.

benefit varied greatly across SNRs. The benefit was the largest (around 30 percentage points) when the SNR was between –6 and 0 dB. Outside this SNR range, DIR benefit decreased considerably. The reason for the reduced benefit is ceiling or floor effect. Specifically, for speech recognition performance with the DIR and OMNI modes, either mode is good when the SNR is high (too easy; ceiling effect), and neither mode is good when the SNR is low (too difficulty; floor effect). Walden et al. further demonstrated that the SNR range in which DIR processing provides the maximum benefit varies considerably across listeners: one listener may achieve maximal DIR benefit at a given SNR while another listener may only obtain minimal benefit at this SNR.

Section Summary

DIR benefit is the benefit provided by DIR processing relative to OMNI processing of

the same hearing aid. It increases as a hearing aid user positions the talker in the front and places noise sources in the rear hemisphere. It also increases as the number of competing noise sources decreases, as the talker-listener distance decreases, as the environment becomes less reverberant, and as the SNR is not too high or too low.

Fitting Factors

Hearing Aid Style

Today, DIR technologies can be implemented on hearing aids of different styles, including BTE, ITE, and ITC styles. It has been suggested that DIR processing may provide less benefit in ITE and ITC devices than the BTEs. This is because the shielding effect of the pinna could interfere with the sound field around the microphone ports of the ITE

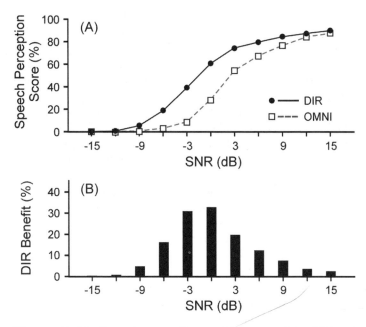

Figure 6–14. Speech recognition performance of the DIR and OMNI modes (**A**) and DIR benefit (**B**) as a function of SNR. Note that DIR benefit is small at very high and very low SNRs. Adapted and republished with permission of American Academy of Audiology, from "Effect of signal-to-noise ratio on directional microphone benefit and preference," by B. E. Walden, R. K. Surr, K. W. Grant, W. Van Summers, M. T. Cord, & O. Dyrlund, *Journal of American Academy of Audiology, 16*(9), 2005; permission conveyed through Copyright Clearance Center, Inc.

and ITC, therefore disturbing the directivity (Agnew, 1996). Data have indicated that for hearing aids with the same processing scheme, the BTE provides greater DIR benefit than the ITE (Pumford, Seewald, Scollie, & Jenstad, 2000; Ricketts, Lindley, & Henry, 2001). For example, Pumford et al. (2000) measured the DIR benefit of 24 adults using the HINT and found that the DIR benefit of the BTE (5.8 dB) was almost twice as large as the ITC (3.8 dB).

Although the BTE may provide larger DIR benefit, two reasons suggest that clinicians do not need to limit their choices to the BTE style when fitting the DIR hearing aid. First, the smaller DIR benefit from the ITE and ITC device can be compensated (augmented) by the natural directivity provided by the pinna. Specifically, the OMNI-aided performance of the ITE is better than that of the BTE because the ITE can utilize pinna directivity. With the natural directivity from the pinna plus the directivity provided by DIR processing, the listener's speech recognition in noise performance is essentially the same for DIR hearing aids with the BTE and ITE styles (Pumford et al., 2000). Second, the effect of the system design and implementation on DIR benefit is greater than that of hearing aid style. A well-designed DIR system in the ITE could provide more DIR benefit than the BTE with a poor design (Ricketts et al., 2001). It is suggested clinicians use the DI as a guideline to choose hearing aids, regardless of hearing aid style (Ricketts et al., 2001). Recent research confirms that ITE and ITC devices could provide considerable DIR benefit (Valente & Mispagel, 2004; Valente, Schuchman, Potts, & Beck, 2000; Wu & Bentler, 2010a).

Venting

A vent is any opening in an earmold or a hearing aid shell that allows air to move in and out of the ear canal. It provides a leakage path for the hearing aid user's own voices, which can be trapped in the ear canal, thus reducing the occlusion effect. The vent also allows sounds below approximately 1 kHz (depending on the vent size) to bypass the hearing aid and arrive at the eardrum. Because hearing aids typically provide smaller gain at low frequencies relative to high frequencies, the vent-transmitted sound usually dominates the low-frequency bands while the hearing aid-processed sound dominates mid- to high-frequency bands. Because the vent-transmitted sounds are not processed by the hearing aid, DIR processing provides less benefit in the low-frequency bands. In general, DIR benefit decreases as the vent size increases. Ricketts (2000a) demonstrated that the AI-DI values are decreased by 1.6 dB from closed earmold to open earmold venting conditions. Kuk, Keenan, and Ludvigsen (2004) also demonstrated a significant negative correlation between vent size and DIR benefit.

Although the DIR benefit decreases as vent size increases, the directivity of DIR hearing aids with vented earmolds is still better than that of OMNI hearing aids. It has been shown that the AI-DI value of hearing aids with open earmolds was greater than that of the aids in the OMNI mode by 4 dB (Ricketts, 2000a). The fact that directivity is still preserved in the aid with open earmolds forms the rationale for using DIR technologies on open-fit hearing aids, which are often preferred to eliminate the occlusion effect. Using an eight loudspeaker sound-field system that reproduces the real-world restaurant sound field in the laboratory, Valente and Mispagel (2008) tested 26 adults and found a 2-dB DIR benefit of open-fit hearing aids relative to OMNI hearing aids. Similarly, Klemp and Dhar (2008) examined listener's speech recognition performance in a diffuse noise sound field and found that the open-fit hearing aids provided a benefit of 2.6 dB

relative to unaided conditions. These findings indicate that although the magnitude of DIR benefit is somewhat smaller than that of hearing aids with closed earmolds, clinicians should not exclude the use of DIR processing in open-fit devices.

As the smaller DIR benefit for hearing aids with vented earmolds is due to vent-transmitted sounds dominating the low-frequency bands, one may ask if DIR benefit could be increased by boosting the low-frequency gain of the hearing aid so that the hearing aid-processed sound could dominate the low-frequency region. This approach has been evaluated in a study by setting the hearing aid gain at low frequencies (250 and 500 Hz) to different levels (Keidser, Carter, Chalupper, & Dillon, 2007). The results indicated that the two settings in which the hearing aid gains were increased to dominate the low-frequency region were not preferred over the setting in which the gain was not increased, regardless of microphone modes (DIR and OMNI). In addition, the amount of low-frequency gain does not have a significant effect on the performance of speech recognition and sound localization, suggesting that the contribution of the low-frequency bands on directivity is limited. Therefore, it is not necessary for clinicians to increase the low-frequency gain in order to maximize DIR benefit.

Low-Frequency Roll-Off

As mentioned previously, the directivity of most DIR hearing aids is achieved by signal subtraction. Note that the subtraction processing occurs for both off-axis signals and, to a lesser degree, on-axis signals. Because part of the on-axis signals will be subtracted out, the gain and output of the DIR hearing aid for the on-axis sound is typically lower relative to the OMNI counterpart (Figure 6–15). The decrease in gain is more significant at lower frequencies because the phases of low-frequency signals are more similar at the two microphone ports. For the same reason, a shorter distance between two microphone ports (e.g., the ITE and ITC devices) causes

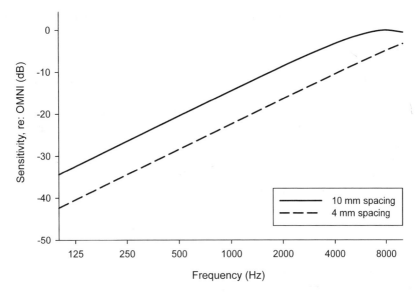

Figure 6–15. Low-frequency roll-off of the DIR system. The figure illustrates the microphone sensitivity of two DIR systems (10 mm and 4 mm microphone port spacing), relative to the sensitivity of an OMNI microphone system. Courtesy of Stephen C. Thompson.

more gain reduction. The low-frequency roll-off can be as high as 20 dB at 1 kHz (Chung, 2004b; Kates, 2008; Thompson, 2002, 2003).

Of concern with DIR processing is the fact that the inherent low-frequency roll-off may reduce the audibility of speech. In order to compensate for the gain reduction, modern hearing aids provide the option to boost the low-frequency gain of the DIR mode so that the gain of the DIR and OMNI modes can be equalized. For DIR hearing aid users with little or no hearing loss at low frequencies, compensating the low-frequency gain may not be necessary. In fact, these listeners may dislike the gain compensation because the increased amplification could make the internal electronic noise of the hearing aid audible.

In contrast, for listeners with moderate or more severe hearing loss in the low-frequency region, the loss of gain in the DIR mode would have a more detrimental effect on audibility of on-axis speech (Freyaldenhoven, Plyler, Thelin, Nabelek, & Burchfield, 2006; Ricketts & Henry, 2002b). As the increased internal noise associated with

low-frequency gain compensation may not be heard by these listeners, gain compensation is generally recommended. It has been suggested that gain compensation should be applied for people with low-frequency hearing loss worse than 40 to 55 dB HL (Freyaldenhoven et al., 2006; Ricketts & Henry, 2002b).

Microphone Port Orientation

Typically, DIR processing is optimized for signals arriving from 0° both in horizon and vertical planes, which is assumed to be the direction of the signal of interest. In order to maximize the DIR benefit, audiologists need to ensure that the axis of microphone ports is on the horizontal plane when the participant's head is comfortably facing forward. (The left or right direction of the microphone axis is generally not adjustable.) Data have shown that if the axis of the BTE is deviated from 0° vertically more than 20°, the AI-DI could decrease by as much as 2.2 dB relative to the optimal orientation (Ricketts, 2000a). The largest directivity reduction occurs when the hearing aid is pointed toward the sky. This is because the microphone ports of the BTE are more shielded by the pinna in this orientation, which could disturb the directivity. Therefore, it is important for clinicians to select the appropriate length of the earmold tube, slim tube, or receiver wire in order to place the microphone port axis on the horizontal plane. Clinicians also need to mark the horizontal line on earmold impressions of ITE/ITCs, so that manufacturers can orient the microphone ports appropriately.

Directivity Pattern

As discussed previously, there are several classical directivity patterns (see Figure 6–8), each of which has a different DI value. If the hearing aid can be programmed only to one directivity pattern, it seems that the hypercardioid and cardioid patterns are reasonable choices because the former has the highest DI values while the latter is the least sensitive behind the listener. Bentler et al. (2004) measured the speech recognition performance and preference of three different polar patterns (cardioid, hypercardioid, and supercardioid) in a diffuse sound field created by eight loudspeakers. They found that the performance of and the preference for the three patterns did not differ significantly from each other. Amlani et al. (2006) measured the speech-clarity judgments of two patterns (cardioid and hypercardioid) in a sound field created using three noise loudspeakers located behind the listener. These investigators found that the clarity judgments were the same for the two directivity patterns across three environments (a sound-treated booth, a simulated living room, and a classroom) and across listeners with different degrees of hearing loss and hearing aid experience. Although the DI value varies across directivity patterns, it seems that the subtle difference among patterns would not considerably affect the DIR benefit and would not be perceived by the listener. Most hearing aids on the market today use either hypercardioid or cardioid patterns as the default directivity pattern.

Adaptive and Automatic Features

Although studies have shown that the listener's performance with and preference for different directivity patterns do not differ significantly, these studies were conducted in sound fields with diffuse or semidiffuse noise. In some special noise configurations, however, one directivity pattern could be better than the other. For example, in an environment with a single noise source located to the listener's side, a dipole pattern would provide better noise attenuation than a super- or hypercardioid pattern. For a single noise presented from behind the listener, a cardioid pattern would be the best (Figure 6–16). Therefore, it could be beneficial if the DIR system can automatically change its directivity pattern according to the location of the noise source.

The idea of automaticity can be expanded to include a simple toggle between DIR and OMNI modes. Specifically, although DIR processing could improve SNR in some noisy environments, full-time use of the DIR microphone is generally not recommended. For example, DIR processing would have a detrimental effect on speech intelligibility when the talker of interest is behind the listener. Field-trial data have confirmed that most listeners prefer being able to switch microphone modes to full-time DIR use (Ricketts, Henry, & Gnewikow, 2003). However, although most modern hearing aids allow users to manually switch between the OMNI and DIR modes, data indicate that approximately one-third of hearing aid users do not switch between microphone modes in their everyday lives regardless of the listening environment, and generally leave the microphone set to the default OMNI mode (Cord, Surr, Walden, & Olson, 2002). The reasons include inability to tell the difference between microphone modes, poor hand dexterity, forgetfulness, and not knowing when or how to switch. Therefore, it would be beneficial if the hearing aid could analyze the characteristics of environments and automatically switch to the appropriate microphone mode.

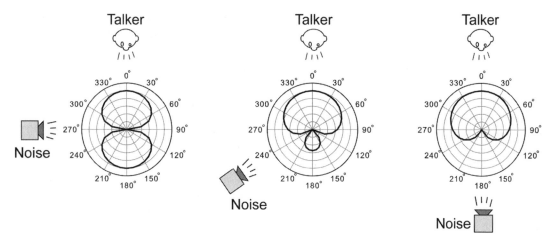

Figure 6–16. The ideal free-field directivity patterns for different noise locations.

In recent years, the automaticity feature of directivity pattern and microphone mode has been implemented in digital hearing aids. Although different terminology is used, in audiological literature, a DIR system that can steer the null of the directivity pattern to the direction of the noise source is typically called an *adaptive* DIR system (e.g., Bentler, Tubbs, Egge, Flamme, & Dittberner, 2004). A system that can automatically switch between OMNI and DIR modes is called an *automatic* system (e.g., Olson, Ioannou, & Trine, 2004). A *fully adaptive system* is sometimes used to indicate a system that has both adaptive and automatic features (e.g., Kuk, Keenan, Lau, & Ludvigsen, 2005).

Adaptive DIR systems can be constructed in many ways. The simplest algorithm uses the output of the microphone system to control the internal delay. The objective of the algorithm is to select an internal delay value that produces the highest degree of noise attenuation or the highest SNR (Kates, 2008). Adaptivity can also be achieved in different frequency bands. This multichannel directivity could be helpful if noises with different frequencies are located at different angles. Note that because adaptive directivity is achieved by changing the parameters such as the internal delay, it can only be implemented on digital DIR systems that use two or more microphones.

The automatic DIR system uses several approaches. The simplest one is based on the overall sound level. The system switches to the DIR mode when the overall sound level is higher than a certain level. A more sophisticated approach uses acoustic scene analyses. For example, hearing aid algorithms may extract the temporal and spectral features of the sound to identify whether the speech and/or noise are present and then estimate the SNR, the location of speech/noise, and the distance between the listener and speech/noise. Based on the acoustic information and some decision rules, the algorithms categorize the listening environment (e.g., speech in quiet, speech in noise, noise only) and then select the best microphone mode. More advanced algorithms have been under development. For example, a recently developed algorithm can estimate the internal representation of the signal in the auditory system or brain and use this information to select the appropriate microphone mode (Grant et al., 2008; Summers et al., 2008).

Although the adaptive/automatic DIR system is theoretically beneficial, the research data reveal mixed results. Several laboratory studies supported the advantage of the adaptive/automatic DIR system over the fixed DIR system (Bentler, Palmer, et al., 2004; Bentler et al., 2006; Blamey, Fiket, & Steele, 2006; Kuk et al., 2005; Ricketts & Henry, 2002a). In general, the advantage is the largest in conditions wherein a single noise source is located outside the polar null of the fixed directivity or in conditions wherein the noise moves. For example, for a single noise source located at 180°, the adaptive system provides 2 dB more advantage than the fixed supercardioid pattern (Blamey et al., 2006). The benefit of the adaptive system decreases when multiple noises exist (Bentler, Tubbs, et al., 2004).

Compared with laboratory data, field data do not overwhelmingly support the advantage of the adaptive/automatic DIR system. Specifically, although Olson et al. (2004) found that the automatic DIR system could pick the correct microphone modes 89% of the time in the real world, in another study 25% of the listeners indicated that the microphone mode was switched either too often or too seldom (Fabry, 2006). Palmer, Bentler, and Meuller (2006) reported that, after trying three microphone systems (OMNI, automatic-adaptive DIR, and automatic-fixed DIR) for 10 days, roughly one-third of the listeners preferred the adaptive or automatic DIR system, while one-third preferred the OMNI mode and one-third could not tell the difference. Bentler, Tubbs et al. (2004) likewise found that listeners did not report any advantages of the adaptive DIR system relative to the fixed cardioid DIR system after two 3-week trials.

It has been suggested that the characteristics of the reverberation and noise configuration in the real world may limit the benefit of the adaptive DIR system over the fixed DIR system (Woods, Merks, Zhang, Fitz, & Edwards, 2010). That is, unlike the single- or moving-noise configurations used in the sound-treated booth or anechoic chamber to demonstrate the difference between the adaptive and fixed DIR systems, most real-world noisy environments are close to a diffuse or semi-diffuse sound field, in which the performances of the two systems are very close. By analyzing the sounds recorded by hearing aids from a variety of everyday environments, these investigators demonstrated that, for more than 95% of the listening time, the benefit of the adaptive system relative to the fixed DIR system is less than 1.2 dB.

Although the benefit is small, one could argue that the adaptive system is still valuable because the SNR improvement afforded by this system is never less than that afforded by the fixed DIR system. However, the benefit of the adaptive DIR system does not come without a cost. For example, the adaptive DIR system could distort the sound localization cues and compromise the localization performance (see the section *Poorer Sound Localization Performance*). Currently, the adaptive and automatic DIR features are available for most modern hearing aids on the market. For clinicians, it seems appropriate to fit DIR hearing aids that implement the adaptive/automatic function, especially on adults who cannot correctly switch the microphone modes. However, clinicians need to bear in mind the limited perceivable benefit and potential disadvantages of the adaptive/automatic DIR system.

Asymmetric Microphone Fitting

Asymmetric microphone fitting, wherein the OMNI mode is used in one ear and the DIR mode in the other, has been suggested as an alternative to resolve the problem that many listeners never switch their microphone modes. Bentler, Egge, et al. (2004) first investigated listeners' performance in the asymmetric fitting. They tested listeners in a diffuse sound field created by presenting diffuse noises from eight loudspeakers. The results showed no significant difference between the asymmetric fitting and the conventional symmetric fitting that set both hearing aids to the DIR mode. It is postulated that in the asymmetric fitting, listeners utilize the information from the ear with better SNR (i.e., the one with the DIR mode) to achieve better performance (e.g., "better ear listening"). Cord et al. (2007) examined 12 listeners' speech recognition performance in the configuration in which the noise sources were placed at 90°, 180°, and 270°. They found that the performance of the asymmetric fitting was slightly lower than that of the bilateral DIR fitting (less than 10 percentage points). However, the difference was not statistically significant.

In contrast, Hornsby and Ricketts (2007) demonstrated that, in a speech-front/noise-diffuse configuration, the performance of the asymmetric fitting was significantly worse than bilateral DIR fitting by 1.5 dB. Similar results have been replicated on school-age children in simulated classroom environments (Ricketts & Picou, 2013). Therefore, it seems that the speech recognition performance of the asymmetric fitting is equal to the bilateral DIR fitting or somewhere between the bilateral OMNI and DIR fittings.

The use of asymmetric microphone fitting is supported by field data. In Cord et al. (2007), listeners were asked to compare bilateral OMNI and asymmetric fittings (DIR + OMNI) in the field for 4 to 6 weeks. The listeners reported that in the environments in which the DIR mode is typically preferred (e.g., speech is close and in front of the listener and noise is not at the listener's front), the rating of ease of listening for the asymmetric fitting is higher than that for the bilateral OMNI fitting. In the environments in which the OMNI mode is typically preferred, the ease of listening rating was the same for the two types of fitting, indicating that the asymmetric fitting did not have a detrimental effect in these environments. These data suggest the feasibility of the asymmetric fitting because at least one of the two hearing aids is in the preferred microphone mode regardless of the listening situation.

In summary, the asymmetric fitting seems a reasonable fitting strategy for listeners who cannot appropriately switch microphone modes. This asymmetric fitting strategy has been incorporated into the fitting software of one manufacturer as a fitting option. However, clinicians should note that, like adaptive directivity, the asymmetric fitting could decrease sound localization performance. This issue will be addressed in the section Poorer Sound Localization Performance.

Section Summary

DIR benefit is negatively affected by large venting and poor microphone port orientation, but less impacted by the choice of hearing aid style and directivity pattern in diffuse noisy environments. The low-frequency gain of DIR processing is lower than OMNI processing and should be compensated for in listeners with a low-frequency hearing loss more than 40 to 55 dB HL. The use of adaptive DIR system could increase the SNR improvement in certain environments, although the improvement in the real world is generally small. For listeners who do not or cannot switch the microphone mode, the use of automatic DIR system and the asymmetric fitting strategy could be beneficial.

Human Factors

Hearing Loss

Listeners with greater hearing loss are generally less able to make use of speech information (e.g., Hogan & Turner, 1998). To investigate if listeners with severe or profound hearing loss could utilize the SNR improvement provided by DIR processing, researchers (Kuhnel, Margolf-Hackl, & Kiessling, 2001) measured the DIR benefit for listeners with hearing loss of 80 to 100 dB HL. In a speech-0°/noise-180° configuration, they found a mean DIR benefit value of 13.7 dB. This large benefit would be expected for a cardioid pattern using the speech-0°/noise-180° configuration. Of interest was that listeners with severe-to-profound hearing loss realized the same benefit as would be expected with a milder loss.

Ricketts and Hornsby (2006) investigated the benefit provided by DIR hearing aids for 20 listeners with 70 to 80 dB HL hearing loss in a moderately reverberant room, wherein speech was presented from 0° and noises were presented from five loudspeakers surrounding the listeners. In contrast with the 13.7 dB-benefit demonstrated by Kuhnel et al. (2001), Ricketts and Hornsby (2006) found that DIR benefit was somewhat small: 5 to 14 percentage points. In another study, Ricketts et al. (2005) measured the DIR benefit for three groups of listeners with different degrees of hearing loss: two groups had mild-to-moderate hearing loss and one group had a hearing loss around 70 dB HL. The former two groups achieved a DIR benefit of around 30 percentage points, while the latter group had only half that amount. These findings suggest that DIR processing provides significant but smaller benefit for listeners with severe hearing loss.

Children

Because children need a better SNR to achieve equivalent speech recognition performance in noise to that of adults (Fallon, Trehub, & Schneider, 2000, 2002) and because the environments in which children acquire knowledge and develop communication skills (e.g., the classroom) can be very noisy (Crandell, 1993; Finitzo-Hieber & Tillman, 1978), fitting hearing aids with DIR technologies on children with hearing loss seems a logical option.

Early data from laboratory experiments support the use of DIR technologies on school-aged children. Kuk et al. (1999) tested 12 children from 7 to 13 years old with mild to moderately severe hearing loss in the speech-0°/noise-180° configuration and found the DIR benefit of from 8 to 19 percentage points. They also found that the degree of hearing loss did not have an effect on the DIR benefits. In another study, researchers (Gravel, Fausel, Liskow, & Chobot, 1999) tested 20 children from 4 to 11 years of age with mild to moderately severe hearing loss in the same speech/noise configuration and found that DIR processing provided a benefit of 4.7 dB over OMNI aided listening.

Recall that the benefit from DIR processing is based on the assumption that listeners can orient their heads toward the talker of interest. Ricketts and Galster (2008) examined whether this assumption holds true in school-age children, by videotaping the head movement of 40 students from 4 to 17 years of age, with and without hearing loss, in school environments. The results revealed that, although children are not always able to—or want to—turn their heads toward the talker of interest, they generally orient their heads with relatively high accuracy. For the 33% of

the time in which the children achieved the highest degree of accuracy, the average error was approximately 15°. These results suggest that children could obtain DIR benefit in the real-world classroom environments.

Using a simulated classroom environment, Ricketts and Galster (2007) examined speech recognition performance for the DIR and OMNI microphone modes in a group of 26 children aged 10 to 17 years in a variety of speech/noise configurations. These researchers observed a significant DIR benefit of 3 dB when the sound source of interest was in the front. However, DIR processing was found to have a detrimental effect on speech recognition performance (around 2 dB) when the sound source of interest was behind the participants. Using a similar methodology, Ching et al. (2009) examined the head orientation of a group of 11 to 78 month old children, with and without hearing loss, in natural environments. The data revealed that more than 40% of the time, children were able to turn their heads toward the primary talkers. The SNR improvement provided by DIR processing was quantified using the Speech Transmission Index (Steeneken & Houtgast, 1980) measure. The data revealed that the DIR benefit is up to 3 dB when the talker is in front of the listener, and −3 dB (i.e., DIR processing is harmful) when the talker is sideways or behind the children. Interesting, the average overall DIR benefit, which was calculated by averaging the time-weighted SNR improvement in each configuration of talker position, was close to 0 dB (no effect) in this study.

These data provide limited support for the use of DIR hearing aids in children. That is, if the primary talkers of interest are mostly located in front of the children or if the microphone mode can be switched to the appropriate mode, either manually or automatically, children with hearing loss could benefit from DIR hearing aids. However, this prerequisite is not always possible. Furthermore, because DIR technologies could have a detrimental effect on incidental learning and warning-sound detection, clinicians need to be very cautious when fitting DIR hearing aids to children with hearing loss.

Older Adults

Compared with younger adults, elderly listeners face greater hearing challenges in noisy environments because they often exhibit poorer speech perception performance in such settings than do younger listeners. This diminished ability is presumed to involve factors ranging from age-related changes in peripheral hearing sensitivity (Humes et al., 1994; Murphy, Daneman, & Schneider, 2006; Schneider, Daneman, Murphy, & KwongSee, 2000), auditory temporal resolution (Fitzgibbons & Gordon-Salant, 1996; Snell, Mapes, Hickman, & Frisina, 2002; Souza & Boike, 2006), and central cognitive abilities (Lunner & Sundewall-Thoren, 2007; Pichora-Fuller, Schneider, & Daneman, 1995; Tun, O'Kane, & Wingfield, 2002). Therefore, fitting DIR hearing aids to older hearing-impaired adults is regarded as a reasonable intervention (Kricos, 2006).

To investigate if the elderly could benefit from DIR processing, Wu (2010) tested a group of 12 older listeners (over 65 years) and a group of 12 younger listeners both in the laboratory and the field. The laboratory results revealed that both younger and older listeners obtained similar DIR benefit and showed similar preference for DIR processing over OMNI processing. However, the field data revealed that older age was significantly associated with a lower preference for the DIR mode, indicating that older users tend to perceive less benefit in the real world than younger users do.

Several reasons may explain why the older listeners perceive less benefit of DIR processing in their everyday lives. First, it has been shown that (older) listeners with reduced cognitive function (e.g., working memory capacity) are less able to detect the differences between hearing aid technologies in real-world complex environments (Lunner, 2003). Second, because older adults generally have social lifestyles that place fewer demands on hearing (i.e., they encounter fewer noisy or loud environments; Wu & Bentler, 2012b), older adults may not obtain DIR benefit very often in their daily environments. Finally, for manually switched DIR hearing aids, Souza (2004) suggests that older listeners may obtain less benefit from DIR processing because of their inability to recognize environments in which switching to the DIR mode might result in the greatest advantage.

Visual Cues

The reader may have noticed that, in this chapter, most cited evidence that supports the benefit of DIR technologies was obtained from studies conducted in contrived laboratory environments. Does DIR processing provide benefit relative to OMNI processing in the real world? Numerous field studies have been conducted to answer this question. Among these studies, some have supported the benefit of the DIR hearing aids (Keidser et al., 2007; Preves et al., 1999; Ricketts et al., 2003). However, more studies were not able to demonstrate the evidence of DIR benefit in the real world (Cord, Surr, Walden, & Dyrlund, 2004; Cord et al., 2002; Gnewikow, Ricketts, Bratt, & Mutchler, 2009; Palmer et al., 2006; Surr, Walden, Cord, & Olson, 2002; Walden et al., 2000; Wu & Bentler, 2010b). For example, in a large scale double-blind study (Gnewikow et al., 2009), 94 hearing aid users were tested in both the laboratory and the real world. The laboratory speech recognition tests indicated that listeners' aided performance with the DIR mode was better than that with the OMNI mode by 2 to 4 dB. However, these listeners did not report a clear advantage of the DIR mode over the OMNI mode, as measured by two self-report questionnaires (Profile of Hearing Aid Benefit [Cox & Rivera, 1992] and Satisfaction with Amplification in Daily Life [Cox & Alexander, 1999]) after using each microphone mode for one month in the real world.

There are many reasons that may explain why DIR benefit has been rarely observed in field studies. One of them is that most self-report questionnaires do not have sufficient sensitivity to detect DIR benefit that is highly dependent on listening situation (Ricketts et al., 2003). For example, DIR processing could improve speech understanding when speech is from in front of the listener, while having a detrimental effect when speech is from the back. Now let's take a look at a situation described in the questionnaire Abbreviated Profile of Hearing Aid Benefit (Cox & Alexander, 1995). "When I am in a crowded grocery store, talking with the cashier, I can follow the conversation." Because the locations of the speech and noises are not specified, DIR processing actually could have a positive, neutral, or even negative effect on speech understanding in this listening situation. If a listener is asked to report his or her average perception in this kind of listening situation using this questionnaire, it is very likely that this listener would report no clear DIR benefit.

Because DIR benefit is highly dependent on the listening situation, laboratory data will not be consistent with real-world results if laboratory testing does not include all factors that could impact DIR benefit. One factor that is common in the real world, but suspiciously absent in many laboratory studies, is visual cues (lipreading). Specifically, in most noisy situations where DIR processing can work effectively (i.e., the talker is in front of and close to the listener), visual cues are almost always available. By utilizing visual cues, the level of a listener's speech recognition performance can increase substantially (Erber, 1969; Hawkins, Montgomery, Mueller, & Sedge, 1988; MacLeod & Summerfield, 1987; Sumby & Pollack, 1954). Now imagine a hearing aid user is in a noisy restaurant. This listener wishes to take advantage of DIR processing, so he sits in front of his friend. Because this listener wants to know to what extent DIR processing could help him, he switches between DIR and OMNI modes during the conversation. Chances are that he will find out that his speech understanding is not very different between the two microphone modes. This is because, with the help of visual cues, the listener's speech understanding with the OMNI mode have already approached his inherent limitation of the speech recognition ability (ceiling). In this case, the listener will not perceive much DIR benefit when switching from OMNI to DIR

mode. Note that this listener may still have a lot of difficulty in this face-to-face conversation because his ceiling performance may not be 100% correct, but rather his maximum attainable performance.

Wu and Bentler (2010a, 2010b) tested 24 adults for the effect of visual cues on DIR benefit. The speech recognition data revealed that listeners obtained significantly less DIR benefit in the audiovisual condition than the auditory-only condition at most SNRs. For SNRs higher than −2 dB, the DIR benefit never exceeded 10 percentage points in audiovisual listening. More importantly, the optimal SNR for DIR benefit in audiovisual listening was below (poorer than) −6 dB, which is not commonly experienced in everyday listening situations. Therefore, although DIR technologies still provide benefit in the real-world audiovisual listening, the benefit is much smaller than what is observed in most auditory-only laboratory testing.

Section Summary

Although DIR hearing aids provide significant benefit to listeners of different ages with varying degree of hearing loss, the benefit decreases as age and hearing loss increase. Children with hearing impairment obtain benefit from DIR processing, but the benefit is available only when children can turn their heads toward the talker of interest (this is also true for adults). While the laboratory data suggest that DIR processing provides considerable benefit, field data rarely show this magnitude of benefit. The availability of visual cues is one reason for this discrepancy as visual cues can increase the performance in the OMNI mode and subsequently reduce DIR benefit.

PERCEPTUAL DISADVANTAGES OF DIRECTIONAL MICROPHONE SYSTEMS

Although DIR processing can improve the performance for speech recognition in noise relative to OMNI processing in certain environments, this benefit is not provided without a cost.

Disadvantages of DIR

Lower Output Level

For several reasons, the DIR system often has a lower output than the OMNI system. First, DIR processing decreases the noise level (and thus improves the SNR). Second, the uncompensated low-frequency roll-off of the DIR mode decreases the level of the on-axis speech. Third, even though the low-frequency roll-off of the DIR system can be compensated to equalize the level of on-axis speech, the speech level in the output of the OMNI mode is still higher than that of the DIR mode because the reflected speech sounds (echoes) that arrive at off-axis angles will be picked up only by the OMNI mode.

The lower speech output level of DIR processing could have a negative impact on speech audibility. The lower output of the off-axis sound in the DIR mode could also have a negative effect because listeners may not want to omit any information from off-axis sounds in the real world. In a study conducted by Smeds et al. (2006), listeners were asked to adjust the volume control of the hearing aid to their preferred level. These investigators found that many listeners made nonspeech sounds very soft in the laboratory, while not doing so in the field. It is speculated that the listeners did not want to miss important soft sounds in the real world. If listeners tend to obtain information from all sounds (including "noises") in the real world and if DIR processing provides only a limited benefit in speech perception (e.g., because of visual cues), listeners may prefer the OMNI mode that has louder (speech and noise) sounds. In fact, instead of detecting an improved SNR in the DIR mode, listeners may believe that DIR processing results in poorer performance because it reduces the sound levels too much. In the field trial, Wu and Bentler (2010b) found that listeners more frequently preferred the OMNI mode than the DIR mode even when the speech/noise configuration favored the DIR mode.

The reported reason that was most associated with the preference for the OMNI was the louder sound in the OMNI mode. It is likely that the louder speech sound in the OMNI mode made listeners believe that speech was more intelligible or clearer in this mode. Therefore, it could be beneficial for clinicians to set the volume of the DIR mode to a higher level, although the higher volume will not change the SNR.

Higher Internal Noise Level

The gain of the DIR mode is inherently lower than the OMNI mode in low-frequency bands (i.e., the low-frequency roll-off). The lower gain in the DIR mode can be compensated electronically. Unfortunately, increasing gain inevitably results in higher internal electrical noise of the microphone system. A well-designed microphone has an equivalent noise level of as low as 25 dB SPL (Kates, 2008). Therefore, if a 20-dB gain is added at low frequencies, the internal noise could be audible by hearing-impaired people in quiet environments. Listeners may report hearing a hissing sound like static or a waterfall. The internal noise will be more problematic in smaller style hearing aids because the low-frequency roll-off is more severe due to the shorter distance between the microphone ports.

It has been argued that the internal noise is not typically a problem because it cannot be heard by hearing aid users in noisy environments, where the DIR mode is supposed to be employed (Kuk et al., 2000). However, many listeners in the field study by Wu and Bentler (2010b) reported the audible internal noise in the DIR mode even in noisy environments. These investigators also demonstrated that the audible internal noise is an important factor resulting in the low preference for the DIR mode in the real world.

Higher Wind Noise Level

When wind passes by the pinna or hearing aid, turbulence in the air flow is created. The hearing aid microphone converts these pressure fluctuations to electrical or digital signals and generates a howling wind noise. Wind noise increases with increases in wind speed and depends on the directions of the wind relative to the head (Thompson, 2002, 2003). Wind noise has a broad spectrum with a low-frequency emphasis. Hearing aid users are more prone to wind noise than people without hearing aids because the hearing aid microphone is not shielded by the pinna and ear canal.

The DIR system generates louder wind noises than the OMNI system. This is because the eddy created by the wind could be treated as a sound source close to the DIR system and the DIR system has a higher sensitivity to the sound source close to the microphone ports (i.e., within 10–20 cm), especially at low frequencies (Thompson, 2002). The wind noise generated by the DIR system is about 20 dB higher than that by the OMNI counterpart. Wind noise will be more problematic if gain is boosted to compensate the low-frequency roll-off inherent in the DIR mode.

Several approaches have been used to resolve the problem of the wind noise. For example, many modern hearing aids have algorithms to detect wind noise. Once the wind noise has been detected, the gain of the low-frequency bands is reduced or the microphone mode is automatically switched to the OMNI mode. Another approach is using the multichannel directivity. That is, the directivity of the low frequency bands can be fixed

in the OMNI mode or automatically switched to the OMNI mode once wind noise is generated. Setting the low-frequency bands to the OMNI mode is also helpful in resolving the problem of the internal noise because gain compensation is no longer necessary. The third way to reduce the level of the wind noise is changing the listener's position relative to the wind. In general, if the listener can orient himself so that the hearing aid faces the direction of the wind or is hidden behind the head (Figure 6–17), the interference from wind noise could be reduced (Chung, McKibben, & Mongeau, 2010; Chung, Mongeau, & McKibben, 2009).

Poorer Sound Localization Performance

Correctly recognizing the direction and location of a sound source is important to communication. For example, the listener needs to localize the direction of warning sounds while walking or driving.

The use of hearing aids could degrade sound localization performance (Van den Bogaert, Klasen, Moonen, Van Duen, & Wouters, 2006) because the location of the microphone and inadequate high-frequency amplification can distort the localization cues. Adaptive DIR systems or asymmetric microphone fittings could further corrupt the localization cues (Keidser et al., 2006; Van den Bogaert,

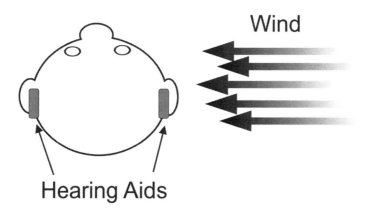

Figure 6–17. The orientation of the listener's head relative to the wind that can reduce the wind noise.

Doclo, Wouters, & Moonen, 2008; Van den Bogaert et al., 2006). This is because the sounds arrive at the two ears with different levels, spectra, and SNRs will be processed differently by the algorithms of the two hearing aids. Van den Bogaert et al. (2006) measured the sound localization performance of bilateral BTE hearing aid users using a 13-loudspeaker array located in the frontal horizontal plane. These investigators found that localization performance in the unaided condition was better than the OMNI-aided condition, which in turn was better than the condition with the adaptive DIR-aided condition. Keidser et al. (2006) tested listeners' localization performance with bilateral BTEs using a 360° speaker array and found that, relative to linear amplification, the amplitude compression and noise reduction algorithms did not have a clinically significant effect on horizontal localization performance. However, asymmetric microphone fitting (fixed cardioid + OMNI, and fixed cardioid + fixed dipole) significantly decreased the localization performance. These findings suggest that clinicians should be aware of the possible disadvantages in localization performance when fitting adaptive DIR hearing aids or using the asymmetric fitting strategy.

Interestingly, a DIR system that has directivity only in high-frequency bands could be used to restore the high-frequency spectra cues and improve localization, often called the "digital pinna effect" (Chalupper, O'Brien, & Hain, 2009). Keidser and her colleagues (Keidser, O'Brien, Hain, McLelland, & Yeend, 2009) found that for stimuli with mid- to high-frequency emphasis, this frequency-dependent directivity could improve localization performance relative to the full-band directivity. However, the field trial of the same study did not reveal significant difference in localization performance reported among OMNI, full-band DIR, and the high-frequency directivity.

CHAPTER SUMMARY

Research data indicate improvements in the speech understanding of listeners with hearing impairment in certain noisy situations by DIR technologies. To obtain the maximum DIR benefit, clinicians need to instruct hearing aid users to choose and arrange appropriate speech/noise configurations. It is equally important for clinicians to consult the listeners regarding the factors that impact DIR benefit and the perceptual disadvantages of DIR technologies.

Today, many new signal processing schemes are being developed to enhance the benefit of DIR technologies. Such schemes include integrating digital noise reduction algorithms to DIR processing to achieve maximum noise attenuation, and using a speech detection algorithm to identify speech location so that the lobe of the directivity pattern can be steered to the talker, even when the talker is behind the listener. Some of these new DIR schemes have shown promise in some listening environments (e.g., Chalupper et al., 2011; Wu et al., 2013). Clinicians should therefore be optimistic about the future development of DIR microphone hearing aids.

REFERENCES

Agnew, J. (1996). Directionality in hearing . . . revisited. *Hearing Review, 3*, 20–25.

American Academy of Audiology. (2006). *Guidelines for the audiologic management of adult hearing impairment.* Retrieved from http://www.audiology.org/resources/documentlibrary/Documents/haguidelines.pdf

American National Standards Institute. (1997). *American National Standard: Methods for the calculation of the speech intelligibility index (ANSI S3.5).* New York, NY: Author.

American National Standards Institute. (2010). *Method of measurement of performance characteristics of hearing aids under simulated in-situ working conditions (ANSI S3.35).* New York, NY: Author.

American Speech-Language-Hearing Association. (1998). *Guidelines for hearing aid fitting for adults.* Retrieved from http://www.asha.org/docs/pdf/GL1998-00012.pdf

Amlani, A. M. (2001). Efficacy of directional microphone hearing aids: A meta-analytic perspective. *Journal of the American Academy of Audiology, 12*(4), 202–214.

Amlani, A. M., Rakerd, B., & Punch, J. L. (2006). Speech-clarity judgments of hearing-aid-processed speech in noise: Differing polar patterns and acoustic environments. *International Journal of Audiology, 45*(6), 319–330.

Bell, S. L., Creek, S. A., & Lutman, M. E. (2010). Measuring real-ear signal-to-noise ratio: Application to directional hearing aids. *International Journal of Audiology, 49*, 238–246.

Bentler, R. A., Egge, J. L., Tubbs, J. L., Dittberner, A. B., & Flamme, G. A. (2004). Quantification of directional benefit across different polar response patterns. *Journal of the American Academy of Audiology, 15*(9), 649–659; quiz 660.

Bentler, R. A., Palmer, C., & Dittberner, A. B. (2004). Hearing-in-noise: Comparison of listeners with normal and (aided) impaired hearing. *Journal of the American Academy of Audiology, 15*, 216–225.

Bentler, R. A., Palmer, C., & Mueller, H. G. (2006). Evaluation of a second-order directional microphone hearing aid: I. Speech perception outcomes. *Journal of the American Academy of Audiology, 27*, 179–189.

Bentler, R. A., Tubbs, J. L., Egge, J. L., Flamme, G. A., & Dittberner, A. (2004). Evaluation of an adaptive directional system in a DSP hearing aid. *American Journal of Audiology, 13*, 73–79.

Beranek, L. L. (1949). *Acoustic measurements.* London, UK: Wiley.

Blamey, P. J., Fiket, H. J., & Steele, B. R. (2006). Improving speech intelligibility in background noise with an adaptive directional microphone. *Journal of the American Academy of Audiology, 17*(7), 519–530.

Boymans, M., & Dreschler, W. A. (2000). Field trials using a digital hearing aid with active noise reduction and dual-microphone directionality. *Audiology, 39*(5), 260–268.

Chalupper, J., O'Brien, A., & Hain, J. (2009). A new technique to improve aided localization. *Hearing Review, 16*, 20–26.

Chalupper, J., Wu, Y. H., & Weber, J. (2011). New algorithm automatically adjusts directional system for special situations. *Hearing Journal, 64*(1), 26–33.

Ching, T. Y. C., O'Brien, A., Dillon, H., Chalupper, J., Hartley, L., Hartley, D., . . . Hain, J. (2009). Directional effects on infants and young children in real life: Implications for amplification. *Journal of Speech, Language, and Hearing Research, 52*, 1241–1254.

Chung, K. (2004a). Challenges and recent developments in hearing aids. Part I. Speech understanding in noise, microphone technologies and noise reduction algorithms. *Trends in Amplification, 8*(3), 83–124.

Chung, K. (2004b). Challenges and recent developments in hearing aids. Part I. Speech understanding in noise, microphone technologies and noise reduction algorithms. *Trends in Amplification, 8*, 83–124.

Chung, K., McKibben, N., & Mongeau, L. (2010). Wind noise in hearing aids with directional and omnidirectional microphones: Polar characteristics of custom-made hearing aids. *Journal of the Acoustical Society of America, 127*, 2529–2542.

Chung, K., Mongeau, L., & McKibben, N. (2009). Wind noise in hearing aids with directional and omnidirectional microphones: Polar characteristics of behind-the-ear hearing aids. *Journal of the Acoustical Society of America, 125*, 2243–2259.

Chung, K., Zeng, F. G., & Acker, K. N. (2006). Effects of directional microphone and adaptive multichannel noise reduction algorithm on cochlear implant performance. *Journal of the Acoustical Society of America, 120*, 2216–2227.

Cord, M. T., Surr, R. K., Walden, B. E., & Dyrlund, O. (2004). Relationship between laboratory measures of directional advantage and everyday success with directional microphone hearing aids. *Journal of the American Academy of Audiology, 15*(5), 353–364.

Cord, M. T., Surr, R. K., Walden, B. E., & Olson, L. (2002). Performance of directional microphone hearing aids in everyday life. *Journal of the American Academy of Audiology, 13*(6), 295–307.

Cord, M. T., Walden, B. E., Surr, R. K., & Dittberner, A. (2007). Field evaluation of an asymmetric directional microphone fitting. *Journal of the American Academy of Audiology, 18*(3), 245–256.

Cox, R. M. (2009). Verification and what to do until your probe-mic system arrives. *Hearing Journal, 62*(9), 10–14.

Cox, R. M., & Alexander, G. C. (1995). The abbreviated profile of hearing aid benefit. *Ear and Hearing, 16*(2), 176–186.

Cox, R. M., & Alexander, G. C. (1999). Measuring satisfaction with amplification in daily life: The SADL scale. *Ear and Hearing, 20*, 306–320.

Cox, R. M., Alexander, G. C., & Gilmore, C. (1987). Development of the connected speech test (CST). *Ear and Hearing, 8*(5 Suppl.), 119S–126S.

Cox, R. M., Alexander, G. C., Gilmore, C., & Pusakulich, K. M. (1988). Use of the connected speech test (CST) with hearing-impaired listeners. *Ear and Hearing, 9*(4), 198–207.

Cox, R. M., & Rivera, I. M. (1992). Predictability and reliability of hearing aid benefit measured using the PHAB. *Journal of the American Academy of Audiology, 3*, 242–254.

Crandell, C. (1993). Speech recognition in noise by children with minimal degrees of sensorineural hearing loss. *Ear and Hearing, 14*, 210–216.

Csermak, B. (2000). A primer on a dual microphone directional system. *Hearing Review, 7*(1), 56–60.

Dillon, H. (2001). *Hearing aids* (1st ed.). New York, NY: Thieme.

Dirks, D. D., Morgan, D. E., & Dubno, J. R. (1982). A procedure for quantifying the effects of noise on speech recognition. *Journal of Speech and Hear Disorders, 47*(2), 114–123.

Dittberner, A. B., & Bentler, R. A. (2007a). Predictive measures of directional benefit Part 1: Estimating the directivity index on a manikin. *Ear and Hearing, 28,* 26–45.

Dittberner, A. B., & Bentler, R. A. (2007b). Predictive measures of directional benefit Part 2: Verification of different approaches to estimating directional benefit. *Ear and Hearing, 28*(1), 46–61.

Dubno, J. R., Dirks, D. D., & Morgan, D. E. (1984). Effects of age and mild hearing loss on speech recognition in noise. *Journal of the Acoustical Society of America, 76*(1), 87–96.

Duquesnoy, A. J., & Plomp, R. (1983). The effect of a hearing aid on the speech-reception threshold of hearing-impaired listeners in quiet and in noise. *Journal of the Acoustical Society of America, 73*(6), 2166–2173.

Edwards, B. (2000). Beyond amplification: Signal processing techniques for improving speech intelligibility in noise with hearing aids. *Seminars in Hearing, 21*(2), 137–156.

Erber, N. P. (1969). Interaction of audition and vision in the recognition of oral speech stimuli. *Journal of Speech, Language, and Hearing Research, 12*(2), 423–425.

Fabry, D. (2006). In one ear and synchronized with the other: Automatic hearing instruments under scrutiny. *Hearing Review, 13,* 36–38.

Fallon, M., Trehub, S. E., & Schneider, B. A. (2000). Children's perception of speech in multitalker babble. *Journal of the Acoustical Society of America, 108*(6), 3023–3029.

Fallon, M., Trehub, S. E., & Schneider, B. A. (2002). Children's use of semantic cues in degraded listening environments. *Journal of the Acoustical Society of America, 111,* 2242–2249.

Finitzo-Hieber, T., & Tillman, T. W. (1978). Room acoustics effects on monosyllabic word discrimination ability for normal and hearing-impaired children. *Journal of Speech, Language, and Hearing Research, 21,* 440–458.

Fitzgibbons, P. J., & Gordon-Salant, S. (1996). Auditory temporal processing in elderly listeners. *Journal of the American Academy of Audiology, 7,* 183–189.

Freyaldenhoven, M. C., Nabelek, A. K., Burchfield, S. B., & Thelin, J. W. (2005). Acceptable noise level as a measure of directional hearing aid benefit. *Journal of the American Academy of Audiology, 16,* 228–236.

Freyaldenhoven, M. C., Plyler, P. N., Thelin, J. W., Nabelek, A. K., & Burchfield, S. B. (2006). The effects of venting and low-frequency gain compensation on performance in noise with directional hearing instruments. *Journal of the American Academy of Audiology, 17*(3), 168–178.

Frye, G. J. (2006). How to verify directional hearing aids in the office. *Hearing Review, 13*(1), 48–57.

Ghent, R. M. (2005). A tutorial on complex sound fields for audiometric testing. *Journal of the American Academy of Audiology, 16,* 18–26.

Gnewikow, D., Ricketts, T., Bratt, G. W., & Mutchler, L. C. (2009). Real-world benefit from directional microphone hearing aids. *Journal of Rehabilitation Research and Development, 46,* 603–618.

Grant, K. W., Elhilali, M., Shamma, S. A., Walden, B. E., Surr, R. K., Cord, M. T., & Summers, V. (2008). An objective measure for selecting microphone modes in OMNI/DIR hearing aid circuits. *Ear and Hearing, 29,* 199–213.

Gravel, J. S., Fausel, N., Liskow, C., & Chobot, J. (1999). Children's speech recognition in noise using omni-directional and dual-microphone hearing aid technology. *Ear and Hearing, 20*(1), 1–11.

Hagerman, B., & Olofsson, A. (2004). A method to measure the effect of noise reduction algorithms using simultaneous speech and noise. *Acta Acoustica, 90,* 356–361.

Hawkins, D. B., Montgomery, A. A., Mueller, H. G., & Sedge, R. (1988). Assessment of speech intelligibility by hearing impaired listeners. In *Noise as a public health problem: Proceedings of the 5th International Congress on Noise as a Public Health Problem, held in Stockholm, August 21–28, 1988* (pp. 241–246). Stockholm: Swedish Council for Building Research.

Hawkins, D. B., & Yacullo, W. S. (1984). Signal-to-noise ratio advantage of binaural hearing aids and directional microphones under different levels of reverberation. *Journal of Speech and Hearing Disorders, 49*(3), 278–286.

Hogan, C. A., & Turner, C. W. (1998). High-frequency audibility: Benefits for hearing-impaired listeners. *Journal of the Acoustical Society of America, 104,* 432–441.

Hornsby, B. W., & Ricketts, T. (2007). Effects of noise source configuration on directional benefit using symmetric and asymmetric directional hearing aid fittings. *Ear and Hearing, 28,* 177–186.

Howell, J., & Saunders, G. (2008). *Directional microphones: Are they functioning properly when issued?* Paper presented at the American Auditory Society Annual Meeting, Scottsdale, Arizona.

Humes, L. E., Watson, B. U., Christensen, L. A., Cokely, C. G., Halling, D., & Lee, L. (1994). Factors associated with individual differences in clinical measures of speech recognition among the elderly. *Journal of Speech, Language, and Hearing Research, 37,* 465–474.

Kates, J. M. (2008). *Digital hearing aids.* San Diego, CA: Plural.

Keidser, G., Carter, L., Chalupper, J., & Dillon, H. (2007). Effect of low-frequency gain and venting effects on the benefit derived from directionality and noise reduction in hearing aids. *International Journal of Audiology, 46,* 554–568.

Keidser, G., O'Brien, A., Hain, J., McLelland, M., & Yeend, I. (2009). The effect of frequency-dependent microphone directionality on horizontal localization performance in hearing-aid users. *Journal of Audiology, 48,* 789–803.

Keidser, G., Rohrseitz, K., Dillon, H., Hamacher, V., Carter, L., Rass, U., & Convery, E. (2006). The effect of multi-channel wide dynamic range compression, noise reduction, and the directional microphone on horizontal localization performance in hearing aid wearers. *Journal of Audiology, 45,* 563–579.

Killion, M. C., Schulien, R., Christensen, L., Fabry, D., Revit, L., Niquette, P., & Chung, K. (1998). Real-world performance of an ITE directional microphone. *Hearing Journal, 51,* 24–38.

Kim, J. S., & Bryan, M. F. (2011). The effects of asymmetric directional microphone fittings on acceptance of background noise. *Journal of Audiology, 50*(5), 290–296.

Klemp, E. J., & Dhar, S. (2008). Speech perception in noise using directional microphones in open-canal hearing aids. *Journal of the American Academy of Audiology,19,* 571–578.

Kricos, P. B. (2006). Audiologic management of older adults with hearing loss and compromised cognitive/psychoacoustic auditory processing capabilities. *Trends in Amplification, 10*(1), 1–28.

Kuhnel, V., Margolf-Hackl, S., & Kiessling, J. (2001). Multi-microphone technology for severe-to-profound hearing loss. *Scandinavian Audiology Supplementum,* (52), 65–68.

Kuk, F., Baekgaard, L., & Ludvigsen, C. (2000). Design considerations in directional microphones. *Hearing Review, 7*(9), 68–73.

Kuk, F., Keenan, D., Lau, C. C., & Ludvigsen, C. (2005). Performance of a fully adaptive directional microphone to signals presented from various azimuths. *Journal of the American Academy of Audiology,16*(6), 333–347.

Kuk, F., Keenan, D., & Ludvigsen, C. (2004). Is real-world directional benefit predictable? *Hearing Review, 11*(12), 18–24.

Kuk, F., Kollofski, C., Brown, S., Melum, A., & Rosenthal, A. (1999). Use of a digital hearing aid with directional microphones in school-aged children. *Journal of the American Academy of Audiology, 10*(10), 535–548.

Latzel, M. (2012). *Binaural VoiceStream Technology— Intelligent binaural algorithms to improve speech understanding.* Retrieved from https://www.phonak pro.com/content/dam/phonak/gc_hq/b2b/en/elearning/publications/insight/2012/Insight_Binaural_VoiceStream_Technology_028-0773.pdf

Lee, L., Lau, C., & Sullivan, D. (1998). The advantage of a low compression threshold in directional microphones. *Hearing Review, 5*(8), 30–32.

Leeuw, A. R., & Dreschler, W. A. (1991). Advantages of directional hearing aid microphones related to room acoustics. *Audiology, 30*(6), 330–344.

Levitt, H. (1971). Transformed up-down methods in psychoacoustics. *Journal of the Acoustical Society of America, 49*(2), 467.

Lunner, T. (2003). Cognitive function in relation to hearing aid use. *International Journal of Audiology, 42*(Suppl 1), S49–58.

Lunner, T., & Sundewall-Thoren, E. (2007). Interactions between cognition, compression, and listening conditions: Effects on speech-in-noise performance in a two-channel hearing aid. *Journal of the American Academy of Audiology, 18,* 604–617.

Lurquin, P., & Rafhay, S. (1996). Intelligibility in noise using multimicrophone hearing aids. *Acta Otorhinolaryngologica Belgica, 50*(2), 103–109.

MacLeod, A., & Summerfield, Q. (1987). Quantifying the contribution of vision to speech perception in noise. *British Journal of Audiology, 21*(2), 131–141.

Murphy, D. R., Daneman, M., & Schneider, B. A. (2006). Why do older adults have difficulty following conversations? *Psychology and Aging, 21,* 49–61.

Nabelek, A. K. (1982). Temporal distortions and noise considerations. In G. Studebaker & F. Bess (Eds.), *The Vanderbilt Hearing-Aid Report.* Upper Darby, PA: Monographs in Contemporary Audiology.

Nabelek, A. K., Freyaldenhoven, M. C., Tampas, J. W., Burchfield, S. B., & Muenchen, R. A. (2006). Acceptable noise level as a predictor of hearing aid use. *Journal of the American Academy of Audiology, 17,* 626–639.

Nabelek, A. K., & Mason, D. (1981). Effect of noise and reverberation on monaural and binaural word identification by subjects with various audiograms. *Journal of Speech, Language, and Hearing Research, 24,* 375–383.

Nabelek, A. K., Tucker, F. M., & Letowski, T. R. (1991). Toleration of background noises: Relationship with patterns of hearing aid use by elderly persons. *Journal of Speech, Language, and Hearing Research, 34,* 679–685.

Nilsson, M., Soli, S. D., & Sullivan, J. A. (1994). Development of the hearing in noise test for the measurement of speech reception thresholds in quiet and in noise. *Journal of the Acoustical Society of America, 95*(2), 1085–1099.

Oeding, K., Valente, M., & Kerckhoff, J. (2010). Effectiveness of the directional microphone in the Baha Divino. *Journal of the American Academy of Audiology, 21*(8), 546–557.

Olson, L., Ioannou, M., & Trine, T. D. (2004). Appraising an automatically switching directional system in the real world. *Hearing Journal, 57*(6), 32–38.

Palmer, C., Bentler, R. A., & Meuller, H. G. (2006). Evaluation of a second-order directional microphone hearing aid: II. Self-report outcomes. *Journal of the American Academy of Audiology, 17*(3), 190–201.

Pichora-Fuller, M. K., Schneider, B. A., & Daneman, M. (1995). How young and old adults listen to and remember speech in noise. *Journal of the Acoustical Society of America, 97,* 593–608.

Plomp, R. (1978). Auditory handicap of hearing impairment and the limited benefit of hearing aids. *Journal of the Acoustical Society of America, 63,* 533–549.

Plomp, R., & Mimpen, A. M. (1979). Improving the reliability of testing the speech reception threshold for sentences. *Audiology, 18*(1), 43–52.

Powers, T. A., & Hamacher, V. (2002). Three-microphone instrument is designed to extend benefits of directionality. *Hearing Journal, 55*, 38–45.

Preves, D. A., Sammeth, C. A., & Wynne, M. K. (1999). Field trial evaluations of a switched directional/omnidirectional in-the-ear hearing instrument. *Journal of the American Academy of Audiology, 10*(5), 273–284.

Puder, H. (2006). Adaptive signal processing for interference cancellation in hearing aids. *Signal Process, 86*, 1239–1253.

Pumford, J. M., Seewald, R. C., Scollie, S. D., & Jenstad, L. M. (2000). Speech recognition with in-the-ear and behind-the-ear dual-microphone hearing instruments. *Journal of the American Academy of Audiology, 11*(1), 23–35.

Ricketts, T. (2000a). Directivity quantification in hearing aids: Fitting and measurement effects. *Ear and Hearing, 21*, 45–58.

Ricketts, T. (2000b). Impact of noise source configuration on directional hearing aid benefit and performance. *Ear and Hearing, 21*(3), 194–205.

Ricketts, T. (2001). Directional hearing aids. *Trends in Amplification, 5*(4), 139–176.

Ricketts, T., & Dittberner, A. B. (2002). Directional amplification for improved signal-to-noise ratio: Strategies, measurement, and limitations. In M. Valente (Ed.), *Strategies for selecting and verifying hearing aid fittings* (2nd ed., pp. 274–346). New York, NY: Thieme.

Ricketts, T., & Galster, J. (2007). Directional benefit in simulated classroom environments. *American Journal of Audiology, 16*, 130–144.

Ricketts, T., & Galster, J. (2008). Head angle and elevation in classroom environments: Implications for amplification. *Journal of Speech, Language, and Hearing Research, 51*, 516–525.

Ricketts, T., & Henry, P. (2002a). Evaluation of an adaptive, directional-microphone hearing aid. *International Journal of Audiology, 41*(2), 100–112.

Ricketts, T., & Henry, P. (2002b). Low-frequency gain compensation in directional hearing aids. *American Journal of Audiology, 11*(1), 29–41.

Ricketts, T., Henry, P., & Gnewikow, D. (2003). Full time directional versus user selectable microphone modes in hearing aids. *Ear and Hearing, 24*(5), 424–439.

Ricketts, T., Henry, P. P., & Hornsby, B. W. (2005). Application of frequency importance functions to directivity for prediction of benefit in uniform fields. *Ear and Hearing, 26*(5), 473–486.

Ricketts, T., & Hornsby, B. W. (2003). Distance and reverberation effects on directional benefit. *Ear and Hearing, 24*(6), 472–484.

Ricketts, T., & Hornsby, B. W. (2006). Directional hearing aid benefit in listeners with severe hearing loss. *International Journal of Audiology, 45*(3), 190–197.

Ricketts, T., Lindley, G., & Henry, P. (2001). Impact of compression and hearing aid style on directional

hearing aid benefit and performance. *Ear and Hearing, 22*(4), 348–361.

Ricketts, T., & Picou, E. M. (2013). Speech recognition for bilaterally asymmetric and asymmetric hearing aid microphone modes in simulated classroom environments. *Ear and Hearing.* Advance online publication.

Schneider, B. A., Daneman, M., Murphy, D. R., & KwongSee, S. (2000). Listening to discourse in distracting settings: The effects of aging. *Psychology and Aging, 15*, 110–125.

Schum, D. J., Matthews, L. J., & Lee, F. S. (1991). Actual and predicted word-recognition performance of elderly hearing-impaired listeners. *Journal of Speech, Language, and Hearing Research, 34*(3), 636–642.

Smeds, K., Keidser, G., Zakis, J., Dillon, H., Leijon, A., Grant, F., . . . Brew, C. (2006). Preferred overall loudness. II: Listening through hearing aids in field and laboratory tests. *International Journal of Audiology, 45*, 12–25.

Snell, K. B., Mapes, F. M., Hickman, E. D., & Frisina, D. R. (2002). Word recognition in competing babble and the effects of age, temporal processing, and absolute sensitivity. *Journal of the Acoustical Society of America, 112*(2), 720–727.

Souza, P. (2004). New hearing aids for older listeners. *Hearing Journal, 57*(3), 10–17.

Souza, P., & Boike, K. (2006). Combining temporal envelope cues across channels: Effects of age and hearing loss. *Journal of Speech, Language, and Hearing Research, 49*, 138–149.

Steeneken, H. J. M., & Houtgast, T. (1980). A physical method for measuring speech transmission quality. *Journal of the Acoustical Society of America, 67*, 318–326.

Sumby, W. H., & Pollack, I. (1954). Visual contribution to speech intelligibility in noise. *Journal of the Acoustical Society of America, 26*(2), 212–215.

Summers, V., Grant, K. W., Walden, B. E., Cord, M. T., Surr, R. K., & Elhilali, M. (2008). Evaluation of a "direct-comparison" approach to automatic switching in omnidirectional/directional hearing aids. *Journal of the American Academy of Audiology, 19*, 708–720.

Surr, R. K., Walden, B. E., Cord, M. T., & Olson, L. (2002). Influence of environmental factors on hearing aid microphone preference. *Journal of the American Academy of Audiology, 13*(6), 308–322.

Takahashi, G., Martinez, C. D., Beamer, S., Bridges, J., Noffsinger, D., Sugiura, K., . . . Williams, D. W. (2007). Subjective measures of hearing aid benefit and satisfaction in the NIDCD/VA follow-up study. *Journal of the American Academy of Audiology, 18*(4), 323–349.

Tchorz, J. (2001). Effects of microphone matching in directional hearing instruments. *Hearing Review, 8*(10), 54–58.

Thompson, S. (2002). Microphone, telecoil, and receiver options: Past, present, and future. In M.

Valente (Ed.), *Hearing aids: Standard, options, and limitations.* New York, NY: Thieme.

Thompson, S. (2003). Tutorial on microphone technologies for directional hearing aids. *Hearing Journal, 56*(11), 14–21.

Tun, P. A., O'Kane, G., & Wingfield, A. (2002). Distraction by competing speech in young and older adult listeners. *Psychology and Aging, 17*(3), 453–467.

Valente, M. (2000). Use of microphone technology to improve user performance in noise. In R. E. Sandlin (Ed.), *Textbook of hearing aid amplification.* San Diego, CA: Singular.

Valente, M., Fabry, D. A., & Potts, L. G. (1995). Recognition of speech in noise with hearing aids using dual microphones. *Journal of the American Academy of Audiology, 6*(6), 440–449.

Valente, M., & Mispagel, K. M. (2004). Performance of an automatic adaptive dual-microphone ITC digital hearing aid. *Hearing Review, 11,* 42–46, 71.

Valente, M., & Mispagel, K. M. (2008). Unaided and aided performance with a directional open-fit hearing aid. *International Journal of Audiology, 47,* 329–336.

Valente, M., Schuchman, G., Potts, L. G., & Beck, L. B. (2000). Performance of dual-microphone in-the-ear hearing aids. *Journal of the American Academy of Audiology, 11*(4), 181–189.

Valente, M., Sweetow, R., Potts, L. G., & Bingea, B. (1999). Digital versus analog signal processing: Effect of directional microphone. *Journal of the American Academy of Audiology, 10*(3), 133–150.

Van den Bogaert, T., Doclo, S., Wouters, J., & Moonen, M. (2008). The effect of multimicrophone noise reduction systems on sound source localization by users of binaural hearing aids. *Journal of the Acoustical Society of America, 124,* 484–497.

Van den Bogaert, T., Klasen, T. J., Moonen, M., Van Duen, L., & Wouters, J. (2006). Horizontal localization with bilateral hearing aids: Without is better than with. *Journal of the Acoustical Society of America, 119,* 515–526.

Walden, B. E., Surr, R. K., Cord, M. T., & Dyrlund, O. (2004). Predicting hearing aid microphone preference in everyday listening. *Journal of the American Academy of Audiology, 15*(5), 365–396.

Walden, B. E., Surr, R. K., Cord, M. T., Edwards, B., & Olson, L. (2000). Comparison of benefits provided by different hearing aid technologies. *Journal of the American Academy of Audiology, 11*(10), 540–560.

Walden, B. E., Surr, R. K., Grant, K. W., Van Summers, W., Cord, M. T., & Dyrlund, O. (2005). Effect of signal-to-noise ratio on directional microphone benefit and preference. *Journal of the American Academy of Audiology, 16*(9), 662–676.

Woods, W. S., Merks, I., Zhang, T., Fitz, K., & Edwards, B. (2010). Assessing the benefit of adaptive null-steering using real-world signals. *International Journal of Audiology, 49,* 434–443.

Wu, Y. H. (2010). Effect of age on directional microphone hearing aid benefit and preference. *Journal of the American Academy of Audiology, 21*(2), 78–89.

Wu, Y. H., & Bentler, R. A. (2007). Using a signal cancellation technique to assess adaptive directivity of hearing aids. *Journal of the Acoustical Society of America, 122*(1), 496–511.

Wu, Y. H., & Bentler, R. A. (2009). Using a signal cancellation technique involving impulse response to assess directivity of hearing aids. *Journal of the Acoustical Society of America, 126*(6), 3214–3226.

Wu, Y. H., & Bentler, R. A. (2010a). Impact of visual cues on directional benefit and preference: Part I —laboratory tests. *Ear and Hearing, 31*(1), 22–34.

Wu, Y. H., & Bentler, R. A. (2010b). Impact of visual cues on directional benefit and preference: Part II —field tests. *Ear and Hearing, 31,* 35–46.

Wu, Y. H., & Bentler, R. A. (2012a). Clinical measures of hearing aid directivity: Assumption, accuracy, and reliability. *Ear and Hearing, 33*(1), 44–56.

Wu, Y. H., & Bentler, R. A. (2012b). Do older adults have social lifestyles that place fewer demands on hearing? *Journal of the American Academy of Audiology, 23*(9), 697–711.

Wu, Y. H., & Bentler, R. A. (2012c). The influence of audiovisual ceiling performance on the relationship between reverberation and directional benefit: perception and prediction. *Ear and Hearing, 33*(5), 604–614.

Wu, Y. H., & Stangl, E. (2013). The effect of hearing aid signal-processing schemes on acceptable noise levels: Perception and prediction. *Ear and Hearing, 34*(3), 333–341.

Wu, Y. H., Stangl, E., & Bentler, R. (in press). Hearing-aid users' voices: A factor that could affect directional benefit. *International Journal of Audiology.*

Wu, Y. H., Stangl, E., Bentler, R., & Stanziola, R. W. (2013). The effect of hearing aid technologies on listening in an automobile. *Journal of the American Academy of Audiology, 24*(6), 474–485.

CHAPTER 7

DSP Hearing Instruments

INGA HOLUBE
HENNING PUDER
THERESE M. VELDE

OUTLINE

Nearly all of today's hearing instruments include digital signal processing. Until the end of the 1980s, hearing health care professionals dispensed analog hearing instruments that were adjusted according to the degree of hearing loss with screwdriver-controlled potentiometer trimmers. Then the advent of integrated circuit chip technology allowed for the development of analog hearing instruments that could be programmed digitally with dedicated programming devices or with personal computers. In 1996, the third type of hearing instrument was introduced; they were digitally programmable and offered digital signal processing. It is this third category of hearing aids that are the focus of this chapter. The first part of this chapter describes the principles of digital technology, and the second part discusses different digital signal processing algorithms. The user benefit of these algorithms is addressed in the respective sections.

PRINCIPLES OF DIGITAL TECHNOLOGY

Analog and Digital Hearing Instruments

Digital hearing instruments have several fundamental differences from analog instruments. Figure 7–1 shows a block diagram of an analog hearing aid. Analog devices consist of a microphone, a preamplifier, a means processor (such as a tone control or an AGC), an amplifier, and a receiver. An acoustic input signal (a sine wave in Figure 7–1) is converted by the microphone to an electronic input signal. This electronic input signal is amplified by the preamplifier, and the frequency response is shaped by the tone control. After this shaping, the signal is again amplified and then converted back to an acoustic output signal by the receiver. Both the acoustic and electronic signals in the processing path are analog.

In analog hearing instruments that are digitally programmable, parameters of the means of processing, such as the tone control or the compression ratio of the AGC, are stored in a memory and can be modified for different hearing instrument users.

Figure 7–2 shows a block diagram of a digital hearing instrument. In contrast with an analog instrument, a digital instrument has an analog-to-digital converter, a digital signal processor, and some method of digital-to-analog conversion. The amplified electronic signals are converted into digitized signals that are processed by the digital signal processor before they are converted back to analog electronic signals. The following section focuses on the difference between analog and digital signals and the principles and advantages of digital signal processing.

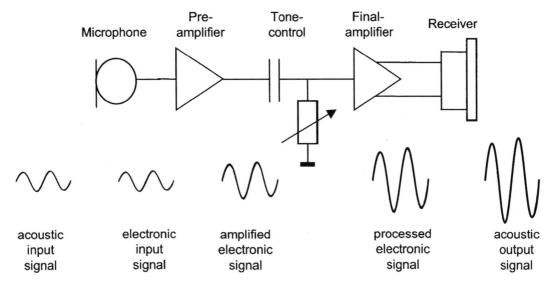

Figure 7–1. Block diagram of an analog hearing instrument.

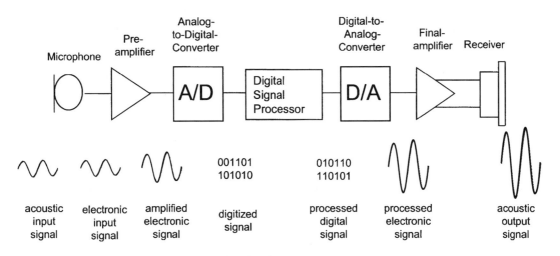

Figure 7–2. Block diagram of a digital hearing instrument.

Analog Signals

All physical signals, such as the sound pressure at the microphone or the voltage of the electronic signal at the receiver of a hearing instrument, are continuous in time and in amplitude. Figure 7–3 shows the time waveform of a sinusoidal electronic signal. Analog signals can have any amplitude value at any particular moment in time, and the level measured at any moment may differ slightly from that immediately preceding or following it. Thus, with this continuously varying signal, there are no "steps" in the signal curve.

Digital Signals

The purpose of the digital signal processor in hearing instruments is to derive, by a series of calculations, an output signal based on the input signal to the instrument. The input

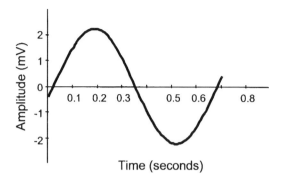

Figure 7–3. An analog signal with different levels at any given point of time.

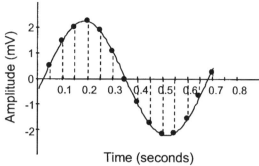

Figure 7–4. An analog signal sampled at discrete points in time.

signal has to be converted into numbers for the calculations, and these numbers can then be added, subtracted, multiplied, or divided. A program that is composed of a series of calculations is called an algorithm. Several reference sources offer a review of digital signal processing (e.g., Lyons, 2011; Oppenheim & Schafer, 1975).

Sampling

The input signal is sampled at discrete points in time. In Figure 7–4, an analog signal is being sampled (e.g., every 0.05 milliseconds), corresponding to a sampling rate of 20 kHz. Only these sampled points or samples are used by the digital signal processor. The rest of the input signal is not considered.

This sampling of the input signal is done in the analog-to-digital (A/D) converter. As is suggested in Figure 7–4, it is important to sample the input signal frequently enough to have a good representation. This requirement is discussed in greater detail later in this chapter.

Quantization

The digital signal processor cannot use numbers with infinite precision for calculation. Therefore, each sample must be either truncated or rounded to a specific precision. This results in a less idealized representation of the analog input signal and is called quan-

tization. The quantized signal is characterized by bit values. A single bit can have two values. These numbers correspond to the two states at its input (i.e., voltage switched on or voltage switched off). In Figure 7–5, we see a digital signal in the upper panel. The signal is either on, with a value of 1, or off, with a value of 0. In the lower panel, the binary code or quantization value corresponding to the signal is given. Numbers that contain only such binary digits (bits) are called binary numbers. The number of bits in a binary number is known as the word length. In this figure, the quantization values are either zero or one. Signals also can be described with greater resolution.

An increase in the word length increases the number of potential values that can be given to a sampled signal. A one-bit A/D converter has 2 (that is, 2^1) values available to assign a sampled point. A two-bit A/D converter has 4 (that is, 2^2) values available to assign to a sampled point. A four-bit A/D converter has 16 (that is, 2^4) values available, and so on.

Figure 7–6 shows the 3-bit digital output (heavy line) for a linear input signal (light line) over time. In this example, the quantization step is 1 mV. When the analog signal is between 0.5 and 1.5 mV, the digital value is 001. Likewise, an analog input signal of 6 mV is converted to the digital value 110. Note that the shape of the digital signal is not linear like the analog signal. Instead, the digital signal

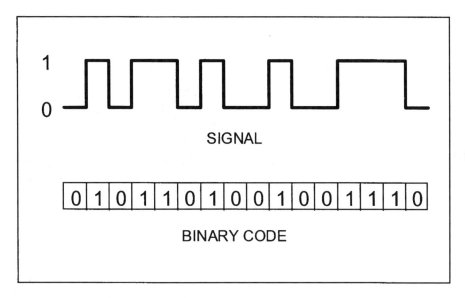

Figure 7–5. A digital signal with only two states, or 1 bit, and its corresponding binary code.

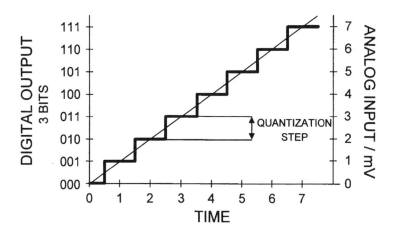

Figure 7–6. Conversion of an analog input signal into a digital signal with 3 bits.

remains at one value until it jumps to the next digital value.

The more bits that are available, the better the analog input signal can be represented by the digital numbers. Figure 7–7 shows two examples of analog signals and their digital representation with different numbers of bits. In panel A, two bits are used. In panel B, four bits are used. The sampled value is held con- stant until the next sample is taken. When a sample is made, the sample is assigned a value. In panel A, only four values are possible to represent the signal because only two bits are used. In panel B, 16 values are possible because four bits are used. The level of the analog signal is rounded to the nearest binary number. The more bits that are used, the smaller the error between the analog and the digital signal.

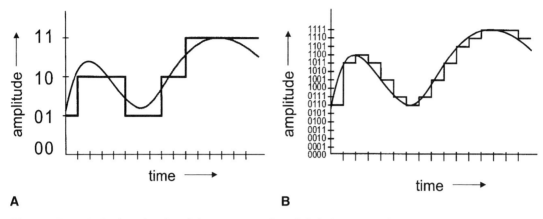

Figure 7–7. A. Analog signal and the corresponding digital signal sampled at 2 bits. **B.** Analog signal and the corresponding digital signal sampled at 4 bits.

Quantization Error

An analog signal and its digitized signal are again shown in Figure 7–8. In panel A, the analog signal was sampled with 3 bits as is indicated by the 8 possible values of the digital signal. The difference between the original and the digitized signal is the quantization error. This error signal is shown in the back waveform. Panel B shows the same original signal and the digitized signal that is sampled with a resolution of 6 bits. Note how the digitized signal more closely approximates the original signal, resulting in the quantization error being nearly zero at all points. The error signal shows that the analog signal is better approximated by the digital signal when more bits are used.

Why is quantization error important to hearing instruments? The quantization error is a random noise with its maximum amplitude at one-half the amplitude of the quantization step. Soft input signals to the hearing instrument, which have smaller amplitude than the amplitude of the quantization noise, cannot be distinguished from the noise. Therefore, the quantization noise determines the noise floor for the digital signal processing. Because the maximum output of the hearing instrument is fixed by the selected receiver, the noise floor determines the dynamic range of the digital system. Each bit increases the dynamic range by 6 dB. A digi-

tal signal processor with 3 bits has a dynamic range of only 18 dB. When using 6 bits, the dynamic range is increased to 36 dB. Audio compact-disc players normally use 16 bits of resolution and, therefore, have a dynamic range of 96 dB.

Aliasing

Let's return to the issue of how frequently a signal is sampled. In addition to the quantization error, a digital system can demonstrate an additional error that is not found in analog systems. This error is related to the sampling frequency of the analog signal. Figure 7–9 shows as an example a sine wave, labeled "input signal" that is sampled at four different discrete points in time. Note that only one or two points are sampled within each cycle. The same four sample points can also represent a different sine wave with a lower frequency, labeled "aliasing signal." This ambiguity results in the presence of a sine wave, which was not present in the original input, at the output of the digital system. This type of error is called aliasing. In an acoustic system, such as a hearing aid, an aliasing error introduces distortions.

A visual example of aliasing error is when automobile wheels appear to rotate backward in movies. The camera samples the wheel's movement at a specific frequency, but the wheel completes a cycle of movement at a

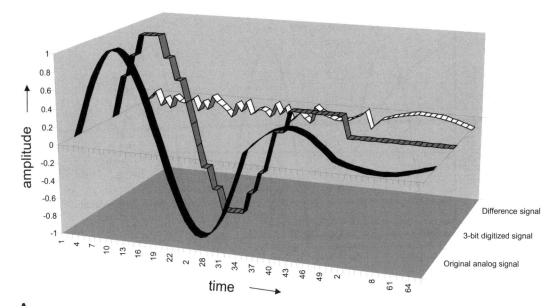

A

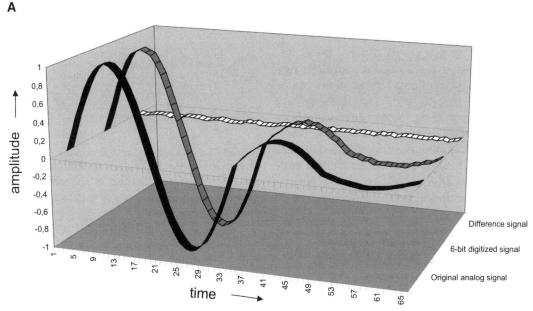

B

Figure 7–8. A. Original signal, digitized signal with 3 bits, and the difference signal. **B.** Original signal, digitized signal with 6 bits, and the difference signal.

frequency faster than the sampling frequency. Our eyes see a lower frequency of movement (as indicated by the wheel turning backward) that fits the camera's samples.

To avoid this aliasing error in a sine wave, it is necessary to sample the input signal with a minimum of two samples per period of the sinusoid. This minimum sample rate is called the Nyquist frequency, named after Nyquist (1928) for his work with telegraph transmission theory. For speech signals, the sampling rate must be at least twice the highest frequency to be processed in a digital system. If an individual wants to hear signals with a

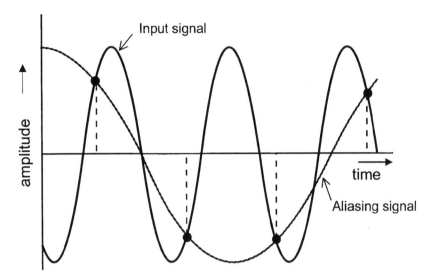

Figure 7–9. Two sine waves of different frequencies that can be represented by the same samples.

frequency content up to 10 kHz, for example, it is necessary to use a sampling rate of 20 kHz. If frequency components above 10 kHz are present in the signal, the person wearing the hearing instrument would hear a false sound. To avoid this aliasing error, the input signal has to be filtered before sampling. This low-pass filter, called an anti-aliasing filter, should have an edge frequency of half the sampling frequency or less.

Principles of Digital Signal Processing

Using the principles we have established in the previous sections about digital signals, we can now examine the digital signal processor. We first describe an A/D converter, and then we discuss some examples of algorithms used in a digital signal processor.

A/D Converter

Figure 7–10 shows the components of an A/D converter. The analog input signal is first low-pass filtered with a cutoff frequency appropriate for a hearing instrument (e.g., 10 kHz). Then, the analog signal is sampled at a rate at least twice the cutoff frequency

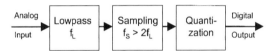

Figure 7–10. Components of an A/D-converter.

of the low-pass filter to avoid aliasing. In this last step, quantization of the samples is dependent on the number of bits available in the A/D converter.

Because each additional bit used in an A/D converter increases the space and the power consumption of a hearing instrument, the maximum number of bits is usually restricted to 16. Therefore, the dynamic range of hearing instruments is 96 dB (16 × 6 dB). The dynamic range in input signals into hearing instruments is greater than 96 dB. Additional precautions to avoid distortion from this difference in dynamic range are discussed later.

Sigma-Delta Converter

One A/D converter commonly used in hearing instruments is a Sigma-Delta converter. In this converter, the analog input signal is not directly converted to a digital signal with 16 bits and a sampling rate of 20 kHz, for example. Instead, the difference in voltage from one sampled point to the next is quantized, as opposed to quantizing the absolute value of the sampled point. In addition, the number of bits is reduced to one, and the sampling rate is increased to a frequency many times greater than the Nyquist frequency used in conventional A/D conversion. For example, a frequency of 1000 kHz (1 MHz) is commonly used for audio applications. By increasing the sampling rate and digitizing only the incremental differences between samples, this system can reduce the inherent noise and increase the dynamic range of a system, even when using only 1 bit for conversion. The increase in the sampling rate is also called oversampling.

Processing Algorithms

After A/D conversion of the input signals, the digital signal processor can now use the digitized signals to process the algorithm with a predefined calculation procedure or algorithm (Figure 7–11).

A simple example of a signal processing algorithm is multiplication of a digital number, resulting in amplification or attenuation of the input signal. For example, multiplication with a factor of 4 results in a gain of 12 dB.

Another example is a digital filter shown in Figure 7–12. In the digital domain, a filter can be constructed by delaying the input signal by a certain time and adding it back to the original signal. By introducing different time delays and multiplying the input signal and the delayed signals by specific values, filters with a variety of characteristics can be created. A high-pass filter can be constructed by subtracting the delayed signal from the input signal, for example. For steady or slowly changing signals, this results in an output that is zero or very small. For fast-changing signals, the difference between the samples is larger, and therefore the output is also larger. This yields a high-pass characteristic.

When processing digital signals, an adequate number of bits should be used in the calculations. In other words, it is important to perform the signal processing calculations with a high word length. This is particularly true for multiplication or division. Within these algorithms, very small binary numbers can be combined with very large binary numbers. To keep a high precision in these calculations, the number of bits (or the word length) within a digital signal processor is often increased relative to the number of bits used in the A/D converter.

Digital-to-Analog Conversion

After creating the desired output by processing the input signal, the digital signal must be converted back to an analog signal. This procedure is called Digital-to-Analog (D/A) conversion. Let us examine two different methods of D/A conversion.

In the first method, the analog signal is derived by converting the digital value into an analog voltage. This voltage is kept constant until the next digital value is presented, resulting in a stepped signal as seen in Figure 7–7. The stepped function is low-pass filtered with a maximum bandwidth of one half of the sampling frequency. Low-pass filtering results in smoothing the steps of the signal, and the analog signal is reconstructed.

The second type of D/A converter is based on similar principles as the Sigma-Delta A/D converter. This method uses short pulses that are output at a fast rate; the digital number of the signal determines the density

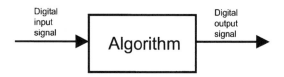

Figure 7–11. Digital signal processor.

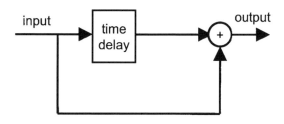

Figure 7–12. Digital filter.

of the pulses. This is shown schematically in Figure 7–13. When this pulsed signal is low-pass filtered, an analog signal is output. When this method is used in hearing instruments, the receiver can act as a low-pass filter. Therefore, an additional low-pass filter may not need to be implemented in the circuit design.

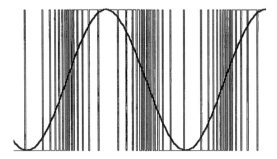

Figure 7–13. Schematic representation of pulse-density modulation. (From "Grundlagen digitaler Signalverarbeitung," by V. Hohmann, 1998, *Zeitschrift für Audiologie, 37*, 124. Copyright 1998 by Median-Verlag. Reprinted with permission.)

Chip Technology

Today's hearing instruments generally contain one integrated circuit chip that contains its electronic parts. These electronic parts are simply small geometric patterns on the chip.

Integrated chips can be characterized by their "structure size," which refers to the spacing between the features. The structure size determines the necessary area on the chip to implement the electronic parts. The smaller the structure size (i.e., the closer the features can be placed), the more electronic parts that can be integrated on the chip; the chip can be smaller but still have the same number of electronic parts. Circuit chips allow digital hearing instruments to be much smaller than analog instruments.

The chips used in hearing instruments must be as small as possible to produce cosmetically desirable instruments. The structure size of the chips has decreased from 3 µ to 65 n within the last 20 years. Figure 7–14 shows progress in miniaturization of the

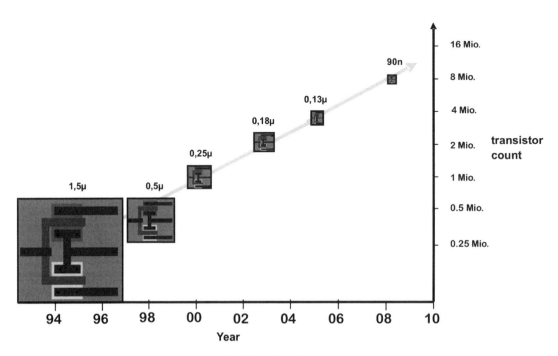

Figure 7–14. Miniaturization progress in chip technology.

integrated circuit chip technology in hearing instruments.

The difference between analog and digital chip technology can be viewed in terms of the complexity of the signal processing algorithms, and therefore in terms of the possible user benefit. This comparison is shown schematically in Figure 7–15. As depicted by the dashed curve, with analog technology, electronic circuits can be manufactured with little effort and low cost. Unfortunately, these electronic circuits permit only rudimentary signal processing features with limited user benefit. As we strive to increase benefit, the complexity of the electronic circuit and the costs increase. With digitally programmable analog technology, illustrated by the dotted curve, the initial effort required to develop new circuits is higher than with analog technology. With this technology, however, meeting the increasingly complex requirements of the signal processing algorithms occurs before the user benefit plateaus. With digital technology, shown by the solid line, the minimum effort and cost for development of simple signal processing algorithms are the highest. The payoff, however, is demonstrated by the small increases in complexity of the circuits that permit large increases in the quality of the processing and potential user benefit. Therefore, high-value modern hearing instruments can be developed with best audiological benefit with digital technology.

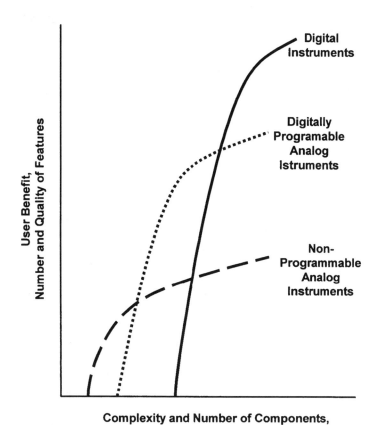

Figure 7–15. Cost versus user benefit for analog and digital hearing instruments. (From "Signalverarbeitungs Algorithmen für digitale Hörgeräte," by I. Holube, 1998, *Zeitschrift für Audiologie, 37,* 177. Copyright 1998 by Median-Verlag. Adapted with permission.)

Advantages of Digital Signal Processing

Digital signal processing has several advantages over analog signal processing including miniaturization, low power consumption, low internal noise, reproducibility, stability, programmability, and signal processing complexity.

1. Miniaturization: Integrated circuit chip technology allows for small-sized digital signal processors. Complex signal processing algorithms can be implemented on a very small chip. This is especially important for the design of cosmetically appealing hearing instruments. If the current signal processing contained in a digital CIC could be implemented using analog technology, the hearing instrument would be the size of a body-worn instrument.

2. Low power consumption: Along with miniaturization comes the advantage of reduced power consumption. For example, a dynamic compression algorithm using digital technology requires only 5 µA, compared with 100 µA for analog instruments. Reduced power consumption permits the use of smaller batteries, which is again advantageous in the design of cosmetically desirable instruments.

3. Low internal noise: The number of bits in the system can control the internal noise of digital signal processors. Internal noise is dependent on word length, not on the algorithms, so with analog technology, internal noise increases with increasing complexity of the signal processing.

4. Reproducibility: In a digital system, signal manipulation is performed with numbers. Thus, the algorithms always perform the same precise calculations, in contrast to analog technology where the output can vary depending on the exact values of the components in the instrument. Analog components can exhibit differences in performance due to discrepancies in the production process.

5. Stability: Digital signal processing is stable because the technology resists external influences. Performance of analog instruments can vary in response to external influences, such as temperature.

6. Programmability: With a single chip, the signal processing and its parameters can be widely altered. In analog technology, such flexibility could only be achieved by changing components.

7. Complexity: Digital signal processing allows implementation of complex signal processing algorithms. One example is the analysis of the input signal and appropriate signal modification based on the result of this analysis. Other examples of processing algorithms are discussed later.

SIGNAL PROCESSING ALGORITHMS

Overview

Figure 7–16 gives an overview of the signal processing algorithms typically included in a high-end digital hearing instrument. Many BTE hearing instruments and also some ITEs contain two microphones for multi-microphone noise reduction and spatial directional filtering. This can be done in different frequency regions. A frequency analysis is also necessary for single microphone noise reduction strategies as well as gain adjustments, dynamic range, and frequency compression. For output signal construction, the different frequency regions are resynthesized. The output of a hearing instrument can reach the microphones causing an unpleasant sound called feedback under certain conditions. Therefore, algorithms for feedback cancellation have been implemented in current hearing instruments. The different processing stages are steered by a classification system that analyzes the listening environment and decides the settings of noise reduction as well as compression stages. Those are also influenced by the binaural link between the two

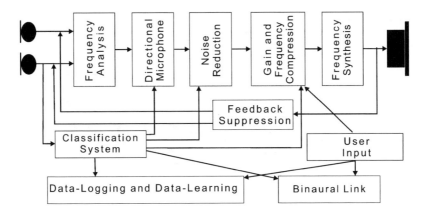

Figure 7–16. Overview of signal processing algorithms within a hearing instrument.

hearing instruments as well as the input of the hearing instrument user and learning algorithms that monitor the preferred settings. The following sections review the processing stages within a typical hearing instrument.

Frequency Analysis

Hearing instruments must be able to separate incoming signals into different frequency regions to compensate for the variety in the frequency configurations seen in hearing impairment in addition to frequency dependent manipulation of the broadband input signal for noise reduction, for example. Thus, the first function performed by the digital signal processor is a frequency analysis of the signal. The wideband input signal is separated into frequency bands, typically done with a bank of filters or a Fast Fourier Transform (FFT). The filter bank is characterized by the number of output channels, the crossover frequencies between the channels, and the steepness of the filter slopes. The more frequency channels, and the steeper the filter slopes are, the finer the control of the signal manipulation in later processing can be. The frequency response function is adjusted by the gain in the frequency channels, allowing for an individualized compensation for a hearing loss.

Dynamic Range Compression

Background

A characteristic of sensorineural hearing loss is reduced dynamic range, which is the intensity range between threshold sensitivity and the loudness discomfort level (LDL). The general goal of a hearing instrument is to amplify soft sounds until they are audible and to amplify loud sounds to be perceived as loud by the individual listener, but not to exceed the listener's LDL. The target amplification is based on a fitting rationale, which may be adapted from published literature, such as DSL m[I/O] (Scollie et al., 2005) or NAL-NL2 (Keidser, Dillon, Carter, & O'Brien, 2012), or it may be proprietary to an instrument's manufacturer.

To compensate for the reduced dynamic range, compression algorithms that automatically adjust the gain for different input levels are implemented. This adjustment is based on the level in individual frequency bands (Figure 7–17). Multichannel compression instruments are commonly used because the reduced dynamic range in most listeners with hearing impairment varies as a function of frequency. In the analog domain, this compression process would be equivalent to having a SPL meter in each frequency band and turning the gain trimmer according to

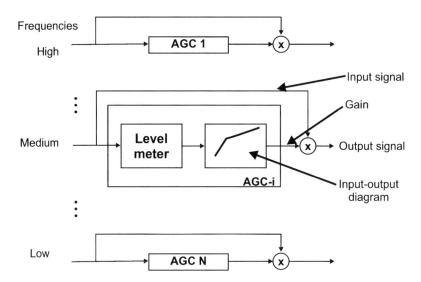

Figure 7–17. Block diagram of a multichannel compression system. Within each frequency channel, the measured input level is converted to a gain dependent on the input-output diagram adjusted for the specific frequency region. The gain is applied to the input signal.

the reading of the SPL meter in real time. For a summary of the research on multichannel compression systems see Braida, Durlach, De Gennaro, Peterson, and Bustamante (1982); Hickson (1994); and Moore (1995).

Settings

The basic setting of the automatic gain control of a dynamic range compression algorithm is characterized by four parameters: two parameters for the static input-output function and two parameters for the dynamic adjustments over time. Figure 7–18 shows an input-output diagram with linear amplification at low levels limited by microphone noise reduction described in a later section. Above the compression threshold, the compression system is active reducing the gain relative to linear amplification resulting in a shallower curve that is described by the compression ratio. The first parameter, the compression threshold, is that level where the shallower curve deviated by 2 dB from the linear amplification function (dashed line in Figure 7–18). The second parameter, the compression ratio, is the ratio between an input level difference to an output level difference and indicates the steepness of the compression curve. A higher compression ratio results in a shallower curve.

Figure 7–19 demonstrates the definition of the two other parameters according to ANSI S3.22. When increasing the level of a sinusoid at the input to a dynamic compression system from 55 to 90 dB and back, the output signal is also increased and reduced. Because of the temporal sluggishness of the system, the gain right after increase of the input signal is too high for 90 dB and has to be reduced. The attack time is defined as that time window starting at the increase of the input signal until the output signal has reached its stationary value for an input level of 90 dB except for a difference of 3 dB. The release time on the other hand is defined as that time window starting at the decrease of the input signal to 55 dB until the output signal has reached its stationary value for an input level of 55 dB except for a difference of 4 dB.

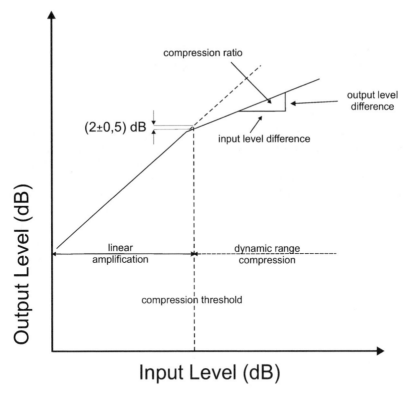

Figure 7–18. Input-output diagram for dynamic range compression. (From *Hearing Instrument Technology for the Hearing Healthcare Professional* (p. 62), by A. Vonlanthen, 2000, Florence, KY: Singular Publishing Group. Copyright 2000 by Singular Publishing Group. Adapted with permission.)

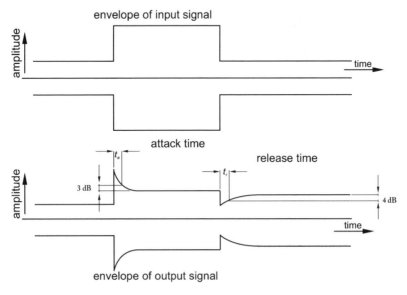

Figure 7–19. Envelope of the input signal with stepwise amplitude modification (*top*) and the respective envelope of the output signal (*bottom*) indicating the definition of the attack and release time. (From *Hearing Instrument Technology for the Hearing Healthcare Professional* (p. 63), by A. Vonlanthen, 2000, Florence, KY: Singular Publishing Group. Copyright 2000 by Singular Publishing Group. Adapted with permission.)

Typically, there are three main approaches to compression in hearing aids (Moore, 1990):

1. Compression limiting is implemented with high compression thresholds, high compression ratios, and short time constants. In this way, the amplification at high levels is restricted.
2. As a means to replace the volume control, automatic volume control (AVC) implements a low compression threshold, low-to-medium compression ratios, and long time constants.
3. Syllabic compression utilizes a low compression threshold, low-to-medium compression ratios, and short time constants to adjust the gain for different speech syllables.

Temporal Behavior

Next, we examine the temporal characteristics of dynamic compression. The time course of compression is characterized by the attack and release time as described. In general, there are two implementations of dynamic compression, syllabic compression and automatic volume control, which differ in their temporal behavior. For a complete review, see Dillon (1996).

The purpose of syllabic compression is to adjust different levels within the syllabic structure of the speech signal. Thus, the attack and release times are very short. With the short attack time, the level of the output signal is reduced quickly when a high input signal arrives. Likewise, with the short release time, the output signal quickly returns to the original level. One advantage of syllabic compression is that it can quickly reduce the gain when sudden loud sounds are presented. In addition, syllabic compression responds to level variations within the speech signal and reduces the dynamic range, which may be advantageous for individuals with a narrow dynamic range. A final advantage is quick recovery from gain reduction when a loud signal is no longer present. The disadvantage of syllabic compression is that the variations within speech are reduced, which might result in poorer speech intelligibility (Plomp, 1988).

Automatic volume control (AVC) has relatively long attack and release times compared with syllabic compression. Consequently, fast changes in the amplitude of the input signal are better preserved because adjustments to the output signal occur over a longer time course.

Whereas syllabic compression responds to the level variations within speech signals, the AVC responds only to the average speech level. This preserves the level variations within speech, which is one advantage over syllabic compression. On the other hand, the disadvantage of AVC is that the LDL may be exceeded because the reduction in gain is slower.

Panels A and B in Figure 7–20 show the effect of syllabic compression and AVC on a single sentence. The syllabic compression algorithm adjusts the signal amplitude in short time slices, increasing the gain during the soft sections and pauses in speech. The AVC algorithm adjusts the volume slowly over long time periods, and the fluctuations of the signal remain nearly unchanged from the original signal.

A compromise combining both compression algorithms is dual compression (Moore, Glasberg, & Stone, 1991). In this algorithm, short and long attack and release times are used depending on the level and time course of the input signal. The dual compression exploits the advantages of both compression procedures. A gain reduction with a short time constant reacts quickly to sudden, loud sounds. The gain quickly turns to the original level after the loud sound is over. Thus, a desired soft signal occurring after a loud sound is not affected. In contrast, if a criterion sound level is present for a longer time, the long time constants are activated. The gain of the hearing instrument is adjusted only to slow changes of the average input level, and the natural loudness variations in speech levels are preserved.

Percentile Analysis

For dual compression and also for other combinations of time constants, depending on

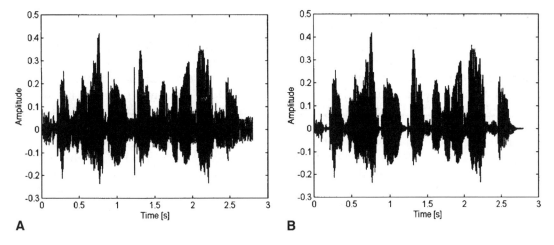

Figure 7–20. A. Effect of syllabic compression on a sentence. **B.** Effect of AVC on a sentence.

current and past input signals used in today's hearing aids, the simple measurement procedure for attack and release time based on level changes of a sinusoidal input is often not applicable. Therefore, fitting software tools offer the possibility of test settings that allow for running all measurements specified in ANSI S3.22. The results can be compared with the data sheet. Nevertheless, an interpretation of the results in respect to speech processing by the individual hearing aid is not possible.

Therefore, a new international standard was developed that describes an International Speech Test Signal (ISTS; Holube, Fredelake, Vlaming, & Kollmeier, 2010), a set of reference audiograms, and a new measurement procedure based on a percentile analysis. The ISTS is meant to be internationally applicable and acceptable since it is composed out of six different languages (Arabic, English, French, German, Mandarin, and Spanish) but shows all temporal and spectral characteristics of one single female speaker. The goal is to apply this signal for measurements in a test box or during probe microphone testing with the hearing aid being in a normal real-world setting with noise reduction and other adaptive algorithms turned on. The result of the measurement is the frequency dependent gain for speech based on the percentile analysis. This analysis is derived by fragmenta-

tion of the ISTS at the input and the output of the hearing aid in time windows with durations of 125 ms in ⅓-octave bands. Speech is a dynamic signal with constantly changing levels. Therefore, the level of each time window will be different from the previous window. The distribution of the levels is used to identify the 30th, 65th, and 99th percentile in dB SPL, indicating the percentage of time windows below the respective level, (e.g., the 65th percentile denotes that level where 65% of all time windows are below and 35% are above). Therefore, the 30th percentile represents the soft parts of speech, and the 99th percentile represents the speech peaks. The percentile analysis is done for the input signal to the hearing aid as well as for its output signal. When comparing the percentiles, gain of the hearing aid can be calculated frequency specific for the soft, medium, and loud parts of speech.

The analysis can also be used to estimate the compression of speech by the hearing instrument. The difference between the 99th and the 30th percentile can be regarded as the dynamic range of speech and is roughly 30 dB at the input to the hearing aid. When comparing this value to the same difference at the output of the hearing instrument, an effective compression ratio for speech can be estimated. This effective compression depends strongly on the active time constants of the compression system. An AVC shows a lower effective compression ratio than syllabic compression even for the same static input output function. Figure 7–21 gives sample results for a simple dynamic compression algorithm with an attack time of 5 ms and a release time of 20 ms (A) and 1000 ms (B). Both results were derived with the same compression ratio for sinusoids of 4:1. The effective compression of the ISTS can be estimated by subtracting the lower limit of the dark gray area (30th percentile) from the upper limit of the light gray area (99th percentile). The difference is smaller in the left panel indicating more compression for the shorter release time than for the right panel derived with the longer release time. Because many of today's hearing instruments use long time constants in listening environments containing speech, the effective compression ratio of speech is typically much smaller than the compression ratio measured with sinusoids and given in the fitting software of the manufacturer.

Reduction of Distortions

As discussed earlier, increasing the number of bits in the A/D converter increases the dynamic range, the size, and the power consumption. Thus, the number of bits is typically reduced to 16. With 16 bits, the dynamic range of the A/D converter is smaller than the dynamic range of the acoustic input signals and the dynamic range of the microphone. To avoid distortions at high input levels, the dynamic range of the input signals is restricted with a high-level compressor. This compressor system has a high compression threshold (e.g., 90 dB) and a high compression ratio (e.g., 10:1). With this high-level compression, input signals up to 110 dB SPL can be processed with minimal distortion.

In conventional analog hearing instruments, the output level of the device was normally restricted by peak clipping, resulting in high distortions of the output signal. In digital hearing instruments, the upper level of the device is restricted by the highest digital number that can be represented by the available number of bits. When the amplification of the hearing instruments exceeds this number, distortions will be audible. The sound quality of these digital distortions is worse than the distortions resulting from peak clipping in analog hearing instruments. Therefore, it is important that an output com-

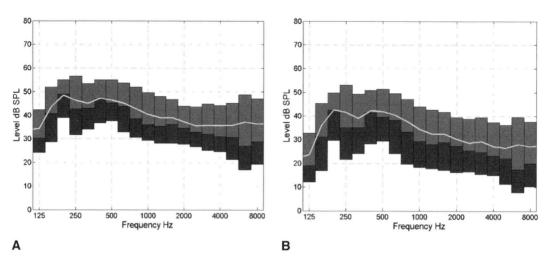

A   **B**

Figure 7–21. A. Percentile analysis for speech at the output of a dynamic compression algorithm with an attack time of 5 ms and a release time of 20 ms. **B.** Same as **A** but with a release time of 1000 ms. The upper limit of the light gray area denotes the 99th percentile, the border between light gray and dark gray denotes the 65th percentile, and the lower limit of the dark gray area denotes the 30th percentile. The white lines give the long-term average speech spectrum.

pression algorithm is also incorporated into digital hearing instruments.

The high-level compressor at both the input and the output compressor have short time constants. The gain must be reduced quickly when loud sounds occur, and the gain must be increased quickly after loud sounds diminish to maintain speech intelligibility.

User Benefit

A primary goal of dynamic compression algorithms is normalization of loudness perception, which can be measured with loudness scaling procedures (e.g., Allen, Hall, & Jeng, 1990; Cox, Alexander, Taylor, & Gray, 1997; Pascoe, 1978). The result of a theoretical loudness scaling procedure is shown in Figure 7–22. For this procedure, listeners are asked to rate the loudness of narrow-band noise on a categorical scale (inaudible, very soft, soft, medium, loud, very loud, too loud). This categorical scale was converted into a numerical scale from 0 to 50 categorical units (CU). Zero CU corresponded to inaudible, and 50 CU corresponded to too loud. A linear function was fit to the loudness ratings for different input levels and defined by two

parameters: the slope and the zero crossing. The zero crossing of this function is an estimation of threshold. The slope and threshold can be used to compare different loudness scaling between listeners with normal hearing and listeners with hearing-impairment and between aided and unaided conditions.

In Figure 7–23, the average slope of the loudness scaling function of 21 listeners with high-frequency hearing loss is shown at 500, 1000, 2000, and 4000 Hz in unaided and aided

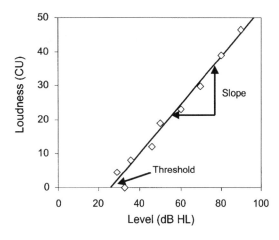

Figure 7–22. Loudness scaling function.

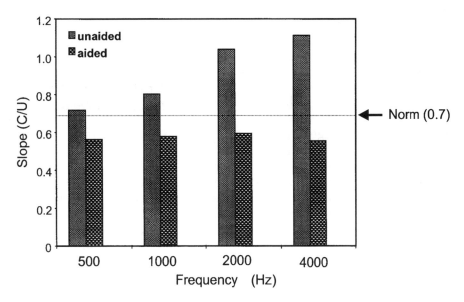

Figure 7–23. Slope of loudness scaling as a function of signal frequency in unaided and aided conditions.

condition. For the unaided condition, the slope increases with increasing frequency. This result is expected because recruitment in the presence of high-frequency hearing loss increases with frequency. When fit with a digital hearing instrument with dynamic compression, the slope differs from the unaided condition dramatically. The aided slope is essentially normalized for all frequencies. The slope of the loudness scaling function of normal-hearing listeners is shown as norm and is independent of the frequency.

Frequency Compression

The right amount of amplification at high frequencies is still under discussion. Fitting formulae based on loudness normalization ask for a high amount of high frequency amplification whereas hearing aid users are often not used to high frequency sounds for decades and criticize a sharp sound quality. In addition, the amount of high-frequency gain is technically limited due to feedback from the hearing aid receiver to the microphone resulting in a nasty whistling sound described later in this chapter. On the other hand, the benefit of high frequency gain for speech intelligibility might be limited for some patients (see e.g., Hogan & Turner, 1998), which is often related to dead regions in the cochlear (see e.g., Baer, Moore, & Kluk, 2002). Several attempts had been made in the past to shift high frequency information to lower frequencies to assure audibility for speech information and to improve speech intelligibility. Simpson (2009) gives an overview of different approaches. In the past, the success was mostly limited mainly because of destruction of inherent speech characteristics.

One algorithm that seems to overcome the drawbacks uses frequency compression, which is illustrated in Figure 7–24. Low frequency information is preserved while high frequencies above a certain cutoff frequency are compressed, that is, higher frequencies are shifted to lower frequencies. This is illustrated in Figure 7–24 by the shallower line

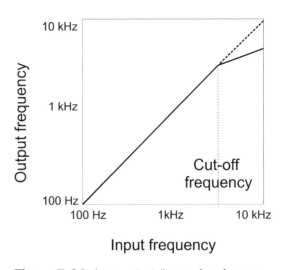

Figure 7–24. Input-output diagram for a frequency compression algorithm. (From S. Launer, 2011, personal communication. Copyright by Phonak AG, 2010. Adapted with permission.)

above the cutoff frequency. Simpson, Hersbach, and McDermott (2005) and also other research groups have investigated this frequency compression algorithm and found improvements for speech intelligibility in quiet. Nevertheless, the benefit seems to be dependent on the hearing loss and the phonemes relevant in the speech test as well as the adjustment of the algorithm parameters that are the cutoff frequency and the compression ratio.

Single-Microphone Noise Reduction

Introduction

Individuals with hearing impairment often report that speech is difficult to understand in listening situations when background noise is present. In the past, a variety of programmable circuits has been developed and evaluated that attempt to improve performance in this difficult listening environment (see e.g., Chung [2004] and Bentler & Chiou [2006] for a review). These circuits have met with varying degrees of success, both in reports of patients' benefit and satisfaction and in terms of commercial success.

In this section, we limit our discussion to digital processing strategies that can be used to tackle the problem of unwanted background noise with a single microphone. Multimicrophone hearing aids have demonstrated that they are an effective solution for improving the signal to noise ratio and thus, improving speech intelligibility in noisy listening environments. A discussion of the design and benefits of multi-microphone directional hearing instruments is reported in the next section.

The introduction of digital hearing instruments has led to the development of unique signal processing that provides advantages over analog instruments. Several manufacturers have introduced signal processing algorithms that detect speech and noise independently and process the two types of signals differently. While the underlying algorithms of these systems may vary, the expected result is the same: improved user listening comfort but only slightly or no improved speech intelligibility in background noise. Additional algorithms identify internal sources of noise, such as microphone noise, and minimize its effects when the user is in a quiet environment. The first algorithm described below is a method of identifying speech and noise based on their modulation spectrum and applying digital control logic to reduce the level of the noise. Second, we discuss an algorithm that filters background noise based on its estimated spectrum. The next two algorithms focus on the detection

and reduction of impulse noise and wind noise. Finally, we review an algorithm that has been found successful in reducing the effects of internal microphone noise.

Modulation-Based Noise Reduction Algorithms

Two important goals in fitting hearing instruments are improving speech intelligibility in noise for individuals with hearing impairment by improving the SNR and improving the quality of the overall signal to make listening more comfortable. One processing strategy that attempts to improve the quality of speech employs the modulation spectrum (Powers, Holube, & Wesselkamp, 1999). In this scheme, the speech and noise are identified according to rules based on the fluctuations of their respective amplitude envelopes. Once identified, the negative impact of the noise can be reduced through frequency-specific gain reduction.

The audible frequency range we typically consider is from 20 Hz to 20 kHz. Auditory signals are some composite of frequencies within that range. Figure 7–25 shows a 1-second segment of a sinusoidal signal. For this signal, the maxima are the same amplitude throughout the sinusoid. When the maxima of the signal change over time, the signal is referred to as amplitude modulated, and this is illustrated by the waveform labeled *A* in Figure 7–26.

The wave form that is defined by the maxima of the sinusoid is called the envelope of the signal, depicted by the wave form

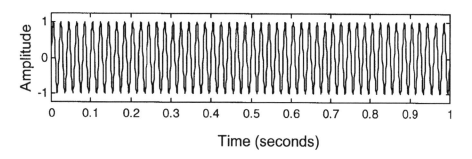

Figure 7–25. Sinusoidal signal.

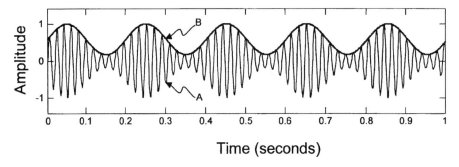

Figure 7–26. Sinusoid modulated at 5 Hz.

labeled B in Figure 7–26. The rate of the change in the signal envelope is the modulation frequency. In this example, the modulation frequency is 5 Hz. Note the modulation frequency is always much lower in value than the original signal frequency.

A sample of speech is shown in Figure 7–27. Typically, the spectrum of speech shows frequency components between 60 Hz and 10 kHz. In addition to the time wave form, this speech signal can be described by its envelope or modulation of the signal amplitude.

The phonemes, syllables, words, sentences, and pauses of speech determine the "envelope" of speech. A human speaker can normally articulate about 12 phonemes, 5 syllables, or 2.5 words per second. A typical sentence is several seconds in duration. The envelope of speech shows a characteristic temporal behavior independent of the speaker or the spoken language. The envelope is an intrinsic and well-defined feature of the speech signal. The importance of the speech envelope has received increasing attention in the speech perception and speech recognition literature (e.g., Drullman, Festen, & Plomp, 1994; Houtgast & Steeneken, 1985). It is only with the advent of the digital signal processing in hearing instruments that this feature has been able to be used to the benefit of the listener with hearing impairment.

The fluctuations of the speech signal envelope define the signal modulation. The envelope is characterized by the modulation frequency and the modulation depth of a sig-

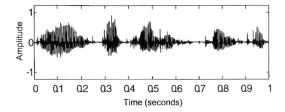

Figure 7–27. Speech signal of a female speaker.

nal. The modulation frequency is defined by the rate of change of the fluctuations. Twelve phonemes per second correspond to a modulation frequency of 12 Hz. Syllables yield a modulation frequency of 5 Hz; words yield a modulation frequency of 2.5 Hz, and sentences a modulation frequency of 0.3 Hz. The modulation depth is the difference between the maxima and the minima of the envelope. The modulation depth of speech is maximum during speech pauses when the signal value is zero.

The modulation spectrum is a plot, which graphically illustrates the relative modulation as a function of the modulation frequency of a signal. Figure 7–28 shows the modulation spectrum calculated from speech of a female speaker (see Ostendorf, Hohmann, & Kollmeier, 1997). In this example, we see the greatest modulation occurring between 3 and 4 Hz.

Plomp (1983) calculated the average modulation spectrum over different listeners. The result was a smoothed curve with a maximum around 3 to 4 Hz. Modulation frequencies of speech are present up to about 15 Hz. His figure is reproduced here as Figure 7–29.

Typically, the modulation spectra for speech and noise are distinctly different. The modulation spectrum of noise shows faster modulations, and thus the maximum modulation is seen at higher modulation frequencies. Figures 7–30 and 7–31 show the time structure of a jet engine noise and its modulation spectrum (Ostendorf et al., 1997). The envelope of the signal in Figure 7–30 does not show the slow fluctuations of the envelope of the speech-time wave form in Figure 7–27. Therefore, little energy is present at low modulation frequencies in the modulation spectrum in Figure 7–31. In this example, the maximum at modulation frequencies of around 30 to 60 Hz is the result of the faster fluctuations in the envelope.

This difference in the modulation spectrum between speech and noise can be used to detect speech and to reduce the noise in the signals. A reduction in noise can result in a more comfortable sound, a reduced listening effort, and increased speech intelligibility. In the application to hearing instruments, the envelope of the signals is analyzed in different frequency channels. If modulation frequencies characteristic of speech are detected (i.e., modulation frequencies of 1 to 12 Hz), the gain in the channel is kept constant. If

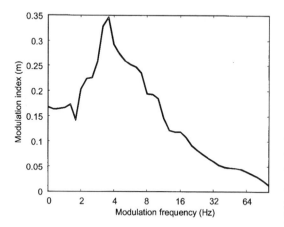

Figure 7–28. Modulation spectrum of a single sentence. (From "Signalverarbeitungsalgorithmen für digitale Hörgeräte" by I. Holube, 1998, *Zeitschrift für Audiologie, 37,* 177. Copyright 1998 by Median-Verlag. Adapted with permission.)

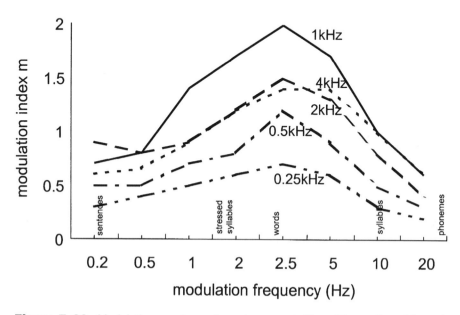

Figure 7–29. Modulation spectrum of running speech (From "Perception of Speech as a Modulated Signal" by R. Plomp, 1983, *Proceedings of the 10th International Congress of Phonetic Sciences.* Copyright by R. Plomp. Adapted with permission.)

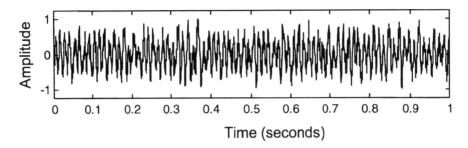

Figure 7–30. Time waveform of jet engine noise.

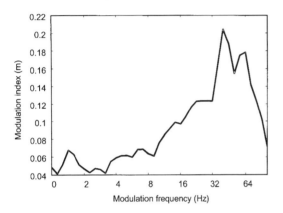

Figure 7–31. Modulation spectrum of jet engine noise. (From "Signalverarbeitungsalgorithmen für digitale Hörgeräte," by I. Holube, 1998, *Zeitschrift für Audiologie, 37*, 177. Copyright 1998 by Median-Verlag. Adapted with permission.)

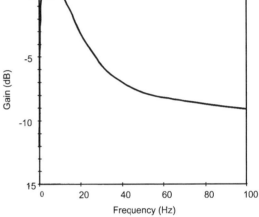

Figure 7–32. Gain reduction as a function of the modulation frequency in modulation-based noise reduction algorithm. (From "The Use of Digital Features to Combat Background Noise," by T. Powers, I. Holube, and M. Wesselkamp, 1999. *Hearing Review Supplement, High Performance Hearing Solutions. Hearing in Noise* (Vol. 3, pp. 36–39). Used with permission from the *Hearing Review*, http://www.hearingreview.com.)

modulation frequencies characteristic of speech are not present in the signal, the gain in that frequency channel is reduced.

The amount of gain reduction is dependent on the modulation frequencies and the modulation depths. Figure 7–32 depicts the change in gain in a given channel as a function of the detected modulation frequency. Figure 7–32 shows that the change in gain is minimal when the modulation frequency is low; with increasing modulation frequency, however, gain is increasingly reduced.

Figure 7–33 depicts the degree of gain reduction as a function of modulation depth. This figure shows that when the modulation depth is low, the reduction in gain is greatest. As the modulation depth increases, the reduction in gain decreases.

The time constant of the modulation detector refers to the duration required to examine the signal for modulation and return the answer to the processor. Recall that the modulation frequencies we are looking for can be as low as 2 Hz. The period of 2 Hz is 0.5 second. Thus, detection of 2 Hz requires a minimum of 0.5 second of sampling. To reliably examine the incoming signal for modulation, the signal processor requires several seconds. To avoid an audible "pumping" effect, the gain reduction should occur within

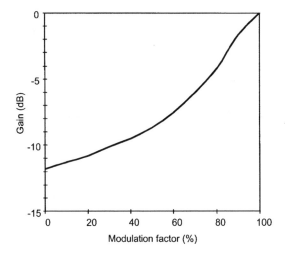

Figure 7–33. Gain reduction as a function of the modulation depth in modulation-based noise reduction algorithm. (From "The Use of Digital Features to Combat Background Noise," by T. Powers, I. Holube, and W. Wesselkamp, 1999. *Hearing Review Supplement, High Performance Hearing Solutions. Hearing in Noise* (Vol. 3, pp. 36–39). Used with permission from the *Hearing Review,* http://www.hearingreview.com.)

approximately 2 to 3 seconds of the onset of the noise signal. If speech is detected as the primary signal, as defined by the modulation spectrum within a given channel, gain should be quickly restored to the original gain values.

There may be some listening situations when a gain reduction is not desired. Some signals processed as "noise" by the hearing aid may indeed be viewed as a "desired signal" by the hearing aid user. One example is music. The modulation spectrum of music is different than the modulation spectrum of speech; therefore, the gain in the channels where the music is present will be reduced. For this type of situation, the hearing aid should deactivate the processing algorithm. This goal is reached by classification algorithms for hearing situations described later is this chapter.

The modulation spectrum provides an effective processing tool for distinguishing between speech and noise signals. In a multichannel system, incoming signals can be broken up into different frequency channels, allowing speech to be distinguished from disturbing noise in specific channels. The gain in the channels without modulations or with modulations at frequencies higher than typical for speech is reduced, reducing the overall noise contained within the complex signal. Presently, the modulation-based algorithms are combined with other noise reduction algorithms described in the next section.

Wiener Filter-Based Approaches

Advanced single channel noise reduction methods exploit the different stationary properties of desired signals, such as speech, and the nondesired noise (i.e., the degree to which the time wave forms of the signals are stationary). Well-established Wiener Filter (Boll, 1979) or related methods (Hänsler & Schmidt, 2004), like the Ephraim-Malah procedure (Ephraim & Malah, 1984, 1985), aim to reduce noise components that are modeled as being stationary longer than speech. This difference to speech concerning the stationary state is fulfilled for a large number of typical noise signals such as car, traffic, or vacuum cleaner noise.

A simplified setup of the Wiener filter is depicted in Figure 7–34. Speech and noise signals superimpose to a noisy signal. The desired output signal of the Wiener filter is an estimate of the clean speech signal.

If the speech and the noise signal are known, the Wiener filter can be calculated based on their respective spectra. In simple words, the Wiener filter attenuates the frequency components according to their SNR. The attenuation is higher, the lower the SNR is in the respective frequency band. For stationary signals (i.e., signals without time variations), the Wiener filter is constant and does not change over time. For nonstationary input signals such as speech, the Wiener filter has to be modified over time. The calculation of the Wiener filter requires estimates of the spectrum of the noisy input signal and of the noise spectrum itself. The input signal spectrum can be easily calculated based on the accessible input signal. The task for estimating the noise spectrum is challenging because the algorithm has to identify which components of the input signal are speech and which ones are noise.

One approach to estimate the noise spectrum is to smooth the input signal during speech pauses and to stop the estimation of the noise during speech activity. This method is based on the assumption that the noise spectrum changes slowly and can be assumed to be static during speech activities.

Alternative approaches for noise spectrum estimation, which do not require a voice activity detection and allow to track noise spectra coarsely also during speech activity,

are mainly based on the minimum statistics approach (Martin, 1994) and related derivatives (Martin, 2001). These approaches profit from the sparseness of speech in the time-frequency domain (i.e., even during speech activity most frequency components are not continuously excited by speech). In the short excitation pauses, the power of the respective frequency components is at a noise level that corresponds to the minimum level of a time frame. This is the prerequisite that such a minimum tracking results in good noise spectrum estimates. In Figure 7–35, the estimated input and noise signal are depicted.

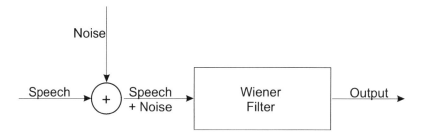

Figure 7–34. Noise reduction model and setup.

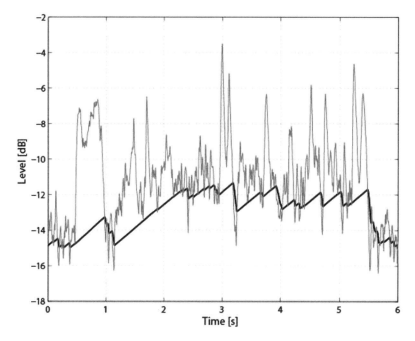

Figure 7–35. Estimated input signal (*gray*) and estimated noise signal (*black*).

The noise and input signal spectra, which are determined based on the procedures sketched above, exhibit different estimation variances due to the different estimation procedures. The estimation of the input signal shows a higher variance (stronger fluctuations over time) as it has to follow the varying speech signal, whereas the estimated noise signal shows a lower variance due to stronger smoothing and further processing such as the estimation stop during speech activity or minimum tracking.

The different estimation variances provoke a rather high variance of the Wiener filter. Accordingly, during pure noise, the Wiener filter varies strongly (Figure 7–36B, upper graph) and provokes tonal artificial noise that is known as "Musical Tones." One possibility to reduce the "Musical Tones" is to overestimate the noise spectrum according to Figures 7–36 and 7–37. The overestimation reduces the filter variance during frames including only noise because the filter generates a stronger attenuation.

Unfortunately low-power speech components are more strongly attenuated by the overestimation that results in a dull sound. A limitation of this unnatural sound is possible by placing a lower limit on the maximum noise reduction with a spectral floor. Of course this modification also limits the noise reduction performance. This means that when performing noise reduction, a balance between the natural sound and the noise reduction has to be found. Especially in hearing aids, it is very important to preserve the natural sound of the desired signal (Hamacher et al., 2005). This is even more important than obtaining a strong noise reduction. The main reason is that hearing impaired people wear hearing aids the whole day and are thus very sensitive to audio signal artifacts.

An example for the noise reduction with Wiener filtering is shown by the comparison of the input and output signal spectra shown in Figure 7–38.

A significant number of studies have investigated the effect of single microphone noise reduction algorithms. A typical result is given by Ricketts and Hornsby (2005). They did not demonstrate a significant improvement in speech intelligibility but proved a subjective preference of signals with noise reduction turned on.

Reduction of Impulse Noise Sources

Short impulsive sounds, such as dish clattering, are annoying for hearing aid users since they typically exhibit a short-term, very high power, but their amplification is not reduced by dynamic compression. The reason is that even time constants that are known as "short" in the context of dynamic compression are too long to compress very short impulses.

The target of the algorithm described in this section is to attenuate impulsive sounds to a comfortable level. It is explicitly not the goal to completely remove transient sounds because they contribute to a natural perception of the acoustic environment. An important constraint is that the algorithm does not harm speech, especially not speech onsets.

As the typical single source noise reduction algorithms described previously, the impulsive signal noise reduction setup also has to rely on different properties of speech and noise concerning stationarity. In this case, the impulsive noise components are regarded as being less stationary than speech. The impulsive noise components, which should be attenuated, show onsets of a few milliseconds. Speech signals in contrast exhibit longer onset periods and can be well modeled to be short-term stationary for frames of 20 to 30 ms.

The algorithm to solve the above described impulsive noise reduction first analyses the signal onsets, detects transient noise components, and then applies an appropriate attenuation. For the detection unit and the routine to calculate the attenuation, several criteria are evaluated: onset time, duration of the onset components, the absolute power of the onset components, and their relative power with respect to the mean power of the current input signal. The detection and the calculation of the impulsive noise reduction are performed in several frequency bands, according to Figure 7–39.

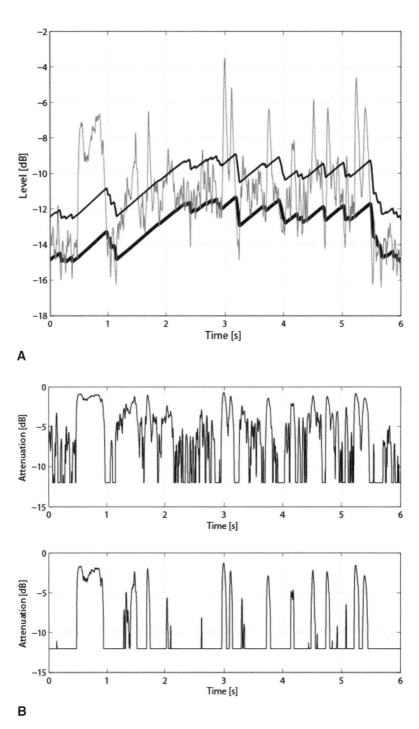

Figure 7–36. A. Noise estimation without (*bold black*) and with (*thin black*) overestimation. **B.** Calculated filter coefficients for the frequency components at 500 Hz without (*top*) and with (*bottom*) overestimation. One observes the severely reduced filter fluctuations during speech pauses.

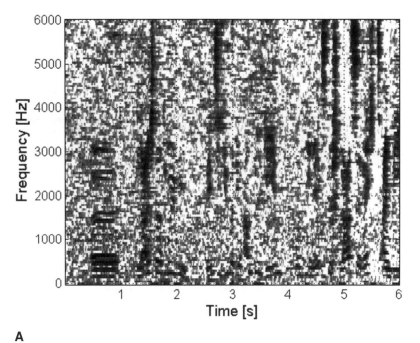

A

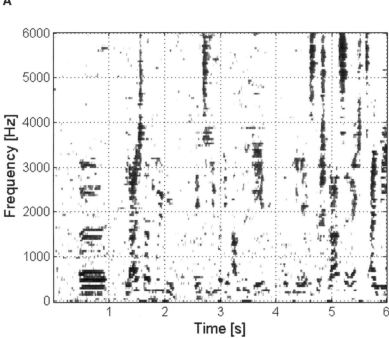

B

Figure 7–37. A. Time-frequency dependent noise reduction filter coefficients, without overestimation. **B.** Same as *A*, but with overestimation. One can well observe that the overestimation strongly reduces the filter coefficient variance during speech pauses.

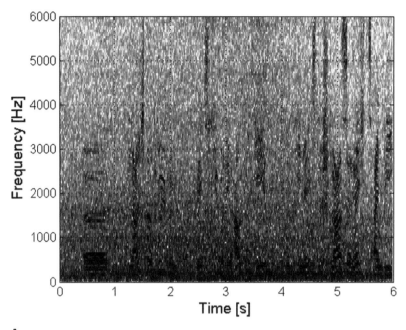

A

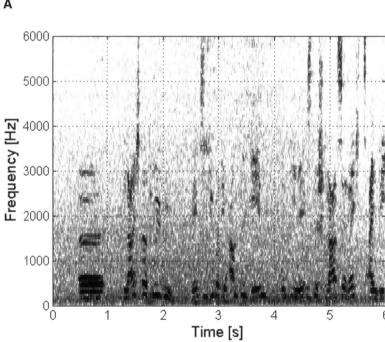

B

Figure 7–38. **A.** Spectrogram of a noisy input signal. **B.** Output signal after noise reduction. The noise floor is reduced whereas the power of the speech components is kept.

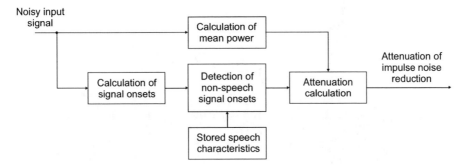

Figure 7–39. Block diagram of the impulsive noise reduction procedure.

Here, two up to eight frequency bands are sufficient. A stronger frequency resolution would harm the time resolution that is necessary for an appropriate impulsive noise reduction. First, the envelope and the mean signal power values are calculated. Comparing the signal envelopes or onsets, respectively, with typical speech envelope characteristics allows to detect transient noise signals.

Only when impulsive components have been detected based on nonspeech onsets, attenuation is applied. The attenuation has to be chosen appropriately in order to preserve a natural sound of the processed signal. Here, the duration and the strength of the attenuation are the two key values.

The attenuation time has to be chosen to suppress the complete signal impulse. A too short attenuation would only target the first part of the impulse and lead to an unnatural reverberant sound impression. On the other hand, the attenuation should not be too long, either. This could provoke a perceived attenuation of the complete acoustic environment. The solution to this problem is—once transient signal components have been detected—to observe the falling signal slopes and to compare its power with the longer term smoothed mean input signal power.

When designing such impulsive noise reduction algorithms, binaural aspects also have to be considered with the target to preserve at least roughly the localization of the attenuated impulsive sounds. Nonfrontal noise pulses are typically perceived louder at one ear, which allows their localization based on the inter-aural level differences (ILDs). After the application of the impulsive noise reduction at both ears, a loudness difference should be preserved that allows to keep the localization of the attenuated signals.

A binaural synchronization of the applied noise attenuation with the result of applying the same attenuation on both hearing aids would solve the problem. However, the binaural synchronization is rather demanding concerning the data rate that has to be transmitted between the hearing aids. The reason is the fast changing impulsive noise attenuation that does not allow a remarkable subsampling (i.e., a conversion to a lower sampling rate for data reduction purposes) of the calculated noise reduction values before the transmission. The solution to this problem is to preserve a certain amount of the signal level differences after the noise reduction.

In Figure 7–40, the spectrograms of a speech signal superimposed with impulse noise and the signal after noise reduction are depicted. The reduction of the impulse components can be well observed.

Many studies have been performed to evaluate the performance of the impulsive noise reduction algorithms. Two main criteria have been considered for the evaluation:

■ Influence on speech intelligibility and
■ User preferences

Speech intelligibility is a consideration because a signal attenuation is always related to the risk of attenuating speech components,

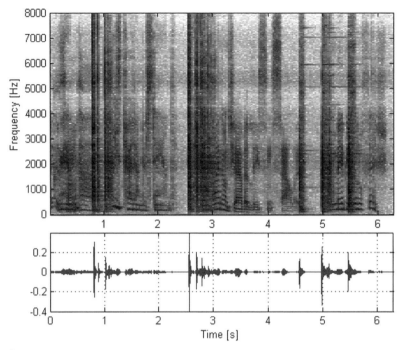

A

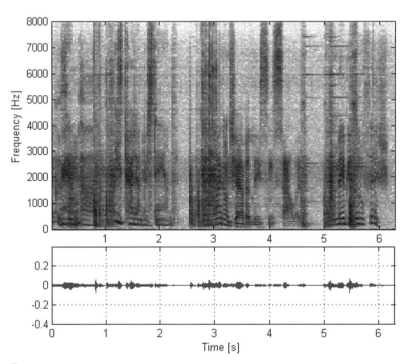

B

Figure 7–40. A. Spectrogram of the noisy input signal. **B.** Spectrogram of the output signal after impulsive noise reduction. Below the time sampled signals are depicted, respectively.

particularly speech onsets, and thereby reducing speech intelligibility. However, tests (Ricketts & Hornsby, 2005) proved the design of the algorithm effective and the possibility to attenuate impulsive noise components without influencing speech onsets: no reduction of speech intelligibility was observed, as shown in Figure 7–41. Concerning the preference, a clear preference of the processed signals has been observed as shown in Figure 7–42.

Wind Noise Reduction

Wind noise is a fluctuating, often high-intensity and low-frequency noise. It occurs when wind blows across the hearing aid microphones in windy environments (e.g. near the sea, when riding bicycles, or during fast walks). For hearing aid users, this kind of noise is typically very annoying. If it occurs during the presence of speech, speech intelligibility is typically severely reduced.

The technical explanation for the occurrence of wind noise is that wind blows across the hearing aid membrane, which is then randomly excited. Typical mechanical wind protection like cotton wool in the mic port can

be used for microphones larger than those in hearing aids. The random and statistically independent excitation of the microphones

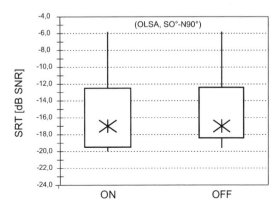

Figure 7–41. Comparison of speech intelligibility (Speech Reception Threshold, SRT) measurements with and without impulsive noise reduction. As desired, the speech intelligibility is not reduced due to impulsive noise attenuation. (From "A novel approach to reduce transient noise in hearing aids: Technical concept and perceptual evaluation," by V. Hamacher, E. Fischer, and M. Latzel, 2006, International Hearing Aid Research Conference, Lake Tahoe, CA. Copyright 2006 by V. Hamacher. Adapted with permission.)

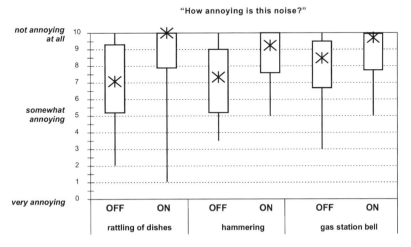

Figure 7–42. Comparison of subjective preference of different impulsive noise sounds with and without impulsive noise reduction. A clear preference of the noise reduced signals can be observed. (From "A novel approach to reduce transient noise in hearing aids: Technical concept and perceptual evaluation," by V. Hamacher, E. Fischer, and M. Latzel, 2006, International Hearing Aid Research Conference, Lake Tahoe, CA. Copyright 2006 by V. Hamacher. Adapted with permission.)

is the basis for a technical solution in two-microphone hearing aid devices. Because nearly all BTE and a large number of ITE devices are equipped with two microphones, a two-microphone based solution targets a high percentage of hearing aid devices.

Analyses show that wind noise is completely uncorrelated at the hearing aid microphones even when they are located closely together, which is in contrast with the acoustic input signals. The latter ones show a very high correlation, even for diffuse acoustic environments. These different correlation properties allow both:

■ A reliable and fast detection of wind noise and
■ Possibilities to determine an appropriate attenuation of wind noise.

In the following, two different possibilities for wind noise detection are sketched. The first is based on the "correlation coefficient" and the second on the "power ratio." Both are explained in the following.

The correlation coefficient describes the similarity between two signals and exhibits values between 0 and 1. For a high correlation, the correlation coefficient shows values near 1 and for a low correlation values near 0. Wind noise with a typical strong signal power for low frequencies cause a low correlation coefficient. A comparison with a certain threshold allows for reliable and fast wind noise detection. A smoothing of the parameter allows for a balance between detection reliability and detection speed.

The power ratio is the ratio between the difference and the sum of the two input signals, and is a frequency dependent quantity. In the case of uncorrelated signals, the power ratio shows values close to the maximum value one, whereas it is severely reduced for correlated audio input signals as shown in Figure 7–43. The power ratio can be utilized to detect wind noise and to determine an appropriate wind noise attenuation. The latter is explained in the following section.

Because the power ratio is frequency dependent, also a frequency dependent detection is theoretically possible. However, typically a frequency independent detection is determined based on a combination of the power ratio values in each frequency band. This approach allows to increase the reliability of the detection. When wind is detected based on the above criterion, a frequency dependent gain is calculated based on the frequency dependent power ratio.

Before, two different criteria have been introduced to detect wind: The frequency independent correlation coefficient and the frequency dependent power ratio. Both can also be utilized to calculate an appropriate attenuation of wind noise.

Once wind has been detected based on the correlation coefficient, this value can be used to set up a simple wind noise reduction approach. Here a high-pass filter is used to attenuate typically low-frequency components of wind noise. The strength or shape of the high-pass filter can be chosen according to the correlation coefficient as depicted in Figure 7–44.

The advantage of this approach is that it is rather robust because it is based on a single value, which typically indicates wind rather reliably. The disadvantage, however, is that is not possible to calculate a frequency variable attenuation.

When target signal components and wind noise are present at the same time, the correlation coefficient only allows for a mean and compromised attenuation. However, a frequency dependent attenuation would allow more effective attenuation of wind and preservation of speech by specifically attenuating frequency components according to their speech-to-wind noise ratio. Such a frequency dependent calculation, described next, is possible with the frequency dependent power ratio.

The power ratio is frequency dependent and allows for a calculation of a frequency variable gain. A simple and efficient method is to use the inverse of the normalized power ratio to determine the wind noise reduction with a lower bound to limit the noise reduction effect and the upper limit 1. The upper limit is 1 (no attenuation) and the lower limit

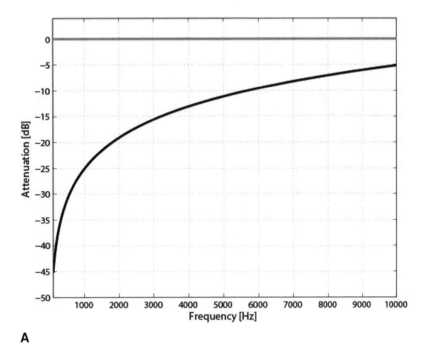

A

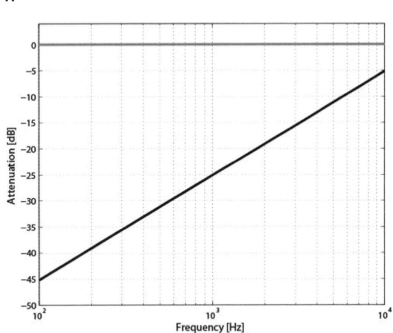

B

Figure 7–43. A. Frequency response of the power ratio for uncorrelated input signals such as wind noise (*gray*) and for correlated signals (*black*), on a linear frequency scale. **B.** Same as *A* but on a logarithmic frequency scale.

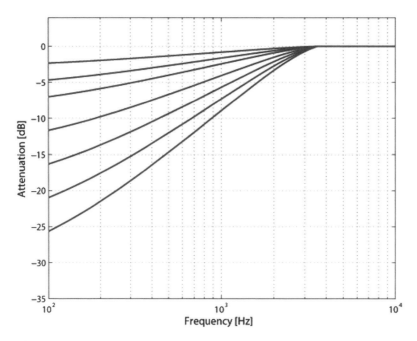

Figure 7–44. Fixed high-pass-shaped wind noise attenuation based on the correlation coefficient.

should be chosen appropriately in order not to disturb desired signal components. This approach allows one to determine for each frequency band an optimal attenuation that allows the best compromise between wind noise attenuation and speech signal preservation. Figure 7–45 gives an example of a spectrogram affected with wind noise and the output signal after applying wind noise reduction.

In Figure 7–46, the block diagrams of both systems, based on the correlation coefficient and on the power ratio, are shown. One can well see that both systems consist of a unit to detect wind and a block to calculate the appropriate wind noise attenuation. In the system based on the correlation coefficient, a single value selects the strength of a high-pass filter, whereas in the power ratio based system, an individual and optimized gain in each frequency band is calculated.

Microphone Noise Reduction

Modern hearing aids use low-noise microphones. Nevertheless, microphone noise, typically described as an unwanted constant

hissing in the hearing aid, would still trouble many hearing instrument users if the microphone noise would not be lowered by an appropriate algorithm. In today's hearing aids, microphone noise is only about 20 dB, but in quiet environments, this can be noticeable for people with hearing thresholds at or near normal for some frequency regions. This complaint could be observed most frequently when minimal venting is used, as this low-level noise cannot escape from the ear canal.

If we consider the input signals to the hearing aid amplifier, we note that both, the input signal to the microphone and microphone noise are present. In most listening environments, the microphone noise will not be audible to the hearing aid user because it is masked when a typically louder input signal is present. Unfortunately, microphone noise may be audible in other mostly quiet situations when no masking signal is present.

Microphone noise reduction is achieved using a squelch function, or a reduction of gain, using nonlinear processing of signals that have intensities below a certain level. If the intensity of the input signal to the micro-

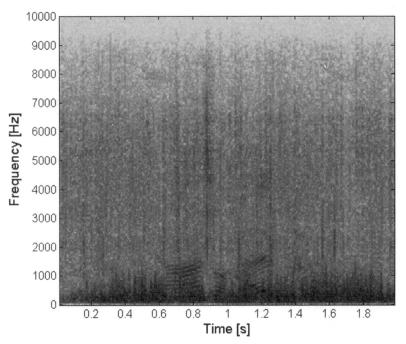

A

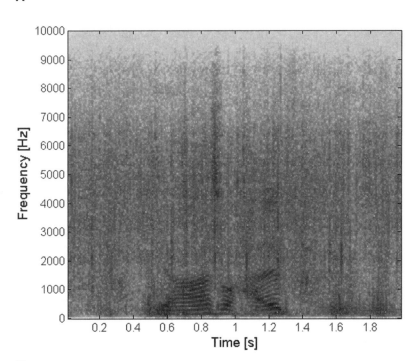

B

Figure 7–45. A. Spectrogram before wind noise reduction. **B.** Spectrogram after wind noise reduction.

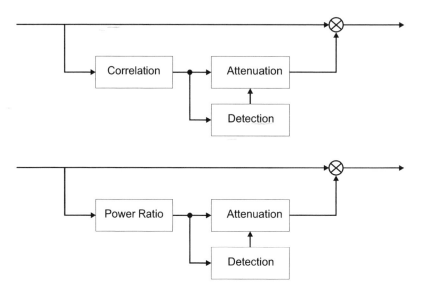

Figure 7–46. Block diagrams of both wind noise reduction approaches described in this section. Above the approach based on the correlation coefficient is shown, and below the approach based on the frequency dependent power ratio.

phone is below a set value, the microphone noise reduction, or squelch, is engaged.

The signal processor continuously monitors intensity of the input signal in each channel of the hearing aid. If the intensity of a signal is below the squelch threshold, the gain of that channel is reduced. The signal processing reduces the remaining low-level microphone noise below the patient's threshold. If the hearing instrument user moves from the quiet environment to one with higher intensity background noise or useful signals, the microphone noise reduction function releases within a short time constant, and the original gain in the channel is returned. Because of the short release time, the user does not miss any components of the useful signal, yet can enjoy a quiet environment.

Multi-Microphone Noise Reduction

Introduction

The algorithms for noise reduction described so far are not able to distinguish between desired and undesired speech signals because most often, the speech one wants to hear and the speech one does not want to hear the same spectrum and the same time structure. Therefore, these algorithms have no benefit in so-called cocktail party situations. To provide benefit in these difficult situations, other options are necessary.

Multi-microphone noise reduction systems are an effective method for improving the intelligibility of speech in noisy situations. They act essentially as spatial noise reduction systems by enhancing the hearing instrument's sensitivity to sound from desired directions over sound from other directions. The sound from "other directions" is normally considered noise and is deemed as not desirable. The general goal of the multi-microphone systems is to improve the SNR.

Directional Microphone Systems

While audibility of the primary signal is essential, SNR (expressed in dB), determines overall intelligibility. Directional microphones, with a primary design aimed at enhancing the SNR, nearly always yield improvements in intelligibility (see e.g., Mueller & Wesselkamp, 1999; Wolf, Hohn, Martin, & Powers, 1999).

Omnidirectional microphones utilize a single microphone and single sound inlet and are equally sensitive to sound from all directions. Directional microphones also utilize a single microphone with two sound inlets and an acoustic damper to shift the phase or to introduce an internal time delay, respectively. In hearing instruments with two omnidirectional microphones, the outputs of the two separate microphones are coupled with time delay and subtraction components. Figure 7–47 shows a block diagram of a possible calculation procedure. Sound inputs to the two microphones differ by an external time delay due to sound traveling from one microphone to the other. The input signal to one microphone is delayed by an internal time delay before both input signals are subtracted. The final stage of the algorithm is a low-pass filter to compensate for the high-pass filter effect comprised in the delay-and-subtract procedure.

Specific directional patterns are determined by the exact values of the time delay corresponding to the microphone distance and the internal time delay. The directionality of a microphone, as shown on a polar plot, can be modified by changing the time delays internally between the two microphones. Figure 7–48 shows the polar plots of different ratios between external and internal time delays, Ti/Te, of the two microphones. In addition, the Directivity Index (DI) is shown. The DI characterizes the strength of the microphone directivity, relating the amplification for the frontal direction and the amplification to all other directions. It suggests the improvement in SNR that can be expected from a microphone system in a diffuse sound field. As can be seen in Figure 7–48, the

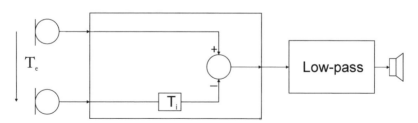

Figure 7–47. Block diagram of a delay-and-subtract algorithm used for directional filtering.

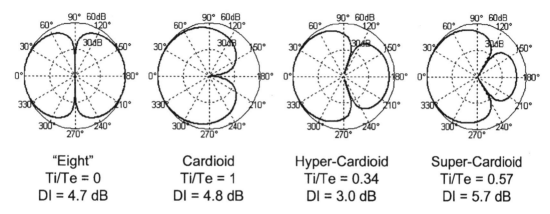

"Eight"	Cardioid	Hyper-Cardioid	Super-Cardioid
Ti/Te = 0	Ti/Te = 1	Ti/Te = 0.34	Ti/Te = 0.57
DI = 4.7 dB	DI = 4.8 dB	DI = 3.0 dB	DI = 5.7 dB

Figure 7–48. Polar plots and DIs for different ratios between internal and external delays in a two-microphone system.

hypercardioid gives the best directionality with a DI of 6 dB.

To achieve the 6 dB advantage in directivity with a two-microphone system, precise matching of the microphones in amplitude and phase is imperative. When a stronger directivity than 6 dB is desired, more than two microphones are necessary.

There is one important advantage of the two-microphone systems over conventional directional microphones. Because it is controlled electronically, the directional effect can be a programmable parameter that can be selected or deleted, depending on the user's needs, for different listening situations. It can even be adaptively steered in different frequency regions dependent on the direction of noise sources.

An alternative solution for a directional microphone implementation is shown in Figure 7–49, which was proposed by Elko and Pong (1995). Both input signals are time delayed and subtracted from each other, whereas a multiplication factor steers the desired polar pattern. This multiplication factor is more easily to handle during adaptive procedures when different polar patterns are required for the spatial directions of disturbing noise. This procedure is duplicated in several frequency channels (Figure 7–50)

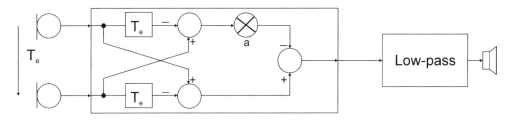

Figure 7–49. Block diagram of an alternative implementation of a directional microphone system.

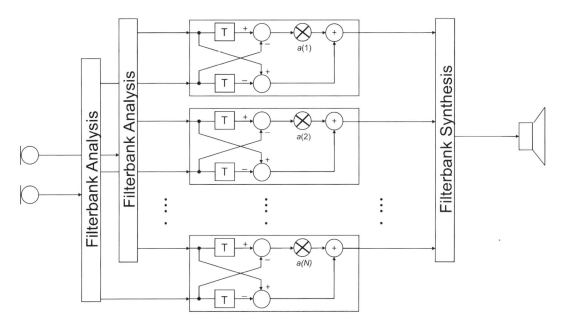

Figure 7–50. Block diagram of frequency dependent directional microphone algorithms.

to potentially reduce noise sources with different frequency content located in various spatial directions.

Figure 7–51 shows an example of a directionality pattern for a two-microphone system mounted to the right ear of the dummy head KEMAR with his nose facing to the top (0°). Compared with Figure 7–48, which shows the behavior in the free field, the KEMAR exhibits a considerable influence on the polar plots due to the head shadow effect. The largest amplification is achieved for signals from the front, whereas signals from the other directions are attenuated relative to the frontal direction.

Figure 7–52 shows results for microphone steering during an adaptive procedure. For the left side of panels A and B, a noise source was located at 120° on the right back side of the head. The source was located at 90° for the right side of both panels. The different colors indicate different frequencies.

Panel A illustrates that not all frequencies meet the target directions precisely. The variation is indicated with a V-notch. Frequency dependent microphone steering allows for a precise adjustment of the directionality pattern (see panel B of Figure 7–52).

Before we discuss the advantages of directional microphone systems, we have to take a look back to the block diagram in Figure 7–49. The last stage consists of a low-pass filter that compensates the high-pass characteristic of the system with a slope of 6 dB per octave. When we do so, the microphone noise spectrum sketched as a black solid line in Figure 7–53 is increased at low frequencies to the black dashed line. The gray line shows a typical spectrum of environmental noise. If the microphone noise is above the environmental noise, it might be detectable especially because hearing losses are typically small at low frequencies. One solution for this problem is to limit directionality at low frequencies.

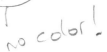

no color!

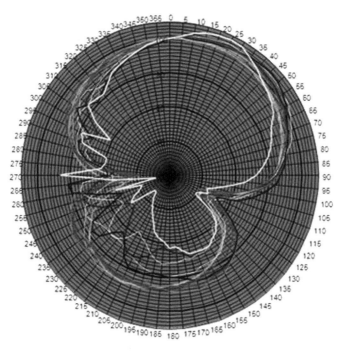

Figure 7–51. Directionality patterns of a two-microphone system mounted on the right ear of KEMAR.

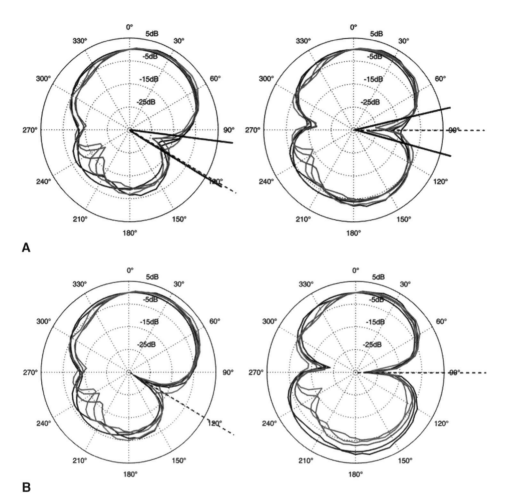

Figure 7–52. A. Directionality patterns for a noise source at 120° (*left*) and 90° (*right*) without frequency dependent microphone steering. **B.** Same as *A*, but with frequency dependent microphone steering.

The technical advantage of directional microphone systems was described above as directivity index. It is calculated from the attenuation of all directions in respect to the frontal direction as average over all frequencies. From the articulation index model, we know that the medium frequencies are most important for speech intelligibility. Therefore, the articulation index weighted directivity index AI-DI includes a respective weighting function into account as shown in Figure 7–54. This figure also gives the results for the AI-DI for an omnidirectional microphone mounted on a head as well as the AI-DI for a natural pinna. The head shadow effect results in an AI-DI for an omnidirectional microphone below, whereas the pinna shows a natural directivity of about 2 dB at high frequencies. The AI-DI of a directional microphone system is about 5 dB. This result is expected to be measured as advantage in SNR in speech tests in background noise.

User Benefit

The benefit of hearing instruments with a directional microphone characteristic has been shown in several studies. To briefly illus-

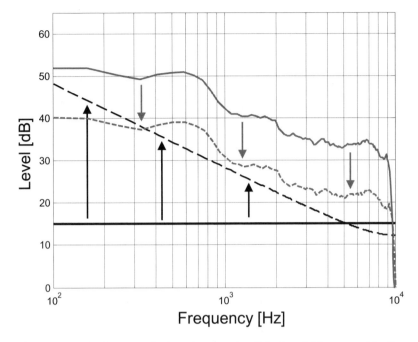

Figure 7–53. Spectra of microphone noise (*black solid*) increased by the low-pass filter of the directional microphone (*black dashed*) and environmental noise (*gray*).

trate the benefits of directional microphone technology, we review one study of speech intelligibility for a hearing instrument with a two microphone directional system in different settings conducted by Hamacher (2006).

The SNR for a speech intelligibility of 50% (speech reception threshold, SRT) was measured in two different situations. In both situations, speech was presented from the frontal direction in a test room with a reverberation time of 300 ms. Different loudspeakers were used to present background noise from various directions. In the first situation, babble noise was presented form 90°, 135°, 180°, and 270° with the loudspeakers oriented to the walls of the test room to simulate diffuse noise conditions. In the second situation, low-frequency traffic noise was presented from the back (180°), and a high-frequency noise, emitted by a food processor, was presented from the left and the right (90° and 270°). Hearing-impaired listeners were tested while the directional microphone system was

in the omnidirectional setting (SH-O), in a static-directional setting with fixed directivity pattern (SH-S) and in an adaptive directional mode (SH-A). The results for normal-hearing listeners (NH) are shown as comparison.

The SRT improves by about 5 dB when using the static directional microphone system compared with the omnidirectional setting. This threshold is not improved in the diffuse noise field (Figure 7–55A) when activating frequency dependent adaptation. Within this situation, noise is coming from all directions. Therefore, none of the directionality patterns improves the SNR over any of the other patterns. Striking is, that the hearing-impaired listeners are already as good as normal hearing listeners in this diffuse field condition. This is different in a directional noise field as shown in Figure 7–55B. The adaptive mode selects that directionality pattern, which attenuates the noise sources from the different directions at most in their respective frequency regions. The result is another

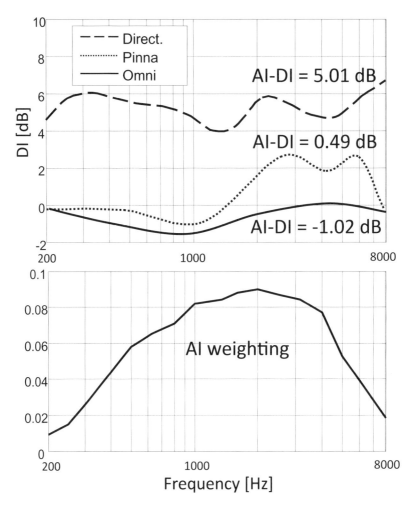

Figure 7–54. Articulation Index weighted directivity index AI-DI for a directional microphone system, the pinna, and an omnidirectional microphone mounted on a head (*top*) as well as the applied AI weighting (*bottom*).

improvement in SRT of about 2 dB. Normal-hearing listeners still have an advantage in background noise, which is demonstrated by their SRT, but some of the hearing impaired listeners are already in the same rage of SRTs when using the adaptive directional microphone system.

Classification systems described in another section of this chapter are able to steer the setting of the directional microphone system dependent on the listening situation. When this steering is done by both hearing aids independently of each other, one hearing aid might be in the directional mode, while the other hearing aid is in omnidirectional mode. The result might be a loss of SRT improvement. Figure 7–56 shows the results of a study conducted by Hornsby and Ricketts (2007). They have used a setting with five different loudspeakers from various directions. The SRT improvement by about 3.5 dB in this setting for directional mode in both hearing aids is reduced to less than 2 dB when one of the hearing aids is in omnidirectional mode. This result motivates for a communication link between the hearing aids,

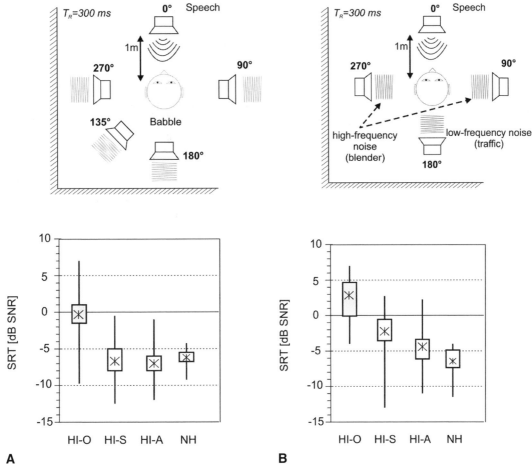

Figure 7–55. A. SRT for hearing-impaired listeners with hearing aid in omnidirectional (SH-O), static-directional (SH-S), and adaptive directional (SH-A) setting as well as for normal-hearing listeners in a diffuse noise field condition. **B.** Same as *A*, but in a directional frequency-dependent noise field. (From "Perzeptive Evaluierung von Methoden zur Sprachverbesserung in modernen digitalen Hörgeräten," by V. Hamacher, 2006, 7. ITG-Fachtagung Sprach-Kommunikation, Christian-Albrechts-Universität, Kiel, Germany. Copyright 2006 by V. Hamacher. Adapted with permission.)

which allows for a common agreement which the microphone setting might be appropriate in the respective listening situation.

Spatial Noise Reduction

In the previous sections, noise reduction procedures have been introduced, which address stationary and transient noise components. Speech as target signal and interfering noise are differentiated by different stationary

properties. Speech is less stationary than typical car or fan noise, whereas speech is more stationary than interfering transients such as the clattering of dishes. The disadvantage of both types of noise reduction is that they do not address interfering sounds with similar stationary properties as speech (e.g., cocktail party noise or all kinds of interfering speakers).

The target and concept of the spatial noise reduction is to utilize criterion other

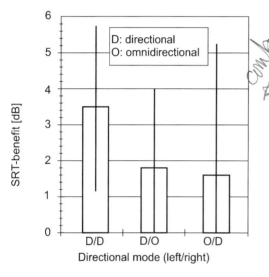

Figure 7–56. Test situation with five loudspeakers and SRT improvement for both hearing aids in directional mode (D/D), left hearing aid directional and right hearing aid directional (D/O), and vise versa (O/D). Data from Hornsby and Ricketts (2007). (From "Perzeptive Evaluierung von Methoden zur Sprachverbesserung in modernen digitalen Hörgeräten," by V. Hamacher, 2006, 7. ITG-Fachtagung Sprach-Kommunikation, Christian-Albrechts-Universität, Kiel, Germany. Copyright 2006 by V. Hamacher. Adapted with permission.)

than the stationary properties to differentiate between target and interfering signals: the direction of arrival. With this approach, the gap between stationary and transient noise reduction is closed. Now, it is possible to attenuate all kinds of noise independent of their stationary properties after the directional microphone system, the so-called beamformer.

The spatial noise reduction concept is still Wiener filter-based as is the stationary noise reduction. However, the power spectral density of the interference is calculated based on an additional beamformer combination of the two hearing aid microphones. A block diagram of the spatial noise reduction concept is shown in Figure 7–57.

Here, one can see that the output of the additional beamformer realizes a cardioid toward the back direction. This means that all nonfrontal signals are considered to be interference. The power of the output signal of the additional beamformer is taken as noise power reference for the Wiener filter-based spatial noise reduction.

For the overall system performance, an effective combination of spatial and stationary noise reduction is optimal. The attenuation for the stationary noise reduction has to be limited to avoid "musical tones" as discussed earlier. However, for a subjectively efficient attenuation of interfering speech, high attenuation values are necessary. The proposed solution is to combine the noise reduction gains via fading based on detection of the stationary characteristics of the signal (Figure 7–58).

When stationary signals are detected, the limited noise reduction for stationary signals is applied whereas in the other case, the higher attenuation for the spatial noise reduction should be used. This allows a subjectively efficient reduction of nonstationary signals such as speech interference.

Speech Focus

When designing a directional system using beamforming for hearing aids, target signals are assumed to originate in the front positions. The performance of the directional system is adapted using the previously described techniques to maximize the SNR. Automatic programs usually activate beamformers in noisy situations, which results in the desired increase of the SNR for front signals.

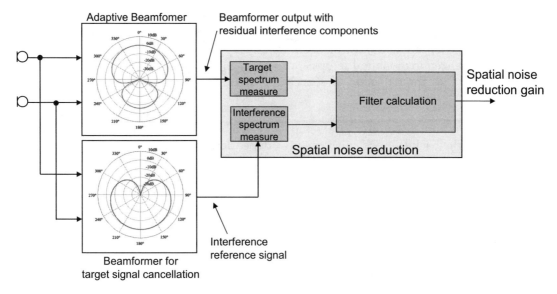

Figure 7–57. Block diagram of the spatial noise reduction concept.

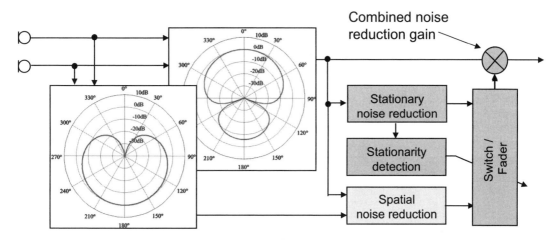

Figure 7–58. Block diagram for a combination of stationary and spatial noise reduction.

However, in situations where the target signal is located in nonfrontal positions, the beamformer activation attenuates the target signal and reduces the SNR, which is not desired. Typical examples are situations of communication in cars, especially when the hearing impaired persons positioned on the front seat try to communicate to persons sitting on the side and back seats. Another example is a conversation of persons walking next to each other on a noisy street. In this case, target signals are coming from the side.

Also here, a directional system with a front focus would degrade the speech intelligibility.

The above-sketched problem can ideally be solved by estimating the direction-of-arrival (DOA) of the speech signal and steering the beam realized by a directional processing toward this direction. Because of the constrained positions of the hearing aid microphone (i.e., a close microphone distance in small housings and the positioning next to the head), an angle-continuous steering of the beam is not possible.

Currently, the speech activity is analyzed with respect to three directions: front, rear, and side. Three different modes of beamforming are realized in monaural setups and activated based on the detection of speech activity. Those are:

■ steering to the front direction (typical setup)
■ steering to the back (flipped microphone settings)
■ omnidirectional processing

where the latter one is used when speech activity at side directions is detected since it is not possible to steer beams to the side with monaural differential beamforming setups. In products, three-directional modes are realized in parallel, as depicted in Figure 7–59.

The output signals are fed to a control unit that analyzes the signals with respect to typical speech characteristics such as the 4 Hz modulation (see section about Acoustic Situation Classification within this chapter). The output with the strongest indication for speech presence is then selected as output signal. Binaural hearing aid systems additionally offer the possibility to steer the beam to side directions by combining the microphone signals of both hearing aids.

True Ear Effect

Directional microphone systems are also used to mimic the directionality of the pinna. In humans, the pinna results in a frequency dependent directionality as shown for the AI-DI in Figure 7–54. This is due to an attenuation of high-frequency components arriving from the back. In a hearing aid's omnidirectional mode, this directionality is lost and localization tasks demonstrate a high number of errors between front and back. One approach to improve localization skills is a fixed directional microphone, which attenuates high-frequency signals from the back as shown in Figure 7–60.

Feedback Cancellation

Introduction

An important design concern for hearing instruments is acoustic feedback. The ringing

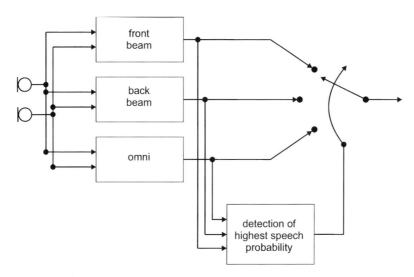

Figure 7–59. Setup of the speech focus system. First three microphone configurations are realized in parallel. The output signals are analyzed with respect to the speech probability. The configuration with the highest probability is chosen as output.

sound that is acoustic feedback is bothersome to hearing instrument users and their conversation partners. Therefore, acoustic feedback and the related whistling is one of the main challenges when developing hearing aids. Generally, acoustic feedback arises when output signal components from the hearing aid receiver are picked up by the hearing aid microphones (Figure 7–61). If the hearing aid amplification is greater than the acoustic attenuation via the feedback path, a closed feedback loop with a loop gain greater than one occurs.

For frequency components where this gain relation and also a certain phase relation occurs, signal components sum up constructively and whistling, called feedback, occurs. Feedback can be extremely annoying to the

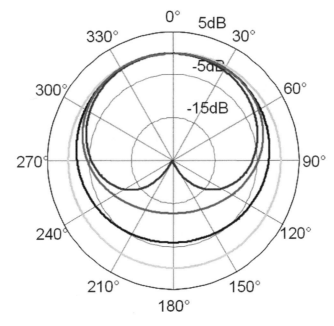

Figure 7–60. Directivity pattern with increased directionality for higher frequencies.

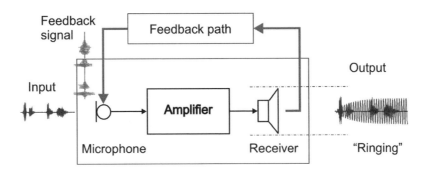

Figure 7–61. Schematic of a condition with acoustic feedback. (From "Hearing Aid Technology," by I. Holube and V. Hamacher, 2005, in J. Blauert (Ed.), *Communication Acoustics*, Springer, p. 270. Copyright 2005 by Springer. Adapted with permission.)

hearing aid user because the intensity of the whistling frequencies is only limited by the receiver power and the compression setting of the hearing aid, respectively.

The tendency to fit hearing aids with open domes and earmolds increases the feedback problem and the challenges to set up high performing feedback cancellation systems. The reason is that for open fitting, receiver signals reach the hearing aid microphones better and feedback loop gain increases.

Feedback Path Analysis

In Figure 7–62, a typical feedback path is shown as impulse response (above) and frequency response (below). One observes a length of 50 to 70 samples for the impulse response at a sampling rate of 20 kHz (equivalent to 2.5 to 3.5 ms), which is typical for acoustic feedback paths in hearing aids. The corresponding frequency response shows a bandpass characteristic with maxima between 1.5 and 5 kHz.

The term "impulse response" can be explained as follows: Transmission paths between a source and a sink typically exhibit a direct path and reflections. For acoustic feedback, the source is the hearing aid receiver, and the sink is the hearing aid microphone. In the case where only the direct path was present, the transmission path could be described by the propagation delay and the attenuation of the sound between the source and the sink. Each reflection component now exhibits an individual delay, which is larger than the delay of the direct path and an individual attenuation. All path components together describe the impulse response. The impulse response can be depicted as in Figure 7–62 upper graph, where the horizontal axis indicates the propagation delay of the path components and the vertical axis indicates their attenuation.

The individual feedback paths depend on different parameters, such as:

■ The vent size for classical earmolds or ITE devices
■ The type and size of the dome for open hearing aid devices
■ The fit of the mold or dome in the ear canal, and
■ Acoustic reflections close to the hearing aid (e.g., provoked by telephone receivers, hands, hats, etc.).

The first two factors are rather static, whereas the second two may vary considerably with time.

In Figure 7–63, examples for typical feedback paths are shown in dependence of the hearing aid type, the vent size, and with reflection instigated by a hand. One observes that moving a hand next to the hearing aid may create a quick increase in the feedback path by more than 20 dB. The following sections describe several means for feedback path suppression.

Gain Reduction—Static or Adaptive

As explained above, a feedback loop gain that is larger than one is a condition for feedback. Thus, feedback can be cancelled by reducing the hearing aid gain, statically or adaptively.

The gain can be limited statically, directly during the fitting session. When applying the

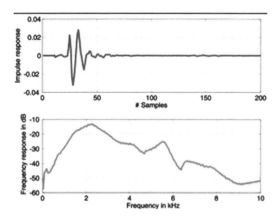

Figure 7–62. Typical impulse response (*above*) and the corresponding frequency response (*below*). (From "Signal Processing in High-End Hearing Aids: State of the Art, Challenges, and Future Trends," by V. Hamacher et al., 2005, *EURASIP Journal on Applied Signal Processing*, *18*, 2924. Copyright 2005 by V. Hamacher. Reproduced with permission.)

gain reduction, a headroom should be considered to avoid the occurrence of feedback due to acoustic reflections close to the hearing aid. Static gain limitation measures typically strongly limit the gain and thus the fitting possibilities of open hearing aids to compensate severe hearing losses.

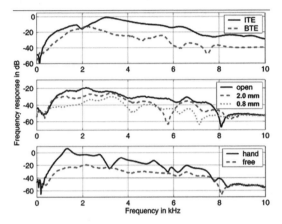

Figure 7–63. Showing the difference of feedback paths dependent on different parameters: hearing aid type (*above*), vent size (*mid*), and moving obstacles (*below*). (From "Signal Processing in High-End Hearing Aids: State of the Art, Challenges, and Future Trends," by V. Hamacher et al., 2005, *EURASIP Journal on Applied Signal Processing*, 18, 2924. Copyright 2005 by V. Hamacher. Reproduced with permission.)

Adaptive gain reduction can reduce the gain limitation problem but not avoid it. The basic idea is to use tonal detectors to detect feedback and the corresponding frequencies. The gain of the feedback frequency band can be reduced or an appropriate notch filter can be applied (Figure 7–64). Once inserted, gain reduction has to be returned after a certain time. Appropriate measures to achieve this have to be found to avoid the reoccurrence of feedback. This adaptive gain reduction limits the possibilities to compensate severe hearing losses. The following adaptive filter approach avoids this side effect.

Adaptive Filters

Typically, the feedback path is modeled by a linear filter as depicted in Figure 7–65 (right). This model is valid under the assumption that hearing aid microphones and receivers are linear systems—an assumption that holds for commonly used hearing aid receivers and microphones.

Suppression of feedback without gain reduction is possible by modeling the acoustic path with an adaptive filter (Figure 7–66). The output signal of the adaptive filter should be equivalent to the acoustic feedback that can be subtracted from the microphone signal to cancel feedback. A gain reduction of

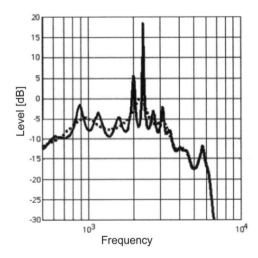

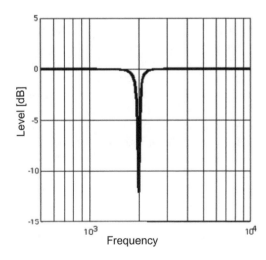

Figure 7–64. Frequency response without (*dotted*) and with (*solid*) feedback (*left*) and notch filter (*right*).

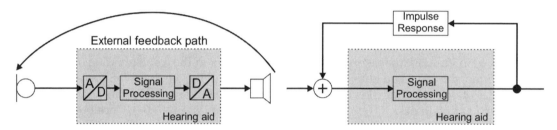

Figure 7–65. Hearing aid scheme with acoustic feedback path (*left*) and a corresponding model (*right*). (From "Signal Processing in High-End Hearing Aids: State of the Art, Challenges, and Future Trends," by V. Hamacher et al., 2005, *EURASIP Journal on Applied Signal Processing, 18*, 2924. Copyright 2005 by V. Hamacher. Adapted with permission.)

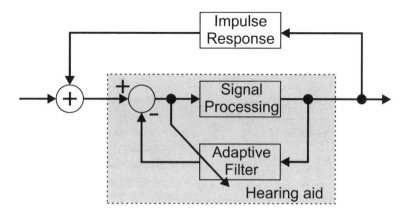

Figure 7–66. Modeling the feedback path with an adaptive filter and subtracting the estimated feedback components. (From "Signal Processing in High-End Hearing Aids: State of the Art, Challenges, and Future Trends," by V. Hamacher et al., 2005, *EURASIP Journal on Applied Signal Processing, 18*, 2924. Copyright 2005 by V. Hamacher. Adapted with permission.)

the hearing aid is not necessary. The amount of feedback reduction is directly related to the precision of the feedback path model. To obtain a high level of precision, an appropriate filter length is required as well as a fast adaptation of the filter to varying acoustic reflections next to the hearing aid. Therefore, adaptive filter techniques have to be applied.

The approach depicted in Figure 7–66 is one application of the "system identification problem" (Haykin, 2002), which can be solved with adaptive filters. The optimal coefficients of the adaptive filter can be obtained based on the minimization of the mean power of the "error" signal, which is the signal after the subtraction of the modeled feedback signal.

The solution to this optimization problem is the Wiener filter.

The adaptive filter is continuously updated to approach the optimal solution. A robust, computation-efficient, and high-performance adaptation is known by the normalized LMS (least mean square) or NLMS (normalized LMS) method (Hänsler & Schmidt, 2004). Within this method, a new filter is calculated based on the previous filter taking the error signal into account. An important value of the adaptation rule is the step-size, which controls the adaptation speed of the adaptation procedure. For the NLMS algorithm, it can be chosen between 0 and 1, being equivalent to a choice of the adaptation speed between an adaptation freeze and the maximal possible adaptation. The input signal to the hearing instrument disturbs the adaptation, because the adaptive filter output should model the feedback signal via the feedback path. The larger the power of the input signal is compared with the feedback signal, the lower the step-size should be chosen.

As mentioned, the desired hearing aid input signal disturbs the feedback cancellation. Additionally, the correlation between the input and the output signal of the hearing aid is typically strong, which plays an important role for feedback cancellation. The correlation provokes the convergence of the adaptive filter to a biased solution, meaning that the filter does not converge on the impulse response of the acoustic feedback path. This may result in the following consequences:

■ Reduced feedback cancellation performance
■ Signal distortion
■ Combined presence of feedback and input signal distortion.

For white noise input signal, the misadaptation is dissolved as well as for signals with low correlation properties. However, signals with strong and especially long autocorrelation functions, generate a strong bias. Those signals are especially tonal signals, instrument signals, and music.

Optimal Feedback Cancellation System

For the optimal design of a feedback cancellation system, the following issues have to be considered:

■ Adaptation disturbance from the presence of the input signal
■ Adaptation bias from the correlation of the hearing aid input and output signal.

For the adaptation disturbances, the relation of the power of the input signal and the feedback signal is especially important. The stronger the relation is, the greater is the adaptation disturbance that is equivalent to the variance of the feedback path estimation. To reduce the estimation variance, the stepsize of the adaptation has to be lowered.

The adaptation bias component is critical because it can provoke a strong misadaptation of the feedback path. Without additional measures, this problem can only be reduced by a complete freeze of the adaptation.

In the following, we describe:

■ A feedback detection method that allows the adaptation only in time frames when feedback is present.
■ A method to cancel the correlation of the hearing aid input and output signal that allows cancellation of the bias of the adaptation.

Both measures are necessary. The feedback detection unit has the target to only adapt the filter when feedback is present. With a high probability and in selected time frames, the relation of feedback and input signal power is high, which reduces the adaptation variance. As the only measure, the feedback detection, however, is not sufficient. Given a feedback path change due to a change of acoustic reflections next to the hearing aid, a filter adaptation would be necessary. When at the same time a music signal is presented as input, the music signal would generate a strong adaptation bias and not allow the adaptation to the correct acoustic path. Without bias reduction, feedback cannot be cancelled.

A reliable feedback detector is important because it decides to freeze or release the feedback adaptation. It is rather complicated to distinguish between feedback and all other types of acoustic input signals. Tonal signals are especially problematic, as they can mimic feedback, and may also arise from music. For desired tonal input signals, the adaptation should not be released since they generate a strong adaptation bias.

For the reliable differentiation of feedback and (tonal) input signals, the so-called fingerprint technology may be possible. The basic idea is to mark the hearing aid output signal acoustically. Analyzing the hearing aid input signal with respect to this mark or fingerprint, allows a distinction between feedback and all other kinds of input signals.

The fingerprint technique has to fulfill the criteria to be:

■ unnoticeable,
■ easily applicable, and
■ easily detectable.

One method that fulfills these criteria applies a slight periodic phase modification at the output signal. A function for detecting this periodic phase modulation analyzes the error signal that is the signal after the subtraction of the modeled feedback path. The presence of the periodic phase modulation is then a strong indication for feedback presence. In Figure 7–67, the block diagram of the feedback cancellation system with phase modulation and the corresponding detection block is shown.

The spectrogram of a typical combined input and feedback signal is depicted in Figure 7–68. One can clearly observe the short presence of the feedback with the phase, respectively, frequency modulated tonal frequency component.

When feedback is detected and the filter adaptation is activated, no bias should disturb the adaptation. To achieve this, no correlation of the input and output signal should be present. The only measure that allows the algorithm to decorrelate the input and output signal components is the application of a nonlinearity to the output signal, as shown in Figure 7–69.

When choosing the nonlinear procedure, the output signal quality should be considered and affected as little as possible. A method that is applicable to hearing aid processing is to apply a frequency shift to the output signal. As a stand-alone method, a frequency shift is already known to enhance the feedback stability (e.g., applied in large speaker systems). Now, combined with adaptive feedback reduction methods, the frequency shift allows for increasing feedback stability since it decorrelates input and output signals and eliminates the bias adaptation.

The signal disturbance, created by the frequency shift, is greater for lower frequency components because it severely disturbs the harmonic signal structure. However, because the feedback path shows a typical bandpass characteristic, and no feedback cancellation is required for low frequency components, no frequency shift is required for low-frequency components. Extensive testing showed that the impact on the signal quality for speech signals is not obvious. For specific music signals with a strong harmonic structure, however, a slight signal roughness can be heard.

The high-pass signal with frequency shifting is generated as follows: First, a split-band filter decomposes the hearing aid output signal into low- and high-pass frequency components. The frequency shift, which is applied to the high-pass components, is then

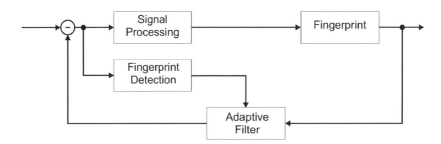

Figure 7–67. Block diagram of a feedback cancellation system with fingerprint technology. The "Fingerprint" module applies a phase modulation to the output signals and the "Fingerprint Detection" module detects the fingerprint and activates the filter adaptation when feedback is detected.

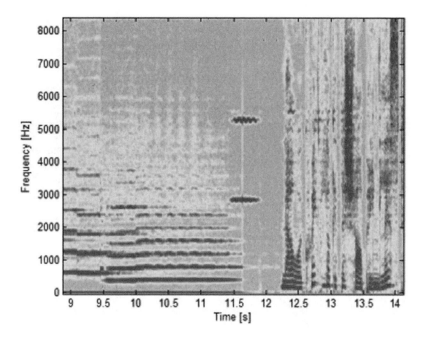

Figure 7–68. Spectrogram of a typical acoustic input of the hearing aid: The first part is music followed by a short feedback signal and a speech signal. One can well observe the phase modulation of the feedback signal between 11.5 and 12 s, which results in a periodic feedback frequency modulation.

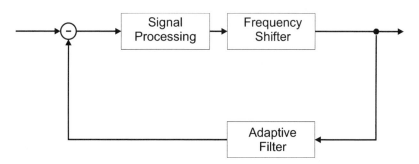

Figure 7–69. The feedback cancellation system with frequency shifter unit to decorrelate the input and output signal components.

realized with a Hilbert transform filter. The Hilbert transformation generates an analytic signal with only positive frequency components. Those are then shifted with respect to the frequency with a simple multiplication with an exponential term. A frequency shift of 20 Hz shows good properties with respect to the desired decorrelation and with respect to a limitation of the signal distortion. A block diagram of the realized frequency shift is shown in Figure 7–70.

Because the split-band filters have no ideal filter slopes, in the frequency region where the high-pass and low-pass frequency components overlap, signal components with and without frequency shift overlap. This doubling of frequency components is shown for a sinusoidal excitation in Figure 7–71.

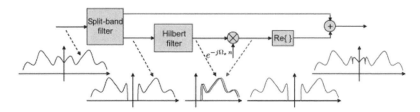

Figure 7–70. Block diagram of the realization of the frequency shift. First a split-band filter separates the high and low frequencies of the input signal. A frequency shift is only applied to the high frequency components. The analytic signal is calculated with a Hilbert filter. This signal is frequency shifted, and the resulting signal is then added to the nonshifted low frequency component.

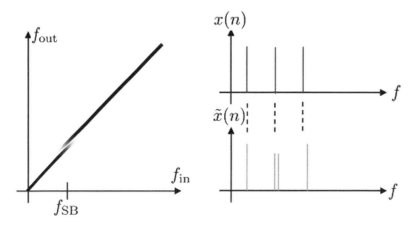

Figure 7–71. *Left:* Frequency input/output relation. *Right:* Three sinusoidal components input signal (*top*) and the corresponding output (*bottom*). Rough sound quality may occur from the doubling of the sinusoidal component near the shifting frequency.

The signal distortion generated by this overlap can be reduced when split band filters are applied with a reduced signal overlap. The sum of the split-band filters results in a frequency response with a narrow dip. Perceptually, the dip disturbs the frequency response much less than the doubling of frequency components.

In Figure 7–72, the block diagram of a complete feedback cancellation system with phase modulation and frequency shift is shown. If the fingerprint generated with the phase modulation is detected, the adaptation of the filter is released. During the adaptation of the feedback cancellation filter, the frequency shift is activated to avoid a biased

adaptation of the filter. When the adaptation is frozen, no frequency shift is applied to limit possible signal distortion from the frequency shift to time periods where it is necessary.

Acoustic Situation Classification

Within this chapter, we have described several signal processing algorithms of today's hearing instruments. Some are more advantageous in certain listening situations, but less advantageous in others, and they might require different situation specific settings. Music, for example, should sound as natural

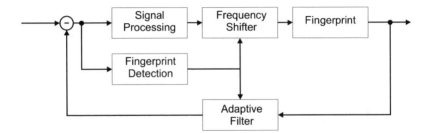

Figure 7–72. Overview of the complete feedback cancellation system with fingerprint and frequency shifter units. The frequency shifter unit is activated when feedback is detected by the fingerprint detection unit to avoid biased adaptation of the filter.

as possible; sound should be amplified from all directions in quiet situations to enable spatial orientation, and directional microphones should be used in noisy environments dependent on the direction of the target speaker. Therefore, different algorithms or different settings are required for different listening situations.

One possible solution is the use of hearing instruments with multiple programs, which have been offered for some time. Unfortunately, this solution requires the hearing aid user to recognize the present listening situation and to select the respective program. A more convenient solution is an automatic classification of the listening situation by the hearing instrument and an automatic selection of the appropriate algorithms and parameter settings.

Today's hearing instruments can distinguish to a certain extent between different listening situations like speech in quiet, speech in noise, noise alone, and music. The general approach of a classification algorithm is shown in Figure 7–73. First, several features are extracted from the input signal and fed into a classification algorithm that compares those features with a stored knowledge about the properties of different acoustic situations. Based on that knowledge, the classifier selects one out of several possible listening situations. The selection is used to choose appropriate algorithms and parameter settings, which are then used within the signal processing stages of the hearing instrument.

This kind of classification system typically influences the single and multi-microphone noise reduction as well as the gain and dynamic compression settings.

Let's have a look to the feature extraction stage. Several features have been proposed to characterize different listening situations. For a detailed analysis see, for example, Kates (2008). One candidate is, for example, the input level at different frequencies because background noises result typically in higher levels at low frequencies. Another example is the dynamic range of an input signal. Stationary background noises cause a narrow dynamic range whereas speech in quiet produces typically a dynamic range of about 30 dB. One feature, shown as an example in Figure 7–74, is the extraction of the envelope of the input signal, described in the section for modulation-based noise reduction. The envelope is filtered in the range of 1 to 4 Hz, and its level is determined. The result is a feature value between 0 and 1. The value is near to one for speech in quiet because of the temporal structure of speech with its characteristic modulation frequencies. Speech in noise and music do not show similar envelope variations, and the modulation based feature results in values close to zero. Therefore, this feature can be used to distinguish between speech in quiet and speech in noise as well as music, but it cannot distinguish between speech in noise and music themselves. Other features (e.g., those based on rhythm) contribute to a more accurate classification.

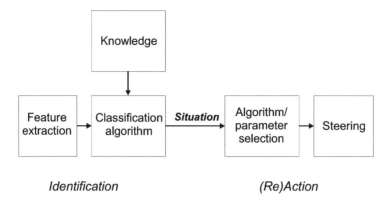

Figure 7-73. Block diagram of an algorithm for acoustic situation classification.

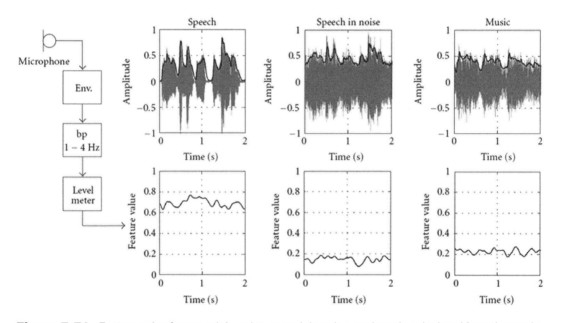

Figure 7-74. Feature value for speech in quiet, speech in noise, and music calculated from the modulations in the range of 1–4 Hz. (From "Signal Processing in High-End Hearing Aids: State of the Art, Challenges, and Future Trends," by V. Hamacher et al., 2005, *EURASIP Journal on Applied Signal Processing, 18*, 2924. Copyright 2005 by V. Hamacher. Reproduced with permission.)

Acoustic situation classification systems extract several features at the same time, and decisions are based on the outcomes of these features. The values of the features are combined to increase the probability of a correct decision. Tools for feature combinations are neural networks known from artificial intelligence research. Other approaches are Bayes classifiers or Hidden Markov Models. A description of these algorithms is beyond the scope of this chapter but are reviewed by Kates (2008).

We now imagine that the classification algorithm has decided for speech in noise and selects the directional microphone as well as a high setting for single-microphone noise reduction. The situation "speech in noise" is difficult to distinguish from music because music often also contains speech and some kind of background. Therefore, in the next phase, the classification algorithm might determine the signal to be music and would therefore deactivate the directional microphone and the single-microphone noise reduction. If the classifier would constantly modify the situation selection and thus abruptly switch between algorithms and parameter settings, the hearing aid user would be confronted with irritating sound impressions. Therefore, commercially available products smear the results of the classifier system over time and smooth the transitions between settings. This results in a robust decision stage preventing classification errors and audible processing changes when moving from one acoustic situation to another one. Figure 7–75 gives an example of a transition between an omnidirectional to a directional setting when the directional microphone system is activated for speech in noise.

In the past years, hearing instruments with a wireless communication link have been introduced. A previous section of this chapter already described the possibility that the directional microphone systems might be in a different setting in both hearing instruments, which might result in reduced speech intelligibility in background noise. Therefore, classification results are transmitted between hearing instruments and analyzed in a common decision-making unit to ensure maximum user benefit in every listening situation. Figure 7–76 gives an example for a decision-making unit. Both hearing instruments are able to classify five listening situations: speech in quiet, speech in noise, stationary noise, nonstationary noise, and music. This information is transmitted to the hearing instrument on the other side of the head. The matrix shows the combined decision. If both hearing instruments agree, then there is no question which situation is classified. If speech in quiet is detected by one hearing instrument, this decision is changed to speech in noise if the other hearing instrument decides for another listening situation. Speech in noise is also decided for, when one hearing instrument classifies this situation and the other hearing instrument classifies any other situation. All other combinations can be seen in Figure 7–76.

Learning Methods

Hearing instruments are fitted to the individual pure-tone audiogram using fitting formulae, which have been derived based on statistical analysis of many fittings, auditory models, and long-term experience. Nevertheless, they will never be able to satisfy every individual hearing aid user due to their individual experiences and expectations. The most important fitting parameter for hearing aid adjustments is the gain that determines loudness perception. Gain is set in frequency dependent bands or broadband by the audiologist via the selected fitting algorithm during the

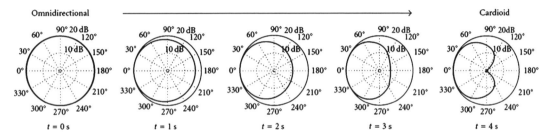

Figure 7–75. Transition from omnidirectional to directional. (From "Signal Processing in High-End Hearing Aids: State of the Art, Challenges, and Future Trends," by V. Hamacher et al., 2005, *EURASIP Journal on Applied Signal Processing, 18*, 2924. Copyright 2005 by V. Hamacher. Reproduced with permission.)

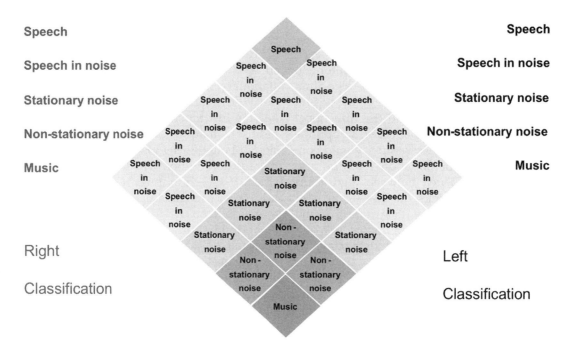

Figure 7–76. Decision-making matrix for coordinating the classified situations of both hearing instruments.

fitting process or it is modified by the hearing aid's volume control by the hearing aid user. Keidser and Dillon (2007) summarize several studies on preferred gain settings relative to the fitting formulae NAL-NL1 and came to the conclusion that about 50% of preferred gain are in a window of +/– 3 dB from NAL-NL1. Also, the preferred gain depends on the initial setting of the volume control leading to less preferred gain for those users fitted with a gain setting below target and a higher preferred gain for those users fitted with a gain setting above target (Mueller, Hornsby, & Weber, 2008).

Hearing aids are typically fitted in a quiet office environment or even a sound proof booth, and are verified using speech in quiet, mostly by talking to the audiologist. Conversations in real life, on the other hand, require a hearing aid setting suitable for speech in noise, reverberation, and at different levels. Also, hearing aid users might adjust their loudness impression over time while using the hearing instrument. Therefore, gain adjustments might be necessary. One approach to adjusting the gain setting individually over time while reduc-

ing the effort for the hearing aid user is the application of a learning method (Chalupper & Powers, 2006). With this kind of method, the hearing aid is trained by analyzing the preferred volume control setting of the individual user. When switching the hearing aid on, the last gain adjustments are analyzed, and a modified gain setting is derived. The goal of this algorithm is to reduce the required gain adjustments over time until the preferred gain setting is reached.

This easy concept is hindered by the requirement of different gain settings for different environments (see e.g., Mueller, Hornsby, & Weber, 2008). Loud sounds, for example, might be too loud and need a lower gain than soft sounds, as per Chalupper, Junius, and Powers (2009). The principle of different gain settings for diferent input levels should be accounted for by the dynamic range compression of the hearing aid described above in this chapter. Nevertheless, the setings of the compression algorithm might not be appropriate for the individual listener in all listening situations and might need modifications.

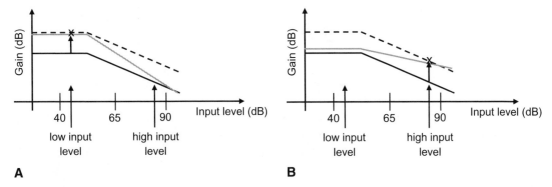

Figure 7–77. Input-dependent gain of the hearing aid (*black line*) and a level independent volume control adjustment (*dotted line*). For low input levels, the preferred setting (*indicated by a cross*) is achieved by increasing the gain and increasing the compression ratio (*panel A*). For high input levels, the compression ratio is decreased (*panel B*).

Figure 7–77 gives an example for the modification of gain and compression ratio dependent on the volume control adjustment at different input levels. After the modification of these parameters, the hearing aid should apply the desired respective gains for all input levels.

Second to overall gain, frequency response settings determine sound quality and speech intelligibility, and therefore satisfaction with hearing instruments. Keidser et al. (2005) have shown that different frequency responses are desired for different listening situations. Other reasons for individual frequency response settings are adaptation processes to long-term hearing impairment without hearing aid use, adaptation to previous hearing aid fittings, or physiological limitation such as dead regions in the cochlea. Individual frequency responses in a trainable hearing aid can be achieved by either direct adjustment of the frequency response when using a treble control, for example, or by indirect frequency response adjustment due to different gain settings in different frequency regions based on the respective signal level. Chalupper et al. (2009) have shown that these learning algorithms can improve users' satisfaction without declining speech intelligibility.

As already mentioned, the hearing aid users might prefer different gain and frequency response settings in different listening situations. Those listening situations deviate not only by their respective frequency dependent level but also by their signal type and listeners' goals and requirements. Speech is normally regarded as a target that has to be understood while noise also contains information and has to be heard, but not more than comfortably loud. Music, on the other hand, often contributes to stress relief that is interpreted very differently by individual listeners resulting in different hearing aid settings. Therefore, varying gain, compression, and frequency response settings are required for different listening environments, even for similar frequency dependent levels. This goal can be achieved by independent learning in the different hearing aid's programs. The drawback of this approach is that the hearing aid user still has to select the program appropriate for the respective listening situation. A more advanced approach to reach this goal is to combine the learning methods with the classification system within the hearing aids as demonstrated in Figure 7–78. Volume control and frequency response changes are allocated to the respective listening situations identified by the classification system, which results in a different setting in the different situations. As soon as one of the situations is classified by the algorithm, the trained parameter setting is automatically applied without program switching.

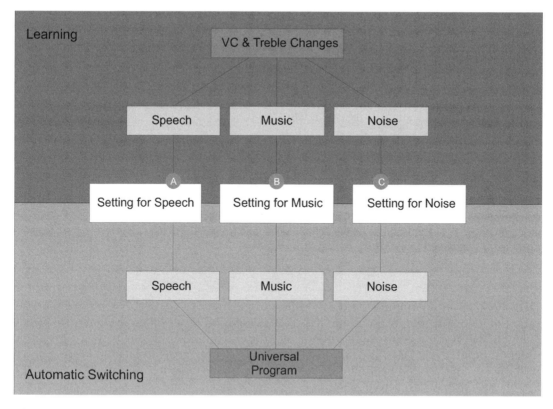

Figure 7–78. Independent learning in different listening environments and respective application of the setting for one universal program. (From "Best Sound Technology Compendium," by Siemens AG, 2010, http://www.siemens.com/hearing. Copyright 2010 by Siemens AG. Adapted with permission.)

INTERACTION OF ALGORITHMS

Hearing aid processing is a combination of several features with each including complicated signal processing: The main important blocks are:

■ Beamforming/directional microphone systems
■ Noise reduction
■ Dynamic compression
■ Feedback cancellation

All of these blocks influence each other. When designing algorithms, this has to be carefully considered. As early as possible interactions have to be analyzed since, based on the results, algorithmic modification may be necessary.

Here we want to consider the main important algorithm interactions in hearing aids without claiming to be exhaustive. These are:

■ Noise reduction and dynamic compression
■ Feedback cancellation and dynamic compression
■ Feedback cancellation and beamforming

Interaction of Noise Reduction and Dynamic Compression

The dynamic compression unit determines a level and frequency dependent gain as described in a previous section of this chapter. The higher the input signal levels in each frequency band are, the more the corresponding hearing aid gains are reduced. The noise reduction algorithm calculates a frequency dependent attenuation with the target to attenuate those frequency bands with low SNR as shown in another section of this chapter.

The noise reduction is typically performed before the dynamic compression. With the combination of these two units, there is a risk that first the noise reduction unit attenuates noise components and the following dynamic compression reduces the noise reduction effect by applying a higher gain due to the lowered input level.

The described combination has to be carefully analyzed when setting up the algorithms in order to avoid the neutralization effect described above. The key to reduce the interactions is to choose appropriate and matched time constants for both algorithms. Time constants should be slower for dynamic compression than for the typical fast acting Wiener filter noise reduction. This choice avoids that during target (typically speech) signal activity, the noise reduction effect is reduced. Noise-only frames are too short such that the dynamic compression could increase the gain when the time constants are chosen appropriately.

Interaction of Feedback Cancellation and Dynamic Compression

Feedback occurs when the loop gain of the hearing aid amplification and the acoustic attenuation between the hearing aid receiver output and the hearing aid microphone inputs is larger than one, as described above. Then typically a loud tonal signal occurs that is limited by the receiver power. When dynamic compression is simultaneously active, the compression limits the output level of the feedback signal. This limitation is equivalent to a hearing aid gain reduction that may lead to a hearing aid loop gain smaller than one and a disappearance of feedback. Without feedback, however, and the corresponding lower signal level, the dynamic compression unit raises the gain and feedback may occur again. Thus, a periodic behavior may occur that is depicted in Figure 7–79.

To avoid this very unpleasant cycle, the choice of the time constants of the dynamic compression plays a major role. Typically, they are fast enough such that a stationary

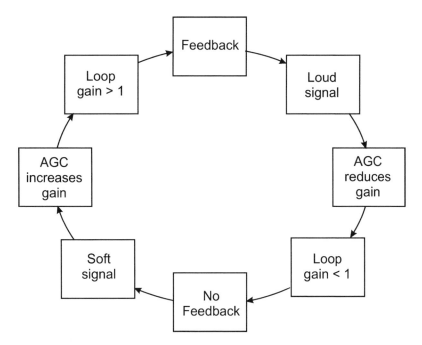

Figure 7–79. Possible vicious circle of an interaction of dynamic compression and feedback cancellation is shown, which may provoke periodically occurring feedback signals.

situation occurs with a lower feedback signal level according to the settings of the dynamic compression.

Feedback detection and the adaptive compensation of feedback is easier to handle when loud rather than soft feedback is present, since the feedback signals are then clearly different from the other acoustic excitation signals. In case feedback cancellation systems have been developed as stand-alone systems, there is a risk that they cannot cope with soft feedback situations. Especially, the interaction with dynamic compression systems exclude the application of the level-based feedback detection systems. The reason is that the feed-

back level heavily depends on the individual settings of the dynamic compression, which may be such that external acoustic excitation can be louder than feedback.

Interaction of Feedback Cancellation and Beamforming

As it can be seen in Figure 7–80, there are two positions of the feedback cancellation system in the hearing system possible: before or after the beamformer. Both have different advantages and disadvantages, and result in differ-

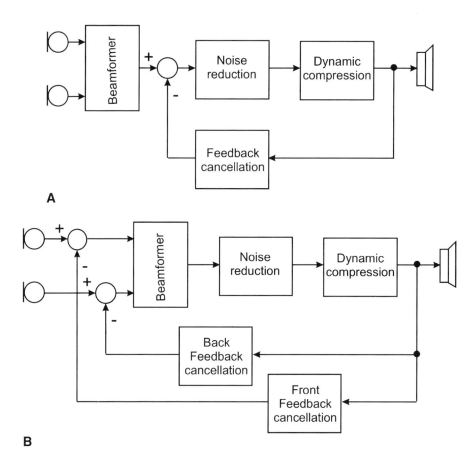

Figure 7–80. Two possible setups for placing the feedback cancellation are shown here. **A.** Feedback cancellation is placed behind the beamformer, with the advantage in computational complexity as only one feedback cancellation has to be realized. **B.** Feedback cancellation independently for each microphone before the beamformer. The advantage here is that the feedback cancellation does not need to model the transfer function of the beamformer which varies for adaptive beamformers and requires a following of the feedback cancellation adaptation.

ent interactions between beamformers and feedback cancellation.

The position of the feedback cancellation after the beamformer has the clear advantage that only one adaptation filter is necessary, which results in a lower overall computational complexity. However, the disadvantage of this setup is that the feedback filter has to model the feedback path and the beamformer processing, because the feedback subtraction point is located after the beamformer. When adaptive beamformers are used, the feedback system has to model the beamformer setup changes and adapt quickly even when no feedback path changes occur. Feedback path adaptation is critical as described in a previous section of this chapter, as there is always the risk to generate signal artifacts. This is a clear disadvantage of the feedback cancellation position after the beamformer.

When positioning the feedback cancellation system before the beamformer, the latter described interaction problem can be avoided since here, the feedback cancellation only models the feedback path. However, in this setup for each microphone signal, feedback has to be subtracted and different feedback paths have to be modeled and estimated. This severely increases the computational complexity.

Also in this position of feedback cancellation and beamforming, interaction occurs which, however, is usually less critical than in the reversed position. This interaction occurs as feedback signals exhibit an incidence direction that is usually a side direction of $+/- 90°$ and may also be reduced or even cancelled by beamformers. When only feedback is present as acoustic excitation, the beamformer adapts to a setting that optimally suppresses the feedback signal by beamforming methods. In case of additional presence of external noise components, the beamformer changes its settings to cancel those signals, and in a reduced way, feedback signals. Very generally speaking, a loop such as described in the interaction of feedback cancellation systems with dynamic compression (see Figure 7–79) may occur. The key to avoid this scenario is to setup well-performing feedback cancellation systems that cancel feedback fast and

efficiently. Then no feedback is present at the beamformer stage. Investigations show that then the risk of interactions with the beamformer is very low.

Concluding the interaction analysis of beamformer and feedback cancellation, feedback cancellation should be positioned before the beamformer, whenever the increased computational complexity can be handled.

FUTURE TRENDS

Several future trends in hearing aids can be expected and as always when trying to predict future developments, not all trends can be foreseen. Here, we want to focus on two trends where already first initial steps were realized in hearing aids. These are binaural processing and learning algorithms.

Binaural Processing

In 2004, Siemens introduced the first binaural hearing system that allowed for exchanging data between the right and left hearing aid by wireless data transmission. A first target was "comfort" by synchronizing volume or hearing aid program changes on one hearing aid between both hearing aids. The second target was a "natural and spatially correct listening experience." Based on the synchronization of the classification results, a first binaural processing hearing aid was designed. The exchange of the classification result offered a synchronized parameterization of the hearing aids. Especially when automatically activating the beamforming based on the classification of a noisy situation, only a synchronous processing allows to ensure a correct spatial perception.

Since that time, all major hearing aid manufacturers introduced binaural processing:

■ Oticon by exchanging data for binaural feedback detection, directional microphone coordination, binaural noise reduction coordination, and binaural dynamic compression.

■ Siemens added a binaurally synchronized automatic beam to different look directions.
■ Phonak was first to introduce a full binaural audio link. One application was to transmit the hearing aid signal with better SNR to the other side with the main focus to in car situations. Recently a binaural beamformer was introduced, which currently still exhibits a limited benefit and high current consumption when it is activated. Nevertheless, this is surely one important future binaural application.

Future binaural hearing aid features will certainly play a major role in different applications where the most important ones may include:

■ Fast binaural feedback detection
■ Binaural dereverberation
■ Binaural beamforming

In all binaural applications, several hearing aid constraints have to be fulfilled. The most important ones are

■ a very low processing latency for the binaural audio transmission and
■ the preservation of the binaural cues.

To limit the latency for the binaural audio signal transmission, low-latency audio and channel coding has to be used. Predictive audio coding schemes such as the G.722 coder (ITU-T, 1988) balance well between computational complexity and latency. The same is valid for convolutive channel coding (Blahut, 1983). For those reasons, both are preferably used in hearing aids.

The preservation of the binaural cues (Blauert, 1996; Eneman et al., 2008; van den Bogeart, 2008) is important for binaural processing as—in contrast with monaural processing where one output signal is generated based on several signals—here the signals for both hearing aids are determined. Binaural cues describe the level and time differences of the acoustic signals of both ears and allow the correct localization of acoustic sources.

In the past, feedback detection systems that require a low binaural data rate have been proposed by Oticon. The low data rate limits such systems to a comparison of local feedback detection results. In case of a full binaural audio transmission, a combined signal analysis of both hearing aid signals is possible such as proposed in a patent (Puder & Rosenkranz, 2009) where the correlation of both signals is determined. Those detection methods are much more reliable and faster. Both are crucial for high quality feedback systems.

Reverberation is created by acoustic reflections of the acoustic environment where the acoustic source and sink, in this case the hearing impaired person, are located. It is known (Bradley, Sato, & Picard, 2003) that a certain amount (approximately 50 ms) of reverberation contributes to a higher speech intelligibility. Higher reverberation, however, continuously reduces the speech intelligibility, mainly for hearing-impaired persons due to higher frequency masking (Jeub, Schäfer, Esch, & Vary, 2010).

Monaural dereverberation techniques are typically based on Wiener-filter theory (Haykin, 2002) where the distorting components from reverberation are estimated based on the reverberation time that is either known or estimated. Estimations of reverberation time typically include the decaying signal components that are longer proportional to the reverberation time.

Binaural techniques explore the coherence of the left and right microphone signals to differentiate between coherent low reverberant components and diffuse high reverberant components (Kuttruff, 2009, Figure 7–81). Because of the distance of ~15 cm between the microphones on both sides of the head, diffuse components are uncorrelated for frequency components above 1000 Hz.

With the coherence value, it is possible to determine the frequency dependent power of the desired component and thus design a Wiener filter (Haykin, 2002) to reduce the noncoherent, for example, reverberant components.

For monaural hearing aid processing, beamforming is state-of-the-art and the currently only known technique that allows to increase the speech intelligibility, proven by

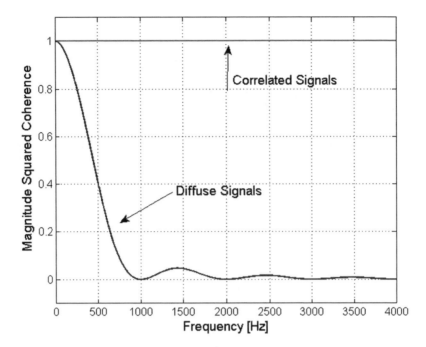

Figure 7–81. Coherence for correlated target signals and diffuse noise reverberation components are depicted for binaural setups with a microphone distance of approximately 15 cm. It can be seen that the coherence measure distinguishes between target signals and reverberation.

objective measurements. Typically, it is possible to attenuate sources of the side or back, meaning in between an angle range of +90°, 180, −90° where the 0°-direction is the direction focused on the speaker. In very noisy environments with competing noise or speech sources at side positions around +/− 45°, a narrower beam would be desirable.

In monaural applications, it is not possible to attenuate sources that are positioned at side positions around +/− 45° due to the physical relation that with closely positioned microphones it is only possible to generate a broad beam. In contrast with monaural applications where typical microphone distances are about 6 to 8 mm in binaural setups, they are at a distance of around 15 cm, the difference between the ears through the head.

The larger distance allows design of beamforming algorithms with a narrower beam. However, the processing methods must be adapted primarily for two reasons:

■ Spatial aliasing occurs for larger microphone distances, when differential methods as described above are used, which generates several beams around the 360°.
■ The signals must be processed to generate two output signals, one for each ear where the binaural cues are preserved.

One possibility for solving the requirements described above is to setup a binaural Wiener filter system. In Figure 7–82, two possibilities (Reindl, Zheng, & Kellermann, 2010) for Wiener filter setups are shown.

Both setups for binaural noise reduction shown here rely on a spectral noise power estimation, which combines the left and the right microphones. Typically, the target source is located in the front position and can be canceled by subtracting both microphone signals. This differential approach allows the spectral noise power estimation. The microphone signals and the estimated noise power

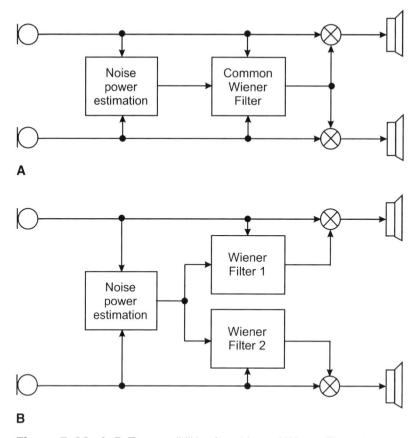

Figure 7–82. A–B. Two possibilities for a binaural Wiener filter setup.

then allow for determining a Wiener filter for nonfrontal interference signals. Here, two setups are possible: A common filter and two different filters, both with advantages and disadvantages. The common filter guarantees the preservation of the spectral cues, whereas the two separate filters allow a better interference reduction.

By subtracting the signals of the left and the right ear microphone signals, a noise reference signal can be generated. This can then be utilized for setting up one common or two separate Wiener filters for suppressing the nondesired signal components in each microphone. Both approaches filter the left and right microphone signals separately, which in general fulfills the requirement of binaural cue preservation. This requirement is fully guaranteed when a common filter is

determined and the filter values are applied to both microphone signals identically.

In Figure 7–83, examples of directional plots for monaural and binaural beamformers are depicted. The clearly narrower beam width of the binaural setup can be observed. Binaural systems also allow to steer the beam to side positions, which is especially advantageous for listening situations, such as the example in the car.

Of course, in a general setup, up to four microphones can be used and combined for an ideal noise suppression. For example, a 4-microphone Wiener-filter (Haykin, 2002) can be designed. This would require the binaural transmission of both microphones of both hearing aids to the other, respectively. Therefore, in typical applications, first a monaural beamformer is calculated, and then

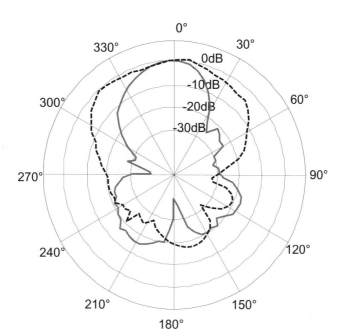

Figure 7–83. Examples for beam pattern for a monaural (*black dashed*) and a binaural (*gray*) beamformer. It can be well observed that the beam toward the frontal direction is much narrower for the binaural approach than for the monaural setup.

based on the single output signals of each left and right beamformer, a binaural beamformer as described above is realized. This approach only requires the transmission of one audio signal between the hearing aids.

Learning Systems

Normally hearing aids are fitted by the hearing care professional and include an optimized adjustment of gains and compression values as well as feature settings. Hearing aid users often have the possibility to adjust their volume or even their frequency shape. After switching the hearing aid off and on again, however, usually the default values set by the professional are restored.

Some years ago, the first hearing aids with a volume-control learning were introduced. Here, the user settings of the volume control are long-term smoothed over time

and stored. In case of consistent adjustments of the hearing aid settings by the hearing aid user, those values may differ from the default settings and are used instead when activating the hearing aid.

Currently Siemens offers advanced learning methods. Here it is possible to learn the hearing aid volume in dependence of the input level and the acoustic environment. This allows a very individualized learning. For example, it is possible to adjust the volume for soft music without changing the preferred settings in all other situations.

In the future, we will certainly see—perhaps starting with a user group that is interested in technical innovations—more options to interact with hearing aids and continuously adjust the hearing aids to optimized individual settings. These individual adjustments and the corresponding learning of the adjusted parameters can be expanded to hearing aid features such as beamforming

:tion. Currently these settings ›y classification systems with ›ing of the classified acoustic situation to the feature settings.

The idea for future learning systems is to link the acoustic environment with preferred settings of specific features in these environments. The learned settings are then applied when these acoustic situations are detected. In a first step, acoustic situations may be identical to the acoustic classes of the fixed and state-of-the-art classification systems. A more general approach also allows learning individual acoustic situations. The advantage would be that these classes would better fit to the individual situations. Examples are the individual acoustic environments where users are active or different preferences of music types. Individual classes allow a very precise detection and the corresponding individual choice of hearing aid settings and parameters.

SUMMARY

This chapter outlines the principles of digital signal processing and processing algorithms for digital hearing instruments, and their benefit for the users of those instruments. Whereas analog signals are continuous in time and in level, digital signals are sampled at discrete points in time and are quantized and represented by binary numbers. Both the sampling and the quantization can result in artifacts, which must be avoided. Several signal processing algorithms can be implemented in digital hearing instruments. They normally include the possibility of frequency specific processing, several possibilities of dynamic range compression, frequency compression, noise reduction, and feedback reduction algorithms. The noise reduction algorithms can be divided into single-microphone systems, which separate speech and noise by their different temporal structure, and multi-microphone systems that separate speech and noise by assumptions about their spatial location. Some of the

algorithms can be adjusted by the audiologist during the fitting process, by the hearing aid users via program switch, or are steered by a situation classifier and learning methods. All algorithms are beneficial for the user of hearing instruments.

REVIEW QUESTIONS

1. An analog sine wave:
   a. Is sampled at 25,000 Hz.
   b. Is continuously varying in amplitude.
   c. Looks like stair steps.
   d. All of the above.

2. A digital sine wave:
   a. May be sampled at 25,000 Hz.
   b. Is not continuous.
   c. Looks like stair steps.
   d. All of the above.

3. Aliasing occurs when:
   a. A 5000 Hz sine wave is sampled at 8000 Hz.
   b. The sampling frequency is less than the Nyquist frequency.
   c. The input signal is sampled at an insufficient number of points.
   d. All of the above.

4. Which was not discussed as a source of error in a digital hearing instrument?
   a. Aliasing.
   b. Quantization.
   c. Integrated chip structure size.
   d. None of these contribute to error.

5. Which statement is true?
   a. In syllabic compression, the attack and release times are short.
   b. Syllabic compression does not affect the dynamic range of speech.
   c. Compared with syllabic compression, automatic volume control has a short attack time and a long release time.
   d. Automatic volume control has a greater effect on the dynamic range of speech than does syllabic compression.

6. The modulation spectrum of speech:
  a. Has a broad peak at 3 kHz.
  b. Has a sharp peak at 30 Hz.
  c. Reflects the frequencies of sentences, words, and speech sounds.
  d. Is an essential measure for the calculation of the directivity index.

7. What is the goal of the following algorithms: microphone noise reduction, directional microphones, and Wiener filtering?
  a. Feedback reduction.
  b. Noise reduction.
  c. Reduction of the occlusion effect.
  d. Instrument size reduction.

8. The relation between the amplification for frontal sounds and the amplification for sounds from all other directions is called:
  a. The squelch effect.
  b. The Nyquist frequency.
  c. The upward spread of masking.
  d. The directivity index.

9. Feedback reduction can be:
  a. Achieved using adaptive filters.
  b. Achieved by modulating the Nyquist frequency.
  c. Achieved with dual compression.
  d. Alas, feedback cannot be affected by digital technology.

10. Name five advantages of hearing instruments with digital technology over hearing instruments with analog technology.
  a.
  b.
  c.
  d.
  e.

Answer Key

1. b
2. d
3. d
4. c
5. a
6. c
7. b
8. d
9. a
10. Miniaturization, low power consumption, low internal noise, reproducibility, stability, programmability, complexity

REFERENCES

Allen, J. B., Hall, J. L., & Jeng, P. S. (1990). Loudness growth in ½-octave bands (LGOB)—A procedure for the assessment of loudness. *Journal of the Acoustical Society of America, 88*, 745–753.

Baer, T., Moore, B. C. J., & Kluk, K. (2002). Effects of low pass filtering on the intelligibility of speech in noise for people with and without dead regions at high frequencies. *Journal of the Acoustical Society of America, 112*, 1133–1144.

Bentler, R., & Chiou, L.-K. (2006). Digital noise reduction: An overview. *Trends in Amplification, 10*(2), 67–82.

Blahut, R. E. (1983). *Theory and practice of error control codes.* Boston, MA: Addison-Wesley.

Blauert, J. (1996). *Spatial hearing—The psychophysics of human sound localization.* Cambridge, MA: MIT Press.

Boll, S. F. (1979). Suppression of acoustic noise in speech using spectral subtraction, *IEEE Transactions on Acoustics, Speech and Signal Processing, 27*(2), 113–120.

Bradley, J. S., Sato, H., & Picard, M. (2003). On the importance of early reflections for speech in rooms. *Journal of Acoustical Society of America, 113*(6), 3233–3244.

Braida, L. D., Durlach, N. I., De Gennaro, S. V., Peterson, P. M., & Bustamante, D. K. (1982). Review of recent research on multiband amplitude compression for the hearing impaired. In G. A. Studebaker & F. H. Bess (Eds.), *The Vanderbilt Hearing-Aid Report* (pp. 122–140). Upper Darby, PA: Monographs in Contemporary Audiology.

Chalupper, J., Junius, D., & Powers, T. A. (2009). Algorithm lets users train aid to optimize compression, frequency shape, and gain. *The Hearing Journal, 62*(8), 26–33.

Chalupper, J., & Powers, T. A. (2006). Changing how gain is selected: The benefits of combining datalogging and a learning VC. *Hearing Review, 13*(13), 46–55.

Chung, K. (2004). Challenges and recent developments in hearing aids part I. Speech understanding in noise, microphone technologies and noise reduction algorithms. *Trends in Amplification, 8*(3), 83–124.

Cox, R. M., Alexander, G. C., Taylor, I. M., & Gray, G. A. (1997). The contour test of loudness perception. *Ear and Hearing, 18*(5), 388–400.

Dillon, H. (1996). Tutorial: Compression? Yes, but for low or high frequencies, for low or high intensities, and with what response times? *Ear and Hearing, 17*(4), 287–307.

Drullman, R., Festen, J. M., & Plomp, R. (1994). Effect of temporal envelope smearing on speech reception. *Journal of the Acoustical Society of America, 95*(2), 1053–1064.

Elko, G. W., & Pong, A. N. (1995). A simple adaptive first-order differential microphone. *Proceedings IEEE Workshop on Applications of Signal Processing to Audio and Acoustics*, 169–172.

Eneman, K., Leijon, A., Doclo, S., Spriet, A., Moonen, M., & Wouters, J. (2008). Auditory-profile-based physical evaluation of multi-microphone noise reduction techniques in hearing instruments. In R. Martin, U. Heute, & C. Antweiler (Eds.), *Advances in digital speech transmission* (pp. 431–458). Chichester, UK: Wiley.

Ephraim, Y., & Malah, D. (1984). Speech enhancement using a minimum mean-square error short-time spectral amplitude estimator. *IEEE Transactions on Acoustics, Speech, and Signal Processing, 32*(6), 1109–1121.

Ephraim, Y., & Malah, D. (1985). Speech enhancement using a minimum mean-square error log-spectral amplitude estimator. *IEEE Transactions on Acoustics, Speech, and Signal Processing 33*(2), 443–445.

Hamacher, V. (2006). Perzeptive Evaluierung von Methoden zur Sprachverbesserung in modernen digitalen Hörgeräten. *Conference ITG-Fachtagung Sprachkommunikation*, Kiel, Germany.

Hamacher, V., Chalupper, J., Eggers, J., Fischer, E., Kornagel, U., Puder, H., & Rass, U. (2005). Signal processing in high-end hearing aids: State of the art, challenges, and future trends. *EURASIP Journal on Applied Signal Processing, 18*, 2915–2929.

Hamacher, V., Fischer, E., & Latzel, M. (2006). A novel approach to reduce transient noise in hearing aids: Technical concept and perceptual evaluation. *International Hearing Aid Research Conference*, Lake Tahoe, CA.

Hänsler, E., & Schmidt, G. (2004). *Acoustic echo and noise control: A practical approach.* Hoboken, NJ: Wiley.

Haykin, S. (2002). *Adaptive filter theory.* Englewood Cliffs, NJ: Prentice-Hall.

Hickson, L. M. H. (1994). Compression amplification in hearing aids. *American Journal of Audiology, 3*, 51–65.

Hogan, C. A., & Turner, C. W. (1998). High-frequency audibility: Benefits for hearing-impaired listeners. *Journal of the Acoustical Society of America, 104*(1), 432–441.

Hohmann, V. (1998). Grundlagen digitaler Signalverarbeitung. *Zeitschrift für Audiologie, 37*, 121–130.

Holube, I. (1998). Signalverarbeitungsalgorithmen für digitale Hörgeräte. *Zeitschrift für Audiologie, 37*, 176–182.

Holube, I., Fredelake, S., Vlaming, M., & Kollmeier, B. (2010). Development and analysis of an International Speech Test Signal (ISTS). *International Journal of Audiology, 49*(12), 891–903.

Holube, I., & Hamacher, V. (2005). Hearing-aid technology. In J. Blauert (Ed.), *Communication acoustics* (pp. 255–276). Berlin, Germany: Springer.

Hornsby, B., & Ricketts, T. A. (2007). Effects of noise source configuration on directional benefit using symmetric and asymmetric directional hearing aid fittings. *Ear and Hearing, 28*(2), 177–186.

Houtgast, T., & Steeneken, H. J. M. (1985). A review of the MTF concept in room acoustics and its use for estimating speech intelligibility in auditoria. *Journal of the Acoustical Society of America, 77*(3), 1069–1077.

ITU-T. (1988). 7 kHz audio-coding within 64 kbits/s. *International Telecommunication Union Recommendation G.722.*

Jeub, M., Schäfer, M., Esch, T., & Vary, P. (2010). Model-based dereverberation preserving binaural cues. *IEEE Transactions on Audio, Speech, and Language Processing, 18*(7), 1732–1745.

Kates, J. (2008). *Digital hearing aids.* San Diego, CA: Plural.

Keidser, G., Brew, C., Brewer, S., Dillon, H., Grant, F., & Storey, L. (2005). The preferred response slopes and two-channel compression ratios in twenty listening conditions by hearing-impaired and normal-hearing listeners and their relationship to the acoustic input. *International Journal of Audiology, 44*(11), 656–670.

Keidser, G., & Dillon, H. (2007). What's new in prescriptive fittings down under? In C. Palmer & R. Seewald (Eds.), *Hearing care for adults* (pp. 133–142). Stäfa, Switzerland: Phonak AG.

Keidser, G., Dillon, H., Carter, L., & O'Brien, A. (2012). NAL-NL2 empirical adjustments. *Trends in Amplification, 16*(4), 211–223.

Kuttruff, H. (2009). *Room acoustics.* Oxon, UK: Spon.

Launer, S., personal communication, May 14, 2011.

Lyons, R. G. (2011). *Understanding digital signal processing.* Upper Saddle River, NJ: Prentice-Hall.

Martin, R. (1994). Spectral subtraction based on minimum statistics. *Proceedings EUSIPCO-1994, Edinburgh, Scotland*, 1182–1185.

Martin, R. (2001). Noise power spectral density estimation based on optimal smoothing and minimum statistics. *IEEE Transactions on Speech and Audio Processing, 9*(5), 504–512.

Moore, B. C. J. (1990). How much do we gain by gain control in hearing aids? *Acta Otolaryngologica, 469*, 250–256.

Moore, B. C. J. (1995). *Perceptual consequences of cochlear damage.* Oxford, UK: Oxford University Press.

Moore, B. C. J., Glasberg, B. R., & Stone, M. A. (1991). Optimization of a slow-acting automatic gain control system for use in hearing aids. *British Journal of Audiology 25*(3), 171–182.

Mueller, H. G., Hornsby, B. W. Y., & Weber, J. E. (2008). Using trainable hearing aids to examine real-world preferred gain. *Journal of the American Academy of Audiology, 19*(10), 758–773.

Mueller, H. G., & Wesselkamp, M. (1999). Ten commonly asked questions about directional microphone fittings. *Hearing Review Supplement, High Performance Hearing Solutions, Hearing in Noise, 3,* 25–30.

Nyquist, H. (1928). Certain topics in telegraph transmission theory. *Transactions of the American Institute of Electrical Engineers, 47*(2), 617–644.

Oppenheim, A. V., & Schafer, R. W. (1975). *Digital signal processing.* Englewood Cliffs, NJ: Prentice -Hall.

Ostendorf, M., Hohmann, V., & Kollmeier, B. (1997). Empirische Klassifizierung verschiedener akustischer Signale und Sprache mittels einer Modulationsfrequenzanalyse [Empirical classification of different acoustic signals and language by means of modulation frequency analysis]. *Fortschritte der Akustik, DAGA-97.*

Pascoe, D. P. (1978). An approach to hearing aid selection. *Hearing Instruments, 29,* 12–16.

Plomp, R. (1983). Perception of speech as a modulated signal. *Proceedings of the 10th International Congress of Phonetic Sciences,* Utrecht, The Netherlands.

Plomp, R. (1988). The negative effect of amplitude compression in multichannel hearing aids in the light of the modulation-transfer function. *Journal of the Acoustical Society of America, 83*(6), 2322–2327.

Powers, T., Holube, I., & Wesselkamp, M. (1999). The use of digital features to combat background noise. *Hearing Review Supplement, High Performance Hearing Solutions, Hearing in Noise, 3,* 36–39.

Puder, H., & Rosenkranz, T. (2009). Method for operating of a hearing device system and hearing device system, U.S. patent application, 2009/0041272 A1.

Reindl, K., Zheng, Y., & Kellermann, W. (2010). Analysis of two generic Wiener filtering concepts for binaural speech enhancement in hearing aids. *Proceedings of the European Signal Processing Conference (EUSIPCO),* pp. 989–993, Aalborg, Denmark.

Ricketts, T. A., & Hornsby, B. W. Y. (2005). Sound quality measures for speech in noise through a commercial hearing aid implementing "Digital Noise Reduction." *Journal of the American Academy of Audiology, 16*(5), 270–277.

Scollie, S., Seewald, R., Cornelisse, L., Moodie, S., Bagatto, M., Laurnagaray, D., . . . Pumford, J. (2005). The desired sensation level multistage input/output algorithm. *Trends in Amplification, 9*(4), 159–197.

Simpson, A. (2009). Frequency-lowering devices for managing high-frequency hearing-loss: A review. *Trends in Amplification, 13*(2), 87–106.

Simpson, A., Hersbach, A. A., & McDermott, H. J. (2005). Improvements in speech perception with an experimental nonlinear frequency compression hearing device. *International Journal of Audiology, 44*(5), 281–292.

van den Bogeart, T. (2008). *Preserving binaural cues in noise reduction algorithms for hearing aids* (PhD dissertation). Katholieke University Leuven, Leuven, Belgium.

Vonlanthen, A. (2000). *Hearing instrument technology for the hearing healthcare professional.* Florence, KY: Singular.

Wolf, R. P., Hohn, W., Martin, R., & Powers, T. A. (1999). Directional microphone hearing instruments: How and why they work. *Hearing Review Supplement, High Performance Hearing Solutions. Hearing in Noise, 3,* 14–25.

CHAPTER 8

From Analog to Digital Hearing Aids

SØREN WESTERMANN
HANNE PERNILLE ANDERSEN
LARS BÆKGAARD

OUTLINE

ACKNOWLEDGMENTS

The authors gratefully acknowledge the contribution of the following people to this chapter:

Anders Holm Jessen

Magnus Nørgaard

Thomas Troelsen

Morten Agerbæk Nordahn

Carsten Paludan-Müller

John Colberg Jensen

Kristian Timm Andersen

Thilo Thiede

Erik Schmidt

Jakob Nielsen

Helge Pontoppidan Föh

Mike Lind Rank

Søren Møllskov Larsen

Martin Mørkebjerg

Anne Vikær Damsgaard

Andreas Kleist Svendsen

This chapter offers an overview of the technical advances in Digital Signal Processing (DSP) hearing instruments since their introduction in 1996 up until the present. The intention is to illustrate how far engineering advances have taken modern digital hearing aids. Advances include Integrated Circuit (IC) technology, Digital Signal Processing (i.e., complex mathematical processing of signals), advanced hearing aid features, wireless communication, and hearing aid programming.

THE TRANSITION FROM FULLY ANALOG TO FULLY DIGITAL HEARING INSTRUMENTS

Up until the mid-1980s, hearing aids were exclusively analog. They were very basic in terms of technology. Incoming sound was amplified by means of a simple amplifier comprising a handful of transistors. The frequency shaping could be modified by means of a few basic filters. Most analog hearing instruments applied linear amplification, which meant that the same amount of amplification was applied to both weak and loud sounds. Output control was achieved by means of limiters or output compressors created from diodes or dedicated transistors. Fine tuning options were restricted to a few manual adjustments made by the audiologist using a screwdriver and trimmers.

In the late 1980s, the first step toward digital hearing aids was taken with the introduction of the first digitally programmable analog hearing instruments (Bernafon Phox, Widex Quattro). Dedicated programmers and later PC-based fitting systems replaced screwdrivers and trimmers, but the actual signal processing was still analog. Programmable hearing aids provided some of the adjustability that characterizes later digital hearing aids. For example, some offered programs for different listening situations. Some also provided greater amounts of amplification for soft sounds, and less amplification for loud sounds (compression). The first radio wave remote controls were also introduced with digitally programmable analog hearing aids.

The first fully digital hearing instruments became commercially available in 1996 (Widex Senso, Oticon Digifocus). Digital hearing aids take advantage of digital signal processing (DSP) technology. The fundamental difference between analog and digital hearing aids is that while analog hearing aids basically just amplify and filter the signal, hearing aids with DSP technology convert the analog microphone signal into a stream of digits by means of an A/D (for analog-to-digital) converter. The digits can then be analyzed, and the desired properties of the signal enhanced by means of sophisticated mathematical formulae (algorithms), before it is converted back to an analog output signal. With the advent of digital hearing aids, existing analog functions could be improved, and new, digital functions, which could not have become reality with analog technology, were introduced.

Digital Implementation of Analog Functions

Basic operations, such as amplification, filtering, compression, and output control are of course still performed by DSP instruments. However, in a modern hearing aid, the performance of those functions may require less than 5% of the DSP's resources. Simple to implement in a DSP, these functions were not the main obstacle to the introduction of digital hearing aids. Rather, it was the development of sufficiently precise A/D and D/A converters that could operate on a small hearing aid battery (1-1.6 V, 1-5 mW), which made the first digital hearing aids possible.

True Digital Features

True digital signal processing opened up for a whole new world of features in hearing instruments. Digital circuits have memory capabilities, and they are able to perform complex calculations of various measures, such as the percentiles or the Speech Intelligibility Index (SII) of a speech signal in noise.

The execution of sequential operations inside the hearing aid is a true digital operation. It allows for in situ measurements performed by the hearing aids, advanced feedback, and occlusion management procedures, data logging during actual use, and wireless synchronization of the behavior of the right and left hearing instruments in a binaural hearing instrument system.

Digital signal processing can also maintain sophisticated simulation models of the acoustic system surrounding the hearing aid. Such models enable the prediction of certain changes in the hearing aid environment, which can be exploited for the prevention of feedback or masking of signals, for instance.

Finally, digital signal processing enables highly sophisticated features, such as controllable/adaptive directional microphone systems and frequency transposition.

DESIGN CONSIDERATIONS

Most aspects of modern living are somehow influenced by microelectronics—the outcome of a revolutionary development started by the invention of the transistor in 1947 and still ongoing. By the early 1960s, other key inventions had helped form the planar silicon integrated circuit (IC or "chip"), which is the cornerstone of modern electronics. Progress has been steady since with roughly a doubling of the number of transistors per chip area every two years. Today the IC industry has grown into a world-dominating industry with multibillion dollar investments into new technologies.

The technologies used by the hearing aid industry have shown similar progress. The first-generation truly digital hearing aids can be exemplified by the Widex Senso. The Senso was designed using a 0.8 μ (micron) technology. With 60,000 transistors, the IC performed 13 million calculations per second. The Senso offered a breakthrough in clarity and ease of adjustment with features that could not have been made with analog technology. In those days, the main challenges in the design process was the low supply voltage because the technology was designed for a much higher supply voltage.

A modern example could be the Widex CLEAR designed using 0.18 μ and 0.13 μ technology. With 6,000,000 transistors, 400 million calculations are performed per second. Today every aspect of the hearing aid has been improved by the technological advances. The sound processing has become extremely advanced to give the user the best combination of comfort, speech comprehension, and overall pleasure of hearing. On top of this, a large number of supporting features have been added. All of this goes beyond what could be achieved using purely analog technologies.

Before entering into a discussion on the various digital features, it is worth contemplating the complex design considerations facing the DSP engineers and integrated circuit designers when developing new DSPs for hearing instruments.

While a new DSP platform may be 10 times more complex than its predecessor, the engineers must still ensure performance with a voltage supply in the range of 1 to 1.6 volt, power consumption at around a milliwatt (mW) and at the same time produce a constant improvement in frequency range, dynamic range, distortion, and other relevant measures. This comprises a tremendous challenge. DSP ICs for hearing aids are, therefore, developed by highly specialized engineers with extensive knowledge of complex math and semiconductor physics.

Complexity and Calculations

A modern hearing aid is typically built around one or more integrated circuits (ICs) containing millions of transistors. Designing such an IC is a challenge that must be broken down into a series of manageable steps. Transistors are combined to form basic logic blocks that are in turn combined to form simple functions such as arithmetic functions or memory. Combinations of simple functions form more complex functions that are in turn combined to form the entire system. Each step in this process must be checked and verified, often with multiple checks.

A number of analog functions must also be designed to perform specific tasks such as analog to digital conversion and radio transmission or reception. Each of these analog functions must be designed specifically for hearing aid usage because the requirements are too specialized for general-purpose building blocks to be usable. A big challenge in this design process is that the electrical properties of modern transistors vary considerably because of the extremely small size.

The manufacturing process for integrated circuits is very costly and typically takes 6 weeks. The manufacture of the first prototype ICs may cost in excess of USD 500,000. Any error in the design will, therefore, result in a considerable expense. This emphasizes the importance of verifying every detail of the design.

Add to this the constraints of limited power available from a single battery. To achieve a reasonable battery lifetime, a CIC hearing aid, which is the smallest and therefore also the least power consuming type of hearing aid, must use less than 1 milliwatt (mW) of power. Yet the performance of the IC inside a modern hearing aid rivals that of many general-purpose systems, such as a PC, with power consumption of 100W or more. The enormously higher efficiency of the hearing aid IC (in the order of 100,000 times) is achieved by carefully designing the ICs to the specific functions they must perform.

The physical constraints of a hearing aid must also be taken into account. Not only is space limited, but the environment may be quite harsh. While the corrosive moist environment is often dealt with by encapsulation, static electricity offers a challenge that must be dealt with during the electronics design.

Application-Specific versus General-Purpose Processors

The vast number of calculations being performed in a hearing aid requires far less power than what would be required by a standard computer. A computer is very versatile, but this comes at a considerable cost in power. Consumer grade computers come with gigabytes of memory even when most uses require far less memory. While computers can perform billions of operations each second, in reality they remain idle most of the time. Yet, to achieve this speed, highly complicated architectures are used that require much power.

When targeting a specific application, the workload can be broken down to small parts, and dedicated processors can be designed that are able to handle each specific task with extreme efficiency. This means that resources can be kept to a minimum. Moreover, operators can be arranged to minimize movement of data, thereby eliminating unneeded power consumption. Spreading the workload on multiple processors reduces the speed requirements, allowing for lower power consumption. Most high-end digital hearing aids are based on such target-specific designs.

A hearing aid manufacturer often uses similar algorithms for different families of hearing aids, and so an integrated circuit may be designed to be shared. It is attractive to make such flexible processors that may be used in several different series of hearing aids. A processor designed for a class of applications will maintain some flexibility, but at the cost of total performance or power. As a general rule, more flexibility will increase power consumption or lower performance. Some companies offer programmable processors targeted for hearing aids. Those processors must necessarily impose limitations on flexibility and on how much processing can be performed. They do, however, offer a solution for designing hearing aids with moderate performance without the considerable additional cost of designing an integrated circuit.

Power Consumption

For many years, the dominant trend in hearing aid design has been invisibility, which has led to the miniaturization of hearing aid components as well as batteries. Achieving the necessary output to compensate for a hearing loss with a small hearing aid battery is no simple matter. High power efficiency is required. Poor efficiency will reduce the battery lifetime, and may also result in reduced sound pressure in the ear of the user. The higher the required sound levels, the larger the receivers, and consequently the battery drain.

From an overall point of view, two processes are responsible for the major part of the power consumption in a hearing aid; viz., the digital signal processing and the final conversion of digital signal into sound. How these processes may be optimized to reduce the power consumption is discussed in the following sections.

Designing for Small Batteries

Meeting the small size and ultra-low power requirements of a modern digital hearing aid cannot be achieved without engineering compromises. In every instance, the user benefit of the signal processing must be weighed against the additional power consumption, and trade-offs involving, for example, performance in noise, dynamic range, bit resolution, or sampling rate have to be taken into account in the design of every single algorithm or subcircuit.

For the most part, textbook solutions are not viable in a hearing aid application. A look inside a hearing aid reveals that practically every component is developed specifically for hearing aid applications. The reason is that, to date, no standard digital signal processors are available, which are capable of running on the supply voltage of a hearing aid battery (1–1.6 V) for a reasonable stretch of time.

Reducing Power Consumption during Digital Signal Processing

Optimizing power efficiency during A/D conversion involves a trade-off between power consumption on the one hand and inherent component noise on the other. The increase in component noise can be reduced to some extent by increasing the physical size of the components, but this will ultimately increase the size of the hearing aid. Another commonly applied method of decreasing the impact of component noise is to increase the amplification of the A/D converter. However, the largest signal level that can be converted is thereby reduced correspondingly. In practice, therefore, the targeted inherent component noise level is only as low as absolutely necessary. An A/D converter with an inherent noise level that is lower than the hearing threshold level of a normal-hearing person would be overdesigned.

In the DSP, power consumption is proportional with the total number of bits changing state (from 0 to 1) each second. So the more calculations the DSP needs to perform per second, the higher the power consumption. Design engineers can, therefore, make a significant contribution toward reducing power consumption by rethinking the principal textbook formulae and finding ways of keeping calculations as simple as possible. Reducing the bit precision is a more direct way of reducing power consumption, as it reduces the number of digits in every calculation. However, this may result in added noise and limited dynamic range. Another direct and easy way of reducing power consumption is to reduce the sampling rate. However, a shortcoming of this method is that it will lead to reduced bandwidth during signal processing.

Choice of DSP IC can also influence the power consumption in a hearing aid. Two types of DSPs are generally used in the hearing aid industry—application specific integrated circuits (ASICs), which are dedicated hardware solutions, and software-based generic or Open Platform DSPs.

The main advantage of Open Platform DSPs is that they offer the manufacturer the flexibility to program different algorithms, and thus base several different hearing aid series on the same DSP IC. As increasingly advanced algorithms are being developed over time, more processing capability, and consequently a new generation DSP will be required at some point. However, if the Open Platform DSP is designed with a certain amount of overcapability to allow for new and more complex algorithms, new generations are not needed so often. On the other hand, overcapability will also make the DSP larger and more power consuming.

ASICs, on the other hand, are dedicated to executing specific algorithms only, so they are generally smaller and more power efficient than Open Platform DSPs. Some flexibility can be included if carefully planned; by using a set of parameters, the actual algorithms can be controlled, but completely new algorithms will need a new ASIC.

Another stage where energy efficiency can be optimized is the output stage where the digitally processed signals are transferred to the receiver. Typically, a so-called Class D amplifier is used in a hearing aid. The signal of the DSP is translated into a digital signal stream and fed to the receiver, where it is converted into an analog signal. The main advantage of using a Class D amplifier is that it has considerably lower power dissipation. In other words, because a Class D amplifier is very efficient, it provides a high level of utilization of the power available from the battery. Class D amplifiers as an integrated part of the digital signal processing were introduced under the name of "Direct Digital Drive" by Widex in 1995.

Sound Fidelity and Precision

Most people would agree that a high sound fidelity is essential for the user's benefit of the hearing aid. So, while designers must make an effort to keep the power consumption at a minimum, it must not be done at the expense of sound fidelity. The question is, though, how to define high sound fidelity.

Providing high fidelity sound in the sense of faithfully reproducing sound to appear natural and unaltered to normal-hearing listeners is hardly a sensible target in connection with hearing aid users, whose sound perception will have changed as a result of their hearing loss. For these people, a faithful reproduction of the original sound requires a deliberate alteration of the signal to compensate for the hearing loss.

A more feasible aim in connection with hearing aid users is to provide a listening experience that is as close as possible to the listening experience they would have had with normal hearing. Normal-hearing persons are capable of hearing frequencies from 20 Hz to 20 kHz and sound levels from 0 dB HL to 120 dB HL. Ideally, therefore, a hearing aid with high fidelity sound should be able to accurately reproduce sounds within these ranges. Important parameters of a hearing aid in this respect are its frequency response and dynamic range. In addition, sounds must be reproduced without artifacts, such as noise, distortion, or unwanted sounds.

Digital signal processing offers the possibility to precisely shape the frequency response using advanced digital filtering. However, design parameters like sampling rate and bit resolution have to be sufficiently optimized to allow an artifact-free signal reproduction. In addition, digital signal processing requires signals to be converted from analog-to-digital and back again by means of A/D and D/A converters. This process may introduce noise and distortion if not carefully designed.

Sampling Rate and Bandwidth

One parameter that affects sound fidelity is bandwidth. An accurate reproduction of the entire frequency range of a normal hearing person requires a bandwidth of at least 20 kHz. However, bandwidth limitations at the high-frequency end are not so critical. Many people may not notice a bandwidth reduction from the 22.05 kHz of a CD to the 15 kHz of an FM radio, for example. On the other hand, most people will notice that a telephone has a thin sound quality as a result of the significantly smaller bandwidth of just 3.4 kHz. In other words, although it may not be worth the effort to achieve a full 20 kHz bandwidth, the lower the upper limit, the greater the consequences for the sound quality.

In digital signal processing, the upper limit of the bandwidth is restricted to one half the sampling rate (i.e., the number of times per second the original analog signal is sampled). This restriction, known as the Nyquist bandwidth, means that in order to be able to reproduce an analog signal, the signal needs to be sampled with sufficient speed. Figure 8–1 illustrates why this is the case. When an analog signal is sampled more than twice per period, the signal frequency can be reproduced from the sampled values without misinterpretations. However, when sampling is done less frequently than twice per period, the number of samples will be too small to ensure that the frequency of the reproduced signal matches that of the original analog signal.

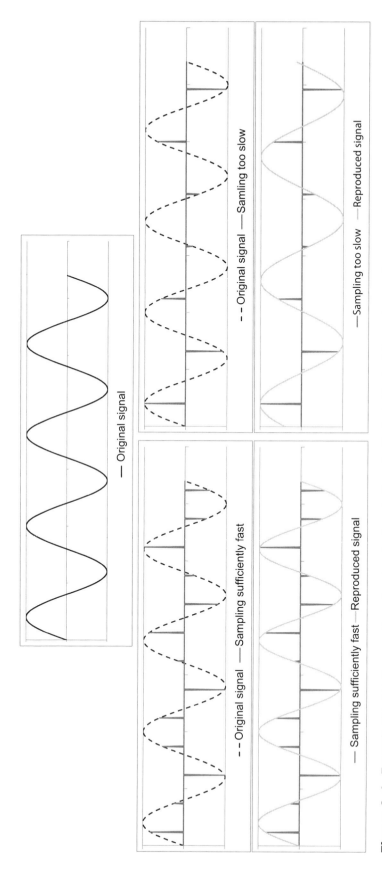

Figure 8-1. Example showing the sampling of a sinus in discrete time. As illustrated in the left panels, a sufficiently fast sampling rate (more than twice the sinus frequency) makes it possible to reproduce the original signal, whereas a sampling rate that is too slow (less than twice the sinus frequency) results in a reproduced signal with a lower frequency than the original (*right panels*).

Since the introduction of digital hearing aids, the sampling rates of digital signal processors for hearing aids have ranged from 16 to 32 kHz, depending on the model and the manufacturer, resulting in corresponding bandwidths of 8 to 16 kHz. The bandwidth of transducers in hearing aids is typically in the range of 10 kHz. A DSP bandwidth of 16 kHz will, therefore, not comprise a limitation, whereas 8 kHz will. In fact, a bandwidth of 8 kHz is less than what could be achieved with analog hearing aid technology.

Bit Precision, Signal Distortion, and Noise

In order to achieve a high sound fidelity, digital signal processing must reproduce signals with a minimum of distortion and noise. Distortion is an alteration of the original signal shape that will make sounds harsh or sharp and reduce the intelligibility of speech signals. Noise, on the other hand, is not related to the original signal. It is an undesired disturbance that may result in the masking of important soft sounds. Distortion and noise will also lead to a reduction of the overall sound quality and user comfort.

The digital signal processing in a hearing aid performs intentional distortion of the original signal by amplifying signals at certain frequencies to compensate for the hearing loss. However, any other kind of distortion that qualitatively changes the signal shape, such as skewing, clipping, or discontinuities, is unintentional and unwanted (Figure 8–2). In order to avoid such distortion, the digital signal processor needs to be able to handle the desired maximum signal level.

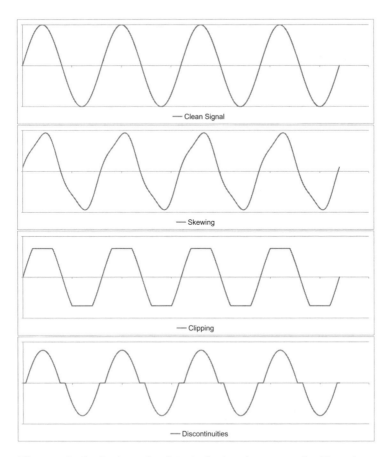

Figure 8–2. A clean (undistorted) signal compared with various types of distortion (skewing, clipping, and discontinuities).

Noise can be introduced intentionally as in the case of tinnitus treatment, but generally noise is an unwanted byproduct introduced by the hearing aid components and signal processing. Usually, it will be heard as continuous static noise. In practice, it is impossible to avoid noise being generated by the hearing aid's components. A feasible target, therefore, is to ensure that the noise remains below the hearing threshold of the user.

In a digital signal processor, signals are represented by bits. Bits must be sufficient in number to represent both the largest and the smallest signals. Insufficient bits will cause distortion for high signal levels and quantization errors, that is, imprecision in the representation of the signal, for low signal levels.

Quantization and noise level are correlated (Figure 8–3). The finer the quantization, the lower the noise level. In other words, noise can be suppressed by introducing smaller quantization steps—using more bits —until the noise is below the HTL of the user and thus becomes inaudible.

The number of bits available for signal representation is termed *bit precision* and is defined by the desired maximum signal level and the required quantization. The bit precision in commercially available hearing aids varies with typical values in the range of 16 to 32 bits. However, these numbers are not necessarily directly comparable. Even though, in principle, a 16-bit precision corresponds to a dynamic range of 96 dB, many algorithms require a higher bit precision locally to ensure an output free from noise and distortion of the available dynamic range.

A simple table of some of the design considerations is seen in Table 8–1. This short chart gives some indication of the "tradeoffs" involved in the design of modern DSP applications in a typical hearing aid.

DIGITAL IMPROVEMENTS OF ANALOG FEATURES

Basic functions, such as amplification, filtering, compression, and output control were already available in analog hearing aids. However, the introduction of digital signal processing meant that these functions could be improved.

Multiple Frequency Bands/Channels

The ability to split the frequency range of the incoming signal into multiple bands, which are then analyzed and processed, is fundamental in the signal processing of digital hearing aids. Multiple frequency bands offer the flexibility of providing different amplification at different frequencies. This is useful in a number of instances, for example, for matching a certain target gain response to the user's hearing loss, or performing more advanced signal processing such as noise reduction or feedback canceling. Generally, the higher the number of frequency bands, the finer the details that can be detected and handled in a given frequency spectrum. However, the cost of this flexibility is increased complexity of the DSP. Moreover, a large number of frequency bands used in conjunction with fast regulation in the compression system may result in the phenomenon known as temporal and spectral smearing, where the amplified signal is stripped of many of the temporal and spectral details used in the identification of speech sounds (Kuk, 2002).

While some hearing aid manufacturers apply individual signal processing in each frequency band, others use the full set of bands for analysis only and combine a number of the frequency bands for the actual signal processing. The bands used during the signal processing are often referred to as frequency channels.

LINEAR AMPLIFICATION

The simplest form of hearing loss compensation is the linear amplification strategy. Linear refers to the 1:1 relationship between input and output signal levels. All signal levels are

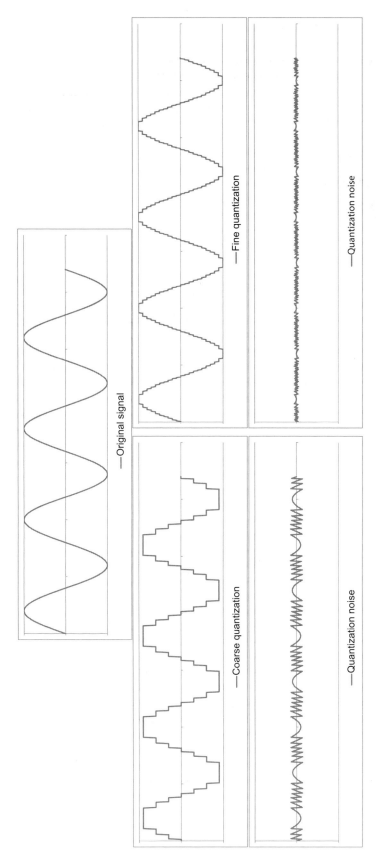

Figure 8–3. Signal representation with limited precision or quantization results in quantization noise, defined as the difference between the quantized signal and the original signal (*illustrated in the left panels*). Finer quantization (smaller steps) result in lower quantization noise (*illustrated in the right panels*).

Table 8–1. Schematic Overview of the Influence of Each Design Factor on the Power Consumption and the Sound Quality of a Hearing Aid

Design Factors	Power Consumption	Sound Quality
Higher number of bits	↑	↑
Higher sampling rate	↑	↑
Smaller chip design technology	↓	—
Dedicated design	↓	—

amplified by the same factor, so an increase in input level will be reflected by the exact same increase in output level.

Linear amplification was the dominant strategy in analog hearing aids. However, with analog electronics, even the application of a large fixed gain factor is a challenge. The amplification process has to be broken down into several stages because of electrical limitations, which may result in noise, distortion, and increased power consumption.

In digital signal processing, the signal and the gain factor are simply numbers to be multiplied, so digital amplification will not introduce noise or artifacts. The end result merely depends on whether the sampling rate and the digital representation (i.e., the number of bits available for each sample) are sufficient to provide a high sound fidelity.

In principle, there is no limit to how much amplification can be achieved in a DSP. The higher the multiplication factor, the higher the gain. For a hearing aid, however, the acoustic amplification achievable is still subject to physical restrictions, most notably the feedback limits imposed by the physical characteristics of the hearing aid and the earmold acoustics. Therefore, digital amplification alone does not offer higher gain possibilities than analog amplification. Even so, one of the major advantages of digital amplification over analog amplification is that it is so simple to implement in a DSP that the design effort can be focused on more advanced features.

COMPRESSION AND TIME CONSTANTS

Until the beginning of the 1970s, amplification in commercially available hearing aids was linear; that is, the same amplification was applied to all sounds—soft or loud. The amplification was typically set to match the target for normal speech, which meant that soft sounds would often be too weak to be audible, while loud sounds would be unpleasantly loud.

Today the vast majority of hearing aids are nonlinear, which means that they use some kind of compression mechanisms. By means of compression, it is possible to match the hearing aid output to the loudness perception of the hearing-impaired user by applying different amounts of gain to soft, moderate, and loud sounds.

Sensorineural hearing loss is typically accompanied by loudness recruitment, which means that a given increase in sound level will be perceived as being far greater by a hearing-impaired person than by a normal-hearing listener. By compressing the amplified signal, it is possible to approximate normal loudness perception for the hearing aid user. The amplification decreases with increased input levels. At very high input levels, little or no amplification is provided as the loudness perception of a person with hearing loss is the same as for a person with normal hearing. This kind of compression is called WDRC (for Wide Dynamic Range Compression), because it is applied over a large part of the dynamic input range. This is illustrated in Figure 8–4.

Modern hearing aids typically have multiple bands to which an equal number of compressors have been assigned, which are able to function according to the individual user's hearing loss. The basis for the gain control performed by the compressor is a measurement of the sound pressure of the input signal.

The regulation time of the compression system is controlled by the frequency with which this measurement is performed. Taken to the extremes, one could imagine a sound pressure measurement device that measured the average sound pressure over a full day. With such a long time constant, the applied gain would never really fit the changing sound environments during the day. The other extreme would be a compressor that responded to every change in sound pressure level as fast as possible always. In this way, gain would constantly change and follow the users hearing loss needs minutely. This might seem like a very good idea, and it has also been tested numerous times. Most of the time, however, the end result is a very poor sound quality and a leveling of important

dynamic features in speech (referred to as temporal and spectral smearing; Kuk, 2002).

The speed with which a hearing aid is able to change its amplification level defines its time constants (or *attack* and *release times*). They refer to the time it takes for the output level of the hearing aid to stabilize in response to a sudden increase or decrease in input level.

Attack and release times have a significant influence on the sound quality of a hearing aid. Attack and release times in a hearing aid with slow time constants (slow-acting compression) are typically longer than 1 second. Time constants in a hearing aid with fast-acting compression (sometimes referred to as instantaneous or syllabic compression) are typically 100 msec or shorter. Studies have shown that hearing aid users generally prefer the sound quality obtained with slow-acting compression (Gatehouse, Naylor, & Elberling, 2006; Neuman, Bakke, Mackersie, Hellman, & Levitt, 1998). However, slow-acting compression will not be beneficial in situations with sudden changes in sound level, for example, when a door suddenly slams in a quiet environment. The compression system must be able to adjust the gain very quickly in response to sudden changes in sound level.

In analog and digitally programmable hearing aids, time constants were controlled by simple resistor-capacitor circuits (RC circuits). Compressors would respond to the *RMS* value of the input signal (a running average of the signal over a given period of time). Therefore, the system would take a little time to respond to a sudden change in the signal. The attack and release times of the compressors were determined by the time constant of the RMS detection circuit.

This is illustrated in Figure 8–5. The left panel shows the appropriate gain reduction in response to a sudden increase in input level. The right panel shows how long it takes two different RC circuits to carry out the gain reduction. The faster circuit (light gray curve) will complete the reduction in 1 second, while the lower circuit (dark gray curve) will only have achieved 75% of the appropriate gain

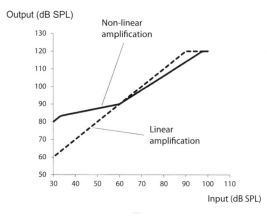

Figure 8–4. Linear versus nonlinear amplification. With nonlinear amplification, proportionally more gain is applied to soft sounds, and less gain is applied to loud sounds to approximate normal loudness perception.

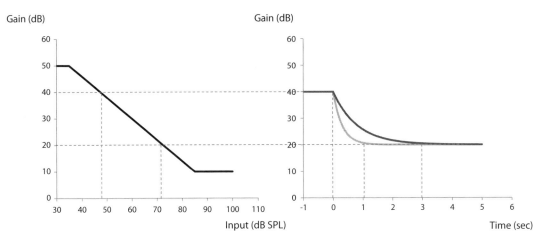

Figure 8–5. The response times of two different RC circuits (*dark and light gray curves, right panel*) with different time constants to a sudden change in input level (*left panel*). Reaching the final gain will take the RC circuit with the longer time constant (*dark gray curve*) more than twice as long as the RC circuit with the shorter time constant (*light gray curve*).

reduction in the same time span. The slower circuit will need 3 seconds to carry out the reduction.

In modern digital hearing aids, time constants can be used in a much more sophisticated manner. Digital devices are not subject to the same limitations as analog instruments, including rigidly defined RC circuits with fixed time constants. In the digital world, one is free to choose whatever method of time constant control is the best match for the compression ratios, and time constants can be combined.

Figure 8–6 shows how different time constants can be combined with different compression ratios. The left panel shows the relationship between gain and input for a compressor with high (CR1) and low (CR2) compression ratios. The right panel shows the regulation times assigned to the two compression ratios. It may be seen that slow regulation (dark gray curve) has been combined with the high compression ratio (CR1), while fast regulation (light gray curve) has been combined with the low compression ratio (CR2).

One example of a sophisticated method for controlling attack and release times is the percentile estimator. Where the RC-circuit

will always stabilize itself to the RMS value of the running signal, a percentile estimator can be set to follow the peak of the signal, the soft part of the signal, the median, or practically any other aspect of the signal. Furthermore, the speed of the estimator can be set to depend on the level, the compression ratio, or any other relevant measure.

Output Control

Providing the right amount of amplification for hearing aid users is no simple matter. On the one hand, some level of amplification is necessary in order to compensate for the hearing loss. On the other hand, the application of too much amplification may result in distortion of the signal and cause the listener considerable discomfort and distress.

A common way of avoiding overamplification is to limit the level of the output signal by means of an Automatic Output Control (AOC) function, sometimes called Automatic Gain Control for Output (AGC-O). A typical AOC will reduce gain quickly when the output signal exceeds a predetermined level and increase it again when the signal is below the

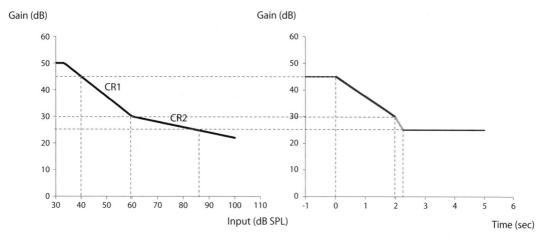

Figure 8–6. In modern digital hearing aids, different compression ratios can be combined with different time constants. In this example, a high compression ratio (CR1) has been combined with slow regulation (*dark gray curve*), while a low compression ratio (CR2) has been combined with fast regulation (*light gray curve*).

critical limit. By setting the permitted maximum output level just below the highest physical output level that the hearing aid is capable of delivering, distortion is avoided.

Limiting the hearing aid output at a specific level can also be used as a tool by the hearing care professional during the fitting process to prevent loud sounds from exceeding the individual user's uncomfortable loudness level (UCL).

A traditional AOC is simple in function and also simple to implement in both analog and digital hearing aids. However, a DSP allows for much more sophisticated methods of output control. These are described in the following.

Advanced Limiters and Intelligent Transient Protection

If loud sounds are amplified to the same extent as sounds produced at normal speech levels, they may be the source of considerable unpleasantness to the hearing aid user. In the past, ensuring an appropriate gain response in connection with sudden loud impulse sounds (transients), such as a slamming door or hammer blows, has proven difficult. As transient sounds are extremely brief in dura-

tion, a slow-acting compression system with attack times of approximately 10 ms reacts far too slowly to be able to avoid gain overshoot. However, the introduction of digital signal processing made it possible to design sophisticated algorithms that are able to identify and handle transient sounds effectively.

Early Implementations

One of the earliest implementations of an advanced output handler in a hearing aid involved a simple identification of impulse sounds based on a comparison of the short-term signal level to the long-term average level of the signal (Widex Senso, 1996). The dynamic range of speech is normally within 15 dB. Thus, when the short-term signal level is above the expected dynamic range, it can be inferred that the signal is most likely nonspeech. This strategy may be beneficial in that it enables an otherwise slow-acting compressor to react with greater speed in response to sudden changes in the signal level. However, even though it will ensure that the prescribed gain level is reached quickly following a sudden increase in sound level, impulse sounds, which, owing to their brevity, do not cause an overall increase in sound level, will slip through.

Identification of Unwanted Transient Sounds

Transient sounds are characterized by being very brief with a steep onset and a fast decay (Figure 8–7). These characteristics are used in modern transient handling algorithms to infer the presence of a transient sound in the incoming signal.

State-of-the-art transient handling algorithms are also able to distinguish between speech sounds and unwanted transient sounds, which enables the preservation of speech cues while attenuating transient sounds. Transient sounds have a very characteristic steep onset and often rise to levels well above the average long-term level of the current sound environment. This means that the identification of transient sounds can be achieved by means of pattern recognition (i.e., a comparison of the properties of transient sounds and speech sounds). And because gain reduction is only triggered by the presence of a transient sound, the audibility and intelligibility of speech are generally not affected in modern, well-designed algorithms.

Some algorithms exploit the tiny processing delay of digital hearings by identifying transient sounds in the broadband signal before it is band-pass filtered and alerting the compression system in advance before the transient sound arrives. Thus, if a transient sound is present in the input signal, the system is able to implement the appropriate gain reduction before the digital signal is converted into an output signal.

The size of the gain reduction needed in connection with transient sounds is individual. Most hearing aid users will be content once the gain overshoot problem is eliminated and the prescribed gain given. However, some hearing aid users suffer from abnormal loudness sensitivity (loudness recruitment, hyperacusis, phonofobia). These people will often prefer a further gain reduction in connection with loud impulse sounds. This option is available in some of the most recent transient handling algorithms.

FFT and Filter Banks

Modern digital hearing aids split the incoming signal into multiple frequency bands to enable a detailed signal processing. A common way of splitting a signal into a large number of frequency bands is to apply the so-called Fast Fourier Transform (FFT) algorithm. Basically, the FFT is used to find the

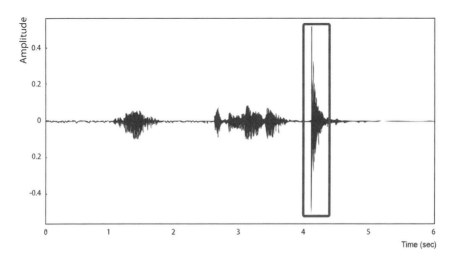

Figure 8–7. Impulse sounds (transients) are characterized by a steep onset, rapid decay, and short duration.

frequency distribution of a signal that has been sampled at evenly-spaced time intervals. In other words, the FFT will show how much of the signal's spectral energy is located in the 500 Hz, 1 kHz, 2 kHz bands, and so on. This is done by transforming a time interval of the signal (i.e., a sample) into a corresponding frequency representation. The resulting number of frequency bands (from 0 Hz to the sampling frequency) will equal the number of signal samples.

Once the signal has been split into bands, signal processing can be applied individually to each frequency band. The ensuing frequency representation will then be transformed back into a time signal by means of a second Fast Fourier Transform (a process known as inverse FFT).

The frequency bands resulting from an FFT are distributed linearly across the entire frequency range. That is, the bandwidth measured in Hz (represented on *x*-axis in Figure 8–8) is the same for all bands. However, it is well known that human auditory perception does not correspond to the equally distributed intervals of the Hz scale. In fact, at frequencies above 1 kHz, human perception of pitch increases logarithmically with frequency (Ellis, 2010; Moore, 2010). From a logarithmic perspective, frequency bands generated by means of an FFT will be wider in the lower end of the frequency range (Figure 8–9). Therefore, the required number of frequency bands is typically determined by the needed bandwidth in the low frequencies. Ideally, this bandwidth should at least correspond to ⅓ octave in order to match the processing of the human ear. However, the larger the number of frequency bands, the larger the number of signal samples that must be transformed. This will increase the processing time of the FFT, and consequently, the overall delay of the digital signal processing. Long processing delays can cause echo effects and lack of synchronization between lips and speech, which will have a negative impact on intelligibility. A trade-off between the frequency selectivity and the overall delay of the signal processing is, therefore, unavoidable.

Another way of separating the signal into frequency bands is to apply a dedicated filter bank. Individual filters can be designed to achieve the precise center frequencies and bandwidths required. The overall processing

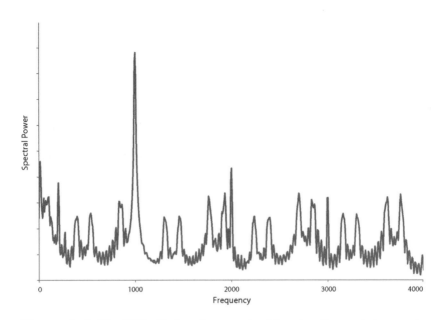

Figure 8–8. The FFT will show how much of the signal's spectral power is located at different frequencies.

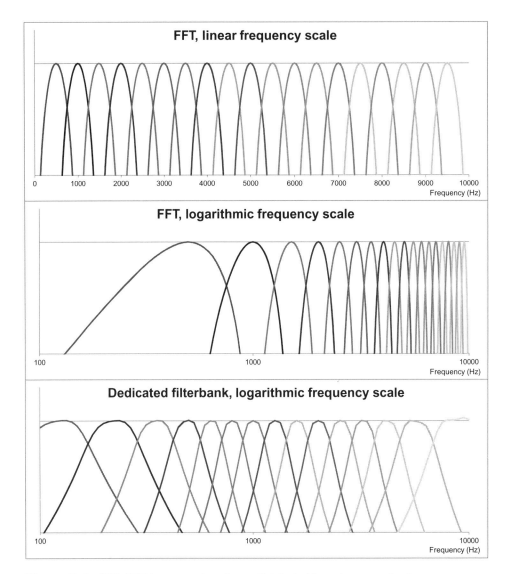

Figure 8–9. With FFT, frequency bands are distributed linearly across the frequency range (*top panel*). On a logarithmic frequency scale (corresponding to the human ear), the frequency bands are widest at the low frequencies and become increasingly narrower with increasing frequencies (*middle panel*). Dedicated filters can be designed freely to match for instance ⅓ octave bands (*bottom panel*).

delay of a filter bank can be kept to a minimum, even though the frequency responses of the individual filters will involve a frequency-dependent delay (known as a group delay), which may be significant in the low frequencies, but will have increasingly less impact toward the higher frequencies. Once the desired signal processing is completed, the signal components in the individual frequency bands can be combined into a complete signal by simply adding them. A dedicated filter bank can provide greater flexibility and a lower overall delay than an FFT solution, but it requires a larger number of specialized filters and may, depending on the actual design, require more processing power from the DSP.

Noise Reduction

It is well-known that normal-hearing listeners' speech intelligibility is adversely affected by noise. There is also plenty of evidence to show that hearing impaired persons' speech intelligibility is affected to an even larger extent in noisy surroundings as a result of their hearing impairment and general deterioration in the auditive system (Humes, 1991; Plomp, 1986).

If the hearing aid user is to derive full benefit from his hearing aids in noise, it is essential that the hearing aid's amplification is adjusted to match the user's ambient sound environment. If the amount of amplification applied is not sufficiently large in noise, speech and other desirable sounds will not be audible. If, on the other hand, the amount of amplification is too great, the user may feel that the noise becomes too loud, and that it drowns out the speech. Too much amplification will have a negative impact on the users' comfort and may cause them to remove their hearing aids.

Typically, the hearing aid's amplification (basic amplification from the compressor) is adjusted to provide optimum amplification of speech in quiet. This applies to the manufacturers' proprietary amplification strategies as well as generic rationales such as NAL and DSL. However, while this amplification strategy will be suitable for speech in quiet or low noise levels, it may not produce the best result in loud noise. The end result may be reduced comfort and speech intelligibility on the part of the listener.

It is in situations with high levels of background noise that noise reduction systems will make a significant difference for the user. The principal task of the noise reduction system is to optimize the hearing aid's amplification in environments with high levels of background noise to ensure the highest possible speech intelligibility and comfort at the same time.

The first noise reduction schemes consisted of simple high pass or low cut filters with a fixed cutoff frequency and a fixed or slightly variable slope. The underlying assumption was that since noise is primarily low-frequent in nature, it can be reduced by removing a predefined range of low frequencies. This assumption is largely correct, but noise can originate from a variety of different sources, so its composition is not necessarily restricted to low-frequency content.

The introduction of digital hearing aids in the mid/late 1990s generated a range of new digital signal processing techniques that could be exploited for a number of purposes. One such purpose was to make the noise reduction systems considerably more sophisticated. Today, noise reduction systems are adaptive, considerably more intelligent, and capable of optimizing their mode of operation according to the ambient noise level in the wearer's surroundings. They are able to distinguish speech signals from noise signals, which in turn allows them to enhance speech and thus increase intelligibility. Some of the most advanced noise reduction systems are able to take the user's hearing loss into account, so that the noise reduction strategy applied is optimized according to the individual hearing loss.

Intelligent Strategies

The introduction of digital hearing aids has enabled the hearing aid companies to develop more sophisticated methods for noise reduction. However, the problem of improving speech intelligibility is extremely complex. Today, a variety of different strategies exist, ranging from the application of a slow overall noise-dependent gain reduction in order to reduce the audibility of the noise, to very fast-acting methods that analyze the incoming signal and quickly adjust the gain when speech is present. A third method involves the formation of beams to filter the signal spatially and attenuate sound coming from a specific direction.

Most state-of-the-art methods split the signal into a number of frequency bands, approximating the critical bands of hearing. The signal is then analyzed in each band and a frequency-dependent gain is applied. This frequency-dependency makes it possible to only alter the signal locally in frequency regions where the speech intelligibility is low, while leaving other parts of the signal, where speech intelligibility is high, unaffected. This also contributes toward achieving a higher overall sound quality.

An important phenomenon in relation to speech perception is simultaneous auditory masking. This occurs when one sound affects the perception of another, simultaneously occurring sound. A commonly experienced example is when a high-level noise signal renders a speech signal partly inaudible. This masking effect, known as upward spread of masking, is asymmetric in frequency, meaning that the masking effect of a given noise signal will spread further upward than downward in frequency. The effect is also highly level-dependent. That is, high-level low-frequency noise will mask signals that are much higher in frequency than low-level low-frequency noise (Moore, 2006). When designing noise reduction systems, it is important to take this masking effect into consideration and reduce gain at frequencies that will generate masking at other frequencies.

Another important aspect when designing noise reduction systems for hearing aids is that people with sensorineural hearing loss have an elevated hearing threshold as well as a reduced dynamic range of hearing. Because the hearing aid provides high levels of amplification to compensate for the elevated hearing threshold, a dynamic speech signal can easily reach the level of loudness discomfort. Reducing the gain for high-level sounds will increase comfort and make the signal more intelligible. On the other hand, as the dynamic range of hearing is reduced, there is a risk of the speech signal ending up below the user's hearing threshold if the amplification is reduced too much. A good compromise is to set the gain so that noise is kept close to the hearing threshold, while the more dynamic speech signal is allowed to peak up into the audible area. An effective measure for quantifying the proportion of speech information that is audible for a listener is the Speech Intelligibility Index (SII; *ANSI S3.5-1997*). This index is essentially a speech-to-noise ratio score that takes both upward spread of masking and speech distortion resulting from too high signal levels into account. The Speech Intelligibility score is calculated in near-critical-bandwidth frequency bands and then summarized into a single value between 0 and 1. In practice, this measure can be used for determining the optimum gain for maximizing speech intelligibility in the ambient background noise.

Another approach to noise reduction involves a fast-acting system that analyzes the incoming signal and changes the gain depending on whether it detects noise or speech. The reasoning behind this strategy is that it is known that most of the information in speech is being carried by amplitude changes in the voice, originating from movements of the mouth cavity, the lips, and the tongue. These amplitude modulations exist in the range from 1 Hz up to around 20 Hz. By amplifying them in the short time intervals they are detected, they will achieve greater audibility than the more stationary background noise. Fast gain reduction can be used to remove reverberation noise, which will improve the dynamic characteristic of the speech and make it more audible.

A third approach, known as beam-forming, uses two or more microphones to spatially filter the signal. Because the microphones are located in different positions and distances from the sources, it is possible to filter out noise coming from another direction than the speech of the dominant speaker. This is, for instance, helpful when the hearing aid user is trying to focus on a speaker standing in front of him while noise or interfering speech from other speakers is coming from behind.

Today, the most advanced hearing aids utilize a combination of all three approaches to obtain the best possible speech intelligibility and overall listening experience.

Multiple Programs, Multi-Memory

For hearing-impaired and normal-hearing listeners alike, moving through the day involves a variety of different listening situations; one-to-one conversations, watching television, telephone conversations, meetings, shopping, driving a car, and so on. The combined need for speech intelligibility and comfort in these situations is seldom fulfilled with just one hearing aid setting. The opportunity to choose between multiple programs, each dedicated to a particular situation, can be a way to address the different needs across multiple sound environments.

Until the mid-1980s, standard user controls were restricted to a volume control and a switch between microphone and telecoil setting on the hearing aid. The volume control permitted the user to increase the amplification in connection with soft sounds and decrease it in connection with loud sounds. In buildings with inductive loop systems, the telecoil setting would provide a better signal-to-noise performance by leaving out most of the unwanted background noise in the room that would otherwise be picked up in the microphone setting. Programs affecting the frequency response consisted of a simple N/H switch on selected aids. The "N" setting (for Normal) was intended for quiet environments. The "H" setting (for High Pass) was intended for noisy environments and would cut away the low frequencies containing the majority of the noise.

With the very first inclusion of digital electronics in hearing aids in the late 1980s came the opportunity of having a number of digitally programmable listening programs, albeit still with analog signal processing. The programs were accessible using a push button on the hearing aid (e.g., 3M Corporation Memory Mate) or via a remote control (e.g., Widex Quattro). Widex Quattro offered four programs, each with programmability of gain, maximum output, low and high-cut filters, plus an additional low-cut filter (the inverse presbycusis adaption filter), compression on/off, microphone/telecoil, and volume control. In total, 8 parameters per program, stored in 20 bits. Each program was independent from the others and as such offered maximum flexibility in setting the fitting parameters. Adjustments were made manually on the basis of charts showing the

response of the hearing aid as each individual setting was altered (Figure 8–10). No real-time visual display was available to allow the hearing care professional to monitor the combined effect of the individual adjustments for the specific client.

When the fully digital era introduced adaptive signal processing with automatic adjustment of gain in multiple frequency channels, it was assumed that with this, more than one program would not be necessary. However, user responses proved this wrong, and subsequent generations of hearing aids, therefore, offered multiple programs also. With each new generation, the complexity of the algorithms in the signal processing increased, as did the number of parameters and the bits necessary to control them.

By 2013, up to 48 frequency channels are state-of-the-art, each with several parameters such as knee-points, compression ratios, and gains. In addition, advanced features such as feedback canceling, noise reduction, frequency transposition, and the generation of sound stimuli for tinnitus relief need control parameters and memory space to store them. The precise number of parameters will depend on the number of channels and activated features and may vary between manufacturers. In the Widex CLEAR440 hearing aid (2010), a typical program requires roughly 200 parameters using a total of 1,100 bits. In addition to this, a little more than 100,000 bits are required by the many factory preset parameters included to optimize the underlying algorithms.

The vast number of parameters makes it practically impossible to allow the hearing care professional to adjust them directly. Instead, the fitting software adjusts the hearing aid on the basis of audiological data such as the user's audiogram and results from various in situ tests performed during the fitting process. In other words, the fitting software utilizes audiological data to set the parameters for the complex algorithms in the digital signal processing. In practice, this means that the programming of the hearing aid can be completed within seconds despite the vast number of adjustable parameters.

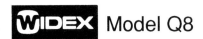

Performance Characteristics

(ANSI S 3.22 - 1987)

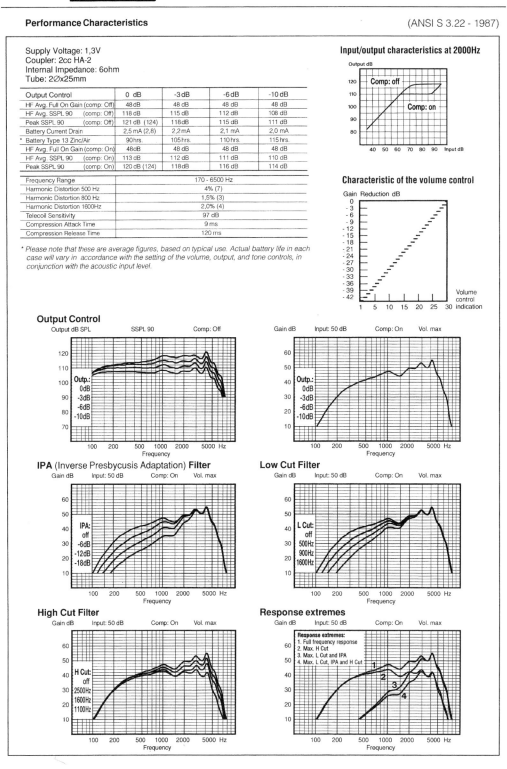

Supply Voltage: 1,3V
Coupler: 2cc HA-2
Internal Impedance: 6ohm
Tube: 2∅x25mm

Output Control	0 dB	-3 dB	-6 dB	-10 dB
HF Avg. Full On Gain (comp: Off)	48dB	48 dB	48 dB	48 dB
HF Avg. SSPL 90 (comp: Off)	118 dB	115 dB	112 dB	108 dB
Peak SSPL 90 (comp: Off)	121 dB (124)	118dB	115 dB	111 dB
Battery Current Drain	2,5 mA (2,8)	2,2mA	2,1 mA	2,0 mA
* Battery Type 13 Zinc/Air	90hrs.	105hrs.	110 hrs.	115 hrs.
HF Avg. Full On Gain (comp: On)	48dB	48 dB	48 dB	48 dB
HF Avg. SSPL 90 (comp: On)	113 dB	112 dB	111 dB	110 dB
Peak SSPL 90 (comp: On)	120 dB (124)	118dB	116 dB	114 dB

Frequency Range	170 - 6500 Hz
Harmonic Distortion 500 Hz	4% (7)
Harmonic Distortion 800 Hz	1,5% (3)
Harmonic Distortion 1600Hz	2,0% (4)
Telecoil Sensitivity	97 dB
Compression Attack Time	9 ms
Compression Release Time	120 ms

Please note that these are average figures, based on typical use. Actual battery life in each case will vary in accordance with the setting of the volume, output, and tone controls, in conjunction with the acoustic input level.

Input/output characteristics at 2000Hz

Characteristic of the volume control

Output Control

IPA (Inverse Presbycusis Adaptation) Filter

Low Cut Filter

High Cut Filter

Response extremes

Figure 8–10. The first digitally programmable hearing aids were adjusted manually from printed charts showing the response of the hearing aid as each parameter is altered.

In addition, for verification and fine tuning purposes, modern fitting software includes graphical illustrations showing the resulting frequency responses and I/O characteristics of the hearing aid. Moreover, fast continuous communication with the hearing aid enables real-time visual display of the signal processing behavior (e.g., the SoundTracker in Widex Compass, Figure 8–11).

TRUE DIGITAL FEATURES

The introduction of digital hearing aid technology opened up endless new possibilities. Developers of hearing devices draw considerable inspiration from other products that also utilize digital technology, for instance computers and cell phones, and new features continue to appear.

The following sections offer a discussion of the most important features that became feasible with the introduction of digital hearing aid technology.

Controllable Sound Generators

One possibility that became available with the introduction of digital technology in hear-

ing aids was the implementation of advanced sound generators that permitted the generation of a wide range of sounds for a number of different purposes.

The possibility of generating sounds was already available in analog hearing aids. However, signal generators (i.e., electronic functions in the amplifier circuit that generate electric signals not originating from the microphone(s) or telecoil) were largely restricted to a very small number of tinnitus masker hearing aids. Typically, white or pink noise was generated by a primitive noise generator and fed to the main amplifier through a separate masker volume control.

In the first fully digital hearing aid from Widex Senso, launched in 1996, sound generation could be exploited for audiometric purposes. The Senso aid had programmable tone generators that could generate tone-complexes for the performance of real ear audiometry (Sensogram). A few years earlier, in 1993, Danavox DFS Genius launched the first hearing aid with feedback cancellation generated test signals to control the feedback cancellation mechanism.

In the beginning, signal generators produced monotonous signals, such as noise and beeps, which could also be utilized for response purposes, for example confirming a

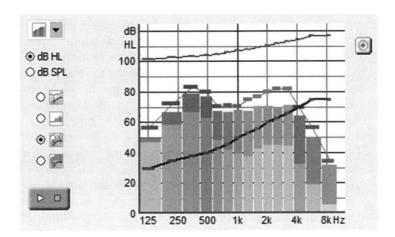

Figure 8–11. Screen shot from Widex Compass showing the SoundTracker. The bars show input + gain in the frequency channels of the hearing aid in real time. The curves indicate the Sensogram threshold and estimated UCL, respectively.

change of program, or a low-battery alarm. Today, it is possible to generate almost any kind of desired signal, for instance sounds known from synthesizers, MP3-players, computers, smart phones, and so on. Moreover, in recent years, storing actual recorded speech messages in the more advanced hearing aids (e.g., Widex mind, CLEAR) has become a possibility. These recorded speech messages can be used to inform users of various hearing aid functions, such as volume adjustment, program change, and battery level in the user's own language by a male or female voice according to the user's preferences. Confirmation of change of program or volume, or warnings of low battery can be much more comprehensible than beeps when presented clearly in the user's own language.

Modern digital hearing aids also permit the integration of extremely sophisticated sound generators for relaxation and tinnitus therapy. Some of those generators can even mimic multiple musical instruments utilizing fractal algorithms to produce harmonic, non-repetitive music patterns (the Zen feature in the Widex mind or CLEAR series).

The different uses of sound generators in hearing aids is discussed in more detail in the following.

Tones and Noise for System Alerts and In Situ Tests

With digital electronics in hearing aids came the opportunity to design artificially generated signals that could be used for a number of different purposes.

The simplest artificial signal shape to produce in a DSP is a square wave (Figure 8–12). Square wave signals are often used for acoustic confirmation of user interactions, such as change of program or activation of volume control, and for system alerts, such as low-battery warnings. The audibility of such signals can be ensured by allowing the amplitude of the signals to be controlled on the basis of the individual hearing threshold and the ambient sound environment.

However, for in situ audiometry, such as Sensogram or in situ RECD measurements,

square wave signals have one major shortcoming; namely distortion (or over-tones). Sinusoids, which are inherently distortion-free, are therefore generally used for audiometric purposes, even though they are considerably more complicated to produce than square waves.

So-called white noise generators are widely used in digital hearing aids, although the term white noise is not strictly correct. Real white noise is generated from a completely random signal, and so is impossible to produce in a digital signal processor, which is inherently deterministic in behavior. However, even though they are not random in nature, white noise signals generated in hearing aids mimic real white noise signals quite closely in that they are characterized by a flat frequency spectrum.

White noise generators are widely used for tinnitus masking and also for initial calibration of feedback cancelling systems in the fitting situation (see the Feedback Management section). When calibrating feedback cancelling systems, it may, in fact, be an advantage not to use real white noise. This is because when the specific noise sequence generated is known, it can be used to calculate physical parameters, such as the delay of the acoustical feedback loop.

Speech Messages

For relatively basic hearing aids with a volume control and a limited number of listening programs, simple beep tones can be sufficient to provide the user with auditory confirmation of changes in the hearing aid settings. However, in modern hearing aids, where dramatic improvements in functionality has led to the inclusion of a variety of different acoustical programs and wireless connectivity options, the necessary number of user control responses and system alerts (such as low battery alert, service reminder, and so on) has increased correspondingly. Speech messages can be a way to make it easier for the user to distinguish between the many acoustic status indicators. Verbal messaging has the advantage of being much less equivocal and prone to misinterpretations than beeps.

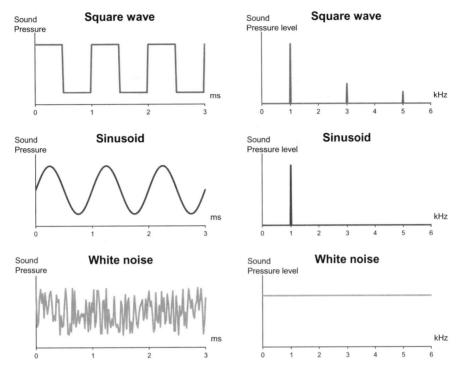

Figure 8–12. Examples of a square wave, sinusoid, and white noise (*left*) with corresponding frequency distributions (*right*). As shown in the frequency domain graphs, square waves consist of a fundamental frequency (1 kHz in this example) and harmonic distortion products at higher frequencies (3 and 5 kHz in this example). Sinusoids, which are only associated with one frequency, are therefore used instead of square waves for audiometric measurements. The spectrum of white noise is distributed evenly across all frequencies.

In order to accommodate the many different users of hearing aids, speech messages have to be language—and in some cases, dialect-specific, and users should also be able to choose the gender of the speaker according to their own preferences. This flexibility requires that all the messages needed to cover the entire set of acoustic indicators be translated into a large number of languages and dialects. Each message must be recorded in high quality with both male and female speakers. Raw recordings of speech messages take up too much memory to be storable in a hearing aid. The messages are, therefore, analyzed and the essential information extracted for encoding (compression in size). This encoded information is stored in the hearing aid memory and decoded for use in a built-in speech synthesizer.

Even with encoding of the speech messages, a hearing aid can have only one version of the speech messages stored at a time. The selection of language and gender must therefore take place during the fitting session, and the chosen version loaded by the fitting program. Speech messages have to be audible to the hearing aid user in every environment. The synthesized speech is therefore amplified according to the configuration of the individual hearing loss and the ambient sound level.

Soothing Sounds for Tinnitus Therapy

Research has shown that as much as 70% to 85% of the hearing-impaired population suffers from tinnitus (Martines et al., 2010). This makes it highly relevant for hearing aid manufacturers to focus on tinnitus therapy in addition to the amplification of sound.

Because the precise mechanisms behind tinnitus are unknown, the only option for the majority of tinnitus sufferers is to learn certain management techniques that may relieve the stress that their tinnitus creates. Most forms of recognized tinnitus therapies involve a combination of counseling, stress reduction, and/or sound therapy (Henry, Zaugg, Myers, & Schechter, 2008).

Some hearing aids can generate sounds that can have a relaxing effect and may be used as a tool in tinnitus therapy.

In the context of tinnitus treatment, the purpose of such background sounds may be:

■ to avoid silence (many tinnitus sufferers cannot tolerate complete silence as their perceived tinnitus may worsen in silence).
■ to distract the hearing aid user's attention from the tinnitus.
■ to mask the tinnitus entirely.

If the tinnitus is to be masked entirely, this is most easily achieved using a steady-state noise signal. However, achieving a complete masking of the tinnitus often requires the noise-masker to be played at a level that is rather uncomfortable in itself.

Thus, distracting the user's attention away from the tinnitus is usually a more desirable approach. For this purpose, a music-like sound can be much more pleasant than a noise signal. Even though prerecorded music could be used to that effect, there are several advantages in using continuously generated music. For example, the length of a prerecorded tune will be limited by the storage capacity in the hearing aid, whereas continuously generated music in principle can go on forever.

Another advantage of continuously generated music is that there is at least some degree of control over important characteristics of the music, for instance speed, frequency range, and level. Tools for sound-based tinnitus management must be able to accommodate variations in individual preferences. People can respond very differently to the same sound stimuli; a sound that is perceived as pleasant by one person may be perceived as annoying by another. However, as a general rule, instrumental music with no lyrics is recommended for tinnitus therapy (Henry et al., 2008).

This type of musical stimuli is generated by the Zen feature that was first offered in 2008 (Widex mind440). The Zen feature uses a music generation algorithm that relies on the mathematical concept of fractals. Specifically, the algorithm generates sequences of predictable, yet unrepetitive music, not unlike classical music. The user has a choice of several preconfigured melodies, and the overall pitch and speed of the music can be adjusted according to the user's individual preferences.

Of course, the music will repeat itself eventually once all involved pseudo random generators have run through all possible states. However, this will take several weeks or months of continuous playing and will, therefore, never be noticeable in practice.

As hearing aids are subject to constraints of limited power, memory, and size, the Zen feature has been designed to generate music with the least possible amount of hardware, memory size, and current consumption. This optimization meant that the feature accounted for less than 5% of the chip area and current consumption when it was introduced in the Widex mind440 series.

In Situ Tests

Acoustic accuracy is instrumental for a successful hearing aid fitting. Without control of the sound produced at the eardrum, hearing aid users may be either insufficiently or overly compensated for their hearing loss, and the benefit of well-designed signal processing features may be diminished. Lack of control with the acoustics may, therefore, significantly reduce the user's hearing ability and comfort.

The performance of the hearing aid when placed in the hearing aid user's ear can be assessed in situ by means of a number of tests. The downside of this is that it takes time and requires the use of specialized audiometric equipment. However, the introduction of sound generators into hearing aids has made it possible to perform a number of these tests using the hearing aids as measurement device.

Threshold Measurements

An audiogram made by means of an audiometer and headphones or earplugs is the standard diagnostic threshold measurement. The audiometer is calibrated to produce a controlled sound pressure at the eardrum of an average adult ear. Thus, no audiogram is completely accurate. The audiometric equipment is calibrated toward average data, and very few real people will match this average ear. If their ears are larger than average, the sound pressure will be weaker. Conversely, if their ears are smaller, the sound pressure will be greater. There is also a difference between the sound pressure applied at the eardrum by headphones or insert earplugs. The audiogram is, therefore, not the perfect basis for making a precise first fitting of a hearing aid.

The possibility of producing tones and more complex sounds via the hearing aid makes it possible to use the hearing aid itself to measure hearing thresholds. The advantage of this is that the hearing loss is measured using the exact same setup and with the exact same acoustic conditions in the ear canal that will later apply when the hearing aid is in use. In other words, measuring hearing thresholds by means of the same system that will be used for amplification will contribute toward a more precise, individualized fitting and calibrate the hearing aid to the individual user. The first in situ audiometry feature to be incorporated into a hearing aid was the Sensogram feature (Widex Senso, 1996).

An important consideration when using a hearing aid for audiometric purposes is what tones should be used. Generally, two types are used for thresholds measurements: pure tones or tone-sweep. A pure tone will reveal the threshold at one specific frequency, whereas a tone-sweep will change in frequency and thereby provide a measurement of the best hearing within the frequency

range that it spans. For diagnostic purposes, the pure-tone threshold will indicate how the threshold changes across specific frequencies (e.g., 500, 1000, 2000, 4000 Hz). For hearing aid calibration though, the measured threshold will be used to set a gain in a frequency range that spans a wider range of frequencies. Using pure tones could, therefore, result in overamplification in one end of the frequency range if the threshold is measured on a slope (as in Figure 8–13). This is where wideband tone-sweeps have their merit.

One of the challenges of measuring hearing thresholds is that the hearing aid has to be able to produce sound in the necessary dynamic range. Very weak tones, which are on the edge of normal-hearing people's threshold, and very loud tones, which are at the limit of the hearing aid's fitting range, must be pure and without noise. Distortion or noise may be audible in regions where the hearing aid user's residual hearing is relatively good, which may lead to an incorrect measure of the hearing threshold.

Loud tones comprise a considerably smaller problem than weak tones. Normally, a hearing aid will be able to produce a sound pressure of up to 90 dB without notable distortion. However, the inherent noise in the hearing aid will be audible to listeners with normal hearing at some frequencies at low sound pressure levels. This is problematic in connection with threshold measurements, and for a long time prevented many hearing aid manufacturers from offering in situ threshold measurement via the hearing aid. The challenge has been overcome by the introduction of an attenuator that reduces the sensitivity of the receiver, which in turn permits the device to produce much softer high-quality tones. The attenuator is controlled by the fitting software. It will be activated when soft tones, barely audible to normal-hearing listeners, are played, but not for louder tones.

In Situ RECD Measurements with the Hearing Aid

The Real Ear to Coupler Difference (RECD) is the difference in decibels, as a function of

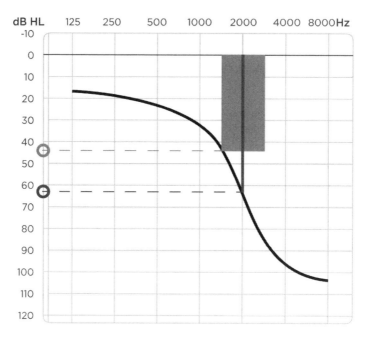

Figure 8–13. The black line shows a sloping hearing loss. A threshold measurement using a pure tone (*dark gray line*) at 2kHz will provide a good indication of the magnitude of the hearing loss at precisely 2 kHz. However, using this threshold to provide gain in a frequency region of one octave around 2 kHz would cause overamplification below 2 kHz where the hearing loss is milder. A sweep measurement (*light gray bar*) in this octave, on the other hand, will reveal the difference in hearing loss configuration at and below 2 kHz, thus reducing the risk of overamplification.

frequency, between the SPL in the ear canal and the SPL in a 2cc coupler, for a specified input signal. In pediatric hearing aid fitting, RECD measurements is a widely applied tool for correcting hearing thresholds and hearing aid output for individual differences in ear canal volume.

During the first years of life, the length of the child's ear canal increases from approximately 14 mm at birth to its adult size of approximately 25 mm (Keefe, Bulen, Campbell, & Burns, 1994; Salvinelli et al., 1991). This has implications for the volume and thus the acoustic properties of the canal. Consequently, fitting rationales used for calculating the hearing aid's gain and output at the eardrum for a given hearing loss include a correction for the difference between an average adult and the child. In this way, overamplification in the

child's small ear can be avoided, and the correct sound pressure will be provided to ensure audibility of speech and environmental sounds. Studies have provided average RECD values from large groups of children (Bagatto et al., 2005; Bagatto, Scollie, Seewald, Moodie, & Hoover, 2002; Feigin, Kopun, Stelmachowicz, & Gorga, 1989). Such data have been incorporated into commercial hearing aid fitting software to predict the RECD for a given age. However, individual RECD values may deviate from the average values by as much as 10 to 15 dB across frequencies. It is, therefore, recommended to always measure the RECD for the individual child and apply these values in the fitting process.

The RECD is typically measured in the clinic using real ear measurement equipment. The real ear response is measured with an insert earphone and a probe microphone positioned close to the eardrum. The 2cc coupler response is then measured with the same insert earphone mounted on a BTE adapter with 25 mm of tubing (Moodie, Seewald, & Sinclair, 1994).

Importantly, the type of transducer used to obtain the measurement will affect the RECD values. The transducer-chain includes the receiver in the insert phone that generates the measurement signal and its coupling to the ear canal or 2cc coupler (e.g., tubing, tip, and coupler adapter). Receivers in insert phones and hearing aids have different frequency responses and, combined with differences in coupling arrangements to the ear canal or 2cc coupler, may cause the measured RECD to vary by as much as 10 to 15 dB in the same ear (Munro & Toal, 2005). When the transducer used for obtaining the RECD is different from the hearing aid transducer that delivers the amplified signal in the ear canal, this may result in an error in the correction of the fitting targets.

However, advances in digital hearing aid technology have made it possible to perform RECD measurements using the hearing aid as both signal generator and measurement tool (Figure 8–14). The real ear measurement is performed with a probe mounted on the hearing aid, and the 2cc coupler response is stored in the hearing aid fitting software (e.g., the In situ RECD procedure for Widex BABY440). In this way, the measured RECD includes all the acoustic characteristics of the hearing aid, its receiver, and its coupling to the ear via the earmold. By using the hearing aid to measure the in situ RECD, the procedure can also be integrated more easily into the hearing aid fitting process. Only a single real ear measurement is needed with the child, and the obtained RECD values are automatically applied to the fitting targets, as well as any in situ thresholds obtained with the hearing aid (e.g., the in situ Sensogram). This allows for a more precise hearing aid fitting that takes into account the uncertainty of the size of the ear canal in young children.

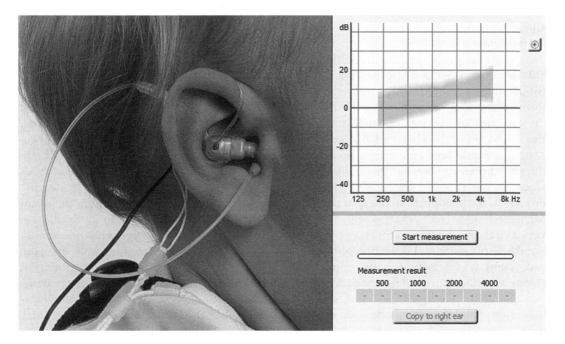

Figure 8–14. Example of the in situ RECD procedure for Widex BABY440. The photograph on the left shows a RITE hearing aid with probe tube mounted for in situ RECD measurement. The corresponding window in the fitting software is shown on the right.

Feedback Management

In all hearing aids—analog as well as digital—insufficient sealing of earmolds or shells will cause sound to leak out of the ear canal to the microphone(s) and result in acoustic feedback (whistling). In analog hearing aids, the usual way of dealing with feedback issues was to manually reduce the high-frequency gain by means of a high cut (also called low pass) filter until the whistling stopped.

The first generation digital hearing aids offered semiautomatic feedback management by including the detection of feedback and a corresponding gain limitation as part of the fitting procedure. A feedback test would find the maximum stable gain (also called the feedback limit) by increasing gain stepwise in each of the frequency channels until feedback occurred. The test had to be performed in a very quiet environment where feedback whistling could be detected by monitoring the signal level at the microphones. Once the maximum stable gain was found, this information was programmed into the hearing aid. The maximum available gain would be set lower than the maximum stable gain to allow for some variation in the ear canal's shape during use.

As signal generators in digital hearing aids improved, so did the feedback tests. Internally generated tones were played through the receiver of the hearing aid into the ear canal of the user. A small portion of this sound, which had been attenuated by the earmold, would reach the microphones, and the sound pressure level at the microphones would be measured by the hearing aid itself. From this, the maximum stable gain could be calculated. This feedback test still required very quiet surroundings to function properly, but the application and detection of tones in each band was less time consuming than stepping up the gain until feedback occurred.

The active feedback canceling systems in modern hearing aids can be used directly in the estimation of the maximum stable gain during fitting. Sound is generated into the ear canal by an internal broadband noise generator in order to create near-optimal conditions for the feedback canceling system. This makes it possible for the feedback system to adapt quickly to the acoustics and the feedback path of the outer ear and estimate the maximum stable gain in each channel. This method is more robust against environmental sounds than the tone based methods and as such is less dependent on very quiet surroundings during testing. Modern hearing aids use a combination of the tone and noise based methods for the feedback test.

Even state-of-the-art feedback canceling systems, which in principle monitor the feedback conditions and continuously adjust themselves accordingly, can benefit from the results of a feedback test at the initial fitting of the hearing aid. The feedback path found during the feedback test provides a good starting point for the active feedback canceling and is also valuable as a nominal solution for situations where adaptation for some reason is not possible.

Feedback Canceling

As mentioned above, feedback may occur if some of the sound that is played by the receiver returns to the microphone through leaks between the ear canal and the hearing aid earmold or through the vent (Figure 8–15). The amplification applied by the hearing aid will not only affect the incoming sound, but also the amount of feedback signal generated. This is not a problem as long as the amplification is less than the attenuation occurring in the loop consisting of hearing aid and feedback path. If the amplification in the hearing aid is greater than the attenuation, the result is an unstable system where an oscillation will build up, resulting in a whistling sound.

Usually, the attenuation and the gain will not be the same across all frequencies, which is why instability usually occurs at one particular frequency. As a consequence, instability will manifest itself as whistling, a tone, or howling. This is illustrated in Figure 8–16. The hearing aid gain and the attenuation in the feedback path are closest to each other

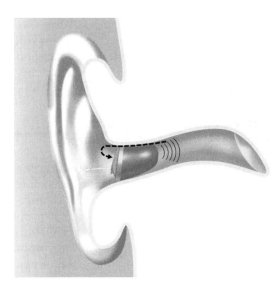

Figure 8–15. Illustration of a feedback path through a leak between the ear canal and the earmold.

at around 5 kHz. Instability is most likely to occur at this frequency, in which case it will result in a 5 kHz tone.

The simplest way to handle problems with feedback is to limit amplification, either manually as in analog hearing aids, or semi-automatically as in digital hearing aids. However, a limitation of the amplification will reduce audibility for the hearing aid user, so ways to suppress feedback without reducing amplification have been pursued since the introduction of the first digital signal processors. Such feedback canceling techniques require an immense number of calculations, and so are not feasible using analog signal processing.

The introduction of digital technology enabled a new, more sophisticated approach to feedback management; viz., feedback canceling. The first product to offer digital

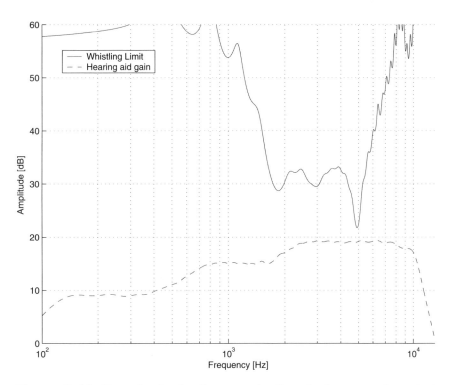

Figure 8–16. Example showing the approximation of a frequency-dependent attenuation of a feedback path (whistling limit) and the amplification of a hearing aid. Feedback is most likely to occur at 5 kHz where the whistling limit and the hearing aid gain are closest.

feedback canceling did in fact rely on analog signal processing (the Danavox DFS Geniuis, launched in 1993), and up until around the year 2000, feedback in fully digital hearing aids was handled by a simple limitation of the amplification. However, advances in the signal processing made it possible to develop a new much more advanced feedback handling method. The new approach involved continuously estimating a model of the feedback path across frequency (FPM). In this way, it is possible to create an artificial feedback path signal, which can be subtracted from the microphone signal (Figure 8–17). Ideally, the real and estimated feedback path signals will cancel each other out, in principle allowing unlimited amplification.

Although much has become possible with the advent of digital signal processing, creating a feedback canceling system that will work perfectly in every situation is by no means a trivial task. For example, the feedback system may mistake systematic sound, such as an alarm or music, for feedback. Moreover, since the head/jaw movements of the user and the surrounding environment constantly change, the feedback path will never be static. The feedback canceling system, therefore, has to adapt fast enough to track those changes without introducing errors. Also, even if a very complex model is applied, it will never be able to reproduce the

actual feedback path in every detail. Even so, a FPM-based feedback canceling system will normally reduce the amount of feedback and consequently increase the maximum available gain.

Strategies for Discriminating Feedback from Ambient Sound

When the ambient sound surrounding the hearing aid is highly unsystematic (e.g., white noise), conditions are particularly advantageous for adaptation of a feedback canceling filter. In this situation, any correlation between the hearing aid output and input must be due to feedback. Conversely, when the ambient sound consists mainly of distinct tonal components, it is particularly difficult to discriminate ambient sound from a feedback signal. There are several ways to deal with the cross-correlation between output and ambient sound, and it is not uncommon to combine more strategies to allow a faster adaptation rate. Below, various strategies are discussed along with the trade-offs involved.

■ *Gain control.* Of course, feedback can always be handled by decreasing the amplification. This will result in reduced audibility, but if a small reduction is sufficient to prevent squealing, a slight loss in audibility for soft sounds may be acceptable.

■ *Inserting a processing delay.* Many correlations are short-time correlations, so insertion of a delay in the signal processing path will generally reduce the correlation between the output of the hearing aid and the surrounding sound. Unfortunately, it takes only a very small processing delay before the user will experience an "echo effect" on his or her own voice. If longer delays are introduced, other people's speech and lip movements will begin to appear unsynchronized.

■ *Addition of probing noise.* Noise can be added to the output, in which case it will appear in the acoustic feedback signal as well as the feedback cancellation signal. The component of feedback driven by

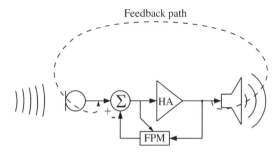

Figure 8–17. Illustration of a feedback canceling system based on a feedback path model (FPM). The idea is to create an artificial feedback path signal, which, when subtracted from the microphone signal, will cancel out the real feedback signal.

the noise will have no correlation with the ambient signal. In this way, the added noise will help discriminating feedback from ambient sound. The noise should be played below the current masking level to prevent audibility. It is common that a short sequence of highly audible noise is used for initializing feedback canceling filters in a fitting situation. This is a fast and accurate means of initializing filters, and in a controlled fitting situation, users generally accept the brief annoyance of this noise.

■ *Amplification of microphone noise.* The compression system in a hearing aid will increasingly amplify sounds as they become softer. When the ambient signal drops below the noise floor of the microphones it is common, however, to reduce amplification to prevent the inherent microphone noise from becoming audible. By ensuring that amplification is only moderately reduced, though, the amplification of the inherent noise will provide an effect similar to that of adding probing noise.

■ *Modulations/time-variations on the output.* By actively modulating the phase, delay, or amplitude of the output signal and demodulating it again at the input, it is possible to distinguish a signal carried by the feedback path from ambient sound. Unfortunately, the time variations affect the output in a somewhat audible fashion, so the variations should be kept small.

■ *Frequency shifting.* A slight shifting or transposition of the frequency spectrum will make the linear correspondence between feedback signal and ambient signal disappear. Frequency discrimination generally deteriorates as a result of hearing loss, but the amount of shifting/transposition must still be moderate to prevent it from becoming audible. For people with severe high-frequency impairment, some hearing aids offer a feature for frequency shifting designed to provide audibility of high-frequency sounds where audibility cannot be provided by amplification (cf. the section on Frequency Transposition). Inciden-

tally, this type of transformation is also a tremendous help in handling feedback.

■ *Slow adaptation.* Decreasing the adaptation rate for somewhat auto-correlated ("systematic") sounds and stopping adaptation altogether when tonal sounds appear is an effective means of avoiding maladjustment of canceling filters. Obviously, this strategy will also reduce the ability to follow fast changes in the feedback path and the handling of feedback "squealing."

When conditions are good, or the system has to track large changes, the adaptation rate can be increased. However, there are situations where large changes occur while conditions for adaptation are poor. These situations can be handled by means of a backup system that will limit the hearing aid gain for a very short stretch of time.

Modern hearing aids often have two microphones to permit focus on sounds coming from a specific direction. Such a directional system comprises an additional challenge to a feedback system because it will be a part of the feedback path (Figure 8–18A). Every time the directional system changes its directional pattern, the feedback path will be affected. The feedback canceling system must, therefore, be able to adapt at the same pace to the change. A solution is to use two feedback canceling systems, one for each microphone. In this way, each feedback canceller can adapt to its own feedback path (Figure 8–18B). Such dual feedback canceling systems were introduced into digital hearing aids in the mid-2000s (Widex Inteo, Gn Resound Metrix).

Open Fittings

Open fittings have become increasingly popular in recent years. They cannot create the necessary sound pressure for people with pronounced (low-frequency) hearing impairment, but for people with mild or mild-to-moderate hearing loss, an open fitting is very attractive. The occluded sound resulting from a blocked ear canal is a major annoyance when low-frequency hearing is relatively

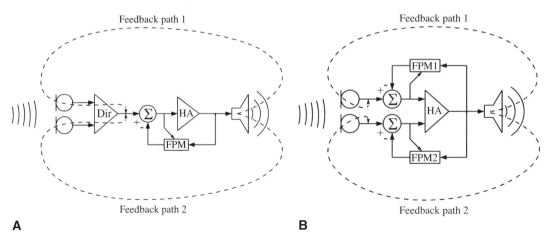

Figure 8–18. A–B. Illustration of a single feedback canceling system with a directional system (Dir) (*left*), and a dual feedback canceling system with the directional system incorporated in the HA block (*right*).

intact, but with an open fitting, occlusion can be avoided. Furthermore, the frequently used soft open ear-tips are barely noticeable when inserted into the ear.

Open fittings will result in more acoustic feedback as more of the receiver output will feed back to the microphones. Recent advances in antifeedback systems have, therefore, made an important contribution to the increased popularity of open fittings. Although performance has greatly improved, there are still limitations to what antifeedback systems can handle. A telephone handset, for instance, is still more likely to generate feedback with an open fitting than with a closed fitting.

Performance and Artifacts

Feedback can always be avoided by reducing amplification. Performance of an antifeedback system should, therefore, be judged by the maximum available stable gain before feedback and the type and amount of sound quality degradation occurring. The complexity of antifeedback systems has increased over the years, and generally users can expect a more stable behavior with fewer artifacts than in earlier products. It is important to note, however, that an effective feedback handling does tend to affect overall sound quality.

The antifeedback system is a feature of modern hearing aids, which is implemented very differently by hearing aid manufacturers. This difference reflects highly different strategies underlying the design of the systems. There is always a trade-off involving efficiency, audibility, and artifacts, and hearing aid users may have very different tolerance of squealing, audible distortion, and reduced audibility. While some hearing aid users feel stigmatized by the occasional squeal, other users may prefer the sound to be as undistorted as possible.

There are many issues to keep in mind when judging feedback performance in a particular hearing aid. The operating range of the antifeedback system can be restricted in different ways and distortions, and artifacts caused by antifeedback handling can take many different forms. Some are described above: large processing delay, frequency shifting, noise, reduced amplification, and so on. Others may be due to the antifeedback system confusing components of the ambient sound with feedback.

Frequency bandwidth varies considerably among hearing aid manufacturers. As feedback is particularly prevalent at higher frequencies, a hearing aid offering a wide bandwidth will also be more subject to feedback and will require a more advanced system. It is common practice that antifeedback systems are active only at higher frequencies because the problem is less pronounced at lower frequencies. In some devices, the starting frequency is 1 kHz, although it is 2 kHz in others. The operating range of the system is rarely advertised by manufacturers. Moreover, there are many different fitting rationales. It is important to keep in mind that a rationale prescribing more amplification will result in increased feedback. The amplification for soft sounds is particularly important in this regard.

Music and alarms can be particularly challenging due to the large number of tonal components. The antifeedback systems may be triggered by the tonal components in the ambient sound, and so many hearing aids offer a special music program, in which the antifeedback system is restricted to static (i.e., nonadaptive) operation, or to operating as a feedback manager (i.e., by limiting amplification) only. Recently, however, some hearing aid manufacturers have succeeded in designing antifeedback systems that are in fact sophisticated enough to work while the user is listening to music.

A few attempts have been made to outline benchmarking procedures for antifeedback systems, that is, procedures for measuring how much stable gain can be provided and the amount of distortion and other artifacts. Early work on benchmarking procedures has been reported by Freed and Soli (2006) and Banerjee, Merks, and Trine (2006). Recently, the development of a black-box measurement method for benchmarking antifeedback performance has been attempted by Spriet, Moonen, and Wouters (2010). Although an interesting first step, this work also reveals that such measurements are not easily obtainable.

Occlusion Management

The phenomenon of the sound of one's own voice changing when the ear is plugged by an earmold is well-known. This effect is also experienced by hearing aid users. Part of the reason is that the amplification of a hearing aid makes a larger number of sounds audible, but the plugging of the ear will also result in the amplification of low frequencies in the ear canal.

When a hearing aid is worn, the sound pressure in the ear will be a result of a combination of different sound sources. One of the sources will be the amplified sound from the hearing aid. Another source will be the sound that travels around the earmold and hearing aid directly into the ear canal. A third significant source will be the sound originating from the vibration of the ear canal wall during one's own speech (Figure 8–19).

The level of the sound from the hearing aid is well under control in modern hearing

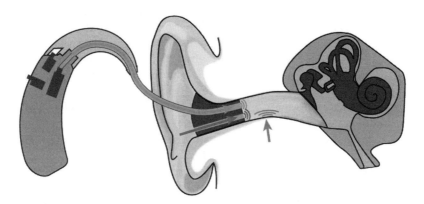

Figure 8–19. Sound may enter the ear canal through three channels: the hearing aid, the vent or other leakages, and via vibrations in the ear canal wall.

aids. In a modern, well-designed hearing aid and fitting rationale, a considerable amount of knowledge of how much sound pressure the hearing aid will deliver in the individual ear canal will have been incorporated into the fitting software.

The level of the direct sound traveling into the ear will be determined by how open or closed the fitting is. The sound pressure will change as a result of leakages and vent design. With a well-fitting earmold, the leak or vent will be more or less identical every time the earmold is put into place. With a mold with a poor fit, on the other hand, the leak may vary from insertion to insertion, and the effect will be more difficult to predict.

The level of the sound generated by one's own voice will be determined by the flexibility and anatomy of the individual ear and by the openness and design of the earmold. A fully closed earmold will provide a much larger bass boost than an open mold. The boost at low frequencies (for example, at 200 Hz) could easily be >20 dB (Killion, 1988; Westermann, 1987). The three sound sources will mix in the ear canal and result in the overall sound pressure present in the user's ear canal.

If a hearing aid user dislikes the quality of his or her own voice, there may be several solutions to this problem. If the hearing loss is mild at low frequencies and the earmold is relatively closed, for example a CIC hearing aid, the sound of the user's own voice may be the louder signal at low frequencies. This is the classic example of the occlusion effect. The standard solution is to introduce a larger vent to provide relief for the low-frequency pressure built up in the ear canal. One thing to bear in mind, though, is that introducing a vent will not only reduce the low frequency power, but also introduce a resonance peak above the low frequency region in question. This may explain why introducing a larger vent does not always solve the problem with the quality of the user's own voice.

If the hearing loss is severe enough in the low frequencies to warrant amplified sound well above the level of the user's own voice, the hearing aid amplification will be the cul-

prit. In this case, the solution will be to alter the amplification to make the sound more comfortable. If the user's voice sounds too boomy, it might be a result of too much sound pressure at the very low frequencies and may be remedied by adjusting gain below 250 Hz. If the user describes his or her voice as sounding artificial, the cause may be a boost around 500 Hz, which is making the sound of the user's own speech metallic.

Trying to solve the above-mentioned problems by the introduction of a larger vent might actually render the artificial sound worse, as the vent can lower the low frequency content and add an extra boost at its resonance frequency at the same time. In fact, if the problem is not caused by occlusion at all, but rather by the user's lack of acclimatization to the new sound of the hearing aid, the introduction of the resonance may render the sound even more unnatural or unpleasant.

Some manufacturers provide a special handle in the fitting software for controlling low frequency gain and the setup of the compression to target problems with the user's own voice.

Directional Microphone Systems

Directional microphones have been used in hearing aids since the 1970s. Despite their name, they are not meant to offer the user an improved sense of directionality. Rather, they function as a spatial noise reduction in the sense that sounds arriving from directions other than the front are attenuated proportionally more. This will provide an increased SNR during conversations in noise.

Until the early 2000s, dedicated directional microphones with two inlets separated by a single diaphragm were commonly used. In the early 2000s, the first hearing aids were introduced with directional behavior based on two omnidirectional microphones. Even though the implementations are different, the underlying principle is the same in the two systems.

A dedicated directional microphone consists of a single diaphragm and two inlet ports. Sound travels from the outside of the hearing aid into the two cavities separated by the diaphragm (Figure 8–20A). If the pressures impinging on the diaphragm from both sides are different, the diaphragm will move in response to the incoming sound, whereby an electrical signal is generated. If, on the other hand, the pressures impinging on the diaphragm from opposite sides are identical, they will cancel each other out, and no electrical signal will be generated. This will ensure that unwanted signals are not picked up and allowed to travel through the hearing aid system.

In order for the signal to be cancelled out, it must arrive at exactly the same time at the two sides of the diaphragm. However, under normal circumstances, a sound signal arriving from the back will reach the rear port a little sooner than it reaches the front port. An acoustic filter is therefore applied in the rear port to delay the signal for as long as it takes for it to travel the distance to the front port.

Similar directional behavior can be achieved with two omnidirectional microphones and digital processing (Figure 8–20B). With this type of system, the delay is applied digitally.

Although the directional behavior achieved by either dedicated directional microphones or multiple microphone techniques

will improve speech understanding in noise, listening in the directional mode also comes at a cost. Inherent in the design of directional microphones is a reduction of acoustical sensitivity at a rate of 6 dB per octave toward the low frequencies. The low-frequency attenuation (or "roll-off") introduced by directional microphone systems makes them less useful in quiet surroundings. This is because the acoustic signal is attenuated below the level of the inherent microphone noise. In quiet situations, therefore, a standard omnidirectional microphone is more beneficial. Historically this has been solved by applying a user-operable slide cover on the rear inlet (Phonak PICS, 1992), or by including a user-operable switch between an omnidirectional and a directional microphone (e.g., Widex Senso Vita, 2004). However, research has shown that a substantial percentage of the hearing aid users who were fitted with switchable omnidirectional/directional hearing aids did not use the directional mode (Cord, Surr, Walden, & Olson, 2002).

Using two (or in principle more) microphones and advanced signal processing, it is possible to adaptively control the change between omnidirectional and directional mode, and hereby relieve the user from having to switch manually. In addition, adaptive signal processing enables the continuous optimization of the directional characteristic to the ambient sound environment. In modern

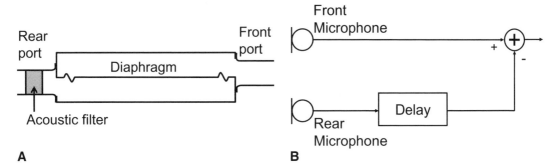

Figure 8–20. A–B. A dedicated directional microphone (*left side*) consists of a single diaphragm and two inlet ports. An acoustic filter is applied in the rear port to delay the signal, so the signal arrives at both sides of the diaphragm at the same time. Similar directional behavior can be achieved with two omnidirectional microphones and digital processing (*right side*, A/D converters are left out for simplicity).

hearing aids, this type of processing has been split in multiple frequency channels. This makes it possible to adapt to and attenuate, for instance, low-frequency noise sources from one direction and high-frequency noise sources from another direction.

In order for the directional behavior to work properly, it is essential that the signals picked up at the front and rear have exactly the same frequency response. When using two single omnidirectional microphones—with production and aging differences to consider—this requires the microphones to be matched, not only during the manufacturing of the hearing aid, but also continuously when the hearing aid is in use.

Adaptive Directional Microphone Systems

With a digital directional system based on two omnidirectional microphones, more flexibility is possible than for an acoustic directional microphone. More types of directional characteristics can be implemented, and the patterns can be varied over frequency or optimized for any sound environment.

Five examples of directional patterns possible with a two-microphone configuration are depicted in Figure 8–21. The omnidirectional pattern (a) is circular, which means it provides the same amount amplification for any direction. The subcardioid (b) attenuates sounds from the rear, and the cardioid (c) has an actual *notch,* which will eliminate sounds straight from the rear. In a diffuse sound field,

the hypercardioid (d) pattern will remove the highest amount of sound (sound from both the rear and the sides). The bidirectional pattern (e) will notch sounds straight from the side. It is possible to notch sounds from the front half-plane as well, but as the directional system inherently assumes that the speaker intuitively will turn to face the speaker (or any other relevant sound source), this is usually not permitted. Usually the bidirectional pattern (e) is the most pronounced filtering permitted. It should be noted that the patterns in Figure 8–21 are ideal "free-field" patterns. In practice, damping and reflections from head and ear will make the patterns look much less smooth.

Directional behavior is important as the spatial noise reduction it performs quite effectively improves speech intelligibility in noise (Valente, Schuchman, Potts, & Beck, 2000). As more ambient noise is attenuated relative to sound from the front, intelligibility will increase accordingly.

Before discussing how to select the *optimal* directional pattern for a given situation, it is necessary to look at the drawbacks of directional filtering. Figure 8–22 shows the *cardioid* filtering patterns achieved for four pure tones of different frequency. The same pattern shape is obtained for each frequency, but as mentioned above increasingly less amplification is obtained at lower frequencies. It is straightforward to implement a digital filter to compensate for the low frequency attenuation. Without this *low-frequency boost* (sometimes referred to as equalization), sounds will

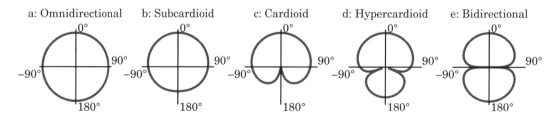

Figure 8–21. Five different polar patterns showing the amplification at the front (0 degrees), rear (180 degrees), right side (+90 degrees), and left side (–90 degrees). The patterns show relative amplification in dB. When the gray curve is far from the center, amplification is high; when it is near the center, amplification is low. It is common in hearing aid processing that amplification is higher for sounds arriving from the front than from other directions.

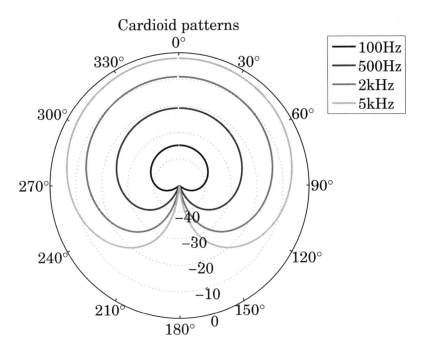

Figure 8–22. Cardioid amplification patterns for four different frequencies. Grid lines show amplification in dB. More amplification is achieved for sounds from the front (0 degrees) than for any other directions. Sounds from the rear (180 degrees) are notched out in this example. Note also that the general level of amplification decreases along with frequency (1 cm microphone distance assumed).

appear "tinny," and audibility may be lost at lower frequencies.

While equalization ensures that the processing results in a natural sound reproduction, the side effect is that microphone noise will be boosted at low frequencies by the same amount of amplification, which is applied to compensate for the low-frequency attenuation. Thus, in quiet surroundings, the directional behavior will, in fact, result in more noise by causing the inherent noise floor of the hearing aid to increase.

Modern hearing aids control the directional characteristic adaptively with the overall target of optimizing SNR in every environment. To design an adaptive procedure, one needs to consider many properties:

■ The directional pattern should minimize ambient noise without resulting in the microphone noise becoming too dominant.

The optimization must also be carried out in a manner that ensures that amplification of sounds from the front is not reduced.

■ As the "optimal pattern" varies over time, optimization must occur continuously. The optimization should not occur too rapidly, as this can lead to annoying "pumping" sound effects if the loudness changes too quickly.

■ In relatively quiet surroundings, an omni-directional pattern is often recommended as it enables the wearer to hear speech from any direction. Directional filtering should, therefore, not be activated until there is a certain amount of noise.

■ Not all sound environments are equally suited for directional filtering. When walking along a busy street, noise level is high, but audibility for all directions is perhaps more important. Also, a directional system can affect the processing of music. Most people will probably enjoy music more without the adaptive filtering constantly altering the frequency spectrum.

◼ In a few situations, it may actually be advantageous to reverse the directional effect in order to zoom backward. For instance, when the user wants to listen to a backseat passenger while driving. This functionality should be restricted to a special listening program in order to prevent behavior confusing the user.

Multiband Directional Microphone Systems

While in the first adaptive directional systems, the same polar pattern was used over the entire frequency range (sometimes referred to as a *wide-band* directional system), it is now customary to optimize the patterns individually in many frequency bands.

The frequency spectrum will often be different for different sound sources, which makes it advantageous to use different patterns for different frequency bands. The most important reason, however, is the above-mentioned equalization, which will amplify microphone noise. As this amplification increases toward the lower frequencies, the ambient low-frequency noise level must be quite high to render the directional mode beneficial. With multiband directional microphone systems, the lower bands can remain in or close to the omnidirectional pattern while more pronounced directionality is allowed for higher frequency bands where microphone noise is not boosted.

Intuitively, one might be concerned that the variation in directional pattern across frequency bands will shape sounds unnaturally when they are not originating from the front. This is generally not noticeable, as room reflections and shadow effects from the head and ear influence the filtering anyway and also prevent that individual sound sources are notched out completely.

Microphone Matching and Calibration

A requirement for achieving the desired directional characteristic using two single microphones is that the microphones are identical with regard to both sensitivity and phase characteristics. If not, it will not be possible to achieve the intended polar pattern. Unfortunately, the matching performed by the microphone manufacturer may not be as accurate as one would hope for. In addition, the microphones will suffer from sensitivity drift because of general aging and exposure to increased temperatures and humidity during use.

Drift in the individual microphones' sensitivity may result in different amplitude responses of the two microphones. An amplitude difference will reduce the directivity, especially in the low frequencies. Figure 8–23 shows the difference between an ideal hypercardioid directional characteristic and the directional characteristic resulting from an amplitude mismatch of 0.25 dB between the microphones.

Differences in phase between the microphones may degrade the directional characteristic further. Figure 8–24 shows the effect on an intended hypercardioid polar pattern (similar to Figure 8–23A) when the phase of the front microphone is 2° less than the rear microphone. The result is a cardioid-like pattern with less directivity. If the phase difference has the opposite sign, the result is more of a "reverse hypercardioid" pattern. That is, the effect is a directional focus toward the rear, which is clearly not a benefit for the user in most circumstances. With aging, the difference can become more pronounced and may ultimately eliminate the directivity in the low frequencies.

Using digital signal processing, it is possible to introduce correction filters that compensate for the differences in amplitude and phase between the two microphones.

Insufficient sensitivity matching at the supplier's and age-related drifting make it necessary to have a matching algorithm that continuously works to ensure the directional performance throughout the lifetime of the hearing aid.

For similar microphones, two parameters are significant for the matching:

◼ Overall sensitivity
◼ Low-frequency roll-off

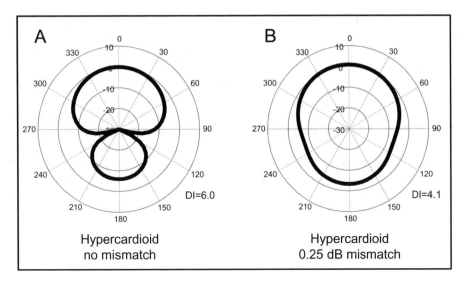

Figure 8–23. Directivity pattern at 250 Hz of a directional unit consisting of two omnidirectional microphones. The distance between the microphone inlets is 10 mm. **A.** The internal delay is adjusted to give a hypercardioid pattern with perfect amplitude and phase match. **B.** Amplitude mismatch of 0.25 dB between microphones.

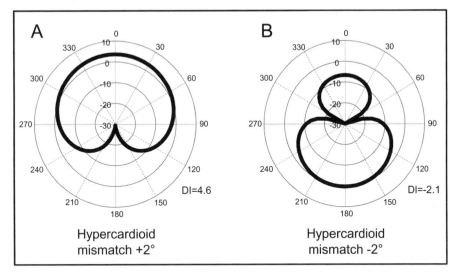

Figure 8–24. Directivity pattern at 250 Hz of a hypercardioid microphone with perfect amplitude match (same as Figure 8–23A), except **A.** Phase mismatch of 2° (rear microphone is delayed); **B.** Phase mismatch of –2° (front microphone is delayed).

A difference in overall sensitivity will affect the entire frequency range if uncompensated, but fortunately it is also the easiest difference to compensate for.

Deviations in the low frequency roll-off significantly affect the phase response in the low frequencies of the audible range. The low-frequency roll-off is needed in the microphone to prevent inaudible sounds from saturating the microphone and A/D converter. As illustrated above, the directional system is very sensitive to phase deviations, so the analysis and correction of deviations in the low-frequency roll-off has to be very precise to ensure directional behavior in the low frequencies. A highly complex algorithm is needed to obtain this degree of precision.

Frequency Lowering

Providing audibility of high-frequency information for people with severe-to-profound or precipitously sloping high-frequency hearing loss is a considerable challenge. In many cases, the high-frequency region in the cochlea is so severely damaged (or "dead") that it is simply not possible to restore audibility by means of conventional amplification (Moore, 2001). This is an important issue, since critical speech cues are located at high frequencies. For example, the spectral energy of the speech sound /s/ is ordinarily located from about 4 kHz and upward (Maniwa, Jongman, & Wade, 2009). Plosive and fricative consonants, such as /s/, /z/, /ʃ/, /t/, /f/, can, therefore, be difficult to perceive for people with high-frequency hearing loss, and their ability to distinguish minimal pairs like "sake," "shake," "take," or "cat," "cats" will consequently be impaired (Flynn, Dowell, & Clark, 1998).

The inability of conventional amplification to secure audibility for people with severe-to-profound high-frequency hearing loss has prompted the hearing aid industry to search for alternative strategies. One such strategy is frequency lowering where high-frequency information is shifted to a lower frequency region with some residual hearing. The first commercially available frequency-lowering hearing aid, a fully analog, rather large bodyworn device, came in 1961 (Oticon TP72). Subsequently, many research trials were conducted with so-called transposers. A large number of strategies were tested, but they all failed on poor sound quality and unwanted artifacts. For a long time, transposition seemed to be at a dead end.

However, three decades later, the first digital device with frequency lowering was introduced (AVR TranSonic). Although digital, the AVR TranSonic was also a rather large, bodyworn device. AVR Sonovation subsequently introduced a BTE with frequency lowering in 1998, but it was not until the latter half of the 2000s, when Widex and later Phonak introduced frequency lowering into their top-range hearing aids, that frequency lowering really caught on.

At the time of writing, frequency lowering devices are available from six hearing aid manufacturers; AVR Sonovation, Widex, Phonak, Starkey, Siemens, and Bernafon.

Timeline:

1961—Oticon TP 72. An analog, bodyworn device.

1993—AVR TranSonic. A digital, bodyworn processor with Digital Frequency Compression. (DFC). Followed by Impact BTE, Impact XP, and Nano XP in 1998–2005.

2006—Widex Inteo. A digital BTE with Audibility Extender (Frequency transposition technique).

2008—Phonak Naida BTE with SoundRecover (Nonlinear Frequency Compression technique).

2011—Starkey Wi BTE with Spectral iQ.

2012—Siemens micon with Frequency Compression.

2013—Bernafon Acriva 9│7 with Frequency Composition.

Current Techniques for Frequency Lowering

The introduction of digital signal processing in hearing aids made it possible to digitally alter the signal to either compress or transpose inaudible frequencies. Below, the four different methods that have been applied in commercially available digital hearing aids longest are described. The remaining two are so recent that in-depth descriptions are not yet available.

■ DFC: This strategy involves the compression of the entire frequency range, which means that none of the original signal will be preserved.

■ SoundRecover:. With this strategy, frequencies above the so-called cutoff frequency (1600 Hz or higher) will be compressed (i.e., squeezed together), while frequencies below the cutoff frequency will be amplified in the conventional manner.

■ Audibility Extender:. This feature performs what is referred to as *linear* frequency shifting. The aim is to preserve the harmonic structure and modulation ratio of the original signal. In the basic mode, it analyzes a source region for spectral peaks and uses this information to shift the most prominent part one octave down to the target region. In the expanded mode, the feature analyzes two source regions and places the most prominent parts of these two at the same octave in the target region. The Audibility Extender selects the source region by a so-called start frequency that can be as low as 630 Hz and as high as 6000 Hz.

■ Spectral IQ:. This feature analyzes the content of the input signal in search for appropriate spectral cues such as /s/ and /t/ sounds, and transposes them to an audible area. When high frequency spectral cues are absent, Spectral IQ is inactive as opposed to the Audibility Extender and SoundRecover, which work continuously. The bandwidth of the total signal is not altered, and thus retains the full bandwidth accessible to the user.

As mentioned in the introduction, the primary motivation for the incorporation of frequency lowering schemes into hearing aids is to render high-frequency speech sounds audible. The majority of the frequency lowering schemes in commercially available hearing aids has been designed to address that specific problem (DFC, SoundRecover, Spectral IQ, Frequency Compression, Frequency Composition).

Environmental sounds such as music, birds chirping, and doorbells often have high frequency content. They typically contain harmonic sounds and may also be frequency and/or amplitude modulated. Because the linear frequency transposition algorithm called the Audibility Extender preserves the harmonic structure and modulation ratio of the original signal, this technique is equally capable of shifting both speech and environmental sound. With the Audibility Extender, birdsong will sound like birdsong, only at a lower pitch.

Research on speech intelligibility has shown that both frequency compression and frequency transposition can improve speech perception and production for hearing aid users (Auriemmo et al., 2009; Simpson, Hersbach, & McDermott, 2006). However, in spite of the efforts of the manufacturers, the sound produced by any of the frequency lowering algorithms will sound unnatural at first and require acclimatization and training. The brain needs time to adapt to a new sound scheme, and this period can be as long as 3 to 6 months. This makes it difficult to test the effectiveness of the algorithms in a laboratory setting, as test subjects rarely benefit from the frequency lowering algorithm at first, but will need time to adapt before being able to exploit the new cues available to them.

Data Logging

Digital technology in hearing aids offers a basis for logging data during use. By means of writeable memory, information about user actions, environmental data, and hearing aid adaptation can be stored and later used by the hearing care professional for fine tuning and counseling purposes. Data are typically collected on usage time, volume control use, program use, and environments the user has been in. The hearing care professional can make use of these data, in combination with subjective input from the user, for improved fine tuning and trouble-shooting complaints, as well as for counseling the user on the basis of his or her individual usage data.

The most basic form of data logging provides simple statistics on usage, collected over weeks or months. This offers the hearing care professional a general picture of how the hearing aid has been used.

Some manufacturers also offer a user-controlled short-term log. This log records environmental data for a very brief stretch of time after being activated by the user. The data logged can be used to analyze specific situations, in which the user is dissatisfied with the performance of the hearing aid.

More sophisticated logging functions are able to monitor the activation of advanced features, such as noise reduction and directional microphone systems. Some manufacturers' fitting software also offers an automatic guidance function that uses the logged usage data to give recommendations for how to improve the hearing aid's settings.

Recent advances in data logging have led to the development of hearing aids that are able to learn from past events. These hearing aids will save the user's preference in different sound environments and exploit these data to make an informed guess on the individual user's preferred settings the next time he or she enters the same acoustic environment.

WIRELESS COMMUNICATION

Wireless technology is common in 21st-century everyday applications. Radios, TVs, cell phones, remote controls, wireless internet, and so on all rely on some kind of radio transmission.

Wireless technology has been applied by the hearing aid industry since the late 1930s and is the backbone of both FM and Telecoil systems. Both types of systems offer direct transmission into the hearing aids of, for example, a sound signal from a microphone worn by a speaker or the sound from a TV set. This can be a distinct advantage for speech comprehension in poor listening conditions, as it improves the SNR by excluding most of the reverberation and noise in the room.

Although it has been possible to change volume and program setting in hearing aids using a wireless remote control since the late

1980s (Widex Quattro, AudioScience Prizm), it was not until 2004 that the first hearing aid was launched that allowed wireless exchange of data between hearing aids for the synchronization of volume control and other features (Siemens Acuris). Since then, many other hearing aid manufacturers have followed suit, and the technology is now also being explored for the exchange of audio between hearing aids.

The reason why the introduction of wireless audio transmission did not happen sooner has to do with the special limitations inherent in hearing aid design. To provide a stable, high-quality connection, radio communication requires space for antennas and transceivers, and power for transmission. Space and power are critical factors in hearing aid design. The following sections explain the background for the introduction of wireless communication in hearing aids and discuss the challenges arising when wireless technology is applied in hearing aids.

Background

As mentioned, space and current drain are two major limiting factors when designing wireless communication for hearing aids. In fact, these two factors will often be decisive for the choice of radio transmission technique.

One vital component of any radio is the antenna. For antennas to be effective, they need to have a certain length. This is easily demonstrated by means of an ordinary transistor radio with a collapsible antenna. The reception is much better when the antenna is at full length than when it is collapsed. It will work at shorter lengths too, but not as effectively. The required length, and thus the necessary space, of a radio antenna is determined by the frequency used for transmission.

This has been clearly reflected in the development of cell phones. Early cell phones were designed for the 450 MHz band. To use these phones, one had to extend the antenna on the phone or have a stationary antenna installed in the car. Modern cell phone technologies use increasingly higher frequencies with the upcoming 4G networks as the current pinnacle with frequencies of up to 8000 MHz (or 8GHz). This development is clearly reflected in the size of today's cell phones. The increase in frequencies has allowed for significantly smaller phones, and antennas are no longer a visible component in the design.

Generally speaking, two different transmission technologies are used in hearing aids today: Radio frequency transmission and near-field inductive transmission.

Near-field inductive transmission has been utilized by the hearing aid industry for many years. It is the technology known from telecoil systems. Telecoil systems basically comprise an inductive loop antenna, which is strung around the perimeter of a room or included in a neck loop, and a coil in the hearing aid which picks up the magnetic field produced by the loop antenna. This type of system only involves a very small battery drain. However, it is only useful for short range communication, and it is very dependent on the actual orientation of the antennas. Experienced users of telecoil systems will know that they lose connection when moving away from the telecoil, and that the loudness of the signal depends on where they sit and which direction the hearing aids are facing.

Radio communication is also known from FM systems. These systems use radio frequency transmission to send signals to a receiver coupled to or built into the hearing aid from a transmitter connected to a microphone. These systems work at higher frequencies and are able to transmit over longer distances than the near-field inductive systems. They also take up more space and use more battery power than telecoil systems.

Most wireless hearing aids use a combination of these two techniques: A short-range lower frequency effective near-field inductive technology for transmission to the hearing aids from a streaming device, and a long-distance high-frequency radio connection between the streaming device and, for example, a transmitter connected to a TV set.

An alternative approach is to aim for a high enough transmission frequency to render the antennas small enough to fit into a hearing aid housing. Some manufacturers have chosen that approach in their most recent products. This allows them to skip the streaming device for some applications and transmit long-range radio signal directly to the hearing aids. The drawbacks of this approach include higher power consumption in the transmitter and a more complicated design to make the receiving unit small enough to fit into the hearing aids. Even so, omission of the streaming device leads to a notable increase in ease of use for the wearer, so it can be expected that hearing aid manufacturers will strive to develop even smaller and more effective radios in the future.

Another benefit of using a higher transmission frequency is that it allows for more transmission bandwidth and, consequently, also for wireless transmission of a greater amount of data.

The trade-offs involved in choosing either of the two transmission technologies in relation to key hearing aid design parameters are listed in Table 8–2.

Table 8–2. Schematic Overview of the Effect of Transmission Technology on a Number of Key Design Parameters in a Hearing Aid

Design Parameter	Near-Field Inductive	Radio Frequency
Size	Smaller	Larger
Optimal frequency range	Lower frequencies	Higher frequencies
Bandwidth	Narrower	Wider
Range	Short range	Long range
Design complexity	Lower	Higher
Power consumption	Lower	Higher

Audio Streaming

As discussed in the previous section, choice of transmission technique is an important aspect to consider when designing wireless communication systems. Another important consideration is what this transmission channel is to be used for. This section discusses one advanced use; viz, real-time streaming of sound directly to the hearing aids.

Direct streaming of sound to the hearing aids is very popular, because it addresses several of the main difficulties experienced by hearing aid users in their daily lives, including watching TV with their families, and talking on a cell phone or landline phone.

The transmission of sound directly to the hearing aids has been possible for many years, using either telecoil loops or dedicated FM systems. However, as both these systems are analog and transmit in mono only, they offer a poorer sound quality than recent systems built on digital transmission.

As high-end hearing aids are digital as standard today, a digital representation of the signal is already available in the hearing aids. However, digital audio data are extremely bulky, so the volume has to be reduced in some manner. The transmission of digital audio data, therefore, involves three steps; compression of the content, transmission, and decompression of the content.

Compression is needed as the amount of raw data is too large to transmit. The greater the amount of data, the greater the required transmission bandwidth and the power consumption. Consequently, some kind of encoding or "packing" of the raw data is done in order to reduce the load. Digital audio data compression is achieved by means of a set of complex algorithms called an audio codec.

The encoded data are sent via the wireless connection. This can be done by means of different techniques (termed the "channel coding"). The design of the channel coding can make the transmission more or less robust toward noise. However, one thing is certain: Transmission errors will occur from time to time, so the system has to be designed to be able to handle such errors.

In the receiving end, the encoded data package is decoded. The similarity of the decoded signal to the raw data will vary depending on the technique chosen for the encoding.

There are many technologies for wireless digital transmission of sound already on the market. Two well-known examples are the technology used in cell phones and Bluetooth technology, which is widely used in wireless headsets or loudspeakers. From an engineering point of view, using one of the existing technologies would be the fastest way to a digital wireless design. However, both technologies have drawbacks that create serious problems in hearing aid applications. Cell phones are quite efficient in terms of compressing the sound to keep the amount of transmitted data low. Unfortunately, however, this is also reflected in the sound quality of cell phones. Focus is generally on the transmission of speech, not on overall sound quality. This makes cell phone compression useless for hearing aid applications.

Bluetooth is designed to transmit sound in an acceptable sound quality and is widely applied in personal audio devices. It is used for playing back recorded music, or in wireless cell phone headsets in situations where the user needs to communicate with someone far away. In both these cases, the inherent audio delay of at least around 150 ms associated with standard Bluetooth technology is of no consequence. Hearing aid users, on the other hand, will often be able to hear both streamed sound from, for example, a TV set and direct acoustic sound in the room picked up by the hearing aid's microphones. In those situations, a delay between transmitted and direct sound of more than 10 ms will result in artifacts; either a metallic sound quality or an echo effect (Figure 8–25). A 150-ms delay would be highly unacceptable.

Hearing aid manufacturers are, therefore, obliged to find ways of tailoring their wireless technologies to meet the special challenges of hearing aid design. It is no simple matter to design a system that can simultaneously maintain high sound quality, low battery drain, and robustness against trans-

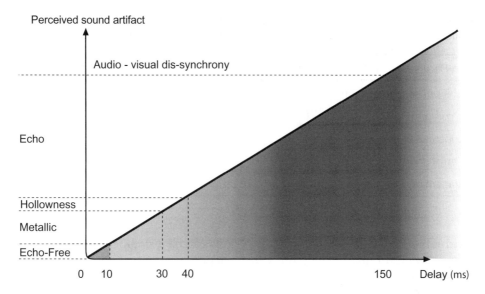

Figure 8–25. The perceptual effect of listening to an original sound mixed with a delayed version of the original. A delay shorter than 10 ms will normally not be audible. A longer delay will result in audible artifacts ranging from a metallic quality to echo. With a delay longer than 100 to150 ms, the synchronization between lip movements and sound will be lost.

mission errors. The design will inevitably involve a choice between possible tradeoffs, as illustrated in Figure 8–26.

A very high sound quality can be obtained by compressing the sound to a very small extent only, or by using a very sophisticated compression technology. The former would result in a large amount of data to be transmitted (measured in kbit/sec), which in turn would lead to a high current drain. A highly sophisticated compression technology could transmit the same sound quality using fewer kbit/sec, but it would also need more processing power and, consequently, also result in a high current drain.

Transmission robustness can be increased by using more power for transmission, or by applying a more efficient error correction. A more efficient error correction requires more calculation power, so both approaches would result in a higher current drain. A third option is to require that data be retransmitted if an error occurs. However, this will lead to a delay in the transmitted sound, and thus to a lower sound quality (Table 8–3).

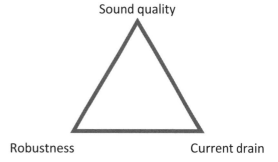

Figure 8–26. Three of the most important factors to consider when designing a wireless technology for hearing aid applications.

Using Hearing Aids as Head Sets

The introduction of wireless hearing aids has led to major changes in the hearing aid industry. Previously, hearing aid manufacturers could concentrate on developing a hearing aid from the point of view of the audiological aspects of compensating for

Table 8–3. The Arrows Indicate an Increase or Decrease in Current Drain, Sound Quality, and Robustness if One Design Parameter Is Changed and the Rest Are Kept Constant

Design Parameter	Current Drain	Sound Quality	Robustness
More kbit per second of sound transmission	↑	↑	—
Higher compression	↑	↓	↓
Stereo instead of mono	↑	↑	—
Better error correction	↑	—	↑
More transmission power	↑	—	↑

the individual user's hearing loss. Nowadays, people expect more from a hearing aid with wireless capabilities. Apart from the hearing aid itself, external devices that enable the user to connect their hearing aid to personal audio devices is a must. What used to be a specialized production of "assistive listening devices" is fast becoming an integral part of a hearing aid company's range of accessories for new hearing aids.

Wireless hearing aids are expected to be able to function as a wireless headset when the user is watching TV or listening to music from a hi-fi. This will allow users to bypass the reverberation and room noise and hear the transmitted sound directly in their hearing aids in a manner that includes compensation for their individual hearing losses.

Another expectation is that wireless transmission of audio can be used to overcome some of the problems of talking on the phone. Getting the phone's loudspeaker sufficiently close to a BTE hearing aid's microphone inlet is not easy. Especially cell phones have very small loudspeakers and are quite small. Insufficient loudness and feedback problems are common experiences for hearing aid users. However, using digital audio streaming to transmit the sound from the phone directly to the hearing aid minimizes those issues.

At the time of writing, a handful of hearing aids are capable of not only receiving streamed sound from external devices, but also of transmitting sound themselves.

This can be a significant advantage during a telephone conversation in that it allows for phone signals picked up by the hearing aid microphone on one side to be transmitted to the other side. It should be noted that while this method provides a clearer telephone sound, it still requires the user to hold the handle close to the hearing aid microphone, and any noise picked up on the transmitting side will be sent to the other hearing aid.

Streaming for Wireless CROS/BiCROS Solutions

Wireless audio transmission is likely to replace the traditional wire used in CROS or BiCROS fittings in a foreseeable future. CROS (Contralateral Routing of Offside Signal) solutions are for people who have normal hearing on one side and unaidable hearing on opposite side. BiCROS solutions are for people with hearing loss on the better side and no aidable hearing on the other side.

In a traditional CROS implementation, a microphone is placed at the unaidable ear. This microphone is connected to a hearing aid on the other ear through a thin wire. The hearing aid will play back the sound from the deaf side to make it easier to communicate without having to constantly worry about keeping the better ear close to the speaker. A BiCROS implementation does the same, but is aimed at people who have hearing loss on the better ear. In this case, the hearing aid will both play back the sound from the unaidable side and provide amplification to compensate for the hearing loss in the better ear.

Even though the wire used in traditional wired CROS/BiCROS solutions (collectively referred to as CROS in the following) have become quite discrete, wearing a thin wire around the neck will cause problems from time to time. It can easily be caught with a hairbrush or damaged otherwise as it is a delicate connection. A wireless CROS would be a great help for the users who are dependent on such solutions.

Wireless CROS systems in digital hearing aids have been on the market for a few years. Common concerns with these first systems have been that users (especially CROS users with normal hearing on one side) will be able to hear the transmission noise. The application of custom-made digital audio transmission techniques may contribute toward reducing the noise level of the transmission, however.

Other concerns apply when designing a digital wireless audio connection for hearing aids. When the hearing aid only has to receive audio data, the unit performing the demanding task of encoding the sound signal can be placed in devices with large batteries, and using a relative power-consuming transmission technology is a viable option.

These considerations are clearly reflected in the range of wireless products offered by the different manufacturers today. Only two use a far-field radio technology to allow transmission directly to the hearing aid from external sources. One product does not allow communication between the hearing aids. The other uses the binaural connection to provide some synchronization of features with an ensuing increase in current drain.

Moreover, at the time of writing, only two hearing aid manufacturers offer direct transmission of sound between hearing aids. Both rely on near-field inductive transmission. However, one manufacturer uses a proprietary coding technology especially designed for hearing aid use, while the other has chosen to rely on commercially available solution. When the proprietary coding tech-

nology designed especially for hearing aid transmission is used, the total current drain is around 1.5 mA in a fully functioning hearing aid. In comparison, the smallest current drain achieved when relying on the commercially available transmission technology is 3.5 mA.

These issues notwithstanding, all of the large hearing aid manufacturing companies have introduced wireless hearing aids within recent years, so even though a number of challenges remain, improvements in the wireless technologies will in all likelihood lead to a greater range of wireless CROS systems in the years to come.

Inter-Ear Functions

The inclusion of wireless technology in hearing aids could be a leap of dimensions similar to the one from analog to digital signal processing in the mid-1990s. Especially the direct exchange of data between two hearing aids (inter-ear communication) makes a significant contribution toward making life easier for hearing aid users.

A simple use of inter-ear communication is the synchronization of user controls (i.e., volume control and program shift). The information that has to be shared is very limited, and transmission of data between the hearing aids is only necessary when controls are actually in use.

The exchange of data can also be exploited for the coordination of more advanced features, such as gain control, directional behavior, feedback canceling, and noise reduction. Although the amount of information to be exchanged is still relatively limited, this functionality requires the hearing aids to communicate regularly (e.g., 20 times per second).

Transmission of live audio signals in high quality from one hearing aid to the other requires much higher data rates and continuous transmission. As mentioned above, inter-ear transmission of audio signals is already used for wireless CROS devices or special programs for telephone conversations. However, the full potential is still waiting to be realized.

Synchronization and Coordination of Features

Wireless exchange of data between hearing aids can lead to a significant increase in ease of use by allowing the synchronization of volume control and change of program. In most cases, hearing aid users will need the same listening program and the same loudness level in both hearing aids. While users wearing uncoordinated hearing aids have to adjust each hearing aid separately every time they need to adjust the volume or change program, one adjustment will produce a simultaneous change in loudness or listening program in a pair of wirelessly coordinated hearing aids. This means that considerably less effort is required to make adjustments.

Another simple feature that may be of great value to the user is the ability to monitor the wireless connection and alert the user if the connection is lost. Physical activity can sometimes result in hearing aids being lost. For example, a hearing aid may be ripped off by a branch while gardening or pushed off by the sidebar of the user's glasses. However, the monitoring of the wireless connection could save the user the inconvenience and expense of having to replace an aid in many cases.

Wireless communication can also be utilized to optimize more advanced features. A digital hearing aid will respond to the ambient sound environment by adjusting for instance gain, noise reduction and directional characteristic to the current situation. A user with independently working hearing aids may experience that sounds from one side trigger a reduction of the level in the nearest hearing aid, while leaving the hearing aid on the far side unaffected. The perceived binaural sound level will be asymmetric and cause the user to feel that the world is skewed. With wireless coordination of the signal processing, advanced features such as compression, noise reduction, and directional microphone systems will no longer react on one-sided input, but on input on the ambient sound environment on both sides of the head.

Feedback canceling has undergone significant improvements since the first gen-

erations and is able to deliver feedback-free performance in many situations. However, with independently working hearing aids, there is still a significant risk of sounds such as sustained tones in music being mistaken for feedback squeals. In such cases, a feedback canceling system will normally attenuate the music. However, feedback squeals are very unlikely to occur in both hearing aids at the exact same frequency. By exchanging information between the hearing aids about the detected sound spectrum, it can be deduced whether it is an external sound rather than a feedback signal that has been detected. In this way, the risk of unnecessary gain regulation resulting from "false positives" can be minimized.

Future Uses

The exploitation of wireless communication between hearing aids is still limited by the typical hearing aid trade-offs of size and power. However, wireless technology is one area where significant leaps of progress are likely to be made in the future.

At present, it is possible to transmit one encoded audio signal from one hearing aid to another. With more efficient radio systems capable of higher communication speed, the continuous exchange of several signals during normal use will become a possibility.

This may, for instance, be used to combine the dual microphone systems in a pair of hearing aids in a quadruple microphone directional system. The use of multiple microphones will offer a better attenuation of noise sources than the dual system typically used today. In addition, if the microphones in the left and right device could be linked freely, directional characteristics could be created that would enable the user to focus in any direction; for instance on a speaker sitting diagonally opposite, and not just in front or behind like at present. The ideal implementation would offer a choice between a user-controllable and an adaptive option.

Last, entirely new processing strategies may arise from the possibility of exchanging audio signals between hearing aids. These may be exploited to create an improved spatial experience, or to enable the user to better distinguish between individual voices. Also, intelligent sharing of the processing power of the two hearing aids may lead to a considerable increase in efficiency. However, most potential uses have not yet been dreamt of.

HEARING AID PROGRAMMING

In the late 1980s, when the first digitally programmable hearing aids came on the market, each manufacturer introduced their own proprietary programming equipment, resulting in a multitude of stand-alone programming units. For the hearing care professionals, it was inconvenient to have to switch programming equipment whenever they wanted to fit hearing aids from a different manufacturer.

Siemens's Programmable Multi-Channel (PMC) unit was one of the earliest attempts to create a universal programming unit that would allow the use of programming modules from different manufacturers. However, in practice, it was mainly used with programmable hearing aids that contained Siemens's own IC platform.

In the early 1990s, some of the large hearing aid manufacturers (ASCOM, GN Danavox, Oticon, Phonak, Resound, Siemens, Starkey, 3M, Unitron, and Widex) joined forces in order to instigate the manufacture of a universal programming unit. The result was the HI PRO box, a programming interface that could connect to a PC and a hearing aid. Manufactured by Madsen Electronics (now GN Otometrics), the HI PRO box was quickly adopted by the majority of hearing care professionals.

The HI PRO collaboration was driven by a need for a common hardware platform. Soon after, the need for a universal software platform that could integrate data from patient databases, audiometric data, and interface with the manufacturers' proprietary software became apparent.

This led to the foundation of the Hearing Instrument Manufacturers' Software Association (HIMSA) in 1993 with the objective of developing a unified system that would allow hearing care professionals to use fitting software from different manufacturers and interface with external audiometric test equipment from different suppliers, while at the same time storing all information in one common database. The resulting NOAH software system has become an industry standard (Figure 8–27). Today, HIMSA is owned by the six largest hearing aid manufacturing companies and has approximately 100 members/licenses (http://www.himsa.com).

In the late 1990s, work began on a new hardware solution that would offer faster data communication to speed up the fitting process and wireless connectivity to computers. The result was the NOAHlink unit, which was a HIMSA product (Figure 8–28).

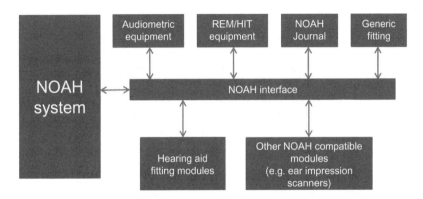

Figure 8–27. The integration framework of the NOAH software system.

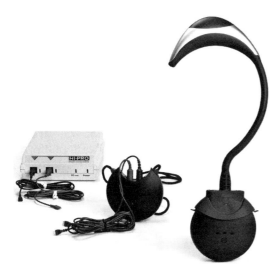

Figure 8–28. A HI-PRO box, a NOAHlink, and a nEARcom hook.

hearing care professionals of the tangle of cables needed if they wanted to have several hearing aid brands at the clinic. Each manufacturer produced their own cables, and often different models from the same manufacturer would require different cables. This generated a market requirement for a unified system that would solve this. To avoid history repeating itself in the shape of a number of proprietary wireless programming systems, Widex, Oticon, and Starkey formed the nEARcom consortium with the object of developing an industry standard solution. However, the nEARcom hook did not become an industry standard in the same manner as the NOAH system. At the present point in time, each manufacturer of wireless hearing aids offers their own proprietary wireless solution.

The NOAHlink used wireless Bluetooth technology to connect to a PC. However, the connection between the hearing aid and the NOAHlink was still established by means of a cable. With the introduction of the NOAHlink, data transmission became nearly 10 times faster. The increased communication speed of the NOAHLink made it possible to add real time interactive functionality for explanatory purposes during fitting and fine tuning, such as Soundtracker in Compass from Widex. While the NOAHlink was able to provide faster transmission of large data packets, the unit did not speed up the entire hearing aid fitting process to any great extent at first, since this process is characterized by the transfer of a large number of small data packets with intermittent exchange of verification data. However, as new hearing aids with increasingly larger amounts of data came on the market, the difference in programming speed with the NOAHlink versus the HI-PRO became more apparent. The total number of NOAHlinks installed amounts to more than 45,000 units worldwide (http://www.himsa.com).

While the introduction of the NOAHlink provided wireless connectivity to the hearing care professional's PC, it did not rid

A GLIMPSE OF THE FUTURE

The number of calculations performed by the processor each second has been rising exponentially ever since the introduction of digital hearing aids (Figure 8–29). This trend, which is characteristic of the development of technology in general (Kurzweil, 2005), is likely to continue for some time yet. Semiconductor technology, however, is already pushing the limits of quantum physics, and a shift in technology will inevitably be required. This shift is generally believed to occur around 2020 (Waldner, 2008). Whether this next technology will be based on nanotubes or diamonds, biology or optics remains to be seen. But as long as there is still a potential for algorithmic inventions that improve life for the hearing impaired, hearing aid chip technology will certainly continue to develop.

In spite of the giant leaps in hearing aid technology so far, challenges still remain. For example, the *cocktail party* problem, which has been studied ever since it was coined by Colin Cherry in 1953 (Cherry, 1953), still remains to be solved successfully. Predicting and optimizing immediate speech perception in noise is not a trivial task, in particular in

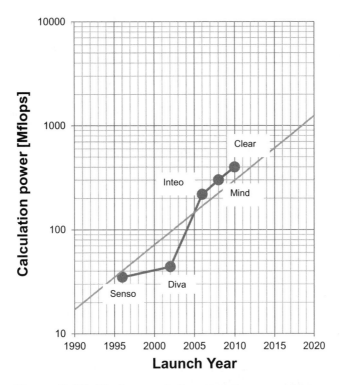

Figure 8–29. The increase in the calculation power of hearing aid processors has risen exponentially since the introduction of the first digital hearing aids in the mid-1990s (exemplified here by Widex hearing aids).

dynamic listening situations with fluctuating noise (such as cocktail parties). Lately, however, the compound scientific effort to understand the properties of individual monaural and binaural hearing has been greatly intensified, and in the near future, psychophysical models can be expected to be integrated into hearing aid signal processing to provide better speech intelligibility for the individual user in adverse conditions (Loizou & Kim, 2011). The integration of these models into hearing aid processing will be a step on the way to solving the cocktail party problem via real-time prediction and optimization of speech intelligibility in the current listening environment.

Whereas single-device processing has evolved significantly since the digital dawn, the exploration of the potential of exchanging information between two hearing aids in a wireless bilateral fitting is still in its infancy. The main challenge of binaural pro-

cessing today, besides the development of sufficiently effective technology to support wireless exchange of information, is that feature effect comes at a price. For example, a super-directional binaural beamformer may be capable of attenuating nonfrontal sound to a much greater degree than single devices, but the price is that the perceptual impression of the room is distorted. For some users, this price may be worth paying in some situations. In the near future, however, the trade-off between binaural feature effect and distortion may be superseded as the potential of our compound knowledge of the individual perceptual system begins to unfold.

Wireless hearing aids already integrate well with technology around us, and the years to come will see a consolidation of the role of hearing aids as the acoustic portal to the technological world around us. Any sound-generating device, be it a cell phone, personal computing device, doorbell, announcement systems, or other, will be able to stream their output directly to the hearing aids. The concept of binaural hearing aids may even extend to include other microphones in the room, either wall-mounted or from hearing aids of other users close by. These wireless sensor networks will integrate with advanced hearing aid signal processing to provide optimum acoustical information to the user.

One thing is certain: the solution to the cocktail party problem will remain one of the main driving forces of hearing aid development for some time yet. But as technology evolves and knowledge of perception expands, the problem will become solved bit by bit until the day that signal processing is so advanced that it will provide even normal-hearing listeners with greater speech intelligibility in adverse listening conditions.

REFERENCES

American National Standards Institute. 1997. *ANSI S3.5-1997. American National Standard Methods for the Calculation of the Speech Intelligibility Index.* New York: Author.

Auriemmo, J., Kuk, F., Lau, C., Marshall, S., Thiele, N., Pikora, M., . . . Stenger, P. (2009). Effect of linear frequency transposition on speech recognition and production of school-age children. *Journal of the American Academy of Audiology, 20*(5), 289–305.

Bagatto, M. P., Moodie, K. S., Scollie, S. D., Seewald, R. C., Moodie, K. S., Pumford, J., & Rachel Liu, K. P. (2005). Clinical protocols for hearing instrument fitting in the desired sensation level method. *Trends in Amplification, 9*(4), 199–226.

Bagatto, M. P., Scollie, S. D., Seewald, R. C., Moodie, K. S., & Hoover, B. M. (2002). Real-ear-to-coupler difference predictions as a function of age for two coupling procedures. *Journal of the American Academy of Audiology, 13,* 407–415.

Banerjee, S., Merks, I., & Trine, T. (2006). Assessing the effectiveness of feedback cancellers in hearing aids. *The Hearing Review, 13*(4), 53–57.

Cherry, E. C. (1953). Some experiments on the recognition of speech, with one and with two ears. *Journal of the Acoustic Society of America, 25*(5), 975–979.

Cord, M. T., Surr, R. K., Walden, B. E., & Olson, L. (2002). Performance of directional microphone hearing aids in everyday life. *Journal of the American Academy of Audiology, 13,* 295–307.

Ellis, D. P. W. (2010). An introduction to signal processing for speech. In W. J Hardcastle, J. Laver, & F. E. Gibbons (Eds.), *The handbook of phonetic sciences* (2nd ed., pp. 757–780). Chichester, UK: Blackwell.

Feigin, J. A., Kopun, J. G., Stelmachowicz, P. G., & Gorga, M. P. (1989). Probe-tube microphone measures of ear-canal sound pressure levels in infants and children. *Ear and Hearing, 10*(4), 254–255.

Flynn, M. C., Dowell, R. C., & Clark, G. M. (1998). Aided speech recognition abilities of adults with a severe or severe-to-profound hearing loss. *Journal of Speech and Hearing Research, 41,* 285–299.

Freed, D. J., & Soli, S. D. (2006). An objective procedure for evaluation of adaptive anti-feedback algorithms in hearing aids. *Ear and Hearing, 27*(4), 382–398.

Gatehouse, S., Naylor, G., & Elberling, C. (2006). Linear and nonlinear hearing aid fittings—1. Patterns of benefit. *International Journal of Audiology, 45*(3), 130–152.

Henry, J. A., Zaugg, T. L., Myers, P. J., & Schechter, M. A. (2008). Using therapeutic sound with progressive audiologic tinnitus management. *Trends in Amplification, 12*(3), 188–209.

Humes, L. E. (1991). Understanding the speech understanding problems of the hearing impaired. *Journal of the American Academy of Audiology, 2,* 59–69.

Keefe, D. H., Bulen, J. C., Campbell, S. L., & Burns, E. M. (1994). Pressure transfer function and absorption cross section from the diffuse field to the human infant ear canal. *Journal of the Acoustical Society of America, 95*(1), 355–371.

Killion, M. C. (1988). *The "hollow voice" occlusion effect.* Proceedings of 13th Danavox Symposium, Chapter 3, 231–241.

Kuk, F. K. (2002). Considerations in modern multichannel nonlinear hearing aids. In M. Valente (Ed.), *Hearing aids: Standards, options, and limitations* (2nd ed., p. 185). New York, NY: Thieme.

Kurzweil, R. (2005). *The singularity is near.* New York, NY: Viking Press.

Loizou, P. G., & Kim. G. (2011). Reasons why current speech-enhancement algorithms do not improve speech intelligibility and suggested solutions. *IEEE Transactions on Audio, Speech and Language Processing, 19*(1), 47–56.

Maniwa, K., Jongman, A., & Wade, T. (2009). Acoustic characteristics of clearly spoken English fricatives. *Journal of the Acoustical Society of America, 125*(6), 3962–3973.

Martines, F., Bentivegna, D., Di Piazza, F., Martines, E., Sciacca, V., & Martinciglio, G. (2010). Investigation of tinnitus patients in Italy: Clinical and audiological characteristics. *International Journal of Otolaryngology, 2010,* Article ID 265861.

Moodie, K. S., Seewald, R. C., & Sinclair, S. T. (1994). Procedure for predicting real-ear hearing aid performance in young children. *American Journal of Audiology, 3*(1), 23–31.

Moore, B. C. J. (2001). Dead regions in the cochlea: Diagnosis, perceptual consequences, and implications for the fitting of hearing aids. *Trends in Amplification, 5*(1), 1–34.

Moore, B. C. J. (2006). *An introduction to the psychology of hearing* (5th ed., 87–91). Amsterdam, Netherlands: Elsevier.

Moore, B. C. J. (2010). Aspects of auditory processing related to speech perception. In W. J Hardcastle, J. Laver, & F. E. Gibbons (Eds.), *The handbook of phonetic sciences* (2nd ed., 454–480). Chichester, UK: Blackwell.

Munro, K. J., & Toal, S. (2005). Measuring the real-ear to coupler difference transfer function with an insert earphone and a hearing instrument: Are they the same? *Ear and Hearing, 26*(1), 27–34.

Neuman, A. C., Bakke, M. H., Mackersie, C., Hellman, S., & Levitt, H. (1998). The effect of compression ratio and release time on the categorical rating of sound quality. *Journal of the Acoustical Society of America, 103*, 2273–2281.

Plomp, R. A. (1986). Signal-to-noise ratio model for the speech-reception threshold of the hearing impaired. *Journal of Speech and Hearing Research, 29*, 146–154.

Salvinelli, F., Maurizi, M., Calamita, S., D'Alatri, L., Capelli, A., & Carbone, A. (1991). The external ear and the tympanic membrane—A three-dimensional study. *Scandinavian Audiology, 20*, 253–256.

Simpson, A., Hersbach, A. A., & McDermott, H. J. (2006). Frequency-compression outcomes in listeners with steeply sloping audiograms. *International Journal of Audiology, 45*, 619–629.

Spriet, A., Moonen, M., & Wouters, J. (2010). Evaluation of feedback reduction techniques in hearing aids based on physical performance measures. *Journal of the Acoustical Society of America, 128*(3), 1245–1261.

Valente, M., Schuchman, G., Potts, L., & Beck, L. (2000). Performance of dual-microphone in-the-ear hearing aids. *Journal of the American Academy of Audiology, 11*, 181–189.

Waldner, J.-B. (2008). *Nanocomputers and swarm intelligence*. London, UK: Wiley.

Westermann, S. (1987). The occlusion effect. *Hearing Instruments, 38*(6), 43. Retrieved from http://www.himsa.com

CHAPTER 9

Technical Considerations for Sound Field Audiometry

GARY WALKER

INTRODUCTION

Audiologists use the term *sound field audiometry* to refer to procedures in which the test signal is presented through a loudspeaker rather than through headphones. Sound field audiometry has long been used to estimate the auditory thresholds of young children and other clients who will not tolerate earphones. In the last decade or so, sound field aided and unaided threshold testing has been used increasingly as part of the hearing aid selection and fitting process. This has followed from the realization that the gain provided by the hearing aid, while being worn by the particular client, is essential information that cannot be accurately estimated from coupler-based measurements. This chapter examines the scientific basis of sound field audiometry as it relates specifically to hearing aid selection, fitting, and evaluation.

ROOM ACOUSTICS

A sound field is any area in which sound waves are present. Sound field audiometry is carried out in a variety of acoustic environments ranging from anechoic chambers, audiometric test booths, and specifically modified rooms to rooms that have little or no special treatment. The sound field is bounded by the walls, floor, and ceiling of the room. The sound field within a room is not uniform, but exhibits different characteristics at different locations. The sound field can be divided into the near and far fields, and the far field can, in turn, be divided into direct and reverberant fields.

If a small sound source is placed in a room and activated, sound waves will move away from it in all directions, with the wave fronts forming a spherical pattern. If sound intensity is measured at 0.5 m and at 1 m from the source, so that the distance of the second measuring point from the source is double that of the first, it will be found that the sound intensity has decreased fourfold. That is, the intensity of the sound is inversely proportional to the square of the distance from its source. The sound is then said to be obeying the inverse square law. A simple rule to remember is that the intensity of such sounds will decrease by 6 dB for each doubling of the distance between the source and the measuring point.

If this rule were to be applied back to the source, the calculations would indicate that an infinite sound pressure level must exist at the source. This is absurd: In fact, the operation of the inverse square law relies on the assumption that the sound's wavefront is spherical. This does not apply in close proximity to the source, and the sound pressure level in this region is almost constant. The term *near field* refers to that area that is so close to the source that the inverse square law does not apply, and the term *far field* refers to all other points in the sound field. At some distance from the source, the spherical wave front becomes so large that, for all practical purposes, it can be considered to be flat. The wave is then described as a *plane wave.*

Up to now, it has been assumed that the sound has traveled directly from its source to the measuring point. In reality, direct sound is by no means the only contributor to the field. When a sound wave strikes an object in a sound field, it may be refracted, reflected, absorbed, or transmitted.

If a large object (e.g., 1 m × 1 m × 2 cm thick) is placed facing a plane sound wave at a frequency of 3 kHz, the successive wave fronts passing the object will be deformed in

Editor's note to the second edition: The chapter submitted by Gary Walker for the first edition of the *Handbook of Hearing Aid Amplification* needs little, if any, modification. Unfortunately, he was unable to revise his excellent chapter. A number of diagnostic procedures conducted in sound field have been greatly expanded over the past decade to assess hearing aid performance. Reverberant sound fields have been utilized to assess the affect on speech recognition as a function of reverberating time. The technical considerations have not changed sufficiently to lessen the contribution of his chapter, however. It is included therefore in the revised edition, as well as in the third edition, as it originally appeared in the first edition.

the manner shown in Figure 9–1. For simplicity, it is assumed that no sound is absorbed or transmitted by the object. The wavelength of a 3 kHz tone is 0.115 m, so the long dimensions of the object are much larger than 1 wavelength.

Waves that pass to the side of the obstacle are diffracted around it. That is, their direction of motion is changed so that some sounds actually reach all points on the back of the obstacle. Because the sound that covers the back comes from wave fronts near the edges, however, the pressure fluctuation reaching most of the back is greatly diminished relative to that at the front, and a "sound shadow" is created.

By contrast, the pressure in front of the obstacle will actually be greater than at its surface. This occurs because waves hitting a solid heavy object reflect off the object and travel back toward the source. Immediately adjacent to the surface of the object, the incoming and reflected waves are still in phase with each other, so their contributions to the total pressure add consecutively (see Figure 9–1). As a result, the pressure is double what it would be if the obstacle was not there, and the sound pressure level (SPL) is thus increased by 6 dB over that in the surrounding field. After the reflected wave has traveled back one quarter of a wavelength

toward the source, it has then traveled a half wavelength farther than the incoming wave it is currently meeting head-on. Consequently, they are 180° out of phase and add destructively, creating a pressure minimum one quarter of a wavelength in front of the obstacle. Thus, the pressure increase observable on the surface exists for only a small fraction of a wavelength in front of the obstacle.

For the opposite situation, when a low-frequency, long-wavelength sound wave hits a very small obstacle, any buildup of pressure on the front surface is prevented because the entire surface of the obstacle is immersed in a relatively large region of uniform pressure. There can be no significant departure from the "natural" pressure of the wave at that point of its travel because there is a sufficient time before the next part of the wave arrives for the molecules to redistribute themselves uniformly around the obstacle. Thus, the pressure on the front, back, and sides of the obstacle is the same as that which would be present in the incoming wave in the absence of the obstacle.

When an incoming sound wave meets a solid obstacle, such as a wall, some sound energy may be transmitted through the obstacle to the far side. This transmission can occur in two ways. First, a genuine acoustic wave

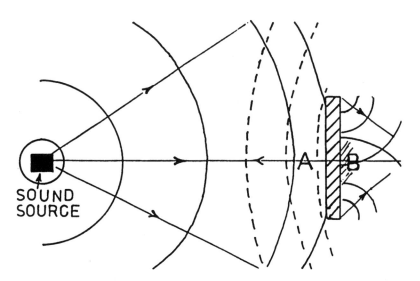

Figure 9–1. Sound propagation.

(i.e., a progression of compressions and rarefactions) can be set up in the obstacle. The magnitude of the sound radiated into the air on the other side of the obstacle by this transmission mechanism is usually insignificant for walls of typical construction. The amount transmitted decreases as the density and thickness of the wall increases and also as the frequency of the incoming wave increases. The second way in which transmission occurs is when the wall as a whole vibrates, much like the diaphragm of a loudspeaker. Just as with acoustic wave transmission, the amount transmitted decreases as the mass of the wall increases and as frequency increases. Thus, irrespective of the type of transmission, the attenuation provided by a wall can be increased by making the wall thicker or by using a denser material. Unfortunately, doubling the mass-per-unit area of a wall (e.g., by doubling the thickness) only results in a 5 or 6 dB decrease in the sound intensity transmitted. It thus quickly becomes uneconomical to continue to increase wall attenuation in this way. An alternative that is usually used when high wall attenuation is required is to use a double wall construction. Provided there is no coupling between the two walls (such as by having them rest on a common, nonabsorbent support or by using too small an air space between them), the total attenuation in dB is twice that of either wall alone. It should be remembered that the attenuation provided by an entire room (such as an audiometric test booth) is often limited by leakage around joints between panels or around windows or doors. That is, air conduction paths provide much better transmission than paths that truly transmit sound through solid obstacles. This occurs because the density of solid objects is many times greater than that of air so that transmission from air to a solid is inefficient. This density change is sometimes described as an impedance mismatch.

Sound, in addition to being reflected from, transmitted through, or diffracted around the obstacle, can also be absorbed at the surface of the obstacle. Soft or porous substances absorb sound more than hard or dense substances. The amount of absorption is characterized by the substance's *absorption coefficient*, which is defined as the proportion of sound intensity that is absorbed when the wave hits a surface. Absorbed sound energy is neither transmitted nor reflected but rather is converted into a small amount of heat energy at the surface of the obstacle. Often the absorption is greater for high frequencies than for low frequencies. When the surface of an obstacle has a high absorption coefficient, the pressure buildup on the front face, which was described earlier, will not occur to the same degree. Recall that the pressure increase occurs when the obstacle is large enough compared with the sound's wavelength to cause a reflected wave to travel back toward the source. It is the in-phase addition of the incident and reflected waves that produces the pressure increase.

If the sound wave is completely absorbed (absorption coefficient = 1.0) by the obstacle, there can be no reflected wave and consequently no pressure increase. The pressure at the surface of the obstacle would then be exactly the same as if the obstacle was not there at all. Intuitively, this seems reasonable because the sound wave travels on past the surface of the obstacle into the absorbent material in just the same way as it would if the absorbent obstacle was absent. For objects with more realistic absorption coefficients (i.e., neither completely absorbing nor completely reflecting), the SPL increase at the surface still occurs, but is of diminished size. It is worth remembering that the SPL increase for a wave hitting a large object wall will always be between 0 dB (for complete absorption) and 6 dB (for complete reflection). From an audiological point of view, the major reason for interest in the pressure increase at the surface of obstacles is that it affects the pressure detected by microphones mounted on the body, such as hearing aid microphones or noise dosimeters.

If a sound source produces a single brief impulse (e.g., a click), an observer will first hear the direct wave, followed shortly by a series of echoes as the sound waves hit the walls of the room and are reflected back into the room, some of them eventually to reach the observer. Because of absorption, each echo will individually be weaker than the direct wave, but the total intensity of all of the reflected sound waves may well be greater than that of the original wave. It is now possible to define the terms *direct* and *reverberant* sound fields. A *direct field* is dominated by directly radiated sound, whereas a reverberant field is dominated by reflected sound. Figure 9–2A, which shows the sound pressure level in a room versus the distance from the sound source, illustrates how the fields combine in a room. The dotted line shows the direct field component, the dashed line the reverberant component, and the solid line the combined field. Note that the logarithmic distance axis used results in a straight-line relationship in the direct field region.

At any particular point in the room, the various reflected waves arriving at that point may tend to add together constructively (i.e., in phase) or may partially or even completely cancel one another out. The combined field is simply the sum of the two individual components (i.e., direct and reverberant). Close to

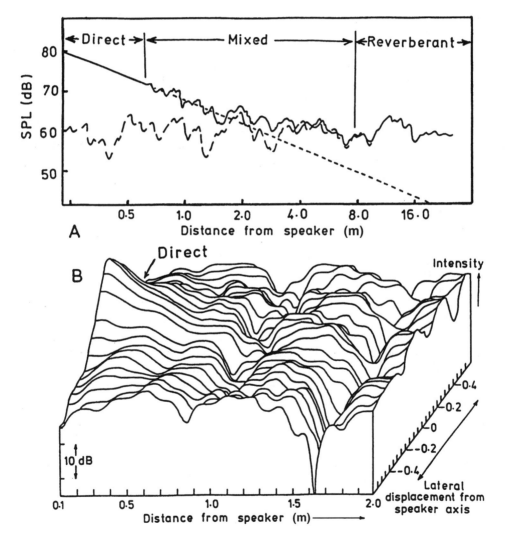

Figure 9–2. Sound fields generated in a room. **A.** The sound pressure level of a pure tone in a room as a function of distance from the sound source. **B.** A three-dimensional (length × width × intensity) representation of a pure-tone sound field generated in a room.

the source, the total field is dominated by the direct component, which varies smoothly by 6 dB for every doubling of distance. Far away from the source, the reverberant field dominates, so small movements by the observer can result in large changes in sound pressure. At intermediate distances, both fields contribute. The distance at which the level of the direct field equals the average level of the reverberant field is called the *critical distance*. In a typical living room with carpets and drapes plus hard and soft furnishings, the critical distance is likely to be less than 1 m. Other rooms, such as kitchens and bathrooms, would typically have more hard surfaces, so their critical distances would be even less. It is concluded, therefore, that in indoor listening situations, the reverberant field is always a significant contributor, and is usually the dominant contributor to the sound field. In panel A of Figure 9–2, maximum variability of the reverberant field is of the order of 6 to 8 dB. For the three-dimensional plot shown in panel B, however, one "trough" in the reverberant field is more than 20 dB "deep." Both parts of Figure 9–2 are based on measurements made in real rooms. The ultimate reverberant field is one in which there is an equal likelihood of the sound arriving at the measurement point from any direction, including above and below. This is called a *diffuse field*.

Two measurements that are basic to architectural acoustics are a room's reverberation time and its absorption coefficient. The *reverberation time* is defined as the time taken for any sound to decay in level by 60 dB. Reverberant sound can have both beneficial and detrimental effects. Although reflected sound can decrease the intelligibility of the original signal by merging one part of the sound into the next, it can add "warmth" to the tonal quality of speech, and, especially, music. Reverberation is often simulated by recording studios for just this purpose. Also, the reverberant sound helps to even out the range of intensities to which people are subjected. Consider what would happen in a lecture theater if only the direct field were

present. Although the audience at the front may only be 2 m from the speaker, those at the back may be 20 m away. This 10:1 distance ratio would mean that those at the front received a signal 20 dB more intense than those at the back. By contrast, the reverberant component of the sound field fills the entire theater uniformly. Thus the people at the back of the theater have the relatively weak direct field considerably augmented by the reverberant sound. Arriving at the correct ratio of direct sound (often described as crisp, clear, or dry) to reverberant sound (often described as smooth, warm, or full) is always a compromise between the conflicting demands of high intelligibility and pleasant tonal quality. It should not be surprising that the optimum amount of reverberant sound depends on the use to which the room or theater is to be put.

SOUND FIELD AUDIOMETRY

When contemplating the practice of sound field audiometry, a number of important questions must be addressed. Walker, Dillon, and Byrne (1984) listed seven such questions:

1. What type of stimulus is most suitable for sound field audiometry?
2. What are the optimal characteristics (e.g., bandwidth) of such a stimulus?
3. What are the relative merits of testing in the direct versus the reverberant field?
4. What test room characteristics are important?
5. How should calibration be performed?
6. What other aspects of testing technique or test room arrangements are important?
7. What limitations apply, and how can they be minimized, if testing has to be performed with a less than optimal stimulus or technique?

Of these questions, the first four are dealt with at length in this chapter, while the others, which are essentially practical, are touched on only briefly.

THE STIMULUS

Problems arise for sound field audiometry as a result of the variation in the sound pressure level of the signal at different places within the room, and because it is impractical to keep the client's ears in exactly the same position for the duration of the test and in exactly the same position assumed during calibration. The problem exists even when the clients are alert and cooperative adults but is much greater when the client is an infant. It is difficult if not impossible to restrain the child's movement without jeopardizing cooperation or inhibiting natural response to the stimulus.

Figure 9–2 should make it clear why pure tones are not considered to be appropriate stimuli for sound field testing in a reverberant field. Small movements of the client's head or drifts in the signal's frequency can result in large variations in the sound pressure level at the test ear. This problem has been noted by many authors (e.g., Morgan, Dirks, & Bower, 1979) and was confirmed by this author and a colleague in an extensive series of measurements (Dillon & Walker, 1982a).

Figure 9–3 shows the sound pressure levels of three tones, 5 Hz apart in frequency, as a function of distance from the sound source. It illustrates how large errors can be introduced by small shifts in the frequency of the tone. It also illustrates how one could be misled regarding the variability of a sound field if judgments are made on the basis of measurements taken at too few frequencies, too few positions in the field, or both.

Dillon and Walker (1982a) listed four attributes that a suitable sound field stimulus should possess:

1. It must be reasonably frequency specific because frequency-specific information is needed for a satisfactory definition of the client's hearing status and amplification needs.
2. The sound pressure level generated in the field must be stable over the whole region that the client's head could occupy during testing.
3. The sound pressure level generated at the client's ear must be stable for small shifts in frequency, such as may occur in an oscillator's output between calibrations.
4. The results obtained in the sound field must be relatable to similar measurements made with pure tones under earphones.

Various complex signals have been promoted as suitable for sound field testing.

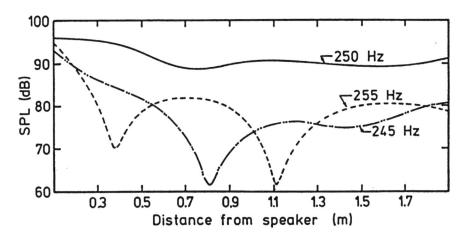

Figure 9–3. The sound pressure levels of three pure tones, 5 Hz apart, as a function of distance from the loudspeaker.

Frequency-modulated (warble) tones and narrow bands of noise are in common clinical use, although their specific parameters vary widely among audiometers. Other stimuli that have been proposed include amplitude-modulated tones (Goldberg, 1979) and damped wavetrains (Victoreen, 1974). The common feature of these stimuli is that they contain energy in a band of frequencies around the nominal frequency. The rationale for their use is that the auditory system averages the sound energy within the pass band, thereby reducing the effects of the energy at any one frequency. The perception of a complex stimulus should, therefore, be relatively unaffected by a null in the room's response if the stimulus contains significant energy within a frequency band that is wider than the null.

Dillon and Walker (1982c) examined the uniformity of sound fields generated by various complex stimuli in a typical audiometric test room. They concluded that, given a rela-

tively uniform distribution of sound energy within its frequency pass band, the factor determining the variability of the sound field generated by a complex stimulus is its bandwidth.

Figure 9–4 shows how the variability of a pure-tone sound field can be reduced by the introduction of frequency modulation. It is clear that the variability of the sound field is inversely related to the bandwidth of the FM tone.

It follows that any comparison of the effectiveness of different types of stimulus must be done with stimuli of equal bandwidths. A number of studies have compared warble tones with bands of noise that were not equal in this respect (e.g., Morgan et al., 1979; Orchik & Rintelmann, 1978; Stephens & Rintelmann, 1978). Their findings and comments may be valid for the particular stimuli investigated, but should not be generalized to include all stimuli of the same type. The noted limitations of the various types of stim-

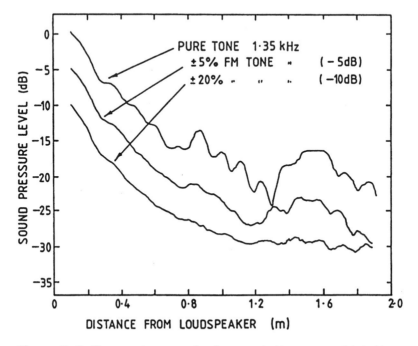

Figure 9–4. The sound pressure levels generated by an unmodulated tone and two modulated tones with the same center frequency but different bandwidths, as a function of distance from the loudspeaker. To facilitate comparison, the overall levels of the tones have been arbitrarily separated by 5 dB.

uli may not apply when they have optimal characteristics.

As all of the types of complex stimulus discussed so far can be produced with a range of bandwidths, this characteristic alone cannot be used to choose between them. Dillon and Walker (1982a) used a variety of grounds to argue against the use of amplitude modulated tones, damped wave trains, and very narrow bands of noise.

Amplitude-modulated tones do not have as uniform a distribution of energy within the pass band as the other candidates and, in the absence of any unique virtue to balance this shortcoming, they were eliminated from further consideration.

Dillon and Walker (1982b) also argued against the use of damped wave trains on the grounds that the results obtained with this type of stimulus cannot be compared with other audiometric data. Audiometry is normally carried out with stimuli whose duration is sufficiently long that it does not affect the results (i.e., >200 ms). Damped wave trains, on the other hand, are exponentially decaying sinusoidal tone bursts in which the number of cycles in each burst remains constant. For practical bandwidths, the stimulus duration is shorter than the integration time of the normal human ear, and the thresholds obtained with them will thus be a function of stimulus duration. The problem is made worse by the fact that the temporal integration function may be grossly disturbed in cases of sensorineural hearing loss (Wright, 1968).

Dillon and Walker's (1982c) results show that band-pass-filtered random noise is inferior to all other stimuli for bandwidths, up to and including 5% of the center frequency. They explained this in terms of the random amplitude fluctuations, which are a characteristic of noise. These fluctuations are relatively slow at the smallest bandwidths and consequently are not smoothed out by the lowpass filter to the same extent that more rapid fluctuations are. For higher center frequencies, the absolute bandwidth of a 5% noise band will be larger. The temporal fluctuations in intensity will, therefore, be faster

and so will increasingly be smoothed by both the ear and the calibrating device.

Audiometric stimuli that contain significant sound energy over a range of frequencies will always underestimate the size of a hearing loss unless that loss is constant across frequencies. The reason is that some of the energy of the stimulus will be at frequencies where the client has better hearing than at the nominal center frequency. This is illustrated in Figure 9–5. Dillon and Walker (1982c) measured the differences between pure-tone and warble tone thresholds as a function of the differences between the pure-tone thresholds for frequencies at the band center and band edge of the warble tone. This revealed that the threshold differences between the pure and warble tones were about 0.75 times the band center to band edge threshold difference. In other words, a broadband stimulus will underestimate a hearing loss in the presence of a sloping threshold curve by an amount equal to three-quarters of the difference between the pure-tone thresholds at frequencies corresponding to the center and band edge of the stimulus. The problem is worse at high frequencies where the thresholds of many people with sensorineural hearing loss change rapidly across frequencies. It is desirable that the stimulus not only have as narrow a bandwidth as practicable, but that energy outside the band limits falls off as rapidly as possible. Orchik and Mosher (1975) demonstrated that filter slopes can have a marked effect on the thresholds obtained with narrow bands of noise. Figure 9–5B shows how the error is increased when the out-of-band slope of the stimulus is less than the slope of the threshold function, but not when it is greater. Threshold functions can be steep. Rosler and Anderson (1978) found slopes as great as 250 dB/octave in the frequency range 2000 to 4000 Hz, whereas Dillon and Walker reported that slopes of 120 dB/octave or more could be expected in this frequency range in 1% of persons with sensorineural hearing loss.

Warble tones do not require filtering for their generation, their spectral slope depending

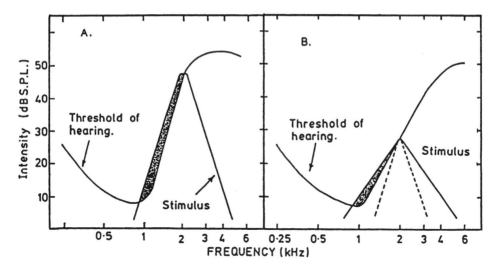

Figure 9–5. A. Shows why the use of complex signals results in underestimation of the threshold. Some of the stimulus energy (*shaded area*) falls at frequencies where the client has better thresholds. **B.** Shows that maximum error will result when the "skirts" of the stimulus are less steep than the threshold (*solid lines*) and minimized when they are steeper than the threshold function (*broken lines*).

on the modulate rate, waveform, and frequency deviation. Very steep slopes can be obtained, especially at the higher frequencies where they are most required. On the other hand, narrow bands of noise with steep filter slopes are not readily available as simple low-order filters will not provide sufficiently steep filter slopes. Furthermore, the use of complex higher order filters is not desirable in a clinical instrument because they require careful alignment. Lippman and Adams (1982), however, have described an inexpensive method of generating suitable noise bands, although the ⅓-octave bandwidth that they suggest would not be optimal for all frequencies. There are also ways of producing bands of noise with the desired characteristics that do not involve bandpass-filtering broadband noise. The noise can be synthesized by adding together a number of discrete components, or it can be produced by means of the modulation technique proposed by Zwislocki (1951). With the advent of microprocessors in audiometers, it is now also possible to generate a noise waveform with any desired spectral properties by cyclically accessing a waveform stored in computer memory.

It is concluded that frequency modulated (warble) tones and suitably generated narrow bands of noise are the stimuli of choice for reverberant sound field audiometry.

The Required Bandwidths of Sound Field Stimuli

The selection of the bandwidths of stimuli for sound field audiometry necessarily involves a compromise. On the one hand, large bandwidths are required to obtain uniform sound fields; on the other hand, small bandwidths are needed to measure a frequency dependent hearing loss. These clearly are conflicting requirements. The size of errors arising from both sources must be quantified before a reasoned decision can be made about the appropriate stimulus for a particular client. If there is reason to believe that the client has a very steep threshold slope, a narrow bandwidth may be chosen for high frequencies, even though this results in a more variable sound field. If the testing is being carried out in an area with poor acoustic characteristics, however, a broader band stimulus may be needed. In this case, the clinician should be aware of the likely size of the introduced error. The author and his colleagues (Dillon & Walker, 1982c; Walker et al., 1984) have considered this issue in detail and have made specific recommendations about the stimuli that should be made available to clinicians.

The Required Modulation Waveform and Modulation Rate of FM Tones

For FM tones, the modulation waveform and rate must also be specified. The modulation waveform describes the manner in which the instantaneous frequency of the signal moves back and forth about the center frequency.

Dillon and Walker (1982b) addressed the question of the most desirable waveform. In electronics, sinusoidal, triangular, ramp, and rectangular (square) waveforms are commonly used. These are shown in Figure 9–6.

Ramp and square wave modulation both involve very rapid frequency changes during their cycles, and this results in a "splattering" of energy to out-of-band frequencies. As can clearly be seen in Figure 9–6, the result is a less-steep, out-of-band characteristic. It is concluded that they are not suitable for use in sound field audiometry. There is little to choose between sinusoidal and triangular modulation. As can be seen in Figure 9–7, sinusoidal modulation produces a steeper "edge" than triangular modulation; however, triangular modulation produces a more

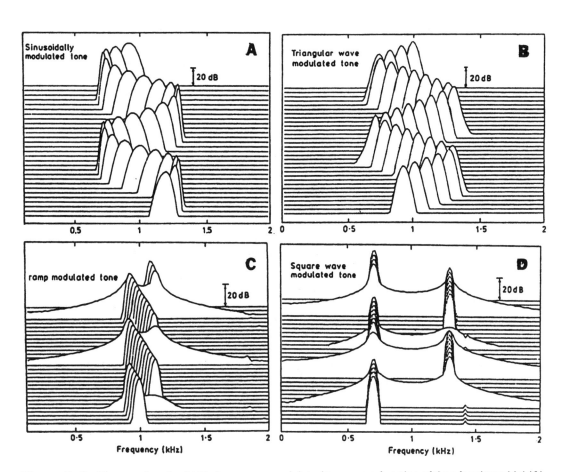

Figure 9–6. The spectra of a 1 kHz frequency modulated tone, as a function of time for sinusoidal (**A**), triangular (**B**), ramp (**C**), and square wave (**D**) modulation.

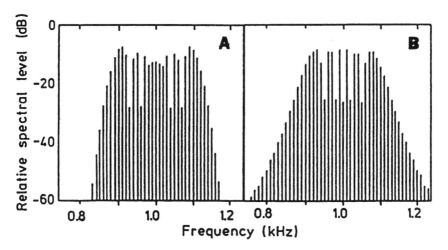

Figure 9–7. Spectra of a sinusoidal modulated tone (**A**) and a triangularly modulated tone (**B**). Note the broader "skirts" but more uniform distribution of energy in *B*.

uniform in-band spectral density (because in sinusoidal modulation, the signal "dwells" longer at the frequency extremes). Both are acceptable, but because triangular modulation has an acceptable out-of-band characteristic and superior in-band characteristic, it is the waveform of choice.

Modulation rate or *modulation frequency* refers to the rate (in Hz) at which the instantaneous frequency is swept across the frequency band. Walker and Dillon (1983) examined the question of which modulation rate or rates are suitable for use in sound field FM tones. Two factors must be considered. First, if the modulation rate is too low, the ear will respond to individual fluctuations as the signal sweeps over the various peaks and troughs in the rooms' response. Consequently, the obtained threshold will depend on the highest peak occurring within the modulation cycle. Second, if the modulation rate is too high, field uniformity will decrease because there will be insufficient spectral components to ensure reasonable averaging within the band. The reason for this is that in the spectrum of an FM tone, the energy of the signal is confined to discrete frequencies, and the spacing between these spectral components is a function of the modulation rate. Hence, for a fixed bandwidth signal,

as the modulation rate increases, fewer and fewer spectral components will fall within the passband. The physical basis of this phenomenon is not discussed here. The important point is that Walker and Dillon's measurements indicate that if, as is usual, the signal bandwidth is a fixed percentage of the center frequency, the upper limit of the range of modulation rates will vary from frequency to frequency. More important, the fall off in energy beyond the band edges of FM tones is partly determined by the modulation rate, being steeper for lower modulation rates. Therefore, the maximum permissible modulation rate is not particularly important because, as steep, out-of-band slopes are very desirable, the modulation rate should be kept as low as possible.

The modulation rate at which individual peaks in the response begin to be perceived will depend on the temporal integration properties of the listening ear. For persons with normal hearing, the threshold and loudness of a pure tone are independent of the duration of the tone as long as that duration is greater than 200 ms. For briefer tones, the threshold of hearing increases with decreasing duration at a rate of about 10 dB per decade of duration. The threshold for a tone of 10-ms duration, for example, will be 10 dB higher than that for the same tone of 100 ms duration. In other words, the normal ear integrates sound energy over a period of about 200 ms (Figure 9–8).

It has been shown by investigators that persons with hearing losses of cochlear origin have abnormal auditory temporal integration with the integration time greatly reduced (e.g., Wright, 1968). The breakpoint in some cases may be as low as 10 ms.

From Walker and Dillon's (1983) measurements, it is clear that although the 5 Hz modulation rate commonly encountered in audiometers may be adequate for persons with normal hearing, it is not adequate for those with sensorineural hearing losses. It is concluded that the preferred modulation rate depends on the center frequency and bandwidth of the tone. For the amplitude fluctuations to be fully integrated by ears with abnormal temporal integration functions, the modulation rate should be at least 20 Hz. As other considerations indicate that the modulation rate be kept as low as possible within

the permissible range, if a single modulation rate is chosen to cover all frequencies, 20 Hz appears to be the best choice.

In summary, the preferred stimuli for reverberant sound field audiometry are triangularly or sinusoidally modulated FM (warble) tones or suitably generated narrow bands of noise. The optimal bandwidth of the stimulus, expressed as a percentage of the center frequency, will vary with frequency, ranging from about 30% at 0.25 kHz to 10% at 4 kHz. Stimuli with longer and smaller bandwidths than this may be needed in some circumstances, however. For FM (warble) tones, the optimum modulation rate will also vary with frequency but, if a single modulation rate is required, 20 Hz is acceptable at all frequencies.

These recommendations have been adopted for use in National Acoustic Laboratory Hearing Centres throughout Australia. Evidence suggests that their use has improved the reliability of sound field audiometry (Byrne & Dillon, 1981; Cichello, 1987).

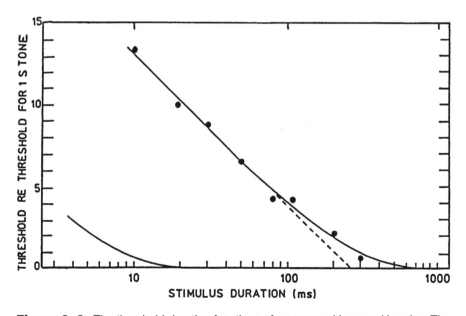

Figure 9–8. The threshold-duration functions of a person with normal hearing. The threshold increases at about 10 dB per decade of time for stimulus durations less than about 200 ms. This indicates that a normal ear integrates sound energy over a 200-ms period. The curve on the left is for a subject with severe sensorineural hearing loss.

Discussion up to this point has been focused on reverberant field testing. It is also possible, of course, to carry out testing in the direct field; that is, in that part of the field where the inverse square law is operating. It has been demonstrated that acceptably reliable results can be obtained from direct field testing, so long as certain precautions are taken (Walker, 1979; Woodford & Tecca, 1985). The crucial question is that of validity. As discussed earlier in this chapter, in most rooms, the direct field would only extend for about 0.5 to 1 m around the sound source. It is argued, therefore, that most listening is carried out under reverberant or mixed field conditions. "Face validity" would seem to favor the reverberant field. It remains an open question as to whether or not direct field testing provides useful information about aided hearing.

In direct field testing, complex stimuli have no advantages over pure tones as stimuli. Because the use of pure tones is convenient and avoids the errors associated with multifrequency stimuli, they are the stimuli of choice. It must be recognized, however, that as soon as the client's head is introduced into the field, it ceases to be a direct field. Thus, for direct field testing, the functional gain and frequency response will be influenced by the azimuth of the incident sound because of head baffle and shadow effects. The choice of testing arrangement (orientation of subject to the loudspeaker) thus becomes a significant issue. Indeed, testing with more than one arrangement may be needed to obtain an adequate description of the performance of hearing aids, especially those with directional microphones or CROS (contralateral routing of signals) fittings.

To minimize errors resulting from small movements of the subject's head toward or away from the sound source, the client should be positioned as far away from the sound source as possible (while staying in the direct field). Even so, a headrest or other restraining device should be used to restrict head movement. Even changes in the positioning of the client's shoulders can result in small changes in the signal reaching the ear (Walker, 1979).

DESIRABLE CHARACTERISTICS OF THE TEST ROOM

In this section, the desirable characteristics of the room in which sound field audiometry is to be conducted is discussed.

Absorption Characteristics

In truly anechoic conditions, the direct field extends throughout the room. Anechoic chambers, therefore, provide the ideal conditions for direct field testing as the test position can be a long way from the sound source, thus minimizing the effects of head movement. Few, if any, clinicians have access to such facilities, however.

If testing is to be carried out in a reverberant field, the question is: Should the room's surfaces be designed to maximize or minimize the amount of reflected energy? Recall the earlier comment that a highly reverberant room reinforces the sound field at the back of the room. Because the answer to the previous question was not clear on theoretical grounds, Dillon and Walker (1981) examined it experimentally. The sound field variability of pure-tone and warble-tone sound fields was measured at a large number of positions within a special room that reverberation time and absorptivity could be systematically varied. As expected for pure tones measured in the reverberant field, the peaks and troughs that occurred at any one frequency sweep became greater in number and amplitude, but lesser in bandwidth as the room was made more reflective. This is illustrated in Figure 9–9, which shows the

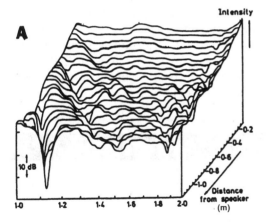

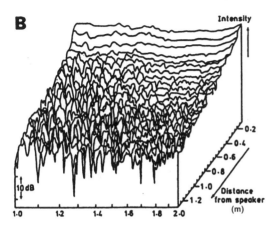

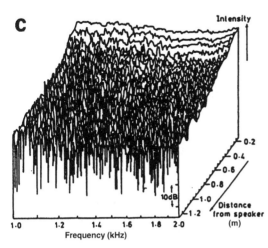

Figure 9–9. Pure-tone frequency response curves for frequencies between 1 and 2 kHz as a function of distance from the sound source for a highly absorbent audiometric test booth (**A**), a moderately reverberant room (**B**), and a highly reverberant room (**C**).

frequency-response curves for frequencies between 1 and 2 kHz as a function of distance from the loudspeaker in rooms having short, moderate, and long reverberation times. This finding supports the theoretical prediction of Schroeder and Kuttruff (1962) that the average frequency spacing between adjacent maxima is equal to 3.9 divided by the reverberation time. Remember that warble tones and bands of noise result in more uniform fields because they average the intensity over the frequencies within their passbands. This averaging is most effective when the troughs are not too deep and when they are narrower in bandwidth than the stimulus. Thus, highly reflecting rooms have the advantage of narrower troughs, but the disadvantage is that these are deep and many. The measurements made with warble tones made two things clear. First, irrespective of the room's reflectivity, the stimuli with the larger bandwidths provided the more uniform fields. Second, the more reflective rooms produced fields that were inferior at all stimulus bandwidths, but particularly for the narrower band stimuli. The obvious practical implication is that the reverberation times of test rooms should be made as short as possible by making all surfaces within them as absorbing as possible.

Background Noise

Various standards specify the maximum background noise that is permissible in audiometric test rooms (e.g., ANSI S3.11977). The aim is to ensure that the background noise does not mask the stimulus and result in spuriously high thresholds. Background noise levels need to be lower for sound field testing than for testing under earphones because the earphones themselves to some extent act as attenuators. As mentioned earlier, complex construction techniques are used by booth manufacturers in order to meet standard specifications, particularly if the test room must be located in a noisy part of the building.

Macrae and Frazer (1980) have pointed out that invalid aided thresholds often result, not because of masking by background noise but because of masking by the internal noise of the hearing aid itself. Valid aided thresholds cannot be obtained if the actual threshold is lower than the equivalent input noise level (EINL) of the aid. Beck (1980) measured the EINLs of 251 different models of hearing aids and reported that the mean EINL averaged over three frequencies (1, 1.6, and 2.5 kHz), was 21.1 dB SPL with a standard deviation of 3.3 dB. Procedures have been developed for checking the validity of aided thresholds (see Macrae, 1981, 1982; Macrae & Frazer, 1980). It should be readily obvious that background noise in the test environment of the EINLs of specific hearing aid models can yield unacceptable threshold measurements.

Size and Shape of the Room

Sound wave patterns are influenced by the shape of the room. Anderson (1979) applied basic acoustic theory to devise two practical sizes for audiometric booths. Walker and colleagues (1984) cautioned, however, that test rooms having optimized dimensions may reduce, but will not eliminate, intensity irregularities in the sound field. They also stated that, to the best of their knowledge, the hypothetical advantages of rooms with such dimensions have never been quantified. They further cautioned that rooms having nonrectangular shapes will not eliminate standing wave effects. So, the only requirement regarding room size and shape is that it must be large enough to permit the subject to be seated at a sufficient distance from the loudspeaker and walls.

Test Arrangements

There are theoretical advantages to placing the loudspeaker in a three-way corner of the room, that is, the conjunction of two walls and floor or ceiling, and this is an arrangement favored by many. It must be cautioned that the advantages would be expected to be small, and several investigations have been unable to demonstrate any advantages at all (Davy, 1981; Walker & Dillon, 1983). It is concluded that the position of the loudspeaker in the room is not critical.

CALIBRATION

A discussion of the practical issues involved in calibration of a sound field does not fall within the scope of this chapter; however, several issues need to be discussed.

Calibration serves two purposes. First, it establishes the relationship between sound pressure level, measured at some point in the field, and the corresponding attenuator setting on the signal generator. Second, it establishes the sound pressure levels corresponding to normal thresholds so that an individual's hearing level may be compared with this standard. This second type of calibration is important for diagnostic audiology but less so for hearing aid evaluation, where interest focuses on the change in threshold that results from the use of a hearing aid and upon the absolute level of sound that can be heard through the aid.

Sound field stimuli have normally been calibrated by measuring the sound pressure levels at the point in the sound field that is later to be occupied by the client's head. With this technique, the acoustic effects resulting from the introduction of the client's head into the field are automatically taken into account when thresholds are measured.

These effects are, to some extent, dependent on the particular test position, however. It can be argued that only those components of head diffraction that are constant across diverse acoustic environments should be included in the measurements. Also, any movement by the client away from the calibration point will result in an error. Use of the complex stimuli discussed in this chapter will minimize such errors, but it will not totally eliminate them. The alternative technique is to place a control microphone on or near the client's head. The output of this microphone is used to automatically control the attenuator of the signal generator in order to maintain an invariant sound pressure level at that point occupied by the microphone. Unfortunately, some error will remain because the control microphone cannot be exactly at the position of interest, that is, the hearing aid microphone post for aided testing or the client's eardrum for unaided testing. Also, head diffraction effects are not included at all in the measurements, so that if one wishes to refer the measurements to the sound pressure level in the undisturbed field, average head diffraction effects must be assumed. Again, errors will be minimized by the use of complex stimuli. Dillon (1982) quantified the errors associated with both calibration procedures and concluded that, on average, the errors were less when the control microphone technique was used.

One other issue remains to be discussed. For all complex stimuli used in sound field testing, intensity at the client's ear will vary with time. Even those stimuli such as warble tones that do not contain temporal intensity fluctuations when generated will do so at the client's ear as a result of peaks and troughs in the room's frequency response being sequentially excited as the tone sweeps across its frequency band. Earlier it was suggested that it is desirable that sound field thresholds be relatable to pure-tone thresholds obtained with audiometric earphones. For this to be achieved, the sound field stimulus must be measured in a way that mimics the temporal integration function of the human ear. From an experiment in which Plomp and Bouman's (1959) "leaky integrator" model of threshold detection was applied, Dillon and Walker (1980) devised just such a method. Unfortunately, this method is not clinically feasible, as it involves the derivation of individual calibration figures for each client. Fortunately, an acceptably accurate approximation can be obtained by reading the peak deflections of a sound level meter in the "RMS fast" mode.

SUMMARY

This chapter has examined the acoustic properties of rooms, with specific reference to the practice of sound field audiometry. A major impediment to accurate audiometric testing in a reverberant or diffuse sound field is the variability of the sound pressure level of the field as a function of both the frequency of the sound and the measurement position in the field. Methods for minimizing these errors have been discussed. Frequency-modulated tones with optimized parameters or suitably generated narrow bands of noise, again with optimized parameters, are proposed as stimuli for reverberant field testing. Direct field sound field audiometry has also been discussed, and it is concluded that in this case, complex stimuli offer no advantages over pure tone. Accurate testing in the direct field is only possible if the client's head can be sufficiently immobilized or if the testing is performed under anechoic conditions, however. Desirable room characteristics and suitable calibration procedures have been considered. If the materials and techniques described in this chapter are employed, it is possible to achieve the same degree of reliability in sound field audiometry as is achieved in traditional audiometry under earphones.

REVIEW QUESTIONS

1. What is sound field audiometry, and why has it come to be more widely used as part of the hearing aid selection and fitting process?

2. What is a reverberant sound field?

3. Describe what happens to a sound wave that is absorbed by an object.

4. Describe the four qualities of a suitable sound field stimulus.

5. What are some of the arguments against the use of damped wave trains as stimuli?

6. Why are ramp and square wave modulation not suitable for use in sound field audiometry?

7. What is the preferred stimuli for reverberant sound field audiometry?

8. Why might the validity of direct sound field audiometry be questioned?

9. Describe the ideal characteristics of the test room in which sound field audiometry is to be conducted.

REFERENCES

American National Standards Institute. (S3.11977). *American standard criteria for background noise in audiometer rooms.* New York, NY: American Standards Association.

Anderson, C. D. (1979). New ideas in sound field systems. *Hearing Instruments, 30,* 12–13, 43.

Beck, L. (Ed.). (1980). *Handbook of hearing aid measurement.* Washington, DC: Veterans Administration.

Byrne, D. J., & Dillon, H. (1981). Comparative reliability of warble tone thresholds under earphones and in sound field. *Australian Journal of Audiology, 3,* 12–14.

Cichello, P. (1987). Sound field visual reinforcement orientation audiometry revisited. *Australian Journal of Audiology, 8,* 12–17.

Davy, J. L. (1981). The relative variance of the transmission function of a reverberation room. *Journal of Sound and Vibration, 77,* 455–479.

Dillon, H. (1982). The use of a control microphone in reverberant sound field audiometric testing. *Journal of the Acoustical Society of America, 72*(Suppl. 1), S108.

Dillon, H., & Walker, G. (1980). The perception of normal hearing persons of intensity fluctuations in narrow band stimuli and its implications for sound field calibration procedures. *Australian Journal of Audiology, 2,* 72–82.

Dillon, H., & Walker, G. (1981). The effect of acoustic environment on the reliability of sound field audiometry. *Australian Journal of Audiology, 3,* 67–72.

Dillon, H., & Walker, G. (1982a). Comparison of stimuli used in sound field audiometric testing. *Journal of the Acoustical Society of America, 71,* 161–172.

Dillon, H., & Walker, G. (1982b). The selection of modulation waveform for frequency modulated sound field stimuli. *Australian Journal of Audiology, 4,* 56–61.

Dillon, H., & Walker, G. (1982c, November). *An optimum bandwidth for audiometric sound field stimuli.* Paper presented at the annual American Speech and Hearing Association convention, Toronto, Canada.

Goldberg, H. (1979, March). Discrete sound field audiometry. *Hearing Journal,* 42–43.

Lippman, R., & Adams, D. (1982). A 1/3 octave band noise generator for soundfield audiometric measurements. *Journal of Speech and Hearing Disorders, 47,* 84–88.

Macrae, H. J. (1981). *Invalid aided thresholds and equivalent input noise levels* (NAL Informal Report No. 81). Sydney, Australia: National Acoustics Laboratories.

Macrae, H. J. (1982). The validity of aided thresholds. *Australian Journal of Audiology, 4,* 48–54.

Macrae, H. J., & Frazer, G. (1980). An investigation of variables affecting aided thresholds. *Australian Journal of Audiology, 2,* 56–62.

Morgan, D. E., Dirks, D. D., & Bower, D. R. (1979). Suggested threshold sound pressure levels for frequency modulated (warble) tones in the sound field. *Journal of Speech and Hearing Disorders, 44,* 37–54.

Orchik, D., & Mosher, N. (1975). Narrow band noise audiometry: The effect of filter slope. *Journal of the American Audiology Society, 1,* 50–53.

Orchik, D., & Rintelmann, W. (1978). Comparison of pure-tone, warble-tone and narrow band noise thresholds of young normal hearing children. *Journal of the American Audiology Society, 3,* 214–220.

Plomp, R., & Bouman, M. (1959). Relation between hearing threshold and duration for tone pulses. *Journal of the Acoustical Society of America, 31,* 749–758.

Rosler, G., & Anderson, H. (1978). Maximum steepness of slopes in hearing threshold curves. *Audiology, 17,* 299–316.

Schroeder, M. R., & Kuttruff, K. H. (1962). On frequency response curves in rooms. Comparison of experimental, theoretical and Monte Carlo results for the average spacing between maxima. *Journal of the Acoustical Society of America, 34,* 76–80.

Stephens, M., & Rintelmann, W. (1978). The influence of audiometric configuration on pure tone, warble-tones, and narrow band noise thresholds of adults with sensorineural hearing losses. *Journal of the American Audiology Society, 3,* 221–226.

Victoreen, J. (1974). Equal loudness pressure determined with a decaying oscillatory waveform. *Journal of the Acoustical Society of America, 55,* 309–312.

Walker, G. (1979). The pure tone in sound field testing. Experimental results and suggested procedures. *Australian Journal of Audiology, 1,* 49–60.

Walker, G., & Dillon, H. (1983). The selection of modulation rates for frequency modulated sound field stimuli. *Scandinavian Audiology, 12,* 151–156.

Walker, G., Dillon, H., & Byrne, D. (1984). Sound field audiometry: Recommended stimuli and procedures. *Ear and Hearing, 5*, 13–21.

Woodford, C. M., & Tecca, J. (1985, June). The use of pure-tone stimuli in a sound field. *Hearing Journal*, 21–27.

Wright, H. H. (1968). The effect of sensorineural hearing loss on threshold-duration functions. *Journal of Speech and Hearing Research, 11*, 842–852.

Zwislocki, J. (1951). Eine verbesserte Ver taubungs-methode für die Audiometric. *Acta Oto-Laryngologica, 39*, 338–356.

CHAPTER 10

Psychology of Individuals with Hearing Impairment

ROBERT W. SWEETOW
JULIE BIER

To maximize success, hearing health care professionals must comprehend the psychology of hearing impairment. As with any other group, individuals with hearing impairment possess a wide range of personalities, desires, and fears. Understanding the factors that influence the thoughts and emotions of these patients can allow the professional to be better equipped to provide appropriate amplification needs.

In this chapter, we analyze the psychology of listeners with hearing impairment, how their behaviors and thoughts are shaped and developed by both internal and external factors and events, and how the hearing health care professional can utilize this knowledge in order to serve this population.

TERMINOLOGY

There may be confusion when discussing certain terms related to persons with hearing impairment. While there is some degree of overlap in these terms, we use the following descriptions:

A. *Hard of hearing:* Disabled to an extent that makes difficult, but does not preclude, the understanding of speech through audition alone, with or without hearing aids.
B. *Deafness:* Disability that precludes understanding speech through the auditory channel alone, with or without the use of hearing aids.
C. *Degree of loss:* Categorized as mild, moderate, severe, or profound.
D. *Disorder:* Disease process or malformation of a physical system.
E. *Impairment:* Loss or abnormality of psychological, physiological, or anatomical structure or function.
F. *Disability:* Activity limitation or lack of ability (resulting from an impairment) to perform an activity in a manner that is considered within the range of normal for a human being
G. *Handicap:* Participation restriction of disadvantage for a given individual, resulting from an impairment or a disability that limits or prevents the fulfillment of a normal role (depending on age, sex, social, and cultural factors).
H. *Benefit:* Decrease in the amount and degree of handicap for an individual.
I. *Satisfaction:* Personal gratification composed of a complex combination of benefit, communication needs, and personality traits.

PSYCHOLOGICAL LEVELS OF HEARING

Ramsdell (1978) proposed that people function in an auditory sense at three different levels: primitive, warning, and symbolic. Each level has a distinct importance, and therefore will be discussed separately.

Primitive Level of Hearing

A major boost in the interest of the psychology and rehabilitation of individuals with hearing impairment occurred following World War II, when army veterans returning home complained of changes in their perception of the auditory world. Ramsdell hypothesized it was not simply the loss of the ability to understanding speech that so adversely affected these veterans, but the loss of background environmental sounds that are heard subconsciously and taken for granted that were sorely missed. Hull (1992) stated that at the primitive level, sound functions as an auditory coupling to the world. People react to the changing background sounds around them without being aware of it. It is this level of hearing that connects us to our environment. A loss of hearing at this primitive level can cause disorientation and even result in an acute state of depression. Because this level of hearing is not at the conscious level, it may be difficult to identify it as the source of depression. Prominent audiologist Dr. Mark Ross noted a practical example of the effect of a loss of hearing at the primitive level. Ross (1999a), who has a long-standing profound hearing loss, contracted an external ear infection and was unable to wear his hearing aids. As a result, sounds and noises that were otherwise taken for granted while wearing his hearing aids were no longer audible, and left him "with a feeling of being cut off from the world."

Signs and Warning Level of Hearing

The next level of hearing goes beyond the realm of background sounds and interprets sounds that serve as warning signals and as signs conveying information. The warning level of hearing provides the listener with essential information about the environment. It is critical because audition can notify us of events that occur outside of the range of the other senses. Alerting sounds have a direct meaning attached to them and require an immediate response. Some examples of alerting sounds include a siren or a smoke alarm. At this level of hearing, not all sounds signal danger, however. Sounds also convey information about objects or events. Examples include a knock at the door or the ring of the telephone. The sound of an alarm clock informs us that it is time to wake up. When hearing is lost at this level, the individual's safety and connection with nonlanguage bearing information is altered. This can lead to feelings of insecurity. Because signal warning hearing and the associated meanings attached to these auditory symbols occur at the conscious level, compensatory strategies can and should be developed. It is also at this level that people utilize hearing as a tool to determine the location of sound, which can provide warning information, information that will provide cues regarding how to position oneself, so that the signal can be most efficiently received, and enhanced understanding in noise due to auditory scene analysis (Bregman, 1990). Additionally, we utilize this stage of hearing to enhance our aesthetic pleasure, for example, when listening to music.

Symbolic Level of Hearing

The highest psychological stage of hearing occurs at the symbolic level. It is here that sound forms the major component of communication and becomes the foundation for language. A loss of hearing at the symbolic level may cause an individual who is hard of hearing to misunderstand certain key words in sentences. Even the emotional content of the spoken message can be lost if linguistic cues inherent in the sentence and prosodic cues bearing information about stress cannot be heard. Loss of hearing at this most identifiable level (communication) with other individuals can cause depression, withdrawal, and isolation.

HEARING LOSS CHARACTERISTICS

The psychological influence and the effect on personality that hearing loss bears on an individual may vary depending on: (1) the degree of the loss, (2) the time at which the loss occurred in the individual's life, and (3) the activity limitations (formerly called disability) and participation restrictions (formerly termed handicap) produced by the structural abnormality (formerly called impairment; World Health Organization, 2001). These factors will influence the choices that the individual will make with regard to the effect the hearing impairment will exert on his or her life.

Degree of Hearing Loss

Individuals who have little or no usable hearing are likely to have a different perspective than individuals who have partial hearing and are able to utilize audition as the primary channel of receptive communication. For individuals with deafness, the realization that they must employ a sensory shift is apparent. For people who are hard of hearing, the propensity to "hold on" to what they have may lead to denial of the problem.

Recognizing inevitable individual variations, certain general statements can be posed regarding the difference in the manner in which individuals with deafness versus those with lesser degrees of hearing loss have historically been viewed and treated by society. As a consequence of this treatment, people with both degrees of hearing loss often face separate struggles and choices revolving around their hearing handicap.

Deafness

Individuals with deafness, as a group, have suffered the indignities of being treated as outsiders or even as people of inferior intellect. Such treatment rose from the historical concepts as discussed by Furth (1966) that thinking could not develop without language, language could not develop without speech, and speech could not develop without hearing, hence the term "deaf mute." It, therefore, was concluded that those who could not hear, could not think. Even Aristotle surmised that those born deaf were also dumb, hence the term "deaf and dumb." Early Greek translators often interchanged the words for speechless and senseless. In the Roman Empire, individuals with hearing impairment who could not speak were stripped of all legal rights. Christians from St. Augustine's era believed that, unlike those with normal hearing, the deaf could not achieve immortality because they could not speak the sacraments. Legal statutes from the 19th-century United States continued to impede the rights of the deaf. In New York, for example, deaf individuals were not allowed to vote. Ship owners arriving in the United States were required to report the names of all deaf persons on board and were obligated to pay exorbitant taxes (Higgins, 1980).

Today, it is the unfortunate reality that individuals with greater degrees of hearing loss frequently continue to be excluded from or avoided by normal-hearing society. This prejudiced attitude is likely an outcome of the lack of education about deafness. The normal-hearing person watching people living with deafness use sign language or who hear their speech may, in fact, be fearful of his or her own inappropriate response to the situation. This is not to imply that the struggles and choices made by a given deaf individual are created only by the reactions of the normal-hearing society. Individuals with deafness do have options. One of the most fundamental choices they can make is whether to attempt to assimilate completely into normal-hearing society with the help of hearing aids or cochlear implants or to assume their role as a member of the "deaf culture." One might argue that selection of the first choice affords a greater number of opportunities, both social and vocational. To do this, however, individuals must be willing to face both intentional and unintentional ridicule, to develop compensation strategies for enhanced communication, and to take chances.

The alternative choice persons living with deafness can make is to separate themselves from the normal-hearing world and enter into a lifestyle often termed "Deaf Culture." One could presume that deaf culture might be selected because the person's role in society might not be accepted by those with normal hearing. In other words, the person with deafness could be considered an outsider due largely to the cultural norms created and controlled by normal-hearing society. On the other hand, a person with deafness who desires to associate primarily with others who share similar struggles and life situations is no different, for example, than people who choose to befriend others who share an interest in art. If individuals desire acceptance into certain deaf cultures, they may be required to accept their values, particularly the use of American Sign Language, associate and identify primarily with other people who have significant degrees of hearing loss (Padden, 1980), and, relevant to this chapter, reject the use of amplification. Conversely, the benefits of this choice of lifestyle are that some of the struggles facing the individual who attempts to fully integrate into "normal-hearing" society may be minimized or eliminated. This individual may be rewarded with the luxury of "letting his or her guard down" and not feeling the need to hide the hearing disability.

Hard of Hearing

A major difference between the person who is hard of hearing and the person with deafness is that the hearing disability may not be as apparent to the rest of society. Therefore, the struggles and choices facing the person with a lesser degree of hearing loss are often quite different than those for the deaf population. Because of learned reactions to disabilities, persons with lesser degrees of hearing loss must contend not only with society's reactions to their disabilities, but also with the internal psychological battle of acceptance of a loss. The choices they make regarding these struggles also will affect their quality and outlook on life.

Similar to people with deafness, persons who are hard of hearing must face the reaction of the normal-hearing society. Society's reactions to disabilities are strange and confusing. Historically, people with disabilities have been viewed in a negative manner and have been faced with severe discrimination and social disadvantage (Barnes, Mercer, & Shakespeare, 2000). Frequently, there are behavioral changes that occur when normal-hearing persons first become aware that the individual they are engaged in a conversation with has a hearing loss. Why does this occur? Perhaps they are surprised by the individual's disability or feel like they were taken advantage of or tricked in some way. These reactions, no matter how inappropriate they may seem, are learned and practiced on almost a daily basis because this is how societal norms are structured. Conversely, when individuals who were once a part of this learned lifestyle recognize they have a hearing loss, they may withdraw or isolate themselves from society in an effort to protect themselves from being discovered. Danhauer, Johnson, Kasten, and Brimacombe (1985) identified the negative attitudes that normal-hearing individuals have when viewing people wearing hearing aids. They defined this as the "hearing aid effect." Many people with hearing loss choose not to pursue hearing aids due to the perceived societal connotation of disability and aging and feel that it is a public admission of hearing loss (Kochkin, 2007). These individuals thus must face a tough choice: to deny their hearing loss or to accept and recognize their "disability" and seek professional advice.

Time of Onset

The individual who acquires hearing loss after developing language may view hearing loss from a different perspective than an individual who has had hearing impairment since birth. To congenitally impaired listeners, their auditory status is their personal norm. Life without hearing has shaped the core of their lives; they only have the life experience of *not* being able to draw information about their environment from their sense of hearing. People who have a congenital hearing loss must face the challenge of learning language via channels that are not the primary route and gathering information about their environment through other means.

For individuals who lose their hearing following the acquisition of language, however, a different set of attitudes occurs. People who had normal hearing may have difficulty reconciling the prejudices and attitudes they developed at an earlier stage of life with their present hearing status. As their hearing loss becomes more conspicuous, this realization can create psychological strife because it becomes evident that they have a disability that will cause modifications to their daily life. As a result, insecurities may develop because of previously learned attitudes regarding hearing disabilities. Individuals who are hard of hearing may suffer from a lack of internal reference. For instance, they may face uncertainty regarding whether the messages being received from improperly functioning sensory organs are being interpreted accurately. They may be concerned that they are violating social rules by speaking at inappropriate loudness levels, asking others to repeat too often, and so forth (Hetu, Jones, & Getty, 1993). The hard of hearing may worry about misunderstandings that occur when they truly do not hear compared with when others incorrectly assume they are engaging in "selective listening." Their initial reaction may be to deny a hearing loss in order to justify remaining an active member of a normal-hearing society and to maintain a certain component of illusion that they do not have a hearing loss. It may be easier, or psychologically less painful, to deny the presence of a hearing loss and the necessity for hearing aids because these issues do not calculate into their perception of self-image (Orlans, 1985). In addition, the longer persons with hearing impairment deny their hearing loss and the longer they live with it, the more they may withdraw socially and develop other compensatory behaviors that may become difficult to break at a later time.

Participation Restrictions and Activity Limitations Produced by the Hearing Disorder

There is little correlation between audiometric threshold data and self-perceived disorder. Palmer, Solodar, Hurley, Byrne, and Williams (2009) point out that an individual with a significant amount of hearing loss may perceive little to no hearing difficulty while someone with only a mild hearing loss may experience a significant handicap (or activity limitations and participation restrictions). Recall that handicap can be defined as a disadvantage for a given individual, resulting from an impairment or a disability that limits or prevents the fulfillment of a normal role (depending on age, sex, and social and cultural factors). Thus, the "handicapping" effects of a hearing impairment are the combined result of the following elements:

■ disorders
■ impairments
■ disabilities
■ resources
■ beliefs
■ perceptions
■ attitudes
■ aptitudes
■ lifestyles
■ behaviors

Therefore, it is critical to recognize that it is the activity limitations and participation restrictions that become the critical issue to address in rehabilitation rather than the disorder. Furthermore, not only does each individual present distinct sets of activity limitations and participation restrictions, but these are constantly changing throughout the course of the psychological adjustment to the hearing loss, as well as the rehabilitation process itself.

PSYCHOLOGICAL ADJUSTMENT TO HEARING LOSS

Kyle, Jones, and Wood (1985) described three phases (awareness, acceptance, and adjustment) that persons with hearing loss must transverse in order to come to terms with their disorder. The length of time a person remains affixed in each stage depends on psychological state, family support, and expectations surrounding the hearing loss.

Awareness Phase

This first phase can last just a few days or as long as a lifetime. Recognition of a hearing loss during the awareness phase may actually begin as an unconscious event. An individual with a gradually progressing mild hearing loss may not even be aware of the deficit because the body and brain may be making the necessary calibration adjustments to compensate. As the hearing loss progresses, it reaches a point at which the individual becomes aware of a change in function. Consequently, compensation strategies are consciously or subconsciously developed to adjust for the change. Eventually, the activity and participation limitations become sufficient so that the person can no longer deny or hide the existence of the hearing loss. When this occurs, the need for remedial help (hearing aids, aural rehabilitation, or both) may be recognized, although not necessarily accepted. As this awareness grows, so does the person's observation of other people's ears and the presence of hearing aids. This increasing awareness is analogous to what one encounters after buying a new car and realizing just how many other drivers own the same model. It occurs because the novelty of the car is in the forefront of the new owner's mind, and it is common to check out who else is driving the same automobile. As the newness wears off, the owner tends to notice the same car less and less because the interest wanes. Similarly, people with hearing loss in the awareness phase may turn their attention to other people's ears to view others wearing hearing aids, the style of device, and so forth. Prior to becoming aware of their own hearing loss, they paid no attention to people's ears, and if they did see someone wearing hearing aids, it was probably by accident. Once awareness of a personal hearing loss is reached, persons with hearing impairment may wish to discover which hearing aids are the most popular and least conspicuous so that they might continue to fit into a normal-hearing society in some capacity. Other individuals may become aware of their hearing loss via external channels. In other words, it may be the frequent remarks of others that will alert an individual that something is awry. Either way, it is necessary to first be aware of the loss before moving to the second stage, acceptance.

Acceptance Phase

The acceptance phase typically lasts a few months following awareness (Kyle et al., 1985). Individuals in this phase come to terms with the fact that they have a hearing loss and are willing to seek professional advice. This is a challenging time for both the hearing health care professional and the patient, as each may have separate goals and objectives they want to address. The hearing health care professional must not dismiss the person's fears of having a hearing loss. We go into greater detail later in this chapter about the clinician's psychological influences in rehabilitation. Kyle et al. (1985) stated, "The diagnosis of decreasing hearing presents a wide range of unpleasant prospects; loss of all hearing, loss of job, independence, and control of social situations; rejection by family and friends; and fear of perceived stigma" (p. 124). It is the responsibility of the clinician to address these fears and gain the trust of patients. Only when this trust is established will patients be willing to accept hearing treatment options, such as amplification or aural rehabilitation.

Acknowledgment is the simple but crucial first step in successfully coping with a hearing loss (Ross, 1999b). The first stage of an effective rehabilitation solution is an admission and acceptance on the part of the individual that he or she has a hearing loss. It is crucial that the person recognize this and begin to explore how it will affect his or her life and the lives of significant others.

Adjustment Phase

It is difficult to determine an average length of time that individuals will spend in the adjustment phase because they are in a constant evolution of change and adjustment to their hearing loss. Adjustment involves establishing control over their activity limitations and participation restrictions and having the power to conform their environment to enhance speech understanding. A loss of power or control can result in an increased awareness of the activity limitations, which can subsequently be transformed into increased restrictions. It is believed that a person's power/powerlessness and ability to control situations is instilled during childhood and reinforced in adulthood (Lerner, 1979). We return to the topic of power and powerlessness later in this chapter in the section discussing the effects of hearing loss on personality. The use of amplification and aural rehabilitation strategies, therefore, can provide the necessary assistance and information in order to institute increased control over personal listening situations.

EFFECTS OF HEARING LOSS ON PERSONALITY

Hearing loss can wield profound effects on aspects of an individual's personality. Three of the most important factors constituting a person's nature are emotions, behaviors, and relationships. These factors influence each other in a type of closed-circle manner. Emotions shape behaviors, behaviors alter relationships, relationships induce emotions, and so on.

Emotions

Negative emotions such as anger, anxiety, guilt, paranoia, embarrassment, frustration, and sadness are not confined to people with hearing loss, but the presence of an impairment certainly can fuel these feelings. People who have difficulty hearing at a cocktail party, for example, may experience a heightened sense of anxiety because they are concerned about responding inappropriately, ignoring someone speaking outside of their visual range, worried about statements others may be making "behind their backs," and so forth. These worries can produce tension, nervousness, irritability, and uncertainty. As stress and anxiety rise, understanding of speech can diminish as the listener tries too hard to distinguish every word and the probability of failure increases. The listener may become frustrated, guilty, or even angry, wondering why he or she has to be in this position. Alternatively, the listener may choose to deflect the blame onto others and suggest it is they who have the "mumbling" problem. In the extreme case, the listener with hearing impairment may develop serious depression (Meadow-Orlans, 1985).

Another force exerting an effect on emotions is the presence of fatigue and increased listening effort (Sarampalis, Kalluri, Edwards, & Hafter, 2009). Normal-hearing individuals do not typically have to expend significant energy to hear in most environments. The impaired listener, on the other hand, may (even without recognizing the effort) need to physically strain to hear during much of the day. Increases in stress and fatigue produce physical changes, such as release of certain hormones and neurotransmitters that can diminish control over emotions. Thus, individuals with hearing impairment may recognize the heightened level of anxiety they experience in adverse listening situations and choose to withdraw and isolate themselves from that environment.

Behaviors

When a person experiences the negative emotions described above, a reaction—likely to take the form of a behavior—is soon to follow. As stated above, anxious, frustrated persons may decide that pain and embarrassment can be minimized or even eliminated by simply removing themselves from anxiety-producing situations. Isolation and withdrawal from social situations is indeed a common defense mechanism. Weiss (1973) describes two types of isolation. Social isolation results from being detached from a social network or community; emotional isolation stems from the loss or absence of an attachment figure. As a person withdraws more from society and social situations, important attachment figures also begin to withdraw from the individual with hearing impairment. Just as it may be easier psychologically for persons with hearing loss to avoid adverse situations and remain at home where they can regulate their listening environment, it may be easier for the normal-hearing person to avoid potentially difficult situations and the negative emotions carried by the anxious or unpleasant associate with hearing impairment. An individual with hearing loss can experience social isolation and emotional isolation simultaneously or separately. These behaviors are typically the result of past experiences and individual reactions toward hearing loss (Surr & Hawkins, 1988). In cases of withdrawal and isolation, persons with hearing losses may develop a certain amount of loneliness. Loneliness is often associated with other emotionally debilitating conditions, such as depression, grief, and anxiety (Dugan & Kivett, 1994).

As discussed earlier, another common behavior associated with psychological adjustment to hearing loss is denial. Kyle et al. (1985) stated that "denial of hearing loss is rational in terms of preserving a self-image, but dysfunctional from a control point of view and will almost certainly lead to rejection of situations that produce the dilemma" (p. 133). Individuals exhibiting this behavior mode are not ready to accept or deal with the effects of hearing loss and tend to make excuses for missed speech information (i.e., "everyone mumbles"). A time will be reached, however, when one's denial of a hearing loss may become intolerable to others who recognize the handicapping nature of the hearing disorder. One of the reasons this occurs is that even though behaviors develop as a consequence of experiences with a hearing loss, it may be difficult for those without these activity limitations and participation restrictions to recognize these behaviors as a normal progression, and they may instead view them as an annoyance. This aspect of how an individual's hearing impairment affects others will be discussed shortly.

Individuals with hearing loss can exert a certain amount of power and control over life's situations to keep themselves feeling secure and unthreatened by society. When listening in background noise, for example, it helps to be familiar with the topic being discussed, the talker's speaking pattern, and to be able to control the environment to increase understanding. Such controls include moving closer to the speaker, moving to a quieter area, positioning the speaker toward the better ear and away from the noise source, and so forth. Every individual's level of power varies based in part on personality, learned strategies, and the effort one will make to manipulate the environment. The person with a hearing loss often finds, however, that with the progression of a hearing loss, the strategies that had once worked so effectively no longer suffice. If the individual's sense of power to control situations becomes unreliable, a sense of powerlessness or learned helplessness develops. The individual's personality may influence how successful the adaptations will become. It is here that people make decisions that ultimately determine the degree to which the activity limitations and participation restrictions become a problem. Here too, the individuals with hearing loss must decide whether or not they will engage in the full course of rehabilitative options made available to them. Frequently, people, despite the negative effects the disorder has on their lives, do not comply with the professionals' therapeutic recommendations (Sweetow & Sabes, 2010).

There are many ways personality can be classified. One classification category that has been shown to be pertinent to hearing impairment is introversion versus extraversion. Persons who are introverted tend to direct their actions or events toward the self, in contrast to extroverted persons who direct actions or events toward the environment (Cox, Alexander, & Gray, 1999). Introverts dealing with the effects of a hearing loss may allow the loss to overtake their lifestyles and could become more withdrawn and isolated. Introverts may find it easier to avoid conflicts related to hearing loss rather than to experience the stress involved in trying to communicate with others. Introverts initially may not be prepared or confident enough to take on the issue of hearing loss by themselves.

Extroverts, on the other hand, use compensation strategies for listening but are not afraid to disclose their loss to a stranger. Extroverts do not easily allow themselves to be dismissed from society; they will do what is necessary to remain active members of the normal-hearing world. This characteristic may include the use of hearing aids to address their hearing disorder.

Cox et al. (1999) reported that individuals' personalities influence their benefits from hearing aids. This research suggests that personality type is correlated with subjects' responses on the subjective Abbreviated Profile of Hearing Aid Benefit (APHAB). "Of the personality variables assessed, the introversion-extroversion dimension was clearly the most salient predictor of hearing aid benefit" (Cox et al., 1999, p. 10). The authors attributed this finding to the extrovert's external locus of control. It is recommended that, as personality can be a possible predictor to successful use of a hearing aid, it should be assessed by the hearing health care professional.

It is also important to keep in mind that benefit from hearing aids does not equate to satisfaction with hearing aids. Cox (1997) estimated that satisfaction is composed of 40% benefit (both psychosocial and acoustic), 25% personal image, 19% service and cost, and 16% negative features. In other words, a person may achieve significant benefit from hearing aid use, in terms of reducing handicap, but may still fail to be satisfied. Here too, personality and attitude play a major role in the final outcome.

Relationships

The effects of a hearing loss and the ensuing psychological adjustment can have damaging effects on interpersonal and family functions. All involved individuals experience separate and distinct issues regarding the hearing loss. "The impaired person experiences the disabilities (and the resulting handicaps) while the unimpaired person experiences the consequences as well as the effects of trying to adjust to these disabilities" (Hetu et al., 1993, p. 364). Embarrassment associated with the inability to understand spoken messages, fatigue from straining to hear, increased irritability and tension, social avoidance and withdrawal, rejection, negativism, and depression can have devastating effects on family relationships (Oyer & Oyer, 1985). It is for this reason that involvement of significant family members or friends is critical to the rehabilitation process. If only the person with hearing loss is involved, the burden of adjustment rests solely on his or her shoulders. The active participation of members in the support structure will provide the necessary information and education about hearing loss, as well as an understanding of the various psychological emotions and behaviors associated with a hearing loss. This knowledge will allow the persons without impairment to experience the consequences of the hearing loss as well as the effects of trying to adjust to disabilities (Hetu et al., 1993). To illustrate this process, let's use a hypothetical example of a couple that has been living together for many years. As one of the members begins to lose hearing, the couple's comfortable and compatible lifestyle begins to change. Communication habits that had worked in the past may no longer be acceptable. Among the difficulties they may experience are understanding each other from separate rooms, carrying on conversations over the telephone, and even conducting discussions at the dinner table. In addition, the need to increase the volume of the television set can lead the couple to move to separate rooms when watching their favorite shows. This may reduce the shared experiences they would normally enjoy discussing together. Also, social situations may become a burden to the couple. Restaurants may seem too loud, and movie or theater dialogue may be difficult to understand. The partner without hearing impairment may find a reduction in the activities he or she can participate in because of the spouse. Frustration may ensue because the normal-hearing spouse has to act as an interpreter and constantly fill in missed information. A modification in communication habits is thus required. If the adjustment process is going to be successful, both parties need to be involved. Each needs to take an active membership in the rehabilitation process in order for healthy adaptation to occur.

The personality characteristics of normal hearing partners can be a significant factor in their reaction to the onset of a hearing loss. The make-up of one's personality is molded and shaped throughout childhood. Personalities are shaped from observations, reactions to various issues, situations, and conversations of parents and family members. Personalities are refined and manipulated through interactions with the world through trial and error.

CULTURAL INFLUENCES OF AGE, ACTIVITY LIMITATIONS AND PARTICIPATION RESTRICTIONS, AND HEARING LOSS

The hearing health care professional needs to be sensitive not only to the auditory limitations of individuals with hearing loss, but must also acknowledge and recognize the effect of cultural background and expectations on psychological impact and subsequent behaviors. Various cultures perceive disabilities in diverse manners. Hearing loss may be perceived as a weakness and, as dubious as the logic may be, an indication of aging. Psychological reaction to aging is also quite diverse and is dictated by many factors including individual feelings, familial expectations, and society's view of the elderly.

Some cultures rely heavily on the elderly for their guidance, experience, and knowledge. The aging process is embraced and valued. Younger individuals in these types of cultures learn the norms of society through the direction and observation of their elders. Other cultures, including our own Western culture, focus more on "the negative, the loss of self-esteem, the weakness, and increasing threats to security" (Busse, 1965, p. 81). Rather than embracing and living out this unique period of life, many people view aging as an inconvenience or a period leading to activity limitations and participation restrictions. The elderly in American culture frequently do not share their experiences because they are left out and because this culture focuses on the value of youth and youthful appearance. As a result, efforts are often made to curb or hide the aging process and the many physical and emotional challenges aging presents. People may try to hide the outward signs of growing old by having plastic surgery or dying their hair. Others may withdraw from social situations that highlight their growing physical limitations. Efforts to hide or delay the aging process may include a denial of health-related issues. The presence of a hearing loss and the need for amplification may be summarily rejected simply because it is associated with aging and the underlining cultural message that the person is becoming weak and a burden on society. Steps need to be taken by the hearing health care professional to address not only the physical but also the psychological needs of the individual with hearing loss. It is the responsibility of the hearing health care professional to address healthy treatment options and strategies for managing the aging process and the person's hearing loss.

Just as cultural and social criteria affect reaction to a disorder, they also may influence the way impairments are addressed and dealt with. For instance, certain cultures may view disabilities as a sign of weakness that reflects a negative image on the entire family. This can lead to an additional emotional challenge for the impaired individual as that person begins to address physical needs through rehabilitation solutions. Thus, these individuals may be torn between their desire to achieve personal goals through rehabilitation and, at the same time, be reluctant to seek help and show outward displays of physical needs (i.e., wearing hearing aids) because of the perceived impact their hearing loss has on the family. It is interesting that some of the cultures that show the greatest respect for the elderly also have difficulty accepting the limitations of the young. Therefore, the key for the hearing health care professional is to acknowledge and understand how the patient's culture may impact the acknowledgement and treatment of a disorder. It is important to work with persons with hearing impairment to explore how their cultural norms and expectations will impact the treatment of their hearing loss.

THE CLINICIAN'S PSYCHOLOGICAL INFLUENCES ON REHABILITATION

Successful rehabilitation requires the collaboration of both the individual with the hearing impairment and the hearing health care professional. Persons with hearing loss are vital to the rehabilitation process in that they must be able to operationally articulate the various barriers and handicaps their hearing disorders are creating in their daily lives. Thus, they must not only recognize the various limitations of their hearing loss, but they must become active participants in the rehabilitation process. Concurrently, the hear-

ing health care professional must be able to utilize counseling skills to break down emotional barriers producing denial, to motivate and to understand the individual's needs, and to convey information in a constructive manner (Sweetow, 1999a). This must be done not only for the patient, but for the family and critical members of the support structure as well.

A primary objective of the clinician in the rehabilitation process is to gain the patient's trust. This is a process that begins at the initial meeting and continues to develop over the course of the professional relationship. While hearing health care professionals focus on the assessment of their patients' hearing needs relevant to their lifestyle and medical background, their patients are developing opinions about the clinician's competence to provide the appropriate treatment and direction for their condition.

Sweetow (1999b) stated that there are three things patients with hearing impairment need to confirm about the hearing health care professional: (1) The professional knows what he or she is talking about, (2) the professional cares about the patient as a person, and (3) the professional has the patient's best interest at heart. He goes on to say that clinicians must establish themselves as having the knowledge, the desire, and the ability to help the patient effect a desired change. Before advice can be offered that is regarded as having great value, the patient must be convinced of the professional's desire to be part of the solution. The patient must believe that the professional not only can help provide the answer to his or her hearing problem, but that the professional is emotionally vested in providing it. In short, the patient must feel that the professional cares.

One of the most effective methods of obtaining trust is through deep listening, creating an atmosphere of security, and identifying and understanding an individual's "salient event" (Hansen, 1998). A "salient event" is what brought the person into the clinic: the individual's own awareness of hearing difficulties or pressures from family or friends. "Salient events" provide the hearing health care professional with a base to understand individuals with hearing impairment and with insight into their emotional needs.

There are three facilitative conditions that must be present if a clinician is to be successful in the rehabilitation process: (1) empathy, (2) respect for the view and feelings of the individual, and (3) a relaxed, friendly attitude toward the person, coupled with an ability to accept criticism and communicate in an understandable manner (Kaplan, 1992). These conditions underscore the fact that each person is different and presents distinctive reactions to hearing loss. The challenge for the hearing health care professional is to recognize these individual characteristics and stages of hearing loss acceptance and to provide the necessary counseling and treatment. Hearing health care professionals should foster the understanding that patients are not alone in their endeavor. The clinician needs to guide patients to view their hearing loss with hope and confidence, so they can address their condition and reduce their activity limitations and participation restrictions.

SUMMARY

- Among the tools a successful hearing health care professional must possess is an understanding of the psychology of the individual with hearing impairment. As with any other group, a wide range of personalities, desires, and fears characterize people with hearing impairment. By understanding the factors exerting influence on the thoughts and emotions of our patients, the professional will be better equipped to meet their amplification needs.
- Humans utilize their auditory sense at three different levels: primitive, warning, and symbolic. Hearing at the primitive level occurs at an unconscious level and produces a connection to the environment; warning conveys information; and symbolic forms the major component of

communication and becomes the foundation for language.

- The psychological influence and the effect on personality that hearing loss bears on an individual may vary depending on the degree of the impairment, how it affects the level of activity limitations, the time at which the loss occurred, and the participation restrictions that result.
- There are three phases of psychological adjustment to hearing loss. The awareness phase is the time during which individuals recognize they have a hearing loss. The acceptance phase occurs when individuals come to terms with the fact that they have a hearing loss. The adjustment phase involves establishing control over their impairment and having the power to modify their environment to enhance speech understanding.
- Hearing loss can exert profound effects on aspects of an individual's personality. Three of the most important factors constituting a person's nature are emotions, behaviors, and relationships. These factors influence each other in a type of closed-circle manner. Specifically, emotions shape behaviors, behaviors alter relationships, relationships induce emotions, and so on.
- The clinician's directives in the rehabilitation process include not only the patient with hearing loss, but also their significant other. A key role the hearing health care professional plays is to develop an atmosphere that allows patients to accept their hearing loss and gives them the confidence to address their needs.

REVIEW QUESTIONS

1. What are the three psychological levels of hearing?

2. What society-based struggles do people with hearing loss face?

3. What choices can people with hearing disorders make with regard to their hearing loss?

4. List the three psychological phases to hearing loss adjustment and identify one important factor that was discussed for each of the phases.

5. During the acceptance phase to psychological adjustment to hearing loss, what is the role of the hearing health care professional?

6. List some of the emotions and behaviors a person with hearing loss might exhibit.

7. What are some of the effects a hearing loss can have on significant others and/or family members?

8. Discuss the importance of personality traits of the individual with hearing loss and how they apply to success with hearing aids.

9. What is the significance of cultural influences on one's reaction to hearing disorders?

10. Name three facilitative conditions to successful rehabilitation.

REFERENCES

Barnes, C., Mercer, G., & Shakespeare, T. (2000). Exploring disability: A sociological introduction. *Sociology, 35*(1), 219–258.

Bregman, A. S. (1990). *Auditory scene analysis: The perceptual organization of sound.* Cambridge, MA: MIT Press.

Busse, E. W. (1965). Research on aging: Some methods and findings. In M. A. Barezin & S. H. Cath (Eds.), *Geriatric psychiatry.* New York, NY: International Universities Press.

Cox, R. (1997). *Satisfaction from Amplification for Daily Living (SADL).* Paper presented at the University of California, San Francisco/International Hearing Aid Seminars Audiology/Amplification Update III, San Francisco, CA.

Cox, R. M., Alexander, G. C., & Gray, G. (1999). Personality and the subjective assessment of hearing aids. *Journal of the American Academy of Audiology, 10*, 1–13.

Danhauer, J. L., Johnson, C. E., Kasten, R. N., & Brimacombe, J. A. (1985). The hearing aid effect—Summary, conclusions and recommendations. *Hearing Journal, 38*, 12–23.

Dugan, E., & Kivett, V. R. (1994). The importance of emotional and social isolation to loneliness among very old rural adults. *The Gerontologist, 34*, 340–346.

Furth, H. G. (1966). *Thinking without language: Psychological implications of deafness.* New York, NY: Free Press.

Hansen, V. (1998). Dealing with the psychological aspects of patient reluctance. *The Hearing Review, 5*, 8–14.

Hetu, R., Jones, L., & Getty, L. (1993). The impact of acquired hearing impairment on intimate relationships: Implications for rehabilitation. *Audiology, 32*, 363–381.

Higgins, P. C. (1980). *Outsiders in a hearing world.* Beverly Hills, CA: Sage.

Hull, R. H. (1992). The impact of hearing loss on older persons: A dialogue. In R. H. Hull (Ed.), *Aural rehabilitation* (2nd ed., pp. 247–256). San Diego, CA: Singular.

Kaplan, H. F. (1992). The impact of hearing impairment and counseling adults who are deaf or hard of hearing. In R. H. Hull (Ed.), *Aural rehabilitation* (2nd ed., pp. 135–148). San Diego, CA: Singular.

Kochkin, S. (2007). MarkeTrak VII: Obstacles to adult non-user adoption of hearing aids. *The Hearing Journal, 60*(4), 7–43.

Kyle, J. G., Jones, L. G., & Wood, P. L. (1985). Adjustment to acquired hearing loss: A working model. In H. Orlans (Ed.), *Adjustment to adult hearing loss* (pp. 119–138). San Diego, CA: College-Hill Press.

Lerner, M. (1979). Surplus powerlessness. *Social policy, 9*, 11–27.

Meadow-Orlans, K. P. (1985). Social and psychological effects of hearing loss in adulthood: A literature review. In H. Orlans (Ed.), *Adjustment to adult hearing loss* (pp. 35–57). San Diego, CA: College-Hill Press.

Orlans, H. (1985). Reflections on adult hearing loss. In H. Orlans (Ed.), *Adjustment to adult hearing loss* (pp. 179–194). San Diego, CA: College-Hill Press.

Oyer, H. J., & Oyer, E. J. (1985). Adult hearing loss and the family. In H. Orlans (Ed.), *Adjustment to adult hearing loss* (pp. 139–154). San Diego, CA: College-Hill Press.

Padden, C. (1980). The deaf community and the culture of deaf people. In C. Baker & R. Battison (Eds.), *Sign language and the deaf community: Essays in honor of William C. Stokoe.* Silver Spring, MD: Aspen.

Palmer, C., Solodar, H., Hurley, W., Byrne, D., & Williams, K. (2009). Relationship between self-perception of hearing ability and hearing aid purchase. *Journal of the American Academy of Audiology, 20*(6), 341–348.

Ramsdell, D. A. (1978). The psychology of the hard of hearing and the deafened adult. In H. Davis & S. R. Silverman (Eds.), *Hearing and deafness* (4th ed., pp. 499–510). New York, NY: Holt, Rinehart and Winston.

Ross, M. (1999a). *My "near deaf" experience* (Unpublished manuscript).

Ross, M. (1999b). *Why people won't wear hearing aids* (Unpublished manuscript).

Sarampalis, A., Kalluri, S., Edwards, B., & Hafter, E. (2009). Objective measures of listening effort: Effects of background noise and noise reduction. *Journal of Speech Language and Hearing Research, 52*, 1230–1240.

Surr, R. K., & Hawkins, D. B. (1988). New hearing aid users' perception of the "hearing aid effect." *Ear and Hearing, 9*, 113–118.

Sweetow, R. W. (1999a). Counseling: It's the key to successful hearing aid fittings. *The Hearing Journal, 52*, 10–17.

Sweetow, R. W. (1999b). Counseling: The secret to successful hearing aid fittings. In R. W. Sweetow (Ed.), *Counseling for hearing aid fittings* (pp. 1–20). San Diego, CA: Singular.

Sweetow, R., & Sabes, J. (2010). Auditory training and challenges associated with participation and compliance. *Journal of American Academy of Audiology, 21*(9), 586–593.

Weiss, R. S. (1973). *Loneliness: The experience of emotional and social isolation*. Cambridge, MA: MIT Press.

World Health Organization. (2001). *International Classification of Functioning, Disability and Health*. Geneva, Switzerland: Author.

CHAPTER 11

Considerations for Selecting and Fitting of Amplification for Geriatric Adults

ROBERT E. NOVAK

The number of persons age 65 years and older with hearing loss significant enough to interfere with communication is growing rapidly. It is estimated that 75 of 1,000 persons aged 65 to 74 years cannot hear and understand normal conversational levels of speech, with this number growing to 150 out of 1,000 (15%) of persons age 75 years and older (Ries, 1994). Others report that, by age 65 years, one-third of the U.S. population develop a hearing loss serious enough to interfere with daily communication (National Ear Care Plan, 1999). As many as 48% or more of older residents of skilled nursing facilities also have hearing thresholds for the speech frequencies (500 Hz–4 KHz) in excess of 40 dB hearing level, (re: ANSI, 1989; Schow & Nerbonne, 1980). Currently, roughly 13% of the U.S. population is 65 years of age and older. The population of 31 million persons over the age of 65 years in 1990 is predicted to increase to 65 million by the year 2030. It is predicted that one in 12 U.S. citizens will be 80 years or older by the year 2050 (Taeuber, 1992). Americans are living longer and generally healthier lives.

The geriatric population is marked by significant heterogeneity as it includes the "young old," for the purposes of this chap-

Editor's note. In 1988, when the first edition of the *Handbook of Hearing Aid Amplification* was published, the combined efforts of Drs. Glorig and Novak resulted in an excellent treatise on hearing problems among the geriatric population. Dr. Glorig was especially instrumental in describing some of the neurophysiological changing associated with the aging process. With the recent death of Dr. Glorig, the task of revising the chapter in both the second and the third editions fell on the ample shoulders of Dr. Novak. Every attempt has been made to maintain the significant contributions of Dr. Glorig, yet offer needed revisions to be consistent with more recent knowledge relating to the aging patient and hearing aid use. One feels certain that Dr. Glorig would approve of the revisions.

ter defined as 65 to 75 years, the old, 76 to 85 years, and the old–old, 86 years and older. Within each of these groups again are a remarkably diverse cohort of people, with great variability in education, socioeconomic status, family support, psychological and physical health, community avocational and ongoing vocational involvement. The over-65 group is also rich in its ethnic and cultural diversity, which affects how they view the need for aural rehabilitation and participate in the rehabilitation process. The majority of the population of persons over age 65 years with hearing impairment still do not seek help for their hearing loss. Seven million cannot afford hearing aids, and nearly 15 million experience prejudice and embarrassment about hearing loss that prevents them from seeking help (Better Hearing Institute, 1999). However, those who do seek amplification share many clinical issues and desired outcomes. The purpose of this chapter is to present a framework for audiologic intervention that emphasizes the desired clinical outcomes shared by the majority of geriatric patients, and to present information that should be considered when designing an amplification system and aural rehabilitation program to achieve these goals.

The process of aging can be divided into three related fields: biologic aging, the physiologic changes that occur at all levels of the individual organism and in all of its functions; psychologic aging, the age-related changes that occur in the behavior of the individual (i.e., perceiving, feeling, thinking, acting, and reacting); and social aging, the changing roles of the individual in society as a result of age-related biologic and psychological changes.

The first part of this chapter is concerned in part with the aging process in the auditory system. Technically, this is defined as hearing loss due to biologic and physiologic changes that are strictly a function of the cell and its organisms. It is impossible to extract age-related cellular changes from changes facilitated by the addition of environmental stressors (e.g., noise, disease, iatrogenesis). The fact that one ages physiologically and biologically also means that there are effects

of changing environments over the aging period. Any study of aging and its effects must assume that the effects that are found are a combination of intrinsic biologic factors and extrinsic environmental factors. At best, the selection of amplification systems is not a simple task, and the probable effects of aging in the selection process should be evaluated. Subsequent portions of the chapter deal with various aspects of the application of hearing aids to the geriatric population with hearing impairment.

PRESBYCUSIS

Physiologic Considerations

High-frequency hearing loss associated with aging was first described in 1891, as was the term presbycusis (Zwaardemaker, 1981). The original spelling was presbycusis; however, presbycusis has become the preferred spelling. Pathologic studies have failed to identify anything pathognomonic of presbycusis. More correctly today, we refer to age-related hearing loss (ARHL) when speaking of "pure" aging effects on hearing as the term presbycusis appears to be a collection of different entities and etiologies other than purely aging (e.g., noise exposure, viral infections, etc.) that occur in various combinations and affect the entire auditory system from the middle ear up to and including the central nervous system. There are predictable changes in function, and such changes require special consideration in the evaluation, selection, and fitting of hearing aid devices.

If one looks at the external ear in the aged, one finds that it has become flabby, the earlobe has become larger and loose, and the ear canal has become quite flexible and sometimes has partially collapsed. These changes are due to changes in the elasticity of the skin as well as in the cartilaginous framework. Cartilaginous changes introduce a special concern when fabricating the earmold impression. The obvious problem presented is that, to make an acceptable impression of the ear canal, one must manipulate the ear in a manner that permits a canal opening adequate to allow the finished earmold, ITE, or canal or CIC aid to pass amplified sound from the hearing aid earphone through the canal bore of the earmold, ITE, or canal hearing aid and, subsequently, to the eardrum.

Insertion of the earmold or hearing aid device into the external canal may produce soreness or irritation at the canal opening due to the sensitivity of the collapsed ear canal tissue when pressure is applied by the physical presence of the earmold or the canal portion of a hearing aid. The impression gun technique, which mixes the agents of the impression material as it is inserted into the ear, is preferred for persons with collapsed canals. The impression material has a liquid consistency as it exits the gun that applies minimal pressure to the canal walls as the impression is being taken. Clients with extremely narrow or collapsed ear canals are not good candidates for ITE aids and should be provided with BTE aids allowing for the use of earmolds that better accommodate the true architecture of the external ear canal. Open ear canal mini-BTE hearing aids with the receiver in the aid or the ear canal and aggressive feedback limiting algorithms are ideal for this population if the amplification requirements of the patients' hearing losses can be accommodated within the limitations of the open ear canal application.

Similar changes may occur in the structures of the middle ear, with associated changes in the sound transmission characteristics of the ossicles. This was demonstrated by Nixon and Glorig (1962) in a study of air- and bone-conduction thresholds as a function of age. They found an air-bone gap at 4000 Hz in many individuals age 55 years and older. Air-bone gaps also were discovered by Rosen, Bergman, Plester, El Mofty, and Sotti (1962) in their study of elderly members of the Mabaan tribe in rural Sudan.

Glorig and Davis (1961) reported that they believed that an air-bone gap of this kind could be caused by an inner ear conductive hearing loss as the result of changes in the basilar partition of the inner ear. These changes, which include the lessening of elastic tissue and the stiffening of the remaining components, have been identified via microscopic analysis. It is unclear what role, if any, these air-bone gap phenomena play in the determination of the recommended frequency-intensity response characteristics of the hearing aid. The presence may account for a higher than expected Most Comfortable Listening level (MCL) at frequencies at which air-bone gaps occur. Higher MCLs may translate into higher gain prescriptions for older adults who have these air-bone gaps compared with other older and younger patients who have similar air-conduction thresholds but an absence of high-frequency air-bone gaps.

Schuknecht (1974) described four types of inner ear loss in presbycusis: sensoripresbycusis, neuropresbycusis, striapresbycuis, and inner ear conductive presbycusis. Glorig and Davis (1961) suggested a similar classification based on their own theoretical constructs.

Sensoripresbycusis is characterized by slowly progressive, bilaterally symmetrical high-frequency sensorineural hearing loss, with good single-syllable word identification. The primary histopathologic finding is an absence or reduction of hair cells, primarily in the basilar portion of the cochlea.

Neuropresbycusis is characterized by high-frequency sensorineural hearing loss with poor single-syllable word identification. Atrophy of the spiral ganglion and nerves of the osseous spiral lamina, mainly in the basal corridor, are the most consistent histopathologic finding with this type of presbycusis.

Striapresbycusis, or metabolic presbycusis, is characterized by a slowly progressive, gradually sloping sensorineural hearing loss (about −8 dB/octave slope) caused by a decrease in the quiescent value of the endocochlear potential (EP) in the scala media even with fairly normal potassium concentration in the endolymph (Schmiedt, 1996), bilaterally symmetrical sensorineural hearing loss starting in the third through sixth decades of life. Single-syllable word identification is good at most comfortable presentation levels. Schuknecht suggested that the pathophysiology of striapresbycusis is related to the atrophy of the stria vascularis and a general reduction in sensitivity of all hair cells due to the metabolic changes of the endolymph. Schmiedt, Lang, Okamura, and Schulte (2002) argues that the metabolic effects (reduced EPs) are the major factor in "pure" age-related hearing loss, more so than sensory or neural effects, which do occur, but are probably more related to noise damage that creates permanent threshold shift and temporary threshold shift. Kujawa and Liberman (2009) suggest that it is the slope of the audiogram that can be a differential diagnostic indicator of metabolic (gradual sloping sensory neural loss) versus sensori (more-preciptitous) presbycusis. Schuknecht and Gacek (1993) expanded on the earlier finding of Schuknecht in discovering that atrophy of the trial tissue was the primary degenerative finding in the temporal bones of older individuals, with the loss of sensori cells being the least important cause of hearing loss associated with aging, once confounding historical factors of noise exposure, drug exposure, and genetic effects are eliminated.

Inner ear conductive presbycusis has been suggested by several authors (Glorig & Davis, 1961; Mayer, 1970; Schuknecht, 1974). Schuknecht (1974) described changes in the cochlear ducts that cause changes in the mass, stiffness, and friction of the moving membranes, thus affecting the transmission of acoustic energy. Mayer (1970) described thickening and hyalinization of the basilar membrane and calcium deposits located mainly in the basal coil. He suggested that the aging process of the basilar membrane causes stiffness and decreased mobility. This hypothesis has not been consistently confirmed. Figures 11–1 through 11–6 are diagrammatic representations of pathology found in microscopic studies of the temporal bones in individuals over 65 years of age. They are accompanied by pure-tone air conduction audiograms and word identification scores obtained by using phonetically balanced (PB)

words. The diagrammatic cochlea shows hair cell rows. Open circles indicate cells that are pathologic. Note the correlation with the dark areas in the organ of Corti shown in the rectangles. Figures 11–1 and 11–2 show findings in patients with primarily cochlear pathology like that found with sensoripresbycusis. Figure 11–3 shows a patient with basal cochlear pathology and significant damage to the spiral ganglion. Note that, although pure-tone thresholds are normal through 2000 Hz, the PB score in quiet is only 82%.

Figure 11–4 shows more diffuse hair cell loss with spiral ganglion damage throughout the cochlea. These findings are consistent with the neuropresbycusis classification. Note the very poor (55%) PB-word identification score and compare it with the relatively good identification score of 80% in Figure 11–2, which depicts similar pure-tone threshold results but minimal spiral ganglion damage (sensori-presbycusis). The loss of central auditory nerve cells also may be related to a loss of synchrony in the central auditory pathways. Such a loss can be detected electrophysiologically by the decreased phase coherence of the middle latency response (MLR) in elderly adults exhibiting central auditory processing disorders (CAPD; Musiek & Rintelmann, 1999). Audiometrically measured CAPD in the geriatric population is independent of peripheral loss of hearing sensitivity (Jerger, Jerger, Oliver, & Priozzolo, 1993), but the decreased speed of information processing created by CAPD can reduce speech discrimination significantly. Jerger et al. (1993) found that CAPD can exist independently of cognitive dysfunction in the elderly. This is the case for most elderly patients who report that reduced conversational rate serves to enhance understanding of what was said.

Figure 11–5 depicts results consistent with the classification of striapresbycusis or metabolic presbycusis: minimum hair cell damage and spiral ganglion pathology but diffuse striavascularis abnormality. Note the excellent PB score (100%), which is consistent with this diagnostic classification.

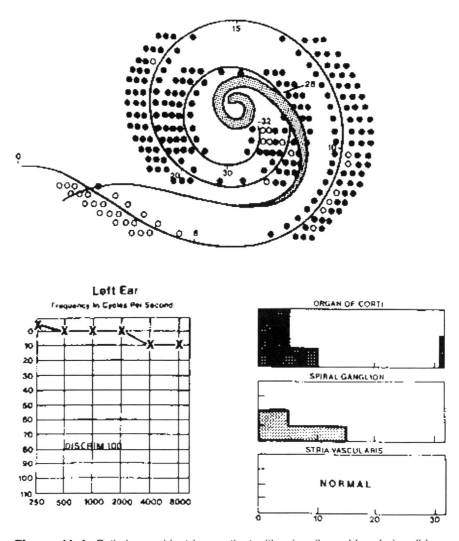

Figure 11–1. Pathology evident in a patient with primarily cochlear hair cell loss. Some damage also is evident in the spiral ganglia. Open circles indicate areas of hair cell loss.

Figure 11–6 depicts the results obtained from a patient with diffuse damage of the organ of corti, spiral ganglia, and stria vascularis (a combination of types of presbycusis). Note the very poor word identification score. Of all the patients described, certainly this individual would have the poorest prognosis for benefit from the use of hearing aid amplification.

Of significance, when one reviews Figures 11–1 through 11–6, is that conventional pure-tone audiometry, in terms of signal detection, MCL, and tolerance discomfort thresholds, may not provide enough information to predict the benefit to be expected in understanding intended verbal messages when hearing aid amplification is provided. Although conventional word identification tests are suspect in ferreting out the best hearing aid device from among several choices, it is readily apparent that some form of speech or speech like assessment is critical to the successful management of the aging patient. For example, the relatively low identification

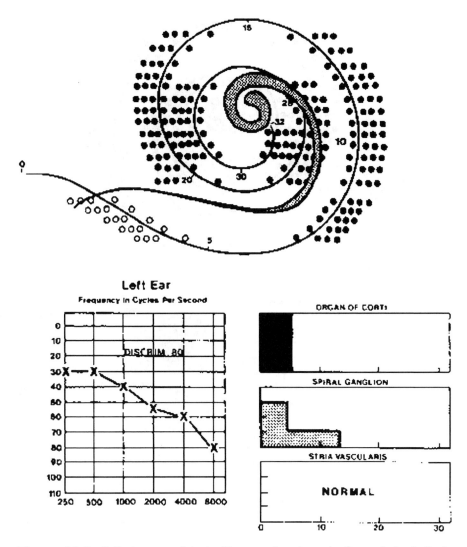

Figure 11–2. Pathology consistent with sensoripresbycusis. Open circles indicate areas of damage in the cochlea.

score shown in Figure 11–4 may suggest that appreciable improvement in speech understanding over time will not differ greatly from the measures obtained initially. Such an observation would have a profound effect on the counseling strategy devised to deal effectively with this patient as a result of the limitations imposed not only by the hearing aid but also by the auditory system itself.

Vasodilation is a common medical treatment for various inner ear diseases, including Ménière's, sudden hearing loss, tinnitus, and presbycusis. The dependence of the inner

ear on a single-ended artery without cross-circulation has led to speculation that vascular insufficiency may, in part, be the cause of these inner ear disorders.

Further understanding of pathologic processes in the internal auditory canal that are responsible for inner ear vascular degeneration and neural loss was contributed by the excellent observations of Krmpotic-Nemanic (1971). She studied 2,600 temporal bones of all ages and demonstrated an apposition of fibrous osteoid and bony material in the fundus of the internal auditory canal

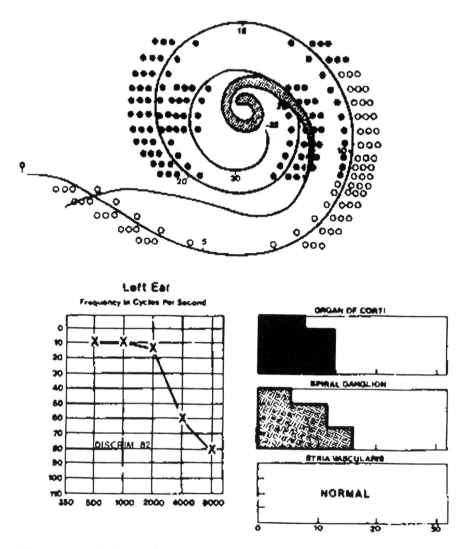

Figure 11–3. Pathology found in a patient with basal cochlear damage and marked changes in the spiral ganglion. Open circles show areas of cochlear damage.

in the region of the spiral tract, beginning at the basal coil. This process reduced the diameter of the hole in the spiral tract through which nerve bundles cross from the inner ear to the internal auditory canal. Hawkins and Johnsson (1985), citing similar findings, called this Hyperstotic Presbycusis. For patients who exhibit severe cochlear-vascular changes, the hearing health care professional should be aware of the pronounced limitations imposed on the probable contributions of the hearing aid.

Extrinsic Etiologic Factors

Hearing loss in the aging ear is believed to be the end result of the cumulative effects of various extrinsic factors in addition to genetically determined patterns of aging. There is a growing interest in environmental factors known to cause hearing loss that can be attenuated or eliminated as part of the overall efforts of hearing conservation. Control of dangerously high sound pressure levels delivered via insert "ear bud" style ear-

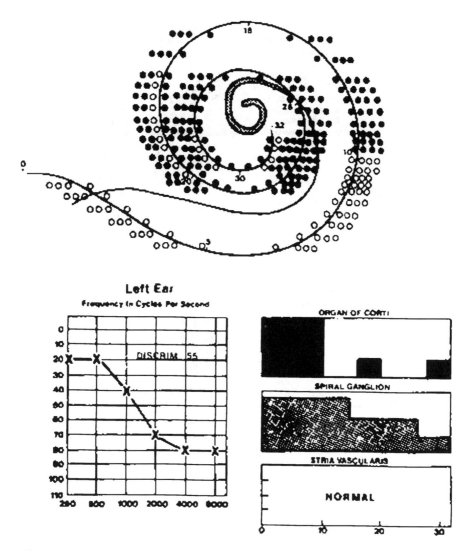

Figure 11–4. Pathologic findings for the patient shown indicate significant hair cell loss as well as spiral ganglion damage. Such findings are consistent with neuropresbycusis. Open circles indicate areas of damage in the cochlea.

phones used with personal listening devices (MP3 players, iPods, etc.) have been identified as of particular concern as an etiology of permanent sensorineural hearing loss in the predominantly younger population regularly using these listening systems. Kujawa and Liberman (2009) examined affects of overexposure of mice to sound intense enough to cause reversible sensory neural loss, on afferent nerve terminals and the cochlear nerve. They found that overexposures to noise causing moderate, but completely reversible threshold elevation leave sensory cells intact, but cause acute loss of afferent nerve terminals and delayed degeneration of the cochlear nerve. They suggest that noise-induced damage to the auditory system has progressive consequences that are considerably more widespread than are indicated by pure-tone threshold testing, and that the neurodegeneration they observed would add to difficulties hearing in noisy environments and could

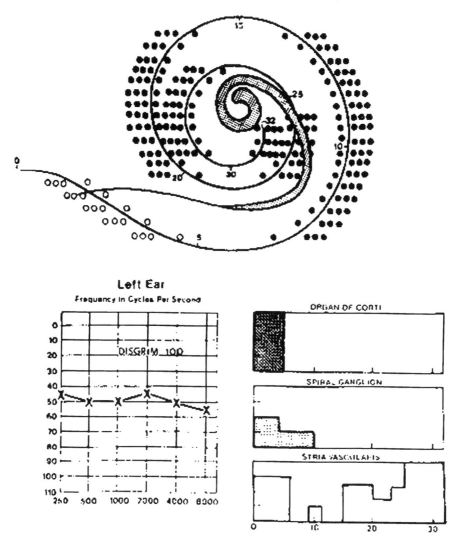

Figure 11–5. Cochlear damage consistent with metabolic presbycusis. Note the excellent word identification score. Open circles indicate areas of damage in the cochlea.

contribute to tinnitus, hyperacusis, and other perceptual anomalies otherwise associated with inner ear damage.

Glorig and Nixon (1962) used the term socioacusis to describe the inevitable effects of daily, nonoccupational noise exposure and the affects of other ototoxic agents (disease, drug therapy, etc.) on hearing throughout the life cycle. The hearing loss of aging, therefore, is the combined result of presbycusis (physiologic aging), socioacusis, and occupational noise.

Relation to Amplification

The end result of the many factors that cause hearing loss in the aged individual is multifaceted and highly complex. Some of these factors affect the application of amplification more than others. The primary biologic factors that limit adapting amplification to the aged ear is related to the pathology in the inner ear and changes in the anatomy and physiology of the central nervous system. Pathology that affects the spiral ganglion causes particular

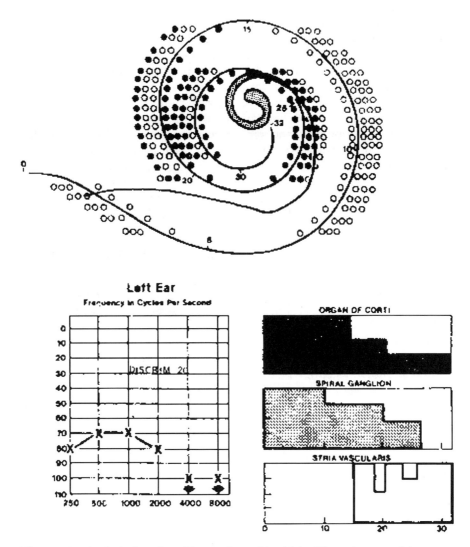

Figure 11–6. Pathology found in a patient with widely diffuse damage of the organ of Corti, spiral ganglion, and stria vascularis. Note the poor word identification score for this patient. Cochlear hair cell loss is indicated by the open circles.

challenges in applying successful amplification. In general, in the absence of causes directly affecting the hair cells, such as noise and ototoxicity, the pathology of aging lies principally in the changes in the spiral ganglion and the neural elements that leave the calyces of the hair cells, and proceed through the auditory nerve to the various stations in the midbrain and cortex.

The cochlea serves as: (1) a coding mechanism in which the hair cells are the center of the coding system and (2) a processor of

information, which is garnered by the hair cells and then transferred to the central nervous system by way of the neural elements.

In the case of abnormal first-order auditory neurons, the neural elements leaving the cochlea are reduced in their ability to process information. The decoding system, the central nervous system, thus receives sparse, poorly coded auditory information. In other words, the principal site of auditory processing is the neural system of the cochlea. If this is faulty, it is difficult to build an extrinsic signal processor (hearing aid device) to correct it. The success of extrinsic signal processing is highly dependent on the degree of pathology in the spiral ganglion and the neural elements that transmit auditory information to the cortex. Differences in amplification results found in patients with similar test data may be explained by differences in cochlear pathology that are not apparent in the test data. In these cases, amplification can be compared with trying to use a public address system with a defective microphone by tailoring the input to the microphone so that the output of the system will be understandable. This has never been done successfully. Good public address systems depend on good microphones or input transducers and highly functional electronic circuits beyond. In the same way, successful use of traditional hearing aids depends on a functioning cochlea (input transducer of the auditory system) with intact "electrical circuits" beyond (central auditory system), which are present in varying degrees in persons with various types of presbycusis.

Independent of the presence of hearing loss and type of presbycusis when hearing loss exists, it has been reported that understanding of speech in noise is more difficult for geriatric patients than for their younger counterparts. The more difficult the speech material becomes, the more favorable the SNR must be for older listeners to achieve the same listening performance as younger listeners. This is true even for older listeners with normal pure-tone sensitivity (Dubno, Dirks, & Morgan, 1984; Schum, Matthews, & Lee, 1991). Difficulty understanding speech in noise is a universal complaint of geriatric patients with hearing impairment and presents a consistent challenge to the design of signal processing algorithms in hearing aids and the matching of these algorithms to the unique needs of each patient with hearing impairment.

In spite of the limitations of the geriatric auditory system, hearing health professionals are increasingly effective in applying appropriately fit amplification to older persons who are potential candidates. With current signal processing/high fidelity hearing aid technology, the prognosis for success can be very good. The challenge for clinicians is to develop assessment procedures that allow the most specific application of amplification to each older hearing-impaired patient and follow-up protocols that maximize acceptance and successful use. To fully appreciate the factors related to hearing aid use in the geriatric population, practitioners also should be aware of the sociological and psychological factors presented by this population of individuals.

PSYCHOLOGICAL AND SOCIOLOGICAL PERSPECTIVES

In addition to changes in sensory and neural auditory processes, aging may be accompanied by modifications in adjustment strategies, problem-solving capacities, and stress-coping responses, emotional states, perception, and memory (Mauldin, 1976). These changes are not consistent across the elderly population with hearing impairments and also may vary as a function of race and culture. The focus of this portion of the chapter is on the relationship these modifications have to the rehabilitation of hearing loss and specifically to the successful fitting of amplification systems in elderly populations.

As with their younger clinical counterparts, successful utilization of amplification by the geriatric population certainly is dependent on the critical audiometric factors of magnitude of loss in threshold sensitivity, reduced tolerance for loud sounds, and the related reduction in speech understanding skills. Although all hearing aid candidates have these problems, many hearing health professionals are not fully aware of other age-related factors that contribute to acceptance and use of amplification systems. Therefore, some of the behaviors manifested by the elderly are reviewed here, and their importance in the consideration of hearing aid use is assessed.

Cultural influences, coupled with the aging process and the changes that accompany it, are often major determinants of the elderly adult's behavior. Social, physical, and economic conditions also may affect attitudes. It is important to assess clients' perception of need for hearing aids, and ability to afford hearing aid use and care for the amplification in the face of other, sometimes more pressing, economic, psychological, and physical realities. The need for hearing amplification is a physical reality. The use and acceptance of any amplification system, however, is tempered by a number of other concerns.

The stereotype of the elderly as physically feeble, severely hearing impaired, partially sighted, and demented fits less than 3% of the aged population. This stereotype would be true if survival to the maximum life span of 110 years was typical (Eisenberg, 1985). Aging can be viewed as both positive and negative, as growth and decline; however, compared with years past, tomorrow's elderly adults will be living longer and healthier lives. The reality also is that the majority of them will be doing it with significant hearing loss, requiring the need for amplification and aural rehabilitation.

Psychology of Adult Onset Hearing Loss

It has been documented that untreated hearing loss in older people can lead to a variety of problems including depression, anxiety, and social isolation (National Council on the Aging, 1999). In a comparison of hearing aid-using and nonusing groups of hearing impaired older people matched for age, gender, and income, the study found hearing-impaired people who do not use hearing aids are more likely to report sadness, depression, worry and anxiety, paranoia, reduced social activity, and emotional turmoil and insecurity. For example, chronic sadness or depression was reported by 14% of hearing aid users versus 23% of nonusers with mild hearing loss. Hearing aid users report improvements in many aspects of their lives, including their family relationships, sense of independence, and sex life. More than 2,000 family members or close friends of the hearing-impaired respondents asked a parallel set of questions also noticed the same improvement in the lives of the hearing-aid users.

Preference for nonuse of hearing aids by the elderly who are candidates for the use of amplification is related to a variety of variables. Popelka et al. (1998) found that the prevalence of hearing aid use among those with a pure-tone average greater than 25 dB HL (average of 500 Hz, 1 kHz, 2 kHz, and 4 kHz) in the poorer ear was 14.6%. The prevalence in a subset of the most severely affected subjects was 55%. Their analysis reveals that current hearing aid use was inversely correlated with word recognition scores, and directly correlated with age, education, severity of loss, self-reported hearing loss, self-perceived hearing handicap, and history of noise exposure. Garstecki and Erler (1998) found that nonuse of hearing aids by those who have been advised to use them by hearing professionals is related to a variety of factors. Female users of hearing aids demonstrated greater hearing loss and poorer word recognition ability, but less hearing handicap, higher internal locus of control, higher ego strength, and fewer depressive tendencies than females who have not obtained recommended hearing aids. Female hearing aid users also assumed responsibility for effective communication. Male users of hearing aids were more accepting of their hearing losses, took responsibility for communication problems, and found hearing aids less stigmatizing than their male nonhearing aid using counterparts.

Seeking help for hearing loss is obviously influenced by economic constraints. Mauldin (1976) observed that certain consequences of aging present problems because they directly impact the older person's consumer needs. Digestive and metabolic changes may require changed diets. Changes in sensory processes, such as eyesight and hearing, may require eyeglasses and hearing aids; physical disabilities may require medical services, medical products, and institutionalization. The hearing health care professional must determine whether the hearing loss is considered a problem by the aged individual and, if it is a problem, where the remediation of hearing loss fits into the older person's priorities of their consumer needs.

Cultural Considerations

In American culture, if one can generalize, the aged often have not been given, or allowed to assume, the esteemed role given to elders in some other societies (e.g., China). Rather, they often are treated with impatience and patronization. Approximately 6% reside in extended care facilities. For a significant subset of the older Americans, as their life expectancy increases, they are given less reason to live (Parenti, 1978). Chinese psychiatrist Wer Chen-1 contended that depression in the elderly is found more often in Western cultures because "the West extrudes older citizens, they lose place in the family, industry, community; their sphere of influence collapses as does their morale, leaving them vulnerable to disability and disease" (Greenblat & Chien, 1983). When hearing loss exists in the older American patient, great potential for depression and low morale must be assessed as possible etiologies of a lack of desire to communicate and to pursue use of amplification and aural rehabilitation.

It is very difficult to make generalizations about older Americans due to the ethnic diversity of the population in the United States and the existence of relatively pure ethnic and cultural subgroups, such as Asians, Native Americans, and "neighborhood" Hispanics and blacks. The sociological ramifications of group membership, sexual differences, and educational and economic levels in each of these subcultures relative to hearing help seeking behaviors of their older members are complex and should be assessed. Although a thorough review of the help-seeking practices of all cultures represented among American elderly is beyond the scope of this chapter, the following is a fairly detailed account of how cultural differences among the Asian elderly may affect hearing aid use.

Cheng (1988, interview) described three subgroups of Asians in America: new immigrants; refugees, including those from Indochina, Vietnam, Laos, and Cambodia; and second-generation Asian-Americans. New immigrants are defined as people who came to the United States as young people after 1950. If they have hearing problems, they are the most likely to seek help. Refugees may rely on remedies from nontraditional health care providers for various ailments, including hearing loss. There are many sheltered, protected, and isolated older people in the refugee subgroup who do not speak English and who live with their extended families. Barriers to the pursuit of hearing health care and hearing aid use in this group include:

- fear of American culture
- illiteracy in their own language and lack of knowledge of English
- lack of knowledge of available help
- psychological maladjustment to life in the United States

The third subgroup is American-born Asians. Cheng described two subgroups within this group. The "Chinatown ghetto" group in which members are born, raised, and never leave the Chinatown area is limited in its understanding of hearing problems and access to audiologic services. On the other hand, individuals who left Chinatown early and established their own lifestyles typically have their own English-speaking physicians and may seek help if they have a hearing problem.

For all groups, Asian cultural themes affect behavior in response to significant hearing loss. A general Asian belief that aging is a natural process that does not require intervention is common. In Asian cultures, for example, the young show respect for adults with hearing impairment either by speaking loudly or nodding to the elder during conversation, even when they cannot hear or understand the speech. In this case, the elders may not feel a need to improve communication because they consistently are acknowledged during family conversations. If they purchase a hearing aid and it does not work satisfactorily, they will simply not wear it rather than seek confrontation. When asked if a problem exists, they will deny it ("How can the audiologist or the dispenser be wrong? It must be me.") Cheng (1988) asserted that these problems will not subside through acculturation in the foreseeable future because increasing numbers of immigrants from Hong Kong and mainland China are expected in the coming years.

Culturally specific issues related to hearing help-seeking behaviors and application of amplification devices in all ethnic subgroups of the American population demand further investigation. The reader is referred to Spector (1996), Purnell and Paulanka (1998), and Geissler (1994) for more detailed information on transcultural issues as they relate to health, illness, and health care, all of which have direct application to the delivery of aural rehabilitative services to elderly members of other cultures.

Sociologic Considerations: The Nursing Home and Multilevel Retirement Community Populations

Of elderly individuals living in the United States at any one time, only 5% to 6% live in intermediate and skilled convalescent care facilities (nursing homes). This aged subpopulation consists of four subgroups:

1. Residents who are in nursing homes for rehabilitation with the realistic expectation of again living independently in the community, depending to various degrees on community-based services and their own resources.
2. Residents who have physical limitations that prevent them from living independently but otherwise are mentally intact.
3. Residents who, like group 2, are limited physically and are also mentally impaired.
4. Residents who are critically and terminally ill.

In addition to the relatively small percentage of single elders living in assisted living/skilled nursing home settings is a growing number of seniors who are electing, often with their living spouse, to give up their single family homes/condominiums/apartments and move into a multilevel retirement community while they are still very physically and socially active. These individuals no longer want the responsibilities of maintaining their own homes and have the resources to voluntarily relocate to these facilities These communities typically have a variety of living options on the same campus, including "independent living" patio homes/cottages and/or apartments located within the main building structure of the community for those who often still have their own cars and do all the things that individuals who are living in their own homes would do; "assisted living" apartments for those individuals who are for the most part able to take care of themselves but need assistance with some activities of daily living, and "skilled nursing or health care" for those requiring more extensive medical/nursing support for physical and/or mental conditions that severely limit their ability to take care of themselves. The first two groups may either fix their own meals in their homes, or take one or more meals in the central dining facility, typically located in the main building on the campus. Meal times for these residents are often the most important socialization time of their day. They are also the residents who take most advantage of many organized social events in the facility. Those in skilled nursing/health care units typically take their meals in their own rooms or in their own smaller dining facility, and often have their own organized social activities focusing on maintaining socialization, and cognitive skills and physical conditioning necessary for their activities of daily living.

Nursing Home Population

Nursing home residents, like many older people, have an increased desire for privacy. The paradox, however, is that institutional living reduces the ability to maintain privacy. For a significant subset of hearing-impaired adults, long-term nursing home residents, hearing loss may be their source of privacy, their insulation from the ever present intrusions on their personal space. Ulatowska (1985) cited gestures, degree of eye contact, gaze, and orientation of body parts as methods used by nonambulatory nursing home residents to declare their territory and desire for solitude. Even a slight movement of the body or chair away from a fellow resident or staff member can indicate the termination of a conversation (Lipman, 1968). With this in mind, the hearing health care professional must ask what maintenance-of-privacy function the hearing loss serves for each of the subgroups of residents, and how truly motivated each group is to improve hearing for purposes of communication.

Specific hearing aid related services that the hearing health care professional might provide for each of these subgroups include the following:

Group One

For rehabilitation patients bound to return to their homes, the goal is to maximize the electroacoustic function of existing hearing aids and assure proper use and application of the hearing aids by the patient and nursing home staff, respectively. Electroacoustically appropriate loaner hearing aids or new hearing aids should be provided in cases in which patients need amplification and do not have their own hearing aids.

Maximum use of residual hearing by members of this group is of paramount importance if they are to have optimum receptive and expressive communication during the rehabilitation process.

Group Two

For permanent residents with good mentation, the goal is to maximize long-term life quality in the nursing home by allowing the hearing-impaired resident the option of using appropriate amplification when they desire to communicate. The ability to succeed in communicating when they desire to and when others must get through is imperative to the quality of life for this population of nursing home residents. The hearing health care professional, therefore, must ensure that:

■ Residents have access to functional and appropriate amplification,
■ Staff participate in regular staff in-service instruction in the use of amplification systems including personal hearing aids and assistive listening devices,
■ They have regular (monthly) follow-up with residents using hearing aids on site,
■ Hearing aid assessment and fitting procedures ensure valid application of amplification (the use of portable hearing aid test box/real-ear equipment is required if the hearing professional is to be able to deliver valid hearing aid services on site),
■ An in-house loaner hearing aid bank exists to ensure access to amplification for new and experienced hearing aid users (hearing aids in the loaner bank can be donated by former residents, their families, and staff members, and electroacoustically analyzed and catalogued for appropriate use. Supportive aural rehabilitation programs and the availability of trained resident peer support and hearing-impaired patient advocate groups also are important for the optimum use of hearing aids by this subgroup), and
■ Assistive devices (e.g., wireless streaming devices that enable hearing aids to communicate with telephones/TV/hand held microphones, and so on [a small percentage of patients may come into the nursing home with this technology]; infrared television listening systems, one-on-one communication systems such as the Pocket Talker, telephone amplifiers, and so on) are available either to augment the residents' hearing aids or to serve as the primary amplifier if personal hearing aids are not used or available.

Group Three

For the cognitively impaired long-term resident with hearing loss, the goal is to maximize functional mentation through the enhancement of meaningful sensory stimulation. The questions that the hearing health care professional must answer for this group include:

- To what degree is inadequate and inconsistent sensory input responsible for the resident's impaired mental health?
- Are the symptoms displayed by this subgroup indicative of true chronic brain degeneration (dementia) or can the symptoms, in part, be described as signs of pseudodementia with the etiology of those symptoms being reduced by increasing the meaning of sensory input (e.g., application of appropriate amplification to increase meaning of auditory input)?

To the extent that the latter is true, the hearing health professional is challenged to fit appropriate amplification and optimize successful use through effective staff involvement and support. The availability of portable auditory brain stem evoked potential equipment and distortion product otoacoustic emission equipment for assessing hearing loss and real-ear probe tube microphone systems for assessing the insertion gain provided by hearing aids, and assistive devices can be very helpful in working with this subgroup. For this group, the use of one-on-one amplification devices such as the Pocket Talker or wireless systems, under supervision when communication is desired may be preferable to the full-time attempted use of personal hearing aids.

Group Four

For the terminally-ill or dying resident, the goal is to support receptive and expressive communication through the final stages of the terminally ill resident's life. The hearing health care professional may be critical in facilitating meaningful communication of the terminally hearing-impaired resident with his or her family physician, clergy, nursing staff, and friends. If hearing-impaired members of this subgroup are not currently hearing aid users, they are logical candidates for use of hearing aids provided from the facility's loaner hearing aid bank or use of institutionally owned assistive listening devices.

The hearing health care professional often must act as a vocal advocate for access of this patient subgroup to hearing aids and assistive listening devices. The Americans with Disabilities Act of 1992 certainly provides legislation to support equal access of residents with hearing impairment in public or corporately owned nursing home facilities. Access by the hearing professional to the hearing-impaired nursing home resident, in most cases, is determined by requests for services by the patient, nursing home staff, patient's physician, or family. Extended care facilities should have nonexclusive contracts with appropriate health care professionals to whom referrals for medical and audiologic intervention can be made. In most states, however, it is only with the consent of the resident's physician that these referrals can be consummated. Therefore, it is imperative for the nursing staff and personal physicians of extended care facility residents to be educated regarding the symptoms that indicate the need for and the potential benefit of appropriate intervention (e.g., hearing aids, assistive listening devices, aural rehabilitation therapy, otologic medical, and surgical treatment) by hearing health care professionals.

Multilevel Retirement Community Population

Multilevel retirement communities will have representatives of all of the populations enumerated above, however in addition, the largest percentage of their residents will be those highly functioning elders (and often their spouses) who have the desire to be socially active, participate in community-based cultural and educational opportunities, often travel nationally and internationally, and just generally want to enjoy their senior years as much as possible. Many of them have hearing loss and may enter the facility with hearing aids supported by their own hearing health care professionals located in the same community. Others may relocate from other areas of the country to be closer to their adult children with no local hearing health professional support, while others still may have undiagnosed or untreated hearing loss, needing active intervention and follow up. The majority of this population with hearing loss (or at least their spouses) realize when a hearing loss is interfering with their social and family life and often want to do something about it (e.g., pursue appropriate medical/audiological intervention including hearing aids/assistive devices if they experience benefit from them). This population of independent seniors with hearing loss living in multilevel retirement communities, given their desire to socialize in a group living environment, their relatively higher level of physical activity and high priority placed on ability to communicate, can be the most motivated and successful users of amplification, assistive communication devices, and beneficiaries of aural rehabilitation services of all subgroups of the elderly population.

Sociological Considerations: Independent Ambulatory Older Adults

Eighty-five percent of the older population live independently in varying stages of wellness and well-being. This group by far contains the majority of aged persons with hearing impairment. Less than 25% of the persons over age 65 with hearing impairment who need and could benefit from amplification, however, have purchased hearing aids (Skafte, 1986). The reasons for this, surmised from clinical experience, include:

■ Lack of acknowledgment of hearing loss as a problem
■ Lack of desire to rehabilitate acknowledged hearing loss
■ Lack of knowledge of available services and technology
■ Lack of appropriate support system and ability to manage use of hearing aids
■ Financial inability to purchase hearing aids

■ Erroneous understanding of what hearing aids can do and dissatisfied testimony from other hearing aid users or their own dissatisfaction with previous hearing aid use
■ Inadequate audiometric and psychosocial assessment of the residual auditory function and communication needs of the aged individual with hearing impairment
■ Amplification that was inappropriately applied because of electroacoustic and personal style preference inappropriateness
■ Lack of or poor supportive aural rehabilitation services for the first-time hearing aid user

Sociological Considerations: Physically Impaired Adults Living at Home

A growing percentage of the elderly individuals who live at home are as functionally impaired as individuals who live in nursing homes. Mutual access of this subgroup of the aged population to the variety of hearing health care services is limited by the individual's motivation to seek help for hearing problems either because of low priority in the list of more fundamental human needs or because of minimal demands for communicative efficacy (i.e., few visitors, no television or radio, no telephone use, or use of communication devices at high volume to compensate for the individual's hearing loss). Access is also limited by the person's ability to get hearing health care services for initial and necessary follow-up appointments. The logistical problems of follow-up may be so overwhelming to the individual that it may seem impossible to overcome them; therefore, the person does not try. Often these individuals are able to stay in their own homes only because of the support/assistance of adult children, or proprietary in-home homemaker/certified nursing assistant/or nursing care. If services are to be provided to this group, they must be more accessible to them than they typically are to the more flexible ambulatory consumer with hearing impairment and coordinated with the individuals who are providing in-home assistance. This population is in most need of in-home hearing health (audiologic) care requiring the audiologist to have the array of portable audiometry, impedance, and computer-based hearing aid test box/real-ear analysis equipment to support the medical referral and follow-up aural rehabilitation process.

Adjustment to Adult Onset Hearing Loss

Kyle, Jones, and Wood (1985) presented a model that described the phases of acquisition and adjustment to adventitious hearing loss in adults. It is important to assess which stage an individual is in when hearing aid assessment and fitting is being attempted. Phase 1, Acquisition of Hearing Loss, is described as the period when the loss is not acknowledged. It may last less than 1 month or go on for 20 years or more. It is the time period between initial onset of loss and the first visit to a hearing health care provider. Up to 75% of the population with acquired hearing loss may be in this phase at any time (Medical Research Council Institute of Hearing Research, 1981). During this phase, the unaided person receives feedback from the environment that he or she is talking too loud, the television or radio is too loud, he or she has misheard important information, and so on. During the initial stages of this phase, the person with hearing impairment ascribes the inability to hear to the faulty speech of others and other problems external to him- or herself. The initial visit to a hearing health care professional for evaluation may be made only in acquiescence to the demands of family members. As realization of the existence of the loss is fundamental to initiation of help-seeking behavior, Kyle and colleagues suggested that when persons are forced to be in situations where they cannot control the volume of speech (e.g., lectures, church), they are apt to more quickly realize the extent of their impairment than if their time is spent in listening activities in which

they can control the volume of speech (e.g., watching television) or ascribe their inability to understand to faulty connections (e.g., using the telephone) may be important. The use of self-assessment scales or hearing handicap inventories at the initial evaluation can help to shorten the duration of Phase 2 by focusing the individual on communication, social, and emotional problems they may be having that are related to their newly identified hearing loss.

Phase 2 is described as the time between first contact with a professional and diagnosis of permanent hearing loss and the receipt of a hearing aid. Kyle and colleagues found that, in England, where hearing aids are provided at no charge, this phase lasted a few months. In the United States, where the cost of hearing aids represents a significant financial investment, this phase may last 1 to 7 years or more. It is marked by uncertainty as to the ramifications of the newly identified hearing loss, and the resolution of this phase in large part is dependent on the accommodation and support of the person's family and friends. The resolution of this phase also is dependent on the person's willingness to accept responsibility for his or her own successful use of assertive communication techniques and speech reading skills taught in supportive aural rehabilitation sessions.

Phase 3 is the period of subsequent accommodation to the hearing loss. This phase is characterized by the individual's realization of the level of control he or she can expect to have in various communication settings. The ultimate goal of hearing aid fitting and supportive rehabilitation is to maximize the independence and control of the hearing-impaired individual in all desired communication environments. Kyle and colleagues cited maladaptive behaviors in this phase as behavioral changes resulting in: (1) excessive introversion and control of conversations with minimal listening, and (2) withdrawal from communication situations that threaten control and independence.

An acceptable resolution of Phase 3 is dependent on how the individual adjusts to the use of the hearing aid in various personal and social situations, vocational and avocational demands, and the dynamics of family life. It also depends on an optimum match between how much control an individual believes they have over the rehabilitation of his or her hearing loss (internal versus external locus of control) versus how much control truly exists. Also fundamental to adjustment to the hearing aid are acceptance of its physical appearance, optimum electroacoustic compatibility with and compensation for the hearing loss, independence in the use of the amplification system, acknowledgment of the use of a less than perfect amplification system to others with whom communication is initiated, and realistic expectations of others regarding the aided benefit the new hearing aid user can derive in a variety of listening environments.

Kyle and Wood (1983) found that, although 89% of their aided respondents had difficulty with street conversations, 79% would not tell people that they had a hearing problem. This also is typical of the reactions of contemporary hearing aid users in the United States. If audiologists and dispensers were able to match perfectly the hearing aid configuration to the psychophysical needs of the patient, there would be no need for public acknowledgment of the loss and the use of hearing aids. However, given the fact that current hearing aids do not fully restore normal hearing function in the damaged cochlea and central auditory pathways, acknowledgment of the hearing loss and use of hearing aids remain critical to the successful resolution of the aural rehabilitation process.

The remainder of this chapter deals with assessment and intervention strategies.

AUDITORY ASSESSMENT FINDINGS IN THE AGED POPULATION

This section concentrates on threshold and suprathreshold auditory function in the aged listener. This information is, of course, most important when considering appropriate assessment and intervention strategies to amplify the older patient with hearing impairment. Marshall (1981) suggested the following hypotheses in the clinical evaluation of the older hearing-impaired listener: (1) Aging listeners are no different than young listeners with equal degrees of hearing loss and (2) aging listeners will show auditory function problems in addition to those shown by younger listeners with similar hearing losses, possibly due to peripheral problems associated with presbycusis, which are not adequately assessed by the pure-tone audiogram, central auditory nervous system degeneration, cognitive differences, or a combination of all of the above.

Assessment Problems Related to Age

The incidence of excessive impacted cerumen is higher in the older versus younger population (Fisch, 1978; Schow, Christensen, Hutchinson, & Nerbonne, 1978). Otoscopy must be performed prior to auditory and hearing aid evaluation, with appropriate intervention.

Collapsing ear canals with the application of earphones also has been found to occur more frequently in older listeners (Schow & Goldbaum, 1980; Zucker & Williams, 1977) and may explain the high incidence of conductive loss cited in several studies (Rosen, Plester, El Mofty, & Rosen, 1970). The implication is to assess the anteroposterior relationship of the tragus to the cavum of the concha and the relative collapsibility of the tragus and cartilaginous portion of the external auditory meatus. Calibrated insert earphones should be used to eliminate this problem. As described earlier, collapsing ear canals also present a challenge for the fabrication of earmolds and ITE hearing aids with open canal mini BTE aids being an appropriate alternative for appropriate candidates.

It has been suggested that aged listeners are more conservative in their threshold criterion than younger listeners when they are asked to respond yes or no to the presence of an auditory signal (Potash & Jones, 1977; Rees & Botwinick, 1971). Clinical observations indicate that aged listeners may be less willing to guess in their discrimination of suprathreshold auditory signals if only a portion of the signal is heard (as with a supra-threshold single-word identification task). This symptom may be representative of older listeners or it may be endemic only to the current aged population as a consequence of low self-esteem and the low value generally placed on the aged by our society. In either case, the implication for the hearing health care professional is to reduce auditory test anxiety and reinstruct the older patient regarding the clinician's expectation that errors in signal identification are expected, and in fact necessary, if an accurate evaluation is to be obtained. Implications for the test procedures include changing the threshold response to a two-interval forced choice task (eliminating the possibility of a nonresponse) and using closed-set, forced choice suprathreshold speech identification tests, such as a Modified Rhyme type test, the Synthetic Sentence Identification Index, or a comparison of closed set (high redundancy) to open-set (low-redundancy) word identification performance using a tool such as the Speech in Noise test (SPIN).

Loudness and Adaptation

Loudness recruitment in the elderly listener with sensorineural hearing loss does exist and is demonstrated by the elevation in hearing thresholds with perceptions of loud sounds that either are similar to or are reduced relative to those for normal hearing listeners. It has been suggested by clinical audiologists that uncomfortable loudness measures using speech and pure tones lack validity as representations of the levels of sound a person will truly accommodate when they are motivated to do so (i.e., in social or vocational situations).

In spite of this perception, it is important to assess frequency-specific tolerance limits, known by various names such as Uncomfort-able Loudness Levels (UCLs), Upper Limits of Comfortable Loudness (ULCL), and Loudness Discomfort Levels (LDLs), in each ear for each subject to make the most appropriate initial decisions regarding the appropriate frequency-specific Saturation Sound Pressure level (SSPL) characteristics of hearing aids.

Adaptation, or reduction in the loudness percept of suprathreshold continuous pure tones, has been assessed in older individuals using Békésy and conventional tone decay tests. Békésy tracings usually are consistent with normal hearing or a cochlear site of lesion (type I or II tracings, respectively; Jerger, 1960; Harbert, Young, & Menduke, 1966), and tone decay is typically less than 30 dB, also consistent with cochlear site of lesion (Ganz, 1976; Olsen & Noffisinger, 1974).

Implications for Amplification

The primary behavioral assessment of recruitment for the aging listener is loudness tolerance for pure-tones, warble tones, or speech. The dynamic range from threshold to these levels is reduced in persons with sensorineural hearing loss. Although the usable auditory dynamic range is not reduced inordinately for aged listeners with hearing impairment as compared with younger listeners with similar hearing loss, they often have a decreased ability to ignore the presence of loud environmental noise. This interferes with their understanding of important auditory input to a greater degree than that experienced by their younger counterparts.

The aided listener with sensorineural hearing loss requires a comparatively wide range of input signal intensities to be amplified to suprathreshold levels and maintained within the compressed suprathreshold dynamic range of the individual. These findings suggest that, if maximum hearing aid benefit is to be achieved for the elderly and all persons with sensorineural hearing loss, SSPL90 values that closely correspond to obtained frequency-specific UCLs must be utilized, while at the same time providing enough gain to boost important auditory stimuli to the person's Most Comfortable

Levels (MCLs). Depending on the separation in dB between the person's MCL and UCL at each frequency, these criteria may be met with the use of a linear amplifier with high-level compression limiting to minimize distortion of high-level inputs and accommodate UCLs. However, as MCLs approach the levels of the UCLs, reducing the dynamic range, it may be possible only to provide adequate gain for lower level input signals to keep all amplified signals below the UCLs. This situation would necessitate the use of a wide dynamic range compression circuit with a low knee-point of compression. Current compression circuits employ the concepts of expansion, compression, unity gain, and high-level output compression limiting. Compression amplifiers that incorporate each of these may have three knee-points, defined as: (1) the input level at which the aid stops increasing in gain for progressively louder soft sounds (expansion) and goes into compression (or gain reduction for successively louder inputs), (2) the input level at which the aid no longer compresses the signal but gives no gain (unity gain) with the output being equal to the input, and (3) output limiting, which is the input level beyond which there is no further increase in output regardless of the change in input.

Multichannel compression circuits give the flexibility to fit a hearing aid that has unique input/output functions for two or more frequency bands. This allows the aid to be programmed to accommodate the unique loudness growth characteristics for each individual in the various frequency bands accommodated by the hearing aid. Although there are aids with as little as two channels and 10 channels or more, it is not clear how many channels are minimally necessary and optimal. The audiologist or the dispenser who uses frequency-specific stimuli to determine MCLs and UCLs also should evaluate whether MCLs and UCLs for more complex signals (e.g., speech and environmental noise) might be somewhat lower due to loudness summation resulting from the simultaneous presentation of the multiple frequency components contained in these stimuli. If this is true, the overall gain of the instrument may

need to be reduced once the independent channels have been set to accommodate the loudness of sounds with complex spectra.

The Independent Hearing Aid Fitting Forum (IHAFF, 1994) proposed a method for assessing loudness growth in a low- and high-frequency band from threshold to perceived uncomfortable loudness. Using the first seven of the loudness levels recommended by Hawkins, Walden, Montgomery, and Prosek (1987), the patient rates the audibility of presented pure-tones at increasing loudness levels typically at 500 Hz and 3000 Hz. With current digitally programmable and programmable true digital signal processing hearing aids, it probably is adequate to assess only threshold and the UCL at each of these frequencies to define the dynamic range accurately. The hearing aid simply will interpolate the appropriate input/output function with associated compression knee points and ratios based on these two end points of the loudness function. In hearing aids with three or more channels, loudness growth using this procedure should be assessed using a frequency at the center of each frequency band included in each channel.

Frequency Discrimination

Reduced frequency selectivity in persons with sensorineural hearing loss has been shown using difference limens for frequency (DLF; Zurek & Formby, 1977). DLFs have been shown to increase with increased magnitude of loss and for low frequencies as well as high frequencies in persons with only high-frequency loss. It has not been established whether aged hearing-impaired listeners have inordinately greater DLFs than their younger counterparts when learning effects and potential age-related criterion effects are controlled (Marshall, 1981).

Psychophysical tuning curves for listeners with sensorineural hearing loss, obtained by fixing the level and frequency of a probe tone and measuring the level of a second tone at various frequencies required to mask the probe, have shown abnormal broadening, abnormal shape, and loss of the tip in regions of hearing loss (Tyler, Fernandes, & Wood, 1984; Zwicker & Shorn, 1978) and abnormality in regions of normal hearing sensitivity (Mills, Gilbert, & Adkins, 1979), especially in the presence of significant high-frequency loss (Nelson, 1979). It is not clear whether these results differ in older versus younger persons with similar audiograms (Marshall, 1981).

It has been suggested that each frequency is surrounded by its own critical bandwidth of frequencies and that all frequencies within the critical band of a probe frequency are processed equally. Thus, formants in the speech signal that are separated by a critical bandwidth are perceived as different frequencies; however, environmental noise located within the critical band of each formant frequency is processed along with the speech signal. A widening of critical bandwidths, or loss of frequency selectivity, has been found with the advent of sensorineural hearing loss (deBoer & Bowmeester, 1974, 1975). The widening of critical bands may be due to cochlear changes (efferent olivocochlear neuron degeneration) not related to afferent input, and frequency discrimination may be independent of loss of pure-tone hearing sensitivity (Bienvenue & Michael, 1979). It has not been shown definitively, however, that the widening of critical bandwidths in aged listeners with sensorineural loss is in excess of that for young hearing-impaired listeners. Bienvenue and Michael (1979) listed four functions of critical bands: (1) to band-limit the effect of background noise on the target signal serving to enhance the SNR, (2) to determine ability to perceive harmonic content and formant content (in the case of speech) of complex signals, (3) to determine ability to perceive phase relationships among tone complexes, and (4) to sharpen frequency discrimination beyond that which can be described by basilar membrane mechanics.

Critical ratios (SNR at masked threshold) and upward spread of masking have been assessed in aged listeners and are a reflection of critical bandwidth. Critical ratios have been demonstrated to increase for higher frequencies in both normal-hearing listeners (Reed & Bilger, 1973) and listeners with high-frequency noise-induced listeners with hearing impairment (Tyler, Fernandes, & Wood, 1984). Margolis and Goldberg (1980) concluded that critical ratios are not a simple reflection of auditory filter bandwidth in aged listeners. Upward spread of masking in aged listeners with hearing impairment has not been shown to be any greater than for younger cochlear hearing-impaired counterparts. Although upward spread of masking has been found to be detrimental to speech discrimination of normal-hearing listeners at high signal intensities (95–100 dB SPL) (Danaher, Osberger, & Pickett, 1973), it has not been shown to be abnormally broad in all listeners with sensorineural hearing loss (Jerger et al., 1960; Leshowitz & Lindstrom, 1979).

Implications for Amplification

It is quite possible that peripheral deterioration of the frequency selectivity of the cochlea accounts in large part for the reduced understanding of speech in noise in the aged listener with hearing impairment. It is also possible that aged persons with different audiometric configurations and etiologies of hearing loss have varying degrees of alteration in critical bandwidths and cochlear-based frequency specificity.

Once a reliable database is established regarding the frequency discrimination of older versus younger hearing-impaired listeners with controls for loss configuration, etiology, and task-response criterion effects, it seems imperative that tasks that assess frequency discrimination be included in the hearing aid assessment process. The information obtained would make it possible to severely band limit the amplified signal, based not only on the audiometric configuration of the pure-tone loss, but also on the extent of abnormality of frequency selectivity across the frequency range, even in the presence of what appear to be normal pure-tone thresholds. This information then could be used to help determine the optimum crossover frequencies in multichannel hearing aids with the steep skirts of digital filters controlling interaction between adjacent frequency bands. This is quite possible with current digital signal-processing technology.

Speech Discrimination

From the previous discussion of the importance of peripheral frequency selectivity to the discrimination of complex signals (speech) in noise, it can be argued that, if population-specific information was available, much of the responsibility for reduction in speech discrimination in noise demonstrated by significant numbers of aged hearing-impaired listeners could be described on the basis of impaired frequency selectivity at the level of the cochlea. If this were true, particularly with the advent of digital-processing technology, algorithms could be designed into the hearing aid to compensate specifically for abnormal cochlear function. An additional portion of the reduction in speech understanding in aged listeners can be explained solely on the basis of inadequate sensation levels, particularly of high-frequency speech sounds and higher formants (F1, F2, and F3) and their transitional cues.

To determine age-only related changes in auditory temporal processing, Blackington, Novak, and Kramer (1988) examined NU-6 word identification in normal-hearing young and elderly subjects with 0% and 60% temporal compression of the speech signals. The authors compared these data with forward masking threshold results using 500 and 2000 Hz as the target stimuli with wide-band noise as the masker. The older subjects, ages 60 to 79 years, obtained 70% correct identification on the compressed speech presented at 40 dB HL compared with 82% correct identification for the young controls. There was no difference in word identification scores between the two groups for noncompressed speech stimuli (97% to 99% for all subjects). Blackington, Novak, and Kramer (1988) also found that, for separations between the masker and target stimuli of 0 to 250 ms, the older subjects required higher tone sensation levels in order to achieve the same 70% correct detection level as their younger counterparts. This was particularly true for the 2000 Hz stimuli.

Implications for Amplification and Aural Rehabilitation

A common clinical observation from aged hearing-impaired listeners is that their understanding of speech improves with a mildly reduced rate of speech. The results of many of the altered speech studies have shown excessively reduced performance in aged hearing-impaired listeners. The results of Blackington, Novak, and Kramer (1988), which showed the same reduction of performance in normal-hearing aged listeners, suggest that the critical causal factors are age-related central factors that are not reflected in changes in pure-tone sensitivity. This has been confirmed more recently by Gordon-Salant and Fitzgibbons (1999). They found that age-related problems for recognition of time-compressed speech are independent of attenuation imposed by hearing loss. This supports the contention that aging, in and of itself, imposes a limitation on the ability to process rapid speech segments. These limitations are believed to be central in nature and most likely associated with deterioration of central timing mechanisms. Although possible, current digital hearing aids are not able to slow the rate of speech being processed in real time. As a result, it is imperative for older listeners to realize that difficulty understanding rapid speech is a common problem of the elderly that is not significantly helped with amplification and that can be reduced simply by asking speakers to slow their rate of speech. The temporal characteristics (attack and release times) of compression circuits also can be a significant factor in reducing the use of temporal and frequency cues in speech. The attack times must be rapid enough to accommodate the loudness of the offending loud sounds while, at the same time, the release times must allow recovery quickly enough to allow for the audibility of the subsequent temporal and frequency cues carried by the softer speech sounds. The selection of appropriate release times is particularly important for the elderly hearing aid user and is deserving of further research.

Binaural Integration

Binaural auditory fusion and release from masking tasks have been used to assess central auditory nervous system integrity. Binaural auditory fusion compares word identification when high- and low-frequency information is presented monaurally versus when high-pass filtered speech is presented to one ear and low-pass filtered speech to the other. Breakdown in the former task can be attributed solely to abnormal cochlear filter effects, whereas breakdown in the dichotic high pass–low pass task can be impaired also by brain stem pathology and bilateral and diffuse cerebral pathology (Lynn & Gilroy, 1976). Investigators have found that the aged listener's binaural fusion ability is not significantly poorer than younger listeners with similar pure-tone thresholds (Harbert et al., 1966; Palva & Jokenen, 1970). In fact, older listeners often perform more poorly on the monaural task than on the dichotic speech fusion task, which is consistent with peripheral auditory system pathology. Franklin (1975) also found this to be true with young (11–23 years) listeners with sensorineural hearing loss.

The binaural Masking Level Difference (MLD) is a psychophysical task that also relies on intact lower brain stem function for maximum MLD results. Many studies that have reported MLD results for presbycusic listeners have concluded that MLDs are generally smaller for the presbycusic population (Olsen, Noffsinger, & Carhart, 1976; Warren, Wagener, & Herman, 1978) in spite of considerable overlap of MLD values between young normal hearing and older hearing-impaired groups. Novak and Anderson (1982) attempted to systematically control for age, degree of hearing loss, bilateral symmetry of loss, shape of loss, and central auditory integ-

rity in the evaluation of the MLD in older hearing-impaired listeners. They found that, for older listeners, MLD magnitudes for 500 Hz were significantly reduced only for the apparent neural presbycusic (Schuknecht, 1964, 1974) group. The authors concluded that central auditory system function as measured by the MLD task was significantly different only for the neural presbycusic group with high-frequency sloping sensorineural hearing loss and single-word identification scores less than 70%. These binaural speech fusion and MLD studies support the contention that binaural integration is intact for many aged hearing-impaired listeners.

Despite these findings, a small percentage of elderly hearing aid users will perform better with monaural than with binaural amplification. Chmiel, Jerger, Murphy, Pirozzolo, and Tooley-Young (1997) studied this phenomenon extensively in one such elderly listener. Their results suggest that age-related changes in interhemispheric transfer of auditory input via corpus callosum may underlie the preference for monaural amplification. These results support the inclusion of behavioral dichotic speech perception tests for older hearing aid candidates to better determine those who may not be successful with binaural amplification.

Implications for Amplification

From the results of the studies cited in the previous two sections, it must be concluded that, although problems of speech understanding in the aged hearing-impaired listener can be attributed in large part to cochlear filtering effects due to pathology at the level of the cochlea, particularly secondary to degenerative changes in the stria vascularis, even older "normal-hearing"(based on audiometric thresholds) listeners show poorer performance than their younger counterparts on temporal masking tasks (compressed speech identification, forward masking signal detection). In this case, age appears to be a critical factor in determining the ability to understand rapid speech. On the basis of the forward-masking data of Blackington, Novak, and Kramer (1988), even normal-hearing older listeners may benefit from mild high-frequency emphasis amplification to improve their detection and processing of rapidly presented auditory information.

In the case of bilaterally symmetrical hearing loss and PB word discrimination scores in excess of 80%, binaural fitting of aids must not be ruled out solely on the basis of concern for inability to binaurally integrate dichotically presented information (typical sound-field listening). Age, in and of itself, does not appear to be a significant factor in reduction of binaural auditory integration or binaural release from masking abilities in the majority of older persons with cochlear-based hearing loss; however, in a small subgroup of hearing aid candidates, monaural speech processing may be better than that achieved with binaural amplification and probably due to higher level central processing problems. For these reasons, the inclusion of central auditory processing tasks such as compressed speech or dichotic listening tasks could allow for better evaluation of hearing aid candidacy and potential hearing aid benefit (Givens, Arnold, & Hume, 1998). These assessment tools could help identify those patients who are going to need more rehabilitative support because of the poor prognosis for successful use of hearing aids in difficult listening situations.

The implications of all of the psychoacoustic findings with aged hearing-impaired listeners are that:

■ The population is indeed composed of subgroups as defined by different peripheral and central auditory system functions.
■ The pure-tone audiogram, in and of itself, is not an adequate descriptor of important auditory psychophysical abilities.
■ The onus is on the audiologist to develop a valid, reliable, and efficient test battery that will delineate cochlear versus retrocochlear function as it relates specifically to the specification of hearing-aid parameters. This test battery must enable the audiologist to assess "hearing aid benefit"

based on both improved auditory function that can be expected based on improved audibility of conversational level speech sounds via "appropriate" amplification versus actual derived benefit based also on psychosocial and motivational parameters unique to each aged listener.

APPLYING HEARING AIDS TO OLDER PATIENTS

The audiologist must apply hearing aids that: (1) have the electroacoustic characteristics most appropriate for the patient's residual auditory function and (2) are acceptable to the patient. Satisfaction of the first requirement does not always ensure satisfaction of the second. Barford (1979) stated that user satisfaction across patients, as measured by speech perception ability, can be high or low with similar sudden significant changes in aided versus unaided auditory sensitivity. High satisfaction results if the additional frequency information provided to the "recognition device" is indeed meaningful and useful. Low satisfaction results when enhanced aided sensitivity for high frequencies relative to low frequencies causes a "mismatch of the recognition device and the input code." A degradation in speech perception ability at the time of initial hearing aid use will result if the latter effect dominates. Barford suggested that, "This mismatch will gradually decrease as a result of adaptation, if adaptation is possible." However, the length of the adaptation is not easily predicted (re: age of patient, type of loss, and a variety of psychosocial variables) for each individual patient and may last from a few days to 6 months or longer. Surr, Cord, and Walden (1998) examined long-term versus short-term hearing aid benefit. This study compared hearing aid benefit obtained 6 weeks and a minimum of 1 year after fitting to determine if changes occurred over time. Fifteen patients were fitted binaurally with a programmable two-channel aid with wide dynamic range compression. The manufacturer's recommended loudness

growth in octave bands, and audiogram programming algorithm and fitting procedures
were used. Following an initial 6-week period
and again following a minimum of one year
of use, the Profile of Hearing Aid Benefit
(PHAB) was administered. Speech recognition performance was tested using the Connected Speech Test (CST) in six-talker speech
babble at 50 dBA, +10 dB SNR, 60dBA, +5 dB
SNR, 70 dBA, +2 dB SNR, and in quiet with
a reverberation time of 0.78 seconds. Significant aided benefit was shown. A comparison
of short-term versus 1-year PHAB and CST
results showed no significant differences
in hearing aid benefit with long-term use.
This suggests that the 6-week acclimatization period evaluated in this investigation
is sufficiently long for clinical trials of this
type of Wide Dynamic Range amplification
supporting the contention that the optimum
trial period prior to final purchase of hearing amplification should be between 30 and
60 days, rather than the typical 30-day period
often dispensed with hearing aids.

Needs and Expectations of the Older Patient

Today, audiologists have the option of recommending hearing aids from a vast array
of real-time, high-fidelity digital signal processing options; with varying numbers of
automatic signal processing options, with
typically higher prices associated with a
greater number of such options. The technology selected should be chosen on the
basis of patient auditory measurements, the
demands of the patients' listening environments, and the importance of functioning
in these environments balanced with the
patients' demand for "the best" technology
the patients' cosmetic demands, desire for
more or less automatic function, and the
patients' financial resources. More and more
of the older patients seeking help for their
hearing loss have the financial resources to
purchase state-of-the art technology. Many
want the best of what is available and expect
that, if they pay the higher price, the hearing

aid will allow them to hear well in all listening environments, with minimal adjustment
or maintenance on their part. In reality, the
expectations of older patients and their families may be unrealistic. However in light of
the high price tag (possible $3,000–$4,000 per
aid) on today's most sophisticated hearing
aids, it is understandable that the patients
and their families may have unrealistic expectations of hearing aid benefit. As audiologists
help their older patients decide between the
various types of technology, it must be determined if the demands of their typical listening situations warrant the expense of the most
sophisticated digital signal processing (DSP)
technology. Hearing aid dispensers often are
prone to encourage their geriatric patients to
purchase the high-end DSP products because
they must be best for the more challenged
auditory processing system of the geriatric
patient. The high cost of high-end DSP technology can encourage the older patient to
have unrealistic expectations of the benefit
they should be receiving from their aids in all
difficult listening environments. Also, to the
extent that the more sophisticated technology
may require greater understanding of its use
and dexterity in its adjustment, there will be
a greater opportunity for failure of the older
patient to use it successfully. Given these
issues and the fact that the older patient often
requires more time for all aspects of hearing
assessment, hearing aid fitting, counseling,
and adjustment to hearing aid use, time, and
attention are critical variables in the design of
an effective hearing aid intervention program
for the elderly patient. MarkeTrakVIII (Kochkin et al., 2010) evaluated "the impact of the
hearing healthcare professional on hearing
aid user success." This study evaluated correlations between dispensing protocols and
successful patient outcomes in the wake of
the ongoing depressing statistics that of the
34.25 million people (most of whom are over
the age of 55 years) with hearing loss, only
approximately 25% own hearing aids, with
the majority of that group having moderate-
to-severe hearing loss with little progress
over this past generation in the proportion of
hearing aid users who are "satisfied" or "very

satisfied" with the use of their hearing aids and approximately 12.4% of individuals with hearing aids (more than one million people) keeping them permanently "in the drawer." Reasons for nonuse of hearing include poor benefit, poor fit with discomfort, and inability to hear in noise any better with the aid than without it. Kochkin (2010) also reports that despite "the digital revolution," more than one half of all patients who own hearing aids would not repurchase their current brand of hearing aids. Kochkin (2007) also asserted that more than four million people who could derive benefit from hearing aids will not purchase them because of bad experiences with hearing aids among their friends and relatives. Major reasons for the return of hearing aids and nonuse include: poor benefit generally and particularly in noisy listening situations, feedback, poor perceived value (benefit/what was paid for the hearing aid), and poor fit/discomfort.

Kochkin et al. (2010) state that the commonsense protocol for fitting hearing aids should include: (1) Physical exam of the ear and review of patient's history, (2) Valid/reliable assessment of the hearing loss, (3) Selection of the correct technology for the patient (including availability of a telecoil), (4) Assessment of client expectations in the context of what is realistic, (5) Assessment of hearing aid performance relative to manufacturer specifications using a hearing aid analyzer PRIOR to fitting of the hearing aid/s, (6) Determination of required valid gain and output prescription and verification of achievement of amplification "targets" across the frequency range using real-ear measurement (REM) with probe microphones, (7) Fine-tuning of the hearing aid acoustical fitting using REM (to monitor discrepancies between aided targets and actual aided benefit created in the fine-tuning process), based on patient input, and patient-specific measures including loudness discomfort level (LDLs), and acceptable noise levels (ANLs) and so on, (8) Validation of hearing aid benefit comparing pre- versus post-measures of speech or sentence comprehension in noise and quiet using real-world performance metrics, and (9) Provision of counseling and aural rehabilitation services relative to the patients needs, including care and maintenance of the aid, insertion of the aids, and instruction on hearing aid features (e.g., effective use of the telecoil) and program options.

In addition to individual counseling, participation in a peer-group aural rehabilitation program (e.g., ReACT: rehabilitative auditory communication training described below) is recommended for seniors who are first-time hearing aid users, or are judged at risk for or are having difficulty adjusting to and learning to use their amplification system.

Christensen and Groth (2008) state that the major errors made by dispensers of hearing aids in rank order include: (1) Failure to verify acoustic fitting using REM, (2) Inappropriate use of open ear canal hearing aid fittings (either not using them when appropriate or using them when they are inappropriate for the degree of hearing loss), (3) Assuming that manufacturer software fitting defaults are achieving appropriate amplification for target frequencies, (4) Not matching client dexterity limitations with the dexterity requirements for successful use of the hearing aid, (5) Not performing appropriate validation measures of hearing aid benefit, (6) Not conducting appropriate and effective counseling, (7) Leaving "first fit" (new hearing aid user acclimatization amplification levels) software settings unchanged over time resulting in a significant gap between target and actual aided REMs with associated poor audibility of target speech sounds (typically voiceless consonants, voiced or voiceless stop consonants, nasal consonants, and second and third vowel formants), (8) Fitting hearing aids on clients unmotivated to use them, (9) Assuming that automatic environmental steering programs (such as adaptive directional microphone switching) are accurate and hearing aids switch appropriately, and (10) Failing to use newer tests (e.g., HINT, Speech Mapping, etc.) to help with selection, fitting, and counseling. The authors emphasize that the "primary mistake . . . was non-use of probe-microphone real-ear measures by audiologists and hearing instrument specialists to objectively quantify the acoustic output of gain of the hearing aids in the patient's ear canal. . . . These measures are critical for assessing audibility, appropriate output for different input levels, and verification of prescriptive algorithms." This was true in 2008 and continues to be true today. There is simply no better way to assess the appropriateness of the amount of amplification being delivered to the eardrum at each frequency in the speech range requiring amplification. It is simply unethical to not use REMs in the fitting of today's sophisticated hearing aid technology.

Selection of Electroacoustic Parameters of Hearing Aids

Auditory Evaluation

It is recommended that, at a minimum, the following parameters should be assessed:

1. Pure-tone thresholds and UCLs under earphones should be obtained to specify general frequency response characteristics and absolute gain and output requirements. Some hearing aid products allow for determination of sound pressure levels required to obtain thresholds and UCLs using the actual hearing aid in the ear as the transducer. For many years, prescriptive methods like POGO II, NAL-R, and DSL 3.0 have been considered the standard approach to identifying target hearing aid insertion or functional gain (Hawkins, 1992; Mueller, 1997). These approaches used threshold data to calculate hearing instrument gain as a function of frequency. Some also calculated a recommended maximum output level of the hearing aid assuming an input of 60 to 65 dB SPL. As these procedures have no way of determining gain appropriate for softer and louder signal input levels, they are not adequate to define the input/output (I/O) gain functions of nonlinear compression aids. The Desired Sensation Level (DSL) I/O algorithm was devel-

oped as an approach for fitting nonlinear compression instruments (Seewald, et al., 1997). To achieve loudness equalization, DSL I/O recommends target output levels for different sound input levels (40, 65, and 95 dB) as a function of frequency. This is the procedure followed in the Speech Mapping approach to real-ear measures. These target output levels are based on the listener's measured thresholds and UCLs. If loudness judgments are not available, DSL I/O will default to predicted data for UCLs, which are about one standard deviation below the mean loudness discomfort levels reported by Pascoe (1988). Loudness equalization should enable the listener to perceive soft sounds as soft, but audible, average conversational sounds should be perceived as comfortable, and loud sounds should be perceived as loud but not uncomfortably loud. This approach is used by a variety of hearing aid manufacturers in their gain and output determination algorithms and is available in several real-ear probe microphone measurement systems. It is appropriate for the fitting of current hearing aid technology in geriatric patients.

2. In applying audiometric data to determinations of frequency response requirements and selection of specific hearing aids, it is important to realize that 2cc coupler values indicated on manufacturers' specification sheets may over represent desired insertion gain (aided versus unaided ear canal sound pressure levels; Hawkins & Schum,1984). This difference will be greater for BTE than for ITE hearing aids, particularly for frequencies above 1000 Hz. Lower insertion gain also will be seen in persons with large ear canal volumes medial to the tip of the hearing aid or the earmold and with very flaccid middle ear systems. This is not so much of a problem when using highly flexible, multichannel digitally programmable aids with adequate "head room" and real-ear probe tube measurements to assess changes in insertion gain or sound

pressure level aided targets, while gain and output parameters of the hearing aid fitting software are manipulated to achieve DSL I/O targets

3. Real-ear unaided response measurements indicating the location and amplitude of the ear canal resonance frequency are helpful in predicting the amount of gain that will be necessary to achieve targets. They should be used to determine if the selected hearing aid has the flexibility to accommodate the gain requirements necessitated by the ear canal resonance values and the target values.

4. Frequency-specific LDLs or UCLs for those frequencies for which amplification is desired should be obtained to specify SSPL90 values to which the aid should be adjusted first. Etymotic insert earphones, available through the Etymotic Research Lab, calibrated in the 2cc coupler are an appropriate transducer for these measurements. LDLs should be obtained for both frequency-specific (at a minimum of one frequency in the center of each of the hearing aid bands for which amplification is required) and broadband stimuli (speech or speech noise) to determine the extent to which loudness summation may necessitate the lowering of the gain and SSPL90 requirements beyond what would have predicted based on frequency specific stimuli only.

5. Dichotic assessment using the Dichotic Digits Test, a test of discrimination of temporally compressed speech, and a test of the discrimination of speech in noise (e.g., Hearing in Noise Test (HINT) should ideally be completed for patients reporting extreme difficulties understanding speech, to assess the prognosis for successful use of binaural amplification, and the need for additional counseling based on unusual difficulty processing rapid speech and speech in noise.

6. Standard single syllable word identification tests should be completed under phones at the patient's MCLs for speech to determine symmetry between ears. Low discrimination scores for this test

should not be a reason for not considering amplification for the geriatric patient. Low discrimination scores in this test condition, particularly for persons with sloping high-frequency losses, are probably a result of inadequate sensation level for high-frequency speech sounds and upward spread of masking of louder low-frequency components in the speech spectrum. If scores are asymmetrical in the presence of symmetrical hearing loss, this should be assessed further to rule out active retrocochlear pathology. Unaided speech discrimination scores (using sentence-level material) also should be obtained in the sound field at 50 dB HL to determine the effect of increased audibility of speech sounds provided by the hearing aid on the aided versus unaided difference score.

In a less than optimal testing environment, such as the nursing home or multilevel retirement community, the effects of background noise are reduced for persons with thresholds of 40 dB HL at or above 500 Hz, particularly if insert earphones are used. Methods utilized include assessment of pure-tone thresholds and UCLs under earphones using a portable audiometer, and identification of recorded words under earphones using recorded speech and an audiometer with speech presentation capabilities. Probe microphone measures are invaluable in allowing a quick and reliable comparison of aided versus unaided ear canal sound pressure levels (insertion gain) or aided sound pressure level targets for various signal input levels, to assess adequacy of hearing aid gain without requiring subjective judgments from the patient. Aided versus unaided speech identification can be assessed in the sound field at a pragmatic distance of 3 feet with the clinician's speech being monitored at 55 to 60 dBA at the patient's location using a sound level meter. The speech stimuli used will vary with the abilities of the patient (standard word lists for more intact patients or abbreviated word lists emphasizing high-frequency words, the Ling-6 Sounds Test incorporated into real words [e.g., shaw, she, shoe, saw, see, sue], or a sentence level test, and more meaningful questions about the patient and his or her environment for less intact patients). Speech testing, aided versus unaided, also should be done with and without the use of lip cues to show the older patient the importance of enhancing hearing aid use by watching the speaker's face.

Assessment of Self-Perceived Handicap Imposed by the Hearing Loss

There are a variety of self-assessment inventories designed to allow patients to rate the psychological, social, vocational, and emotional handicaps imposed by their hearing losses.

Use of the Hearing Handicap Inventory for the Elderly-Screening Version (Ventry & Weinstein, 1982; Weinstein & Ventry, 1983) is recommended because it has been used and validated with hearing-impaired older persons typically seen in speech and hearing clinics. It is relatively short and assesses the critical concerns of the emotional, social, and situational effects of the hearing loss. Weinstein and Ventry found that older patients with pure-tone averages of 0 to 25 dB HL (500, 1000, 2000 Hz) almost never described their hearing losses as handicapping. Half of the patients with pure-tone averages of 26 to 40 dB HL perceived the hearing loss as a handicap and half did not. Older patients with hearing losses greater than 41 dB HL very often (88–92%) perceived their hearing loss as handicapping. There was, however, considerable variability even for the greater-than-40-dB loss group in the degree (mild to significant) of perceived handicap. Results for older persons were very similar to the results for younger persons, and audiometric data (e.g., pure-tone averages, speech reception thresholds, and speech discrimination scores) accounted for less than 50% of the variance in self-assessed hearing handicap. These results are consistent with the recommendation that, although pure-tone thresholds are important

for the description of the desired hearing aid electroacoustic parameters, they do not adequately describe the functional deficits imposed by a given hearing loss, particularly for losses less than 40 dB HL for the three high-frequency (1K Hz, 2kHz, and 4kHz) pure-tone average.

The Better Hearing Institute (BHI) Quick Hearing Check is a 15-item, 4-point Likert-scaled (0 = strongly disagree and 5 = strongly agree) hearing loss inventory based on the revised American Academy of Otolaryngology-Head and Neck Surgery (AAO-HNS) 5-minute hearing test is also an excellent tool for clients to determine their need for hearing help. Kochkin and Bentler (2010) report that it has excellent "face" validity as the items assess common problems of people with hearing loss that are generally accepted as signs of hearing loss by hearing care practitioners. The test is available to download on the BHI website (http://www.betterhearing.org) and can either be administered to clients or self-administered by them to determine how their perceptions of their hearing ability compare with others with confirmed hearing loss, how the significant others of others with similar hearing difficulty would describe the client's communication difficulty, and whether pursuit of a "hearing solution" (e.g., hearing aids/counseling) might be needed. Kochkin and Bentler report high validity (as compared with objective measures of hearing loss) and reliability of this instrument, and recommend it as "a tool (which) can be used for effectively providing consumers with more information about their hearing loss and moving those with hearing loss closer to seeking a hearing solution."

Mueller, Hawkins, and Sedge (1984) suggested that, for the majority of the hearing-impaired population who have potential for bilateral amplification, it is preferable to use compression, directional microphones, and binaural fitting. If the patient is over 70 years of age and a first-time hearing aid user, the recommendation for binaural fitting might be qualified, based on the person's ability to physically and mentally cope with, at first, just one new hearing aid and then, at a later time, possibly a second hearing aid. This must be weighed with the potential for a less than optimum experience with a unilateral fitting, because of the elimination of the client's access to the benefits of binaural aided signal processing (sound localization, ability to better "pick target speech" out of a background of noise (three-dimensional hearing), and the ability to "squelch" the affects of the noise by head movements that take advantage of differential amplified phase cues of sounds being delivered to each ear. Digital signal processing that enables binaurally fit hearing aids to "communicate with each," in order to maintain the relative loudness of amplified signals based on their actual differential phase and intensity cues have the potential to improve binaural hearing in noise over totally independent, binaurally fit hearing aids that may in fact use their compression systems to erroneously overcompress the gain in the aid closest to the sound (because it has a higher sound pressure level) possibly leaving the contralateral aid uncompressed, resulting in the sound in the aid closest to the sound being softer than that in the contralateral ear. Although the advantages of coordinated binaural hearing aid systems seem obvious, the challenge is to measure whether they are actually working using REMs as the obvious tool.

Prediction of Ability to Successfully Use Amplification

The Rupp Feasibility Scale for Predicting Hearing Aid Use (Rupp, Higgins, & Maurer, 1977) differentially weights factors of motivation, fault, initial impression, age, vision, significant others, self assessment, functional gain for speech, adaptability, manual dexterity, and financial resources and, accordingly, allows for scoring of each patient from poor (0) to excellent (100) prognosis for successful use of hearing aids. Hosford-Dunn and Baxter (1985) found that, in a group of 95 patients (mean age, 65 years) with mild-to-severe hearing losses at 1000 to 4000 Hz, clinician-assessed "motivation" and "initial subjective impressions of amplification" to be the two best predictors of long-term (first 3 months of aid use) satisfaction. As Hosford-Dunn and Baxter suggested, for patients older than 70 years of age, other factors of this instrument (e.g., assessment of digital dexterity, eye/hand coordination, and visual acuity) have predictive value as well and should not be eliminated for that population.

Verification of Hearing Aid Benefit

Whether the prescriptive approach is used with a presetting of the hearing instrument, or whether the instrument is adjusted to match prescribed amplification targets, it is important to remember that achievement of the targets cannot be assumed from manufacturer software predictions and must be measured. As stated previously, two verification methods are recommended: (1) probe-microphone measurements, and (2) aided loudness scaling.

Sound pressure level-based fitting algorithms display the DSL I/O targets on the screen of the real-ear system. Real-ear aided sound pressure level measurements then can be taken to determine closeness of fit of the actual aided sound pressure level measures to the DSL I/O targets. The aid then can be adjusted while the signal is present to bring the output levels within target values for the various input levels of 40 dB, 65 dB, and 90 dB. Probe microphone measurements can also be useful in assessing the effect of noise reduction algorithms when they are engaged, and the effectiveness of directional microphones using aided sound pressure level measures to determine if REM aided levels change significantly with changes in the location of the sound source. Real-ear probe microphone measures are comforting to the older patient in that their use builds trust with the dispenser. The patient is able to see targets for amplification represented on the equipment screen, the closeness of fit of the obtained real-ear data, and the relationship between changes in measures of real-ear insertion gain on the screen and changes in their perception of speech and other environmental sounds. Aided Speech Mapping is a particularly useful tool, as it enables the client to see how changes in amplified hearing levels will improve their ability to detect the presence of otherwise hard-to-hear speech sounds comparing amplified versus unamplified hearing levels using the "speech banana" or Articulation Index that predicts ability to understand speech (0–100%) based on the audibility of the range of speech frequencies.

Aided loudness scaling can be used to verify that desired gain is delivered across a wide range of input levels. Narrowband signals for three or more different frequencies can be used to assure that loudness is restored across frequencies for different inputs. With multichannel instruments, it is recommended that at least one frequency lies within each channel. Some hearing care professionals use a modified scaling technique for the aided speech testing modeled after the Independent Hearing Aid Fitting Forum (IHAFF) verification guidelines (Valente & Van Vliet, 1997). Speech inputs at three different levels (45, 65, and 85 dB SPL) are presented, and the patient is required to rate these speech inputs as "soft," "comfortable," and "loud but okay" (Zelisko, Wolf, & Burton, 1999). Other time-honored methods of loudness assessment include tolerance for clapping, sudden loud sounds such as keys dropping on a table top, a door slamming, and live-voice loud-speech at a 6-foot distance from the speaker.

Fine Tuning

Following verification of the performance of the hearing aids on each ear, the patient then can participate in the fine tuning of the hearing aid(s). Realear probe tube measurements using a composite signal provide the best method for real-time assessment of the effects of changes in such parameters as gain for soft, medium, and loud sounds in each channel, and channel specific compression thresholds and ratios. Unfortunately, as ques-

tionnaire inventories reveal, many dispensers avoid using real-ear measurements because they believe they take too much time, they think they "know" the hearing aids and the benefit being delivered, they don't have the equipment, or they are just too lazy. Real-ear probe tube measures are certainly less time-consuming than sound field functional gain measures, provide much more information, give the patient a means to monitor the effects of changes in hearing aid settings, and minimize the need for fine tuning beyond the weekly monitoring conducted during the trial period. As stated earlier, with the complexity of today's digital signal processing hearing aid technology, there is no better way for the hearing aid dispenser to determine if the appropriate amount of sound amplification is being delivered than through the use of REMs. To not use REMs in fitting hearing aids is a disservice to our clients, and borders on being unethical.

Validation Through Self-Assessment Inventories

On completion of the verification measures and fine-tuning adjustments, subjective validation of the effectiveness of the fitting is an essential component to the fitting and follow-up protocol. There are a variety of scales that can be used for this purpose. It is best to have the patient complete the scale at least twice, once prior to the fitting of the instrument(s) and at the completion of the trial period. Regardless of the instruments used, it is important that they be completed under the supervision of the clinician with the audiologist presenting each scale item in an interview context. The older patients often appreciate ongoing explanation of the rating scale and interpretation of the questions to minimize the chance for confusion during the completion of the inventory. Although there are many outcome scales available, the following are ones that have good utility with senior patients:

Hearing Handicap Inventory for the Elderly-Screening Version (HHIE-S; Ventry & Weinstein,

1982). This 10-item tool assesses both social and emotional handicap that is created by the hearing loss and the reduction of the handicap as a result of utilization of the hearing aid(s).

The Better Hearing Institute (BHI) Quick Hearing Check: 15-item, 4-point Likert-scaled (0 = strongly disagree and 5 = strongly agree) hearing loss inventory based on the revised American Academy of Otolarygnology-Head and Neck Surgery (AAO-HNS) 5-minute hearing test is also an excellent tool for clients to determine their need for hearing help. It assesses common problems of people with hearing loss that are generally accepted as signs of hearing loss by hearing care practitioners. The test is available to download on the BHI website (http://www.betterhearing.org) and can either be administered to clients or self-administered by them to determine how their perceptions of their hearing ability compare with others with confirmed hearing loss, how the significant others of others with similar hearing difficulty would describe the client's communication difficulty, and whether pursuit of a "hearing solution" (e.g., hearing aids/counseling) might be needed. It can be used for effectively providing consumers with more information about their hearing loss and serve as a pre-post test to assess benefit derived from the use of amplification and associated aural rehabilitation counseling.

Client Oriented Scale of Improvement (COSI; Dillon & Ginis, 1997). The COSI is a self-assessment scale in which, prior to hearing aid fitting, the patient selects and rank orders up to five communication settings/goals that are important to him or her. The scale then is readministered during the trial period and rehabilitation program, and at each visit, allows the patient to indicate the degree of change on a five-item scale from "worse" to "much better." This scale focuses the patients on their most important amplification goals and allows them to reassess the importance of these goals throughout the trial period.

Profile of Aided Loudness (PAL; Mueller & Palmer, 1998). The PAL is designed to assess if normal loudness restoration has been established. Patients rate their loudness perceptions for 12 real-world sounds (e.g., a door slamming, an electric razor, their own breathing, etc.) and also rate their satisfaction with the loudness levels of each ("just right" to "not good at all"). The results are compared with similar loudness ratings provided by normal-hearing listeners. This can be completed also by the normal-hearing spouse as a second assessment for the actual noises being rated by this patient in his or her environment (e.g., a barking dog, a clothes dryer that may be unusually loud in a given environment and not "typical").

As appropriate, the patient and his or her spouse should complete these questionnaires to triangulate what the patient is saying, with what the clinician is observing, and what a third party living in the patient's environment also is observing.

Participation in a Group Aural Rehabilitation Program (ReACT) During the Trial Period

It is essentially unethical to dispense amplification to elderly patients without the benefit of a structured individual or group follow-up aural rehabilitation program during the trial period with their new hearing aid(s). This is true of both new and experienced users, as experienced users typically are graduating to more sophisticated technology and can benefit from the technical support, the ongoing audiological assessment, and the social support of their peers. Northern and Beyer (1999) reported the hearing aid return rate was 3% for patients who attended a group aural rehabilitation (AR) program and 9% for those who did not. Other clinics have also reported a 3% return rate when using group AR program (Katz, 2002). Abrams, Chislom, and McArdle (2002) also found that dispensing a group aural rehabilitation program with a hearing aid fitting nearly doubled the cost effectiveness of their time spent when compared with fitting the hearing aid alone. Chisolm, Abrams, and McArdle (2004) found that noted improvements in patient's self-perception of their communication performance measured after the completion of a group AR program remained stable until follow-up testing a year later. Novak has titled his group AR program, "Rehabilitative Auditory Communication Training" (ReACT). It is helpful to have a meaningful acronym for the rehab program, so that it can be referred to easily both in advertisement ("Do you think you have a hearing loss . . . ReACT!") and discussion with the patient. This program is dispensed with the hearing aid, and the cost is bundled into the cost of the aid(s). It includes the attendance of the spouse, friend, or significant other of the person receiving the aids and typically is limited to about eight people per session. ReACT is a 3- or 2-hour per week family-centered program. The ultimate goal is to enable successful adjustment to and use of hearing amplification and reduce the hearing loss from the status of a handicapping condition to an inconvenience fully managed by the elderly patient and his or her family. Components of ReACT include:

■ Education of the patient regarding his or her hearing loss, the probable etiology, and other hearing disorders common to the elderly population,

■ Development of educated consumers regarding effective use of their new hearing aids and other assistive listening devices,

■ Development of new assertive communication skills, speech-reading skills, and an understanding of the commonality of communication, social, and emotional issues shared by seniors with hearing loss,

■ Use of the group process to seek solutions to hearing loss-related problems and, as a laboratory, to practice assertive communication techniques and communication repair strategies,

■ Ongoing electroacoustic fine tuning of the hearing aids using real-ear probe microphone measurements and modification of the physical characteristics of the earmold or ITE aids as needed according to the feedback from each patient, and

■ Gradual adjustment of the hearing aid electroacoustic parameters of the hearing aids

to achieve ultimate target goals as tolerated by the patient during the trial period.

The best schedule for ReACT for the elderly patient population is typically late morning or early afternoon. Saturday clinics are also an option. The majority of older patients do not want to drive at night and do not like early morning appointments or appointments that require driving in "rush hour" traffic or that interfere with traditional meal times.

SUMMARY

The aged hearing-impaired population presents infinitely complex diagnostic and rehabilitative challenges to hearing health care professionals. Older hearing aid candidates may have a variety of physical changes in addition to hearing loss that provide a complicated backdrop to problems created by hearing loss, or hearing loss may be their only significant disorder. Aged patients may present themselves alone with no one to assist in the aural rehabilitation process, or they may be warmly supported by a child, a spouse, or a friend in their adaptation to the use of hearing aids and new assertive communication skills. They may have predominantly cochlear-based sensorineural hearing loss and seem minimally different from their younger counterparts, or more typically they may have more difficulty understanding aided speech than would be predicted on the basis of their pure-tone audiograms. They may present themselves at hearing aid clinics because they truly realize the extent of their disability and desire rehabilitation or may come only to appease a significant other with no acknowledgment of responsibility for the communication problems they are having.

Knowledge of appropriate psychophysical data necessary to describe discretely the auditory function of presbycusic subgroups is incomplete. Our ability to model "normal" auditory function in each aged hearing-impaired patient with uniquely appropriate amplification is, therefore, also imperfect. The procedures that are used in the assessment of the aged client for use of amplification should specifically define unique cochlear versus central auditory function in presbycusic subgroups. The resultant data should be adaptable to a prescriptive approach for the fitting of state-of-the art hearing aids in a way that minimizes the time spent in hearing aid evaluation and fitting and maximizes time spent in counseling and family-centered aural rehabilitation.

In the final analysis, the clinician is best advised to listen to elderly clients and to understand, as much as possible, the perspective (cultural, social, psychological) of the client with respect to the hearing aid and aural rehabilitation process. Successful aural rehabilitation of the older client is possible only if there is mutual respect and honesty between the client and the hearing health care professional with sincere motivation of the client to fully participate in and ultimately take responsibility for their aural rehabilitation The onus is on the individual hearing health care professional to recommend the most appropriate hearing aid or aids and appropriately validate their function and benefit to the older client, provide supportive family-centered aural rehabilitation counseling, and involve the patient in a manner that will maximize independent use of all of the equipment and communication strategies offered.

REVIEW QUESTIONS

1. What are the various types of presbycusis, the bases for their classification, and the audiometric patterns unique to each?

2. What audiometric data are recommended to provide the basis for hearing aid selection for elderly patients?

3. Why are cultural considerations important when attempting to provide hearing aids to older patients whose culture identity is other than American.

4. How would you uniquely approach Asian Elders from the various subgroups described in this chapter, and how might these considerations apply to the aural rehabilitation of elderly clients from other cultures

5. Are two hearing aids always better than one for geriatric patients? How would you determine this in your patients, particularly when low communication demands and economics encourage consideration of monaural amplification?

6. Should today's complex digital signal processing hearing amplification systems ever be fit to a client or adjusted based on client feedback without the use of real-ear probe tube microphone (REM) measurements?

7. How would you take into consideration the concepts discussed in this chapter in counseling your geriatric patients about selecting from the array of hearing aid and assistive device technology that exists and that are described in greater detail elsewhere in this text?

8. Is there a relationship between the cost of the hearing aid and the expectations for success of the elderly hearing aid user?

9. Do the elderly have greater needs for support services than younger adult patients?

10. What methods would you propose to assess the patient's ability to manipulate the hearing aid that you are recommending?

11. What are the recommended steps in the Geriatric Hearing Aid Evaluation and Orientation Process?

12. Should hearing aids ever be delivered to first-time geriatric hearing aid users

without the support of initial and follow-up individual counseling or a group aural rehabilitation program conducted during the trial period?

REFERENCES

Abrams, H., Chisolm, T., & McArdle, R. (2002). A cost-utility analysis of adult group audiologic rehabilitation: Are the benefits worth the cost? *Journal of Rehabilitation Research and Development, 39*(5), 549–558.

Barford, J. (1979). Speech perception processes and fitting of hearing aids. *Audiology, 18,* 430–441.

Better Hearing Institute. (1999, June). Retrieved from http://www.betterhearing.org/demograp.htm

Bienvenue, G., & Michael, P. (1979). Digital processing techniques in speech discrimination testing (critical bandwidth measurements for use in hearing aid testing). In P. Yaneck (Ed.), *Rehabilitative strategies for sensorineural hearing loss.* New York, NY: Grune & Stratton.

Blackington, B., Novak, R. E., & Kramer, S. A. (1988). *Temporal masking effects for speech and pure-tone stimuli in normal hearing aged subjects* (Unpublished master's thesis). San Diego State University, San Diego, CA.

Cheng, L. R. (1988). Personal interview with R. E Novak. San Diego, CA.

Chmiel, R., Jerger, J., Murphy, E., Pirozzolo, F., & Tooley-Young, C. (1997). Unsuccessful use of binaural amplification by an elderly person. *Journal of the American Academy of Audiology, 8,* 1–10.

Chisolm, T., Abrams, H., & McArdle, R. (2004). Short and long-term outcomes of adult audiologic rehabilitation. *Ear and Hearing, 25*(5), 464–477.

Christensen, L., & Groth, J. (2008). *Top ten clinician mistakes in geriatric hearing aid fitting.* Seminar presented at American Academy of Audiology, Dallas, TX.

Danaher, E. N., Osberger, M., & Pickett, J. (1973). Discrimination of formant frequency transitions in synthetic vowels. *Journal of Speech and Hearing Research, 16,* 439–451.

deBoer, E., & Bowmeester, J. (1974). Critical bands and sensorineural hearing loss. *Audiology, 13,* 236–259.

deBoer, E., & Bowmeester, J. (1975). Clinical psychophysics. *Audiology, 14,* 274–299.

Dillon, H. J., & Ginis, J. (1997). Patient oriented scale of improvement (COSI) and its relationship to other means of benefit and satisfaction provided by hearing aids. *Journal of the American Academy of Audiology, 8,* 27–43.

Dubno, J. R., Dirks, D. D., & Morgan, D. E. (1984). Effects of age and mild hearing loss on speech rec-ognition in noise. *Journal of the Acoustical Society of America, 76,* 87–96.

Eisenberg, S. (1985). Communication with elderly patients: The effects of illness and medication on mentation, memory, and communication. In H. K. Ulatowska (Ed.), *The aging brain and communication in the elderly.* Boston, MA: College-Hill Press.

Fisch, L. (1978). Special senses: The aging auditory system. In J. C. Brocklehurst (Ed.), *Textbook of geriatric medicine and gerontology.* New York, NY: Churchill Livingstone.

Franklin, B. (1975). The effects of combining low- and high-frequency pass bands on consonant recognition in the hearing impaired. *Journal of Speech and Hearing Research, 18,* 719–727.

Ganz, R. P. (1976). The effects of aging on the diagnostic utility of the rollover phenomenon. *Journal of Speech and Hearing Disorders, 41,* 63–69.

Garstecki, D. C., & Erler, S. F. (1998). Hearing loss, control and demographic factors influencing hearing aid use among older adults. *Journal of Speech, Language and Hearing Research, 41,* 527–537.

Geissler, E. M. (1994). *Pocket guide to cultural assessment.* St. Louis, MO: Mosby.

Givens, G. D., Arnold, T., & Hume, W. G. (1998). Auditory processing skills and hearing aid satisfaction in a sample of older adults. *Perceptual and Motor Skills, 86,* 795–801.

Glorig, A., & Davis, H. (1961). Age, noise and hearing loss. *Annals of Otology, 70,* 556–571.

Glorig, A., & Nixon, H. L. (1962). Hearing loss as a function of age. *Laryngoscope, 27,* 1596–1610.

Gordon-Salant, S., & Fitzgibbons, P. J. (1999). Profile of auditory temporal processing in older listeners. *Journal of Speech-Language-Hearing Research, 42,* 300–311.

Greenblatt, N., & Chien, C. (1983). Depression in the elderly. In L. Breslau & M. Haug (Eds.), *Depression and aging—Causes, care and consequences.* New York, NY: Springer-Verlag.

Harbert, R., Young, J., & Menduke, H. (1966). Audiological findings in presbycusis. *Journal of Auditory Research, 6,* 297–312.

Hawkins, D. B. (1992). Prescriptive approaches to selection of gain and frequency response. In H. G. Mueller, D. B. Hawkins, & J. L. Northern (Eds.), *Probe microphone measurements.* San Diego, CA: Singular.

Hawkins, D. B., & Schum, D. J. (1984). Relationship among various measures of hearing aid gain. *Journal of Speech and Hearing Disorders, 49,* 94–97.

Hawkins, D. B., Walden, B., Montgomery, A., & Prosek, R. (1987). Description and validation of an LDL procedure designed to select SSPL90. *Ear and Hearing, 8,* 162–169.

Hawkins, J. E., Jr., & Johnsson, L. G. (1985). Otopathological changes associated with presbyacusis. *Seminars in Hearing, 6,* 115–132.

Hosford-Dunn, H., & Baxter, J. H. (1985). Prediction and validation of hearing aid wearer benefit: Preliminary findings. *Hearing Instruments, 36,* 34–41.

IHAFF unveils fitting protocol at Jackson Hole Rendezvous. (1994). *The Hearing Review, 9.*

Jerger, J. (1960). Békésy audiometry in analysis of auditory disorders. *Journal of Speech and Hearing Research, 3,* 275–287.

Jerger, J., Jerger, S., Oliver, T., & Pirozzolo, F. (1993). Speech understanding in the elderly. In B. R. Alford & S. Jerger (Eds.), *Clinical audiology: The Jerger perspective.* San Diego, CA: Singular.

Jerger, J., Tillman, T. W., & Peterson, J. L. (1960). Masking by octave bands of noise in normal and impaired ears. *Journal of the Acoustical Society of America, 32,* 385–390.

Katz, J. (2002). *Handbook of clinical audiology* (5th ed.). Baltimore, MD: Lippincott Williams and Wilkins.

Kochkin, S. (2007). MarkeTrak VII: Obstacles to adult nonuser adoption of hearing aids. *Hearing Journal, 60*(4), 27–43.

Kochkin, S. (2010). MarkeTrak VIII: Customer satisfaction with hearing aids is slowly increasing. *Hearing Journal, 63*(1), 11–19.

Kochkin, S., Beck, D., Christensen, L., Compton Conley, C., Fligor, B., Kricos, P., . . . Turner, R. (2010). MarkeTrak VIII: The impact of the hearing healthcare professional on hearing aid user success. *The Hearing Review,* 12–34.

Kochkin, S., & Bentler, R. (2010). The validity and reliability of the BHI Quick Hearing Check: An existing tool that can help guide more consumers to hearing help. *The Hearing Review, 17*(12), 12–28.

Krmpotic-Nemanic, J. (1971). A new concept of the pathogenesis of presbycusis. *Archives of Otolaryngology, 93,* 161–166.

Kujawa, S., & Liberman, C. (2009). Adding insult to injury: Cochlear nerve degeneration after "temporary" noise-induced hearing loss. *The Journal of Neuroscience, 29*(45), 14077–14085.

Kyle, J. G., Jones, L. G., & Wood, P. L. (1985). Adjustment to acquired hearing loss: A working model. In H. Orlans (Ed.), *Adjustment to adult hearing loss.* Boston, MA: College-Hill Press.

Kyle, J. G., & Wood, P. L. (1983). *Social and vocational aspects of acquired hearing loss.* Final report to MSC School of Education, Bristol. (Reported in Kyle, J. G., Jones, L. G., & Wood, P. L. [1985]. Adjustment to acquired hearing loss: A working model. In H. Orlans [Ed.], *Adjustment to adult hearing loss.* Boston, MA: College-Hill Press.)

Leshowitz, B., & Lindstrom, R. (1979) Masking and speech-to-noise ratio. *Audiology and Deaf Education, 6,* 5–8.

Lipman, A. (1968). A socio-architectural view of life in three homes for older people. *Gerontologica Clinica, 10,* 88–101.

Lynn, G. E., & Gilroy, J. (1976). Central aspects of audition. In J. Northern (Ed.), *Hearing disorders.* Boston, MA: Little, Brown.

Margolis, R., & Goldberg, S. (1980). Auditory frequency selectivity in normal and presbycusic subjects. *Journal of Speech and Hearing Research, 23,* 603–613.

Marshall, L. (1981). Auditory processing in aging listeners. *Journal of Speech and Hearing Disorders, 46,* 226–236.

Mauldin, C. R. (1976). Communication and the aging consumer. In H. J. Oyer & E. J. Oyer (Eds.), *Aging and communication.* Baltimore, MD: University Park Press.

Mayer, O. (1970). Das anatomische Substrat der Altersschwerhörigkeit [The anatomical substrate of old-age deafness]. *Archiv Ohren-Nasen-und Kehlkopf Heilkunde, 105,* 1313.

Medical Research Council Institute of Hearing Research. (1981). Population study of hearing disorders in adults. *Journal of the Royal Society of Medicine, 74,* 819–827.

Mills, J. H., Gilbert, R. M., & Adkins, W. V. (1979, February). *Some effects of noise on auditory sensitivity, temporal integration and psychophysical tuning curves.* Paper presented at Second Midwinter Research Meeting of the Association for Research in Otolaryngology, St. Petersburg, FL.

Mueller, H. G. (1997). Prescriptive fitting methods: The next generation. *Hearing Journal, 50,* 10–16.

Mueller, H. G., Hawkins, D., & Sedge, R. K. (1984). Three important variables in hearing aid selection. *Hearing Instruments, 35.*

Mueller, H. G., & Palmer, C. V. (1998). The profile of aided loudness: A new "PAL" for '98. *Hearing Journal, 51,* 10–16.

Musiek, F., & Rintelmann, W. (1999). *Contemporary perspectives in hearing assessment.* Boston, MA: Allyn & Bacon.

National Council on the Aging. (1999). *Survey of hard of hearing hearing aid users and non-users and their families.* Washington, DC: Author.

National Ear Care Plan. (1999, June). Retrieved from http://www.necp.com/hrstats.htm

Nelson, D. A. (1979, February). *Frequency selectivity in listeners with sensorineural hearing loss.* Paper presented at Second Midwinter Research Meeting of the Association for Research in Otolaryngology, St. Petersburg, FL.

Nixon, J. C., & Glorig, A. (1962). Changes in air and bone conduction thresholds as a function of age. *Journal of Laryngology, 76,* 288–292.

Northern, J., & Beyer, C. (1999). Reducing hearing aid returns through patient education. *Audiology Today, 20,* 143–150.

Novak, R. E., & Anderson, C. V. (1982). The differentiation of types of presbycusis using the masking level difference. *Journal of Speech and Hearing Research, 25,* 504–508.

Olsen, W. O., & Noffsinger, D. (1974). Comparison of one new and three old tests of auditory adaptation. *Archives of Otolaryngology, 99*, 94.

Olsen, W., Noffsinger, D., & Carhart, R. (1976). Masking level difference encountered in clinical populations. *Audiology, 15*, 287–301.

Palva, A., & Jokenen, H. (1970). Presbycusis v. filtered speech test. *Acta Otolaryngologica, 70*, 232–241.

Parenti, M. (1978). *Power and powerlessness*. New York, NY: St. Martin's Press.

Pascoe, D. (1988). Clinical measurements of the auditory dynamic range and their relation to formulas for hearing aid gain. In J. H. Jensen (Ed.), *Hearing aid fitting: Theoretical and practical views*. Copenhagen: Stougaard/Jensen.

Popelka, M. M., Cruickshanks, K. J., Wiley, T. L., Tweed, T. S., Klein, B. E., & Klein, R. (1998). Low prevalence of hearing aid use among older adults with hearing loss: The epidemiology of hearing loss study. *Journal of the American Geriatric Society, 46*, 1075–1078.

Potash, M., & Jones, B. (1977). Aging and decision criteria for the detection of tones in noise. *Journal of Gerontology, 32*, 436–440.

Purnell, L. D., & Paulanka, B. J. (1998). *Transcultural health care: A culturally competent approach*. Philadelphia, PA: F. A. Davis.

Reed, C. M., & Bilger, R. C. (1973). A comparative study of S/NO and E/NO. *Journal of the Acoustical Society of America, 53*, 1039–1044.

Rees, J. N., & Botwinick, J. (1971). Detection and decision factors in auditory behavior of the elderly. *Journal of Gerontology, 26*, 133–136.

Ries, P. W. (1994). Prevalence and characteristics of persons with hearing trouble: United States, 1990–91. National Center for Health Statistics. *Vital Health Statistics, 10*(188).

Rosen, S., Bergman, M., Plester, D., El Mofty, A., & Sotti, M. (1962). Presbycuses study of a relatively noise free population in the Sudan. *Annals of Otolaryngology, 71*, 727–743.

Rupp, R., Higgins, J., & Maurer, J. F. (1977). A feasibility scale for predicting hearing aid use (FSPHAU) with older individuals. *Journal of the Auditory Rehabilitation Association, 10*, 81–194.

Schmiedt, R. (1996). Effects of gaining on potassium homeostasis and the endocochlear potential in the gerbil. *Hearing Research, 102*, 125–132.

Schmiedt, R., Lang, H., Okamura, H., & Schulte, B. (2002). Effects of furosemide applied chronically to the round window: A model of metabolic presbyacusis. *The Journal of Neuroscience, 22*(21), 9643–9650.

Schow, R. L., Christensen, J. M., Hutchinson, J. M., & Nerbonne, M. A. (1978*). Communicative disorders of the aged*. Baltimore, MD: University Park Press.

Schow, R. L., & Goldbaum, D. E. (1980). Collapsed ear canals in the elderly nursing home population. *Journal of Speech and Hearing Disorders, 45*, 259–267.

Schow, R. L., & Nerbonne, M. A. (1980). Hearing levels among elderly nursing home residents. *Journal of Speech and Hearing Disorders, 45*, 124–132.

Schuknecht, H. F. (1964). Further observations on the pathology of presbycusis. *Archives of Otolaryngology, 80*, 369–382.

Schuknecht, H. F. (1974). *Pathology of the ear*. Cambridge, MA: Harvard University Press.

Schuknecht, H. F., & Gacek, M. R. (1993). Cochlear pathology in presbycusis. *Annals of Otology, Rhinology, and Laryngology, 102*, 1–16.

Seewald, R. C., Cornelisse, L. E., Ramji, K. V., Sinclair, S. T., Moddie, K. S., & Jamieson, D. G. (1997). DSL V 4 1a for Windows. A software implementation of the desired sensation level DSL i/o method for fitting linear gain and wide dynamic range compression hearing instruments. London, ON: University of Western Ontario.

Skafte, M. (1986). Communicate for a longer life. *Hearing Instruments, 37*, 4.

Spector, R. E. (1996). *Cultural diversity in health and illness*. Stamford, CT: Appleton & Lange.

Surr, R. K., Cord, M. T., & Walden, B. E. (1998). Long term versus short-term hearing aid benefit. *Journal of the American Academy of Audiology, 9*(3), 165–171.

Taeuber, C. (1992). *Sixty-five plus in America*. Washington, DC: U.S. Department of Commerce, Economics and Statistics Administration. Bureau of the Census.

Tyler, R. S., Fernandes, M., & Wood, E. J. (1984). Masking temporal integration and speech intelligibility in individuals with noise induced hearing loss. In G. Taylor (Ed.), *Disorders of auditory function III*. New York, NY: Academic Press.

Ulatowska, H. K. (1985). *The aging brain: Communication in the elderly*. Boston, MA: College-Hill Press.

Valente, M., & Van Vliet, D. (1997). The IHAFF protocol. *Trends in Amplification, 2*.

Ventry, L. M., & Weinstein, B. E. (1982). The hearing handicap inventory for the elderly: A new tool. *Ear and Hearing, 3*, 128–134.

Warren, L. R., Wagener, J., & Herman, G. (1978). Binaural analysis in the aging auditory system. *Journal of Gerontology, 33*, 731–736.

Weinstein, B. E., & Ventry, L. M. (1983). Audiometric correlates of the hearing handicap inventory for the elderly. *Journal of Speech and Hearing Disorders, 84*, 379–383.

Zelisko, D., Wolf, R., & Burton, P. (1999). Matching new technology to patient's needs. *The Hearing Review, 6*.

Zucker, K., & Williams, P. S. (1977, November). *Audiological services in extended care facilities*. Paper presented at the American Speech and Hearing Convention, Chicago, IL.

Zurek, P., & Formby, C. (1977). *Frequency discriminability of sensorineural listeners*. Paper presented at the Second Midwinter Research Meeting of the American Speech and Hearing Association, Chicago, IL.

Zwaardemaker, H. (1981). Der verlust an horen tonen mit zunehemendum alter: Ein neues gesetz [The loss to hear tone with increasing age: A new law]. *Arch Ohr Nas-Kehlk-Heilk, 32*, 53.

Zwicker, E., & Shorn, K. (1978). Psychoacoustical tuning curves in audiology. *Audiology, 17*, 120–140.

CHAPTER 12

Hearing Technology for Children

JACE WOLFE
SARA NEUMANN

**SELECTION OF APPROPRIATE HEARING AID
CHARACTERISTICS FOR CHILDREN**
Earmolds
Digital Signal Processing and Other Advanced
    Technology Features
Directional Microphones
Extended Bandwidth Technology
Frequency Lowering Technology
Binaural Signal Processing
Direct Auditory Input/Telecoil/Wireless Streaming
Prescriptive Methods for Selection of Real Ear
    Aided Gain and Maximum Output for Children
    Using Hearing Aids

**VERIFICATION TO ENSURE HEARING TECHNOLOGY
IS APPROPRIATE FOR THE PEDIATRIC WEARER**
Tips for Successful RECD Measurements
Real Ear Probe Microphone Measurements
SII/SHARP
Cortical Auditory Evoked Potentials
Aided Testing
Aided Speech Perception Testing

**PRACTICAL ISSUES TO ENSURE REAL-WORLD
SUCCESS**
Hearing Aid Orientation
Eyes Open, Ears On: Wear Time
Device Use in Older Children
Management and Follow-Up Care
Mentoring and Working with Families
Hearing Assistance Technology
Digital Radio Frequency Transmission
Adaptive RF Personal Systems
Additional Hearing Assistance Technology

**VALIDATION TO ENSURE THE PEDIATRIC HEARING
AID WEARER IS MEETING AGE-APPROPRIATE
GOALS AND EXPECTATIONS**
Monitoring Speech/Language Evaluations/Staffing

CONCLUSION

REFERENCES

INTRODUCTION

Because of the success of early hearing detection and intervention programs (i.e., universal newborn hearing screening and follow-up diagnostic services), children with hearing loss are typically identified within the first few weeks of the newborn period. Pediatric audiologists are faced with the challenge of providing hearing aids that provide consistent audibility for a wide range of speech sounds as well as other signals of interest, while also ensuring that the output of the hearing aids is safe and comfortable. This task is critically important as it is well established that optimal development of auditory and spoken language abilities are predicated upon consistent access of intelligible speech during the first 2 to 3 years of life (e.g., the critical period of speech and language development; Sharma, Dorman, & Spahr, 2002; Yoshinaga-Itano, Sedey, Coulter, & Mehl, 1998). Additionally, as children transition from the newborn period through the toddler years and eventually through the school-aged period and young adulthood, pediatric audiologists must be prepared to assist the child and family in addressing the unique obstacles encountered at each phase.

The goal of this chapter is to familiarize the reader with evidenced-based practices that seek to optimize the success that a child with hearing loss and his or her family achieve with hearing aids. The chapter is organized into five sections:

1. Assessment of auditory function and determination of candidacy for hearing technology.
2. Selection of appropriate hearing aid characteristics for children.
3. Verification to ensure hearing technology is appropriate for the pediatric wearer.
4. Practical issues to ensure real-world success.
5. Validation to ensure the pediatric hearing aid wearer is meeting age-appropriate goals and expectations.

The American Academy of Audiology (AAA) Task Force on Pediatric Amplification Guidelines recently drafted a document to provide a collection of evidence-based recommendations and practices to guide clinicians in providing best practices specific to the provision of amplification with the goal of meeting the comprehensive needs of children with hearing loss (AAA, 2013). In the AAA Clinical Practice Guideline on Pediatric Amplification, the task force states that the purpose of amplification is "to provide to an infant or child with impaired hearing, the opportunity to have access to as much of the auditory environment, and in particular speech, as feasible. Provision of appropriately amplified auditory input to the child with hearing loss maximizes the opportunities for the child to develop age-appropriate receptive and expressive oral communication, language development, literacy skills, and psychosocial skills." Furthermore, the Task Force defines the primary goal of amplification as the provision of audibility, "to the degree possible given the hearing loss and limitations of hearing aid amplification, across the long-term average speech spectrum (LTASS), without delivering any signal that is of an intensity that would either be uncomfortable or unsafe. Goals of amplification also include minimal distortion, appropriate signal-processing strategies for the listener, to provide features that maximize audibility of the desired signal and insofar as possible, provide a reduction of undesired signals (noise), to offer flexibility and ease of connection to external devices, and to facilitate physical comfort such that consistent, daily use is possible." These goals, along with the AAA Clinical Practice Guideline on Pediatric Amplification in general, serve as the overriding foundation on which the information presented in this chapter resides.

ASSESSMENT OF AUDITORY FUNCTION AND DETERMINATION OF HEARING TECHNOLOGY CANDIDACY

In order to provide appropriate amplification for young children, the audiologist must obtain a frequency-specific assessment of auditory function of both ears. Specifically, this assessment should determine the type, degree, and configuration of the child's hearing function for each ear. Professional guidelines indicate that a comprehensive evaluation of a child's auditory function should include otoscopy, a measure/estimate of air-conduction and bone-conduction hearing sensitivity for at least two frequencies, assessment of middle ear function, assessments of otoacoustic emissions, and a case history (ASHA, 2004; Joint Committee on Infant Hearing, 2007).

Electrophysiologic Assessment of Auditory Function: Factors Influencing Hearing Aid Fitting in Infants

The Joint Committee on Infant Hearing (2007) indicates that newborn hearing screening should be completed by 1 month of age; diagnostic audiologic assessment should be completed by 3 months for children who do not pass their newborn hearing screening, and intervention should be provided by 6 months for children who are identified with significant hearing deficits. For infants at risk for hearing loss, clinicians must rely on frequency-specific tone-burst ABR (tb-ABR; or auditory steady-state response [ASSR]) to obtain an ear-specific and frequency-specific assessment of auditory function. The interested reader is referred to these cited references for excellent information regarding the practical application of electrophysiologic assessment of auditory function in infants (British Columbia Early Hearing Program, 2008; Hall & Swanepoel, 2010; Newborn

Hearing Screening Programme, 2010; Stapells, 2011).

Research has demonstrated a strong correlation between infants' tb-ABR thresholds and behavioral thresholds (Stapells, 2011; Stapells, Gravel, & Martin, 1995). In general, tb-ABR provides a better approximation of behavioral threshold for higher frequency stimuli (e.g., 4000 Hz) than lower frequency stimuli (e.g., 500 Hz). Also, for the most part (65% of the time), infant tb-ABR thresholds (dB nHL) are generally 5 to 10 dB higher than behavioral thresholds (measured in dB HL). However, it is possible, albeit rare, that differences of 25 dB may exist between behavioral and tb-ABR thresholds. Conservative, frequency-specific correction factors have been proposed to estimate behavioral hearing sensitivity from tb-ABR thresholds (Table 12–1; Stapells, 2011).

These correction factors are subtracted from the tb-ABR threshold (db nHL) to obtain an estimated hearing level (dB eHL):

Equation 12–1:
tb-ABR threshold (db nHL) – correction factor (dB) = estimated behavioral hearing level (dB eHL).

For example, if the tb-ABR threshold at 2000 Hz is 60 dB nHL, then the 5 dB correction factor is subtracted to provide an estimated behavioral threshold of 55 dB eHL. It should be noted that these correction factors were developed from research studies conducted by David Stapells (Stapells, 2000, 2011; Stapells et al., 1995). In order for these correction factors to be applied to clinical tb-ABR information in a valid manner, the clinician should utilize ABR test parameters and acquisition methods similar to those

Table 12–1. Frequency-Specific Correction Factors to Estimate Behavioral Audiometric Thresholds (e.g., dB eHL) from tb-ABR Thresholds (dB nHL)

Frequency (Hz)	500	1000	2000	4000
Correction Factor (dB)	15	10	5	0

used by Stapells and colleagues whose work generated the correction factors. The reader is referred to Stapells (2011) for an excellent review of contemporary practices in electrophysiologic assessment of auditory function. Additionally, it should be noted that these correction factors are intended to be taken into account by the Desired Sensation Level Multistage Input/Output algorithm version 5.0 (DSL m[i/o] v5.0). Specifically, in some fitting platforms (e.g., Audioscan Verifit), the correction factors are automatically applied when the clinician specifies that the audiometric information being entered into the Verifit system are tb-ABR thresholds in dB nHL. Conceivably, one clinician could conduct ABR assessment and apply correction factors to provide an estimated audiogram in dB eHL to a second audiologist who will fit the child's hearing aids. Then, the second clinician could take those estimated hearing levels and erroneously apply the correction factors a second time resulting in an inaccurate estimate of hearing sensitivity. As such, it is important that clinicians who are providing services for a child with hearing loss must develop a protocol so that the correction factors used to arrive at dB eHL are only applied one time during the assessment and hearing aid fitting process. Details of the DSL m[i/o] v 5.0 fitting method are discussed later in this chapter.

The ASSR has also received a great deal of interest as a tool to estimate hearing sensitivity in infants (Rance, 2008). However, the ASSR does possess a few limitations relative to tb-ABR for the assessment of auditory function in infants. First, the ASSR frequently possesses a small amplitude in newborns, which may make it difficult to identify at levels consistent with behavioral threshold (John et al., 2004). Second, unlike the tb-ABR, there are no universally accepted correction factors to estimate behavioral thresholds from ASSR thresholds in newborns. Finally, more research is needed to determine a better understanding of the bone conduction ASSR in infants. It is possible that additional development of ASSR stimulus parameters and response acquisition techniques along with further research will eliminate the aforementioned limitations of ASSR and subsequently result in the routine inclusion of ASSR as a tool to estimate infants' hearing sensitivity.

Behavioral Assessment of Auditory Function: Factors Influencing Hearing Aid Fitting in Infants

Once an infant reaches 6 to 9 months developmental age, it is generally possible to evaluate the child's hearing sensitivity via visual reinforcement audiometry (VRA). It is important for the clinician to have a thorough appreciation for best practices associated with VRA assessment in order to avoid the attainment of insufficient and/or inaccurate information during VRA evaluation. The reader is referred to additional sources for an excellent review of best practices related to VRA assessment (Gravel, 2000; Widen, 1993).

Many experts suggest that VRA assessment is appropriate for use between the ages of 6 to 24 months (Gravel, 2000; Widen, 1993). However, the authors' anecdotal experience suggests that many infants and young children with hearing loss become uninterested in the VRA test paradigm after multiple applications to evaluate unaided and aided auditory function. As such, the authors encourage the auditory-verbal therapists with whom we work to begin practicing on a conditioned play audiometry response in the child's therapy sessions shortly after the child's first birthday. It is fairly common for children to develop a reliable conditioned play response by the time they are 18 months of age, a fact that greatly enhances the amount of diagnostic information clinicians may obtain in the infant and toddler years. For younger children, it is imperative that the clinician is equipped with a large number of engaging conditioned play audiometry tasks to acquire and maintain the child's attention throughout the test session. Figure 12–1 provides an example of some of the conditioned play tasks the authors have found to be successful in facilitating conditioned play response in young children.

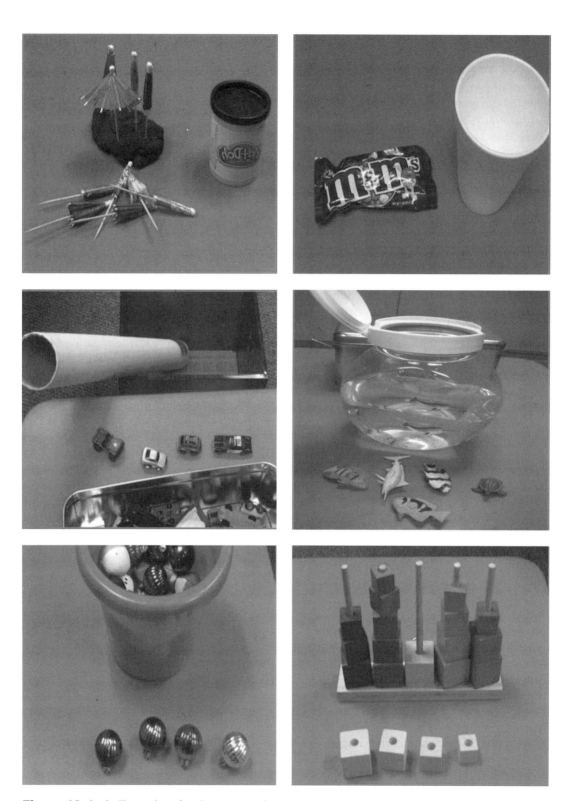

Figure 12–1. An illustration of various toys and games used to facilitate for conditioned play audiometry.

For both VRA and CPA unaided assessment, it is imperative to use insert earphones to present test signals. Presentation of test signals in the sound field does not allow for an ear-specific assessment of auditory function. The general audiometric advantages of insert earphones over supra-aural earphones are well documented, but particularly in the case of fitting hearing aids for children, the conversion of behavioral thresholds from dB HL to dB SPL at the tympanic membrane is more straightforward with the use of insert earphones relative to assessment with supra-aural earphones.

Although it is ideal to evaluate hearing sensitivity with insert earphones coupled to foam eartips, many infants and young children are reluctant to tolerate the insertion of the foam tips. To overcome this obstacle, Bagatto and Moodie (2007) described a clever solution in which the insert earphones are coupled to the child's personal earmolds. The clinician should attempt to attach the earmolds to the child's clothing so that the insert cartridges and tubing are out of the child's sight and reach (Figure 12–2).

In some cases, the tubing of the earmold will have been stretched out by the earhook of the child's hearing aid and cannot be not firmly coupled to the insert earphones. If this problem occurs, the clinician may place a small piece of tubing from a standard insert earphone foam tip onto the nipple connector of the insert earphones. This step should facilitate an intimate connection between the insert earphone and the child's earmold. It is important to note that the clinician should document whether a foam tip or an earmold was used for audiometric assessment, as the choice of coupling option will influence the sound pressure level that corresponds to threshold during testing. The same coupling option (e.g., earmold or foam tip) that is used for audiologic assessment should also be used for real-ear-to-coupler (RECD) measurement during the hearing aid fitting/verification. The RECD is discussed in detail later in this chapter including the impact the RECD has on audiometric threshold data.

Determining Candidacy for Hearing Technology

The Pediatric Working Group on Amplification for Children with Auditory Deficits stated that children who have thresholds equal to or poorer than 25 dB HL may be considered as candidates for amplification of some form (Pediatric Working Group, 1996). The AAA Clinical Practice Guideline on Pediatric Amplification (2013) states that some form of amplification system should be considered for "any type or degree of hearing loss that could possibly interfere with normal developmental processes."

Auditory Capabilities of Children with Hearing Loss

When considering whether hearing technology should be provided for a child with a hearing deficit, the clinician should consider the unique listening needs of young children. First, children do not have a lifetime of experience with language as adults do, and consequently, children are less able to take

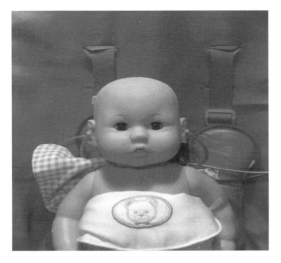

Figure 12–2. An illustration of proper placement of insert earphone cartridges and tubing for infants.

advantage of linguistic and contextual cues to extract information from an auditory signal. Instead, young children must rely on being able to faithfully decode the acoustical phonemic elements of speech to comprehend the auditory message.

Furthermore, children with normal hearing require a more favorable SNR than adults with normal hearing in order to adequately comprehend speech in the presence of competing noise. Likewise, children with hearing loss require a more favorable SNR than children with normal hearing in order to sufficiently understand speech in the presence of noise (Boothroyd, 1997). The ASHA guidelines state that children with hearing loss should be provided with a +15 dB SNR in order to effectively understand speech in the midst of competing noise (ASHA, 2005). Unfortunately, the SNR in typical classroom settings is often +5 dB or poorer (Sanders, 1965).

Additionally, children with hearing loss require greater sensation levels in order to comprehend low-level (e.g., soft) speech (Scollie et al., 2005). Nozza (1988) reported that infants with hearing loss require a sensation level that is 20 dB higher than adults in order to achieve similar understanding for soft-level speech. In contrast, studies do show that children with hearing loss have a similar threshold of discomfort for high-level sounds as adults with hearing loss (Kawell, Kopun, & Stelmachowicz, 1988). The provision of a higher level output for low-level (e.g., soft) inputs is particularly an important consideration as it is well known that a great deal of what children learn about speech and language arises from their access to speech that is not directly intended for the child but rather arrives incidentally. Incidental listening refers to the act in which a child listens in on or "overhears" the conversation of two bystanders in the room. Researchers have suggested that as much as 60 to 90% of a child's speech and language development is contingent upon incidental listening (Ching, 2009; Cole & Flexer, 2007). Incidental listening often occurs to a speech signal that has originated from across the room from the child, and as a result, the signal is low in level

by the time it reaches the child. As such, it is critical for children to have full-time and sufficient audibility for low-level sounds.

Relatively recent research has also shown that children with hearing loss also require a wider bandwidth in order to optimize their ability to understand speech. Stelmachowicz and colleagues (2002) conducted an elegant study in which they examined speech understanding for low-pass filtered speech tokens (/isi/, /ithi/, /ihi/), and determined that adults required a bandwidth extending to 6000 Hz in order to reach asymptotic performance levels. In contrast, children with hearing loss required a bandwidth extending to 9000 Hz to optimize understanding of high-frequency phonemes such as /s/. This finding is important, because high-frequency phonemes contribute a great deal to the clarity and meaning of speech. For instance, the phoneme /s/ is the third most frequent used phoneme is English speech, and possesses an important semantic and grammatical role in English speech, including the signification of plurality, verb tense, and possessiveness. These findings are also of great concern, because young children often spend the majority of their days listening to the speech of other children and women, both of which possess a considerable amount of information in the high frequencies.

The question of whether to recommend hearing technology for children is straightforward for children who have bilateral hearing loss that is moderate in degree or poorer and whose families want their child to listen and talk. These children will develop significant delays in auditory and spoken language abilities without consistent use of appropriate hearing technology. The question of whether hearing technology should be provided for a child with an auditory deficit becomes more complicated for children with unilateral hearing loss, minimal/mild hearing loss, rising hearing loss, discrete high-frequency hearing loss in the presence of normal low- and mid-frequency hearing, and auditory neuropathy spectrum disorder. Because each of these situations is unique, the proceeding discussion addresses these items separately.

Children with Minimal to Mild Hearing Loss

Bess, Dodd-Murphy, and Parker (1998) defined minimal and mild hearing loss as a bilateral sensorineural hearing loss with average pure-tone thresholds in the 20 to 40 dB range. Numerous studies have shown that children with mild hearing loss experience significant difficulties in multiple domains (e.g., communication, psychosocial, emotional, academic, etc.) when compared with children with normal hearing. For instance, Ross and Giolas (1971) measured monosyllabic word recognition for phonetically balanced words presented at 65 dB SPL to children with mild hearing loss and with normal hearing, and reported mean scores of 46% correct and 91% for the hearing-impaired and normal-hearing children, respectively. Additionally, Crandell (1993) evaluated sentence recognition in noise for 20 children with normal hearing and 20 children with slight to mild hearing loss and found poorer speech recognition in noise for the children with minimal hearing loss.

Research has also shown that children with mild hearing loss are at significant risk for academic difficulties, language disorders, increased stress, emotional and behavioral problems, as well as fatigue from increased listening effort (Bess, Dodd-Murphy, & Parker, 1998; Davis, Elfenbein, Schum, & Bentler, 1986). Bess and colleagues (1998) evaluated audiologic, psychosocial, and education outcomes of 1,228 children in grades 3, 6, and 9 from the Nashville Metropolitan School District. Of the children in this sample who were identified with mild hearing loss, 37% failed at least one grade, compared with less than a 3% failure rate for children with normal hearing. Additionally, third-grade students with mild hearing loss scored significantly poorer than normal hearing children on the CTBS/4 subtests for reading vocabulary, reading total, language mechanics, word analysis, basic battery, spelling, and science.

Sixth- and ninth-grade children in the Bess et al. (1998) study also completed the COOP Adolescent Method (COOP) assessment to evaluate potential difficulty in the physical, social, and emotional domains. Children with mild hearing loss reported lower energy levels and self-esteem, and higher stress when compared with children with normal hearing.

Furthermore, Bourland-Hicks and Tharpe (2002) examined listening effort and fatigue while children with normal hearing and mild hearing loss listened to speech in quiet and in a variety of SNRs. Although no differences were observed in fatigue experienced by the two groups, the children with mild hearing loss did require greater listening effort when asked to simultaneously attend to a visual and auditory stimulus. Specifically, children were asked to repeat words in the presence of noise while also pushing a button any time an LED light appeared on a screen positioned in front of them. The children with hearing loss required a longer amount of time to push the button when the light appeared indicating that more effort and cognitive facilities were being assigned to the listening task.

Finally, Elfenbein et al. (1994) examined oral communication aptitude in a group of elementary-aged children with a range of hearing loss, and concluded that children with mild hearing loss possessed more articulation errors and pragmatic mistakes, which may be attributed to reduced access to morphological markers in speech. Children with mild hearing loss in the study also reported that they perceived errors in their own speech and experienced difficulty producing intelligible speech.

In their landmark study of children with minimal to mild hearing loss, Bess and colleagues (1998) reported that to their knowledge, none of the children with mild hearing loss used hearing aids and noted that "additional research is needed on the efficacy of amplification" for children with mild hearing loss. The sentiment that there is no consensus of appropriate amplification technology for children with mild hearing loss was reiterated in a review of amplification considerations for children with mild hearing loss by McKay, Gravel, and Tharpe (2008), who suggested that more studies are needed to determine appropriate hearing aid technologies for children with minimal and mild hearing loss.

Although there is a paucity of studies demonstrating the benefits of hearing technology for children with mild hearing loss, the AAA Clinical Practice Guideline on Pediatric Amplification (2013) does state that "children with minimal and mild hearing loss are at high risk for experiencing academic difficulty and may be considered candidates for amplification systems." Given the aforementioned difficulties and limitations associated with pediatric minimal and mild hearing loss, the authors of this chapter routinely recommend amplification for children with mild hearing loss. This decision should be made with the family in order to determine that the medical (i.e., additional disabilities), communication, social-emotional, and academic needs that are unique to each child as managed is a manner that is satisfactory for the child and family.

Children with Unilateral Hearing Loss

Unilateral hearing loss is identified as a pure-tone average of at least 20 dB HL or pure-tone thresholds of at least 25 dB HL at two or more frequencies above 2000 Hz in the affected ear with an average pure-tone threshold in the good ear of no more than 15 dB HL. It is well-known that unilateral hearing loss results in difficulty understanding speech that originates from the side of the poorer ear (e.g., head shadow effect; Ruscetta, Arjmand, & Pratt, 2005), difficulty understanding speech in noise (Bess, Tharpe, & Gibler, 1986), and difficulty localizing the origin of a sound (Bess, Tharpe, & Gibler, 1986).

Numerous studies have also shown that children with unilateral hearing loss experience considerable difficulties with communication and academic challenges (Bess et al., 1998; Bess et al., 1986). Research suggests that children with unilateral hearing loss are 10 times more likely to fail a grade than children with normal hearing (Bess et al., 1998; Oyler, 1988). An additional 13% to 60% will require special services to succeed in school settings (Bess & Tharpe, 1984; Tharpe, 2008),

and children with unilateral hearing loss typically have more behavior problems and report higher levels of stress and lower self-esteem than their counterparts with normal hearing (Bess et al., 1998).

Because of the difficulties discussed above, the AAA Clinical Practice Guideline on Pediatric Amplification states that "children with aidable unilateral hearing loss should be considered candidates for amplification in the impaired ear." The AAA Clinical Practice Guideline on Pediatric Amplification also suggests that amplification should be considered for children with severe-to-profound hearing loss in the poorer ear as long as the child's age and ability allow for them to control their environment based on what they receive from their hearing technology. Various amplification options for children with unilateral hearing loss are discussed later in this chapter. It should be noted that the AAA Clinical Practice Guideline on Pediatric Amplification states that there are not enough data available to inform clinicians sufficiently about how we should proceed with selecting amplification for children with unilateral hearing loss. Furthermore, research has produced mixed results regarding the efficacy of amplification in reducing the deleterious effects of unilateral hearing loss in children (Tharpe, 2007).

Children with Permanent Conductive Hearing Loss

Children with permanent conductive hearing loss are certainly at risk for speech and language delays, and as such, they should be fitted with amplification to optimize access to speech and environmental sounds. Air-conduction hearing aids may be considered if the child's anatomy allows for the use of a behind-the-ear hearing aid (i.e., sufficient auricle and external ear canal to allow for hearing aid retention). Bone-conduction hearing devices are particularly appealing for children with aural atresia because of the obvious complications associated with hearing aid retention. However, research has suggested that bone-conduction hearing devices may provide better sound quality and performance than air-conduction hearing aids when the air-bone gap exceeds 30 dB (Mylanus, Van der Pouw, Snik, & Cremers, 1998). Surgically implanted bone-anchored hearing devices are not typically considered for use in children until 5 years of age. However, the bone-conduction hearing device processor may be worn on a softband by infants and young children.

Children with Auditory Neuropathy Spectrum Disorder

Controversy has existed over whether children with auditory neuropathy spectrum disorder (ANSD) benefit from hearing aids. Berlin and colleagues have suggested that children with ANSD typically do not receive significant benefit from hearing aids (Berlin et al., 2009), whereas others have suggested that some children with ANSD receive substantial benefit from hearing aid use (Rance, 2005; Roush, Frymark, Venediktov, & Wang, 2011). A recent meta-analysis by Patricia Roush and colleagues (2011) indicated that about one half of children who had ANSD and were fitted with hearing aids experienced significant improvement in their speech understanding (Roush et al., 2011), while the other one-half showed little to no open-set speech recognition with the use of hearing aids.

The AAA Clinical Practice Guideline on Pediatric Amplification (2013) states that children with ANSD "should have a trial with amplification as soon as it can be established that hearing sensitivity is sufficiently poor that speech conversational levels will not be easily audible." Hearing aids are typically fitted for children with ANSD on the basis of behavioral audiometric thresholds and fine-tuned on the basis of follow-up audiologic assessment and information derived from standardized questionnaires completed by the child's family.

Sharma and colleagues (2011) have shown that early provision of amplification results in better auditory brain development and auditory skill development for children with ANSD. As such, it is desirable to fit hearing aids as early as possible for children who have ANSD and have limited access to speech. However, it is often impossible to obtain a reliable behavioral audiogram in this population until at least 6 to 9 months of age. Some researchers have explored the cortical auditory evoked potential (CAEP) as a tool to determine whether hearing aids should be fitted for children with ANSD, and if so, how the hearing aids should be programmed (Pearce, Golding, & Dillon, 2007). Once hearing aids are fitted, the clinician should also administer standardized questionnaires to determine whether the goals of amplification have been met (see the section on validation in this chapter). It should be noted that children with ANSD secondary to Otoferlin mutations typically do not receive benefit from hearing aid use, because the impairment that exists at the synapse between inner hair cells and auditory nerve fibers (Berlin et al., 2009).

Cochlear implants (CI) are often considered for children who have ANSD with speech and language delays and who do not benefit from hearing aids. Roush and colleagues (2011) did report that CIs typically provide considerable benefit for children with ANSD, but they also noted that as many as 27% of children with ANSD achieve open-set speech recognition scores of less that 30% after implantation. Poor performance with a CI is likely related to the etiology of the ANSD or to a late age at implantation. Research has shown poorer CI outcomes for children who were born without auditory nerves (Buchman et al., 2006). Considering this, the managing CI surgeon should obtain an magnetic resonance imaging (MRI) scan using the cochlear nerve protocol to evaluate the integrity of the auditory nerve prior to cochlear implantation. Cochlear implant outcomes may also be poor if ABR abnormalities are attributed to brainstem dysfunction rather than a site of lesion in the cochlea, at the synapse, or with the auditory nerve (Gibson & Sanli, 2007). Finally, provision of cochlear implantation after the cessation of the critical period of language development would also quite likely result in a poorer outcome for a child with ANSD much in the same way that late implantation affects all children who have hearing loss and who are not exposed to intelligible speech during the first few years of life.

Routing of Signal

Once the hearing loss has been identified, the provider needs to determine how the sound of interest will be transmitted from the child's personal hearing technology to the child's auditory system; this is referred to as routing of the signal. Options include air conduction, bone conduction, electrical stimulation, or a combination of any of these routing options (AAA Clinical Practice Guideline on Pediatric Amplification, 2013). The choice of how to route the signal is influenced by several factors including whether the hearing impairment is unilateral or bilateral, as well as the degree, configuration, and type of hearing loss. When hearing loss occurs in both ears, bilateral amplification is typically the standard of care. However, there are times, when bilateral amplification may not be the optimal choice (i.e., binaural amplification results in poorer speech recognition than use of a hearing aid on the better ear alone (binaural interference); physical abnormalities such as atresia or other outer ear anomalies.

Considering the type and degree of loss allows you to determine what type of hearing aid should be selected or if a cochlear implant or other implantable hearing technology may be an option. Digital air-conduction BTE hearing aids are ideal for most children with mild-to-moderate sensorineural hearing loss.

Alternatives to Bilateral Air-Conduction Hearing Aids

There are times, however, when air conduction devices are contraindicated or do not represent the ideal choice of hearing technology for a child with a hearing impairment.

In these cases, other devices may be recommended. For children that have chronically draining ears or other outer or middle ear anomaly (e.g., atresia, microtia, cholesteatoma, congenital ossicular chain defect, etc.), wearing air conduction hearing aids may be difficult or impossible. For these cases, a suitable alternative is bone-anchored hearing aids (BAHAs). BAHAs route the signal of interest to the cochlea via bone conduction, essentially bypassing the affected outer or middle ear. BAHA devices are typically the gold standard hearing technology for children with bilateral aural atresia and are often the only option to allow these children access to intelligible speech for listening and spoken language development. Furthermore, research has suggested that BAHA devices provide better performance than air-conduction hearing aids for persons with a conductive component (i.e., air-bone gap) exceeding 30 dB (Hol, Snik, Mylanus, & Cremers, 2005; Snik et al., 2005).

Additionally, BAHA devices may also be considered for children with single-sided deafness. The BAHA device is placed on the side of the poorer ear, and the signal it captures is transmitted via bone conduction to the better hearing ear on the contralateral side.

The BAHA system is designed for a titanium abutment to be implanted into the skull. The BAHA processor is coupled to the abutment so that vibrations from the processor are transmitted directly to the implanted abutment. Because the skull is not sufficiently thick during the first few years of life, the implanted abutment is not commercially approved by the U.S. FDA for children under 5 years of age. For children under 5 years of age, the BAHA processor may be held to the head by a headband (e.g., softband). Those children typically wear the processor on the softband until they are 5 years old and/or their skull is thick enough to undergo the surgical procedure. It should be noted that the signal is attenuated by about 15 dB when the processor is worn on the skin rather than the abutment (Hakansson, Tjellstrom, & Rosenhall, 1984).

Another option for children with single-sided deafness is a contralateral routing of signal (CROS) hearing aid. In the case of a wireless CROS fitting, a receiver or microphone (cased in a device that looks like a BTE or ITE hearing aid) sits on or in the affected ear, and the signal is wirelessly delivered via radio frequency transmission to an air-conduction hearing aid positioned on the better. In a CROS system, the hearing aid on the better ear is programmed to provide little to no gain, so that is essentially transparent to the unaided condition. In the case where the better ear also has some hearing loss, a bilateral CROS (BICROS) may be considered. A BICROS is similar in function to a CROS except for the fact that the gain/output of the device on the better hearing ear is programmed to match a generic prescriptive target in order to overcome the hearing loss of that ear.

CROS hearing aids have been shown to overcome the head shadow effect (Punch, 1988). However, it is unlikely CROS hearing aids will improve localization for a child with asymmetrical hearing loss, and speech recognition may actually decrease with CROS use when the signal of interest originates from the side of the better ear and the competing noise is dominant at the poorer ear (Valente, Sweetow, Potts, & Bingea, 1999). In such a case, older children and adults should be instructed to turn off the microphone/transmitter on the side of the poorer ear. Because young children are unlikely to be able to follow through with this instruction, a CROS is not an ideal option for infants and toddlers with hearing loss. Furthermore, because all children with asymmetrical hearing loss or single-sided deafness or asymmetrical hearing loss are likely to experience difficulty understanding speech in the presence of noise, audiologists should routinely consider wireless remote microphone technology (e.g., personal digital radio frequency/FM system) for this group.

Electrical Stimulation

Cochlear implantation may be considered for children with severe-to-profound hearing loss. In fact, cochlear implantation is likely the ideal hearing technology for children with profound hearing loss. Some children with severe hearing loss will receive satisfactory benefit and performance from hearing aids, while others will require cochlear implantation for at least one ear to facilitate adequate speech, language, and auditory skill development. It is imperative for the audiologist to partner with an auditory verbal therapist or speech-language pathologist who is well-acquainted with typical auditory and spoken language development in order to determine whether an infant or young child is making age-appropriate progress in auditory, speech, and language development. Cochlear implantation should be considered when progress is significantly poorer than what would be expected for a child of similar corrected age and nonverbal IQ. It should be noted that cochlear implants are not commercially approved by the FDA for children under 1 year of age. However, an emerging trend in pediatric hearing health care is the provision of cochlear implants prior to 1 year of age for children with profound hearing loss.

Many children with bilateral severe-to-profound hearing loss use two cochlear implants. Children who receive one cochlear implant should continue to use a hearing aid on the opposite ear, unless the clinicians' assessment indicates that contralateral hearing aid use is detrimental. In such a case, bilateral cochlear implantation should be considered.

For patients with precipitously sloping hearing losses, where better low-frequency hearing sensitivity is in the normal to moderate range, and high-frequency hearing is in the severe to profound range, electro-acoustic (EAS) stimulation (e.g., hybrid cochlear implant) may be the best option. This is achieved by providing amplification for low-frequency sounds via a hearing aid and providing electrical stimulation for high-frequency sounds via a cochlear implant. The efficacy of hybrid cochlear implants is currently being investigated in FDA clinical trials, but at the time of this writing, hybrid cochlear implants are not commercially available for adults or children in the United States. Hybrid cochlear implants are commercially available in most European countries.

Special Considerations for Children with Unilateral Hearing Loss

Children with unilateral hearing loss are known to struggle in background noise, experience difficulty with sound localization, and are more likely to repeat a grade in school (Bess et al., 1998). However, it is important to note that there is a paucity of evidence describing the efficacy of different hearing technologies for children with unilateral hearing loss, and consequently, there is no standard recommendation in regards to the ideal amplification solution for this group. If an infant or young child is diagnosed with a conductive or sensory hearing loss that is moderate in degree or better, then amplification should be considered to reduce the chances of auditory deprivation and insufficient development of the auditory nervous system contralateral to the ear with hearing loss (Ponton, Eggermont, Kwong, & Don, 2000; Sharma et al., 2002). For children with mild-to-moderate sensory or conductive unilateral hearing loss, amplification of the poor ear is likely to be beneficial, and as a result, it should be considered shortly after the diagnosis of the hearing impairment. However, for children with severe to profound unilateral hearing loss, the provision of amplification for the poorer ear may possibly result in binaural interference, either from distortion introduced by the poorer ear or from crossover of the high-gain amplified signal to the better hearing ear. As such, the audiologist should exercise caution when deciding whether to recommend amplification for children with severe-to-profound hearing loss. As previously mentioned, the type of hearing technology suggested for children with unilateral hearing loss may range from a traditional BTE hearing aid, a personal wireless remote microphone system, a CROS hearing aid, or a BAHA device. Additionally, some reports are suggesting that cochlear implantation may be beneficial for persons with single-sided deafness (Arndt et al., 2011; Baguley, 2010; Buechner et al., 2010). Because each child is different and may or may not benefit from a device, a trial with amplification is always recommended. Feedback from the child, parents, as well as the child's therapists and teachers will help determine the best solution for each child.

Regardless of the decision to provide hearing technology, the clinician must closely monitor the speech, language, and auditory development of children with unilateral hearing loss. The authors of this chapter recommend using a monitoring protocol beginning at the time the child is identified with a unilateral hearing loss. A suggested protocol includes routine audiological monitoring every 3 months up to age 5 years, and every 6 months thereafter. Speech and language development should also be closely monitored. If the child does not make 6 months progress in a 6-month time interval, then auditory verbal therapy or speech-language therapy should be considered. In this case, the provision of hearing technology should also be considered.

SELECTION OF APPROPRIATE HEARING AID CHARACTERISTICS FOR CHILDREN

Once the degree, type, and configuration of hearing loss are determined, the most appropriate hearing technology may be selected for the child. There are many considerations when selecting a hearing aid for a child (i.e., type, power level, technology features, and safety). A BTE hearing aid model is recommended for young children primarily because it can accommodate continuous changes in ear growth by using a replaceable earmold. The BTE hearing aid comes in many different sizes and power levels to address varying degrees of hearing loss. Historically, BTE hearing aids have been large and cumbersome, but as technology continues to improve and become miniaturized, BTE hearing aids continue to get smaller without compromising on technology features. This is especially helpful for retention in very young children. It is important, however, that the audiologist selects a hearing aid based on the child's hearing loss and power needs, not on cosmetics. This can also be part of the counseling process for parents to understand why a specific hearing aid is selected. With that said, the audiologist should resist the temptation to select a hearing aid with a greater fitting range than is necessary to meet the needs of the child. Hearing aids with exceptionally high gain and output capabilities may possess higher internal noise levels that may degrade the sound quality of the signal for a child with lesser degrees of hearing loss.

Additionally, many BTE hearing aids come with direct audio input (DAI) capabilities, which should be considered as a mandatory feature of pediatric hearing technology. DAI allows for use of personal frequency modulated (FM)/digitally modulated (DM) systems, which are necessary to optimize young children's performance in noisy and reverberant environments as well as when the primary of signal of interest originates for a more than a few feet from the child. Furthermore, telecoils, tamperproof battery doors, and pediatric earhooks should be selected for hearing aids fitted to children. Also, the ability to deactivate volume and program controls in the software is necessary. Recently, hearing aids have also become increasingly water-resistant with some even claiming to be waterproof. Water resistance is certainly an attractive feature for infants who put their hearing aids in their mouth and for older children who are active in sports and water activities.

An ITE hearing aid is contraindicated for infants and young children for many reasons including but not limited to: (1) small size can present a choking hazard, (2) the device cannot be easily modified/changed as a child grows, and (3) the hard shell can put a child at risk for trauma to the ear from blows to the head. In addition, ITE hearing aids do not often have many of the features necessary for children, including DAI compatibility for hearing assistance technology (HAT), built in wireless, and telecoils. The growth of the external ear slows considerably by about 8 years of age, so an ITE hearing aid may be considered at that time. However, the potential for trauma to the ear during sports, as well as the lack of optimal access to HAT remain.

Additional options for hearing aids that were previously only recommended for adults include an acoustic slim-tube configuration with a BTE or a BTE aid with a receiver in the canal (RIC) hearing aid. A standard or mini BTE can be coupled to the ear by an acoustic thin tube with a dome or traditional type of earmold (AAA Clinical Practice Guideline on Pediatric Amplification, 2013). Thin tube devices will likely decrease the output of the hearing aid relative to a traditional earmold. As such, real ear verification measures are imperative to ensure appropriate output for low-level, conversational-level, and high-level speech.

Receiver in the canal (RIC) hearing aids, created with the receiver in the ear canal rather than within the BTE, allow for a smaller device while maintaining the power of a larger device. If these models are to be selected, it is important to consider whether the child's ear is large enough to accommodate the receiver size. Also, the clinician should keep in mind the fact that placement of the receiver in the ear canal makes it more susceptible to damage from cerumen, moisture, and so on. Finally, many RIC devices are quite small and may possess DAI or a telecoil, and may not allow for personal FM/DM use or access to HAT.

Earmolds

It is fairly typical for children identified in the first months of life to require in excess of 15 to 20 new earmolds during their first year of life. This is especially true for children with severe high-frequency hearing loss. Earmolds often must be replaced weekly during the first 3 to 4 months of life, and every other week from 4 to 6 months of age. External ear growth begins to taper off between 6 to 12 months of age, and as a result, earmold remakes are not required nearly as frequently after the child's first year.

Style and Material

A full-shell earmold with a helix lock should be used with infants, while preschool and early elementary aged children may use a full-shell or skeleton style earmold. A helix lock may not be necessary for children who are of preschool age and older. Alternative earmold styles (e.g., half-shell, canal, etc.) may be selected for older children (≥ 6 years of age).

Earmolds come in acrylic, vinyl, and silicone material. Earmold material should be soft. Vinyl earmolds are usually ideal for children during the first 6 months of life, because medical grade silicone material is often too pliable, making it difficult to insert into the soft external ear of an infant. Medical grade silicone material should be considered for children 7 months and older. In some cases, hypoallergenic earmold materials may be necessary to prevent a reaction to the earmold. Materials that are considered hypoallergenic include: polyethylene, implant grade silicone, and poly methyl methacrylate (Microsonic Earmold Laboratories, 2006). Although it is rare, it should be noted that color dyes may increase the chances of an allergic reaction in some children. Longer earmold canal stalks may be beneficial for children as the longer canal portion may: (1) potentially reduce the chances of feedback, (2) increase the sound pressure level at the eardrum without need to increase the electrocscoustic gain, and (3) enhance sound quality (AAA Clinical Practice Guideline on Pediatric Amplification, 2013). Additionally, because young children often pull their hearing aids out of their ears by grabbing the earmold tubing, the clinician should request that the earmold laboratory couples the tubing to the mold via tubing cement or a sturdy adhesive.

Earmold Acoustics

Earmold configuration and acoustics are an often neglected area of audiology. Rather than relying on the digital signal processing to do all of the work in delivering the acoustic signal to the ear, an earmold should be acoustically designed to complement the hearing aid processing. The selection of an appropriate earmold style and features will help ensure that prescriptive targets can be met for a particular child with a given hearing configuration. The earmold acoustics should also be reflected within the hearing aid software for appropriate fitting guidelines to be incorporated into the fitting. In general, venting influences low-frequency sound transmission, damping influences mid-frequencies, and horn influences high-frequency transmission (Microsonic Earmold Laboratories, 2006). Of course, a large vent will limit the amount of available gain before feedback across all frequencies. The authors provide the following recommendations for ideal earmold fit and satisfaction in children (See Table 12–2 for a comprehensive chart regarding earmold features and uses). The reader is referred to Chapter 3 in this text for additional information regarding earmolds.

As ear size allows, the clinician should attempt to provide a large sound bore (e.g., 3 mm horn) when hearing loss from 2000 to 4000 Hz is between 30 to 80 dB HL. Size 13 tubing should be considered for remaining cases. For very young children, it is important to confirm that the earmold tubing is not crimped or collapsing within the earmold. This may effectively block transmission of sound through the earmold or create a "reverse-horn effect," which results in attenuation of high-frequency output. Of course, in some cases, the size of the child's ear canal may make it possible to avoid a reverse-horn effect. The AAA Clinical Practice Guideline on Pediatric Amplification (2013) recommends using an electroacoustic measure with the earmold coupled to the hearing aid to determine the acoustic influence of the earmold on the output of the hearing aid.

Venting is often essential in adult fittings to avoid occlusion effect complaints (Kuk, Keenan, & Lau, 2005). Venting should also be considered in children, as research has shown that localization and speech recognition in

Table 12–2. Earmold Features Along with the Effect Feature Has on Hearing Aid Function

Earmold Feature	Purpose
Large Soundbore	Prevents sound from becoming pinched as it moves through the tubing; increases high frequencies (>3000 Hz)
Standard Soundbore	Decreases high-frequency emphasis, moves peak to lower freuqency
Choke, Small, Reverse	Can cut off high-frequency sounds
Parallel Vent	Allows low-frequency sounds to escape, allowing for a more natural sound quality when hearing is normal
Angle/Diagnonal Vent	When the vent intersects with the soundbore as close to the end of the canal as possible. Less ideal, but may be necessary in the case of a small ear canal. May reduce high-frequency emphasis and cause feedback problems.
Size 13 Tubing	Standard tubing size
3-mm (Libby) Horn Tubing	Increases high-frequency response by as much as 10–12 dB; Produces boost in signal above 2000 Hz
Reverse Horn	Rolls off high-frequency sounds
Dry Tubing	Denser tubing material that helps reduce moisture buildup in the tubing
CFA (continuous flow adapter) Tubing	Different configurations of tubing and sound bores that can be used to address high-frequency hearing losses, especially "ski-slope" or reverse slope hearing losses. Refer to your earmold manufacturer's manual for selection of the correct CFA type.
Tube Lock	Helps with tubing retention, essentially "locking" tube in place. Helpful for tubing that comes out easily.
Damped Earhook	Smooths the frequency response, especially in the mid frequencies: 1000–4000 Hz

Source: Data adapted from Microsonic Custom Earmold Manual, 2006.

noise will likely be impaired if children with normal low-frequency hearing are fitted with occluding earmolds (Johnstone & Robertson, 2010). Venting is largely unnecessary and possibly undesirable when low-frequency (e.g., 500 Hz) thresholds exceed 40 dB HL. For children with normal hearing or mild low-frequency hearing loss, vent diameter should be selected based on the goal of achieving a balance between avoiding occlusion while also ensuring optimal audibility for mid- and high-frequency speech sounds that are critical for speech intelligibility. For young children who have normal low-frequency hearing sensitivity (or mild low-frequency hearing loss)

and are developing language, the primary goal is to provide consistent audibility for speech. As such, the vent diameter should be selected with the first consideration being the largest vent that will still allow the hearing aid output to meet generic prescriptive targets for low-level speech.

Parallel venting (with the vent parallel to the soundbore) is the recommended vent configuration for children, as diagonal vents may increase the likelihood of acoustic feedback and/or reduce high-frequency gain (Microsonic Earmold Laboratories, 2006). However, when a child's ears are not large enough to accommodate a parallel vent, an angle/diagonal vent may be required (AAA Clinical Practice Guideline on Pediatric Amplification, 2013).

For children who have normal or near-normal hearing thresholds in the low frequencies and who are old enough to keep the hearing aids consistent, open fit earmolds may be used. This also applies to children with unilateral hearing loss as Johnstone and colleagues' research (2010) have found improved sound localization and spatial hearing with open fit earmolds, and children reported improved sound quality and improved localization abilities.

To select the most appropriate earmold for a child, the clinician should be familiar with the materials, mold styles, and options available from each manufacturer they work with, as these characteristics differ between earmold manufacturers.

Additional Considerations Related to BTE and Earmold Use in Children

As part of the counseling and hearing aid orientation process, the family should be made aware of several safety hazards associated with hearing aid use. The audiologist should order hearing aids in which the small parts (e.g., earhooks, earmolds, batteries, etc.) are designed to be tamper-proof and safe for the child. Interestingly, parents have identified safety as more important than device use when the child could not be closely attended to, such as riding in the car (Moeller, Hoover, Peterson, & Stelmachowicz, 2009). At hearing aid checkups, the audiologist should inspect the integrity of all parts (earhooks, connection between tubing and earmold, battery boor, etc.) to ensure the child cannot dismantle the device and ingest the individual components.

Although it is obvious to most clinicians to select pediatric tonehooks, tamper-proof battery doors, and so on when initially completing an order form for hearing aids for a child, the clinician must also consider necessary modifications when ordering accessory equipment. For instance, it is also necessary to ensure safety when ordering integrated FM/DM receivers (with which it is often nec-

essary to change the battery door to accommodate the integrated receiver) or FM/DM boots. At the time of publication, the International Electrotechnical Commission (IEC) had issued a new standard that all pediatric hearing aids, for children under 36 months of age, use a tamper-proof battery door lock in addition to the battery lock/retention system to prevent accidental swallowing of the battery. The FDA is also working on a standard for this as well, but it is not yet in effect at the time of publication. These devices are designed to enhance safety by not only keeping the battery in the correct place, but also by keeping the battery door itself from being opened (International Electrotechnical Commission, 2013; Phonak, 2013).

The audiologist must also assist the family in facilitating hearing aid retention on the small ears of a child. Products are available to support device retention and keep them from becoming a choking hazard. See Figure 12–3 for photos of specific retention devices. Although it seems like a fairly mundane consideration, pediatric-designed earhooks should be selected for use in small children, as they are smaller and designed in such a way that allows the hearing aids to sit closer to the child's head. In addition, double sided toupee or clothing tape and/or clown glue are also recommended to keep the hearing aids firmly secured behind the ears, making it harder for young children to remove them. In extreme cases in which a child consistently grabs at his or her hearing aids, the audiologist may recommend use of a bonnet or aviator cap to prevent the child from removing the hearing aids. Of course, in these cases, the audiologist should also rule out that the child is not removing the hearing aids because the output is uncomfortably high (or insufficient).

Digital Signal Processing and Other Advanced Technology Features

The AAA Clinical Practice Guideline on Pediatric Amplification (2013) identifies five fun-

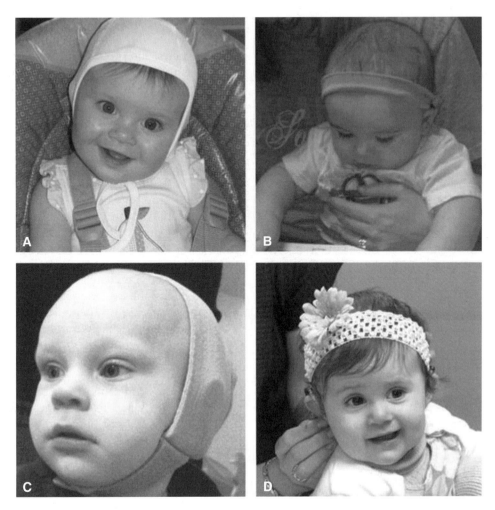

Figure 12–3. Hearing aid retention options **A.** Pilots cap (available at http://www.hannaandersson.com/) **B.** Hearing aid headband **C.** Hearing halo **D.** Traditional headband, repurposed to retain hearing aids.

damental requirements for hearing aid audio signal processing including:

1. The system should avoid unnecessary distortion.
2. The system should allow sufficient frequency shaping to meet the prescriptive requirements of the hearing loss configuration.
3. The system should allow sufficient frequency shaping to allow one to match frequency-specific targets.
4. The system should employ amplitude compression that offers the flexibility to

restore audibility for low level inputs while maintaining comfort for high level inputs.
5. Output limiting must be sufficient to avoid exposure to loud sounds while minimizing electroacoustic distortion.

A number of advanced hearing aid processing schemes and features may be used to assist the clinician in meeting these fundamental requirements. The application of these features in the pediatric population will be discussed in the proceeding section. However, the reader is referred to Chapters 7 and 8 in this text for detailed information pertaining to advanced signal processing.

Digital Signal Processing

Digital signal processing (DSP) is routinely used in hearing aids fitted for children. DSP is required to implement in a wearable device many of the advanced signal processing features that are instrumental in meeting the aforementioned fundamental requirements for hearing aid audio signal processing. As discussed in Chapter 7 and 8 of this text, the benefits of DSP have largely rendered analog hearing aids as obsolete, a fact that is particularly a reality in provision of contemporary hearing aid technology for children.

Amplitude Compression/Expansion

Of all signal processing features available in hearing aids today, amplitude compression is quite possibly the most important signal processing feature to imperatively include in a pediatric hearing aid fitting. As previously mentioned, a fundamental objective of amplification for children with hearing loss is to restore audibility of low-level speech, optimize the sensation level for average-level speech, and ensure that high-level sounds are not uncomfortable for the child. Also, it is desirable to approximate loudness normalization if possible, so that the child experiences the same range of loudness as a child with normal hearing. It is impossible to achieve these goals without the use of amplitude compression processing.

Numerous studies have shown that wide dynamic range compression generally improves children's speech recognition for low-level sounds while maintaining comfort for moderate and high-level sounds (Jenstad, Pumford, Seewald, & Cornelisse, 2000; Jenstad, Seewald, Cornelisse, & Shantz, 1999). The AAA Clinical Practice Guideline on Pediatric Amplification (2013) explicitly states that children's hearing aids should employ amplitude compression.

In spite of the universal acknowledgement that the use of wide dynamic range compression is imperative for children, there is, however, no consensus for what compression parameters are ideal for children. Specifically, there is no protocol for the selection of basic amplitude compression parameters such as compression threshold, compression ratio, or compression attack and release times. The authors suggest that compression parameters should be determined on the basis of what is required to match DSL v 5.0 or NAL-NL2 targets speech inputs for 55, 65, and 75 dB SPL speech inputs, and a high-level swept pure tone (e.g., 90 dB SPL) does not exceed maximum output targets of an independent prescriptive method. Furthermore, the clinician should strive to pursue aided thresholds of no more than 25 dB HL from 250 to 8000 Hz. There is not enough evidence to justify the use of a particular set of attack and release times. Theoretically, longer release times may help preserve amplitude cues when high compression ratios are used to position a large range of acoustic inputs into the child's dynamic range. In reality, dual-action time constants are probably ideal so that fast attack and release times may be used to quickly restore audibility after compression, whereas slow release times may be used to preserve amplitude cues as within the wearer's reduced dynamic range of hearing (Dillon, 2012).

Expansion processing increases gain with increases in the input level. Expansion is used for very low-level inputs to improve listening comfort for low-level noise. However, it is important for the clinician to ensure that expansion does not limit a child's access to low-level speech. The reader is referred to sections addressing verification and validation in this chapter for information pertaining to tools clinicians may use to verify a child has adequate access to low-level speech.

Multiple Channels

Most modern hearing aids typically include multiple channels to allow for compression to be optimized across the frequency range when hearing loss varies as a function of hearing loss. For instance, a relatively greater amount of compression is required in the high-frequency range with little to no compression in the low-frequency range for persons with near-normal low-frequency hearing and a sloping high-frequency hearing loss. Several studies have shown improved speech recognition with multiple channel compression when compared with performance with single-channel compression (Aahz & Moore, 2007; Woods, Van Tasell, Rickert, & Trine, 2006). Also, multiple channels may be advantageous for the implementation of frequency specific digital noise reduction and directional amplification. However, the clinician should exercise caution when using multiple channel compression in conjunction with high compression ratios and fast release time, which is a combination that may reduce the natural intensity contrasts that exist between low-frequency (e.g., vowels) and high-frequency (e.g., sibilants) phonemes.

Multiple Bands

A frequency band describes a frequency region over which the clinician may adjust

the gain/output in the programmable hearing aid software. Multiple bands are imperative to allow the clinician to adjust the frequency response of the child's hearing aid to match an independent prescriptive target at multiple input levels (Figure 12–4). The AAA Clinical Practice Guideline on Pediatric Amplification (2013) states that children should be fitted with hearing aids that possess at least four to seven clinician-adjustable software bands and also states that there should be no disadvantage to increasing the number of bands beyond seven.

Output Limiting

Peak clipping and output limiting are two methods to limit the maximum output of a hearing aid. Peak clipping introduces distortion to the hearing aid output and results in poor sound quality and speech recognition for high-level inputs and/or for high-gain hearing aids (Dillon, 2012; Hawkins & Naidoo, 1993). As a result, peak clipping is generally

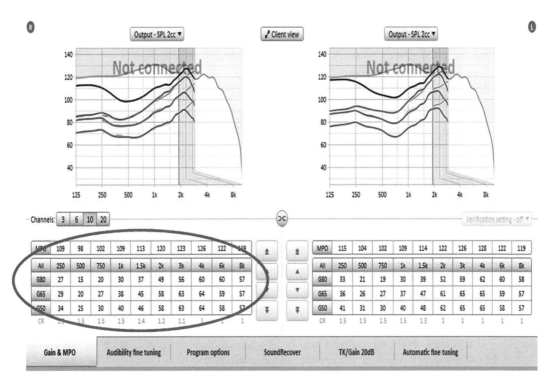

Figure 12–4. An illustration of a hearing aid that provides multiple bands for input level and frequency-specific adjustment of gain and MPO.

not used as a method of output limiting in modern hearing aids.

Compression output limiting should be used to limit the output at a level that maximizes the headroom of the hearing aid while also avoiding discomfort and high-level sound-induced hearing loss. Real ear or simulated real ear electroacoustic measures should be conducted to make certain that compression output limiting is set appropriately for each individual child. More detail pertaining to the selection of compression output limiting parameters is provided in the section in this chapter addressing hearing aid verification for children.

Acoustic Feedback Cancellation

Acoustic feedback limits the amount of available gain that may be provided by a hearing aid, and it obviously hinders sound quality. Acoustic feedback is a potential problem for all hearing aid wearers, but it is particularly a challenge for infants and toddlers, because it is difficult to maintain tight-fitting earmolds when their ears grow very quickly. Acoustic feedback cancellation has the potential to increase the available gain before feedback. This may extend the life of an earmold (i.e., the amount of time between ear impressions to make new earmolds), and it also may allow for the provision of larger vents for older children whose ear size can accommodate the presence of a vent.

The consensus among experts is that acoustic feedback cancellation should be used in hearing aids for children (AAA Clinical Practice Guideline on Pediatric Amplification, 2013; Dillon, 2012; Johnson, Ricketts, & Hornsby, 2007). The clinician should keep a few important considerations in mind regarding acoustic feedback cancellation. First, there are various methods that can be used to eliminate acoustic feedback. Some methods, such as a low-level, high-frequency cut or notch filtering, simply reduce audibility for low-level sounds, while other methods, namely acoustic feedback cancellation via phase inversion and cancellation, eliminate feedback without sacrificing gain. Clinicians are responsible for

understanding the method used in the hearing aid they are fitting for children. In general, the clinician should determine whether the hearing aid uses gain reduction or filtering to avoid feedback. If so, then the acoustic feedback cancellation system may sacrifice audibility and should be avoided. The clinician should also inquire about the typical addition in gain before feedback that may be expected from the acoustic feedback system.

Another practical consideration is the fact that clinicians should conduct verification after the acoustic feedback test is run in the hearing aid fitting software. It is common for available gain to be limited during the feedback test, and as such, the clinician should verify the gain/output of a child's hearing aid after the available gain has been determined by the feedback test. Finally, it may be helpful for the clinician to determine whether prescriptive targets can be met without the use of acoustic feedback cancellation. If the hearing aid output is substantially shy of the prescriptive target when encountering acoustic feedback without the use of acoustic feedback canceller, then it is quite possible that the hearing aid will produce intermittent feedback and/or entrainment artifacts when fitted to target with acoustic feedback cancellation enabled. In this case, it may be wise to obtain a better fitting earmold for the child.

Digital Noise Reduction

Digital noise reduction (DNR) is a form of hearing aid audio signal processing that reduces the gain of the device when the input primarily consists of noise. Numerous studies have shown that DNR typically offers little to no improvement in speech recognition in noise for adults (for a review, see Bentler, 2005). However, research with adults does suggest that DNR offers significant improvement in listening comfort in noise and noise tolerance as well as a reduction in annoyance and cognitive load and that adult hearing aid wearers consider DNR to be a very valuable feature of their hearing aids (Boymans & Dreschler, 2000; Mueller, Weber, & Hornsby, 2006; Ricketts & Hornsby, 2005; Sarampalis, Kalluri, Edwards, & Hafter, 2009; Walden, Surr, Cord, Edwards, & Olson, 2000).

There is an emerging body of publications describing results of studies that have examined the benefits of DNR for children. For example, Stelmachowicz et al. (2010) evaluated speech recognition in noise both with and without DNR for 16 children with mild to moderately severe hearing loss. On average, there was no difference in speech recognition in noise between the DNR on and off conditions. Other researchers have also shown no deterioration in speech recognition in noise with the use of DNR (Auriemmo et al., 2009a; Pittman, 2011).

Specifically, Andrea Pittman (2011) conducted a novel study in which she compared the ability of children with hearing loss to learn new words both with and without DNR. She evaluated 41 children with normal hearing, and 26 children with mild to moderately severe hearing loss. The children were divided into two age groups: (1) 8 to 9 years-old and (2) 11 to 12 years-old. For the younger children with hearing loss, there was no difference between the DNR on and off conditions in the ability to learn new words. However, the older children with hearing loss were better able to learn new words with the use of DNR relative to their performance without DNR. Pittman (2011) concluded that use of DNR may result in reduced cognitive load, which may facilitate for efficient vocabulary development for children with hearing loss.

The AAA Clinical Practice Guideline on Pediatric Amplification (2013) notes the aforementioned benefits of DNR for adults, while also acknowledging that use of DNR typically does not result in a reduction in speech recognition in noise for children. However, the AAA Clinical Practice Guideline on Pediatric Amplification does wisely point out that clinicians should be aware that selection of a manufacturer's more aggressive DNR option designed to prioritize comfort may negatively impact speech recognition in noise.

Ryan McCreery (2010) has provided an excellent protocol for evaluating the potential effect of DNR. McCreery noted that pediatric audiologists should ensure that DNR does not reduce gain when a positive SNR exists. He notes that many hearing aid electroacoustic analyzers are capable of measuring the output of a hearing aid to a calibrated, combined speech-in-noise signal. He suggested that pediatric audiologists should evaluate the output of hearing aids to a combined speech-in-noise with a positive SNR (e.g., +3 dB) with both DNR disabled and enabled. Ideally, there should be no difference in the output recorded for the two conditions indicating that the DNR does not reduce hearing aid gain when speech is present (Figure 12–5). Additionally, the clinician may also measure the output of the hearing to a steady-state noise signal for both the DNR off and on conditions. These measurements will allow the clinician to observe the effect of DNR when only noise is present.

It should be noted that research does suggest that DNR of contemporary hearing aids across and within manufacturers vary quite substantially in their implementation of DNR. Furthermore, within a hearing aid model, the DNR may behave differently dependent upon the degree of hearing loss of the user. The astute clinician should objectively measure the DNR for each user to fully understand its effect on the signal a child receives.

Directional Microphones

Aside from remote microphone hearing assistance technology, directional microphone technology has been shown to be the most effective means to improve speech recognition in noise (see Bentler [2005] for a review). The reader is referred to Chapter 6 for a detailed discussion on microphone technology. As noted in Chapter 6, most modern hearing aids allow for switching between omnidirectional and directional modes. This switching can occur manually (i.e., the wearer pushes a button or switch to deliberately switch between omni-directional and directional modes), or it may occur automatically. Furthermore, most contemporary automatic directional aids also adaptively change the directional polar plot pattern, so that the null

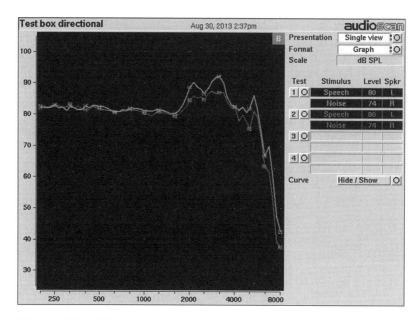

Figure 12–5. Illustration of a verification measure confirming that digital noise reduction (DNR) did not reduce gain when speech and noise were both present (+6 dB SNR). It is not readily evident, but the output of the hearing aid was measured with DNR enabled (#1) and disabled (#2). Because DNR did not reduce gain when speech and noise were both present, the tracings of each measurement completely overlap one another.

is positioned to coincide with the direction of arrival for the most intense noise source. Additionally, some hearing aids will position the maximal lobe of sensitivity toward the direction in which the most favorable SNR exists. Many of these hearing aids will not attenuate microphone sensitivity in the front hemisphere when speech with a positive SNR resides in front of the user. Several differences are likely to exist in the criteria manufacturers employ to determine whether a hearing aid should be in omnidirectional or directional mode. It is the clinician's responsibility to understand the parameters the hearing uses to determine directionality and also to counsel the child and/or the child's caregivers regarding proper use of directional amplification.

Numerous studies have shown that directional microphones typically provide a 3 to 8 dB improvement in the SNR (Dillon, 2012; Preves, Sammeth, & Wynne, 1999; Ricketts & Hornsby, 2003; Valente, Fabry, &

Potts, 1995; Valente et al., 1999). The magnitude of SNR improvement depends on a number of factors. Directional hearing aids are more effective in environments with low reverberation and when the signal of interest arrives from in front of the hearing aid user and the noise arrives from behind the user. Also, directional microphone technology is ideal when the hearing aid wearer is in close proximity to the source of the signal of interest, and the signal source must be spatially separated from the competing noise. Initial studies of directional microphone benefit for adults were conducted in sound-treated test booths (which are obviously relatively low in reverberation), and the signal of interest was positioned in the front of the user, while the competing noise source was positioned directly behind the user. These studies showed considerable improvement in the SNR required for 50% correct performance (approximately 8 dB SNR improvement) (Valente et al., 1995; Valente et al., 1999).

Later research that evaluated directional performance in reverberant environments with multiple noise sources surrounding the hearing aid wearer showed much smaller improvement in the SNR required for 50% correct performance, but nevertheless, directional microphones still provided approximately 2 to 3 dB improvement in the SNR (Ricketts & Hornsby, 2003). Given the fact that each 1 dB improvement in the SNR typically results in about a 10% increase in speech recognition, the 2 to 3 dB improvement in SNR provided by directional microphones can be quite beneficial. Numerous studies have shown that directional amplification has the potential to significantly improve speech recognition in noise for pediatric hearing aid wearers (Auriemmo et al., 2009a; Ching et al., 2009; Gravel, Fausel, Liskow, & Chobot, 1999; Ricketts & Galster, 2008; Ricketts, Galster, & Tharpe, 2007). Additionally, research has shown that children with hearing loss may be more likely to orient toward a signal of interest (Ricketts & Galster, 2008).

Although directional hearing aids can improve speech recognition in noise, there is an understandable reticence toward recommending directional technology with children. The primary concern stems from the potential for directional hearing aids to limit a child's access to important speech and environmental sounds arriving from behind or to the side of the child. Incidental listening refers to a listener's ability to attend to a message that is not directly intended to the listener. For instance, incidental listening occurs while a child is sitting in the corner of the room playing with a toy while also passively listening to a conversation his parents are having across the room. Estimates suggest that incidental listening accounts for 60% to 90% of what children learn about language (Ching et al., 2009; Cole & Flexer, 2007). If directional amplification limited access to incidental sounds arriving from behind a child, then the child's model for language development may be compromised. Also, directional amplification may potentially hinder audibility for warning sounds arriving from behind (e.g., a car horn).

Indeed, there are research studies that indicate that directional amplification can be detrimental to a child's speech understanding ability when the signal of interest arrives from behind the child (Ching et al., 2009; Ricketts, Galster, & Tharpe, 2007). Ricketts and colleagues (2007) evaluated the speech recognition in noise of 26 children who ranged in age from 10 to 17 years old and used hearing aids capable of switching between omnidirectional and directional mode. The evaluation was completed in a classroom environment, and the noise was presented from four loudspeakers located in the corners of the classroom. Speech recognition in noise was assessed while the signal of interest arrived from the front of and also from behind the child. Compared with performance in the omnidirectional mode, children received a 2 dB improvement in the SNR with directional amplification when the signal of interest arrived from the front. However, when the signal of interest arrived from behind the children, the SNR required for 50% correct performance was 2 dB poorer in the directional mode. Ricketts et al. (2007) concluded that children should only use directional amplification when the signal of interest is located in the front hemisphere, and that hearing aids should be equipped with the ability to switch between directional and omnidirectional modes.

Ching and colleagues (2009) at the National Acoustic Laboratories of Australia (NAL) also conducted a study with the intent to determine whether directional amplification is appropriate for children with hearing loss. Twenty-seven children (11 with normal hearing and 16 with hearing loss) ranging in age from 11 to 78 months of age participated in the study in which video recordings were made of children as they resided in "naturalistic" settings. These settings included: (a) the child directly interacting with an adult/caregiver in a play situation, (b) the child playing while two adults interacted with one another, (c) the child was indoors with other children and adults, and (d), the child was outdoors with other children and adults. Examiners reviewed the video of the children in each of the aforementioned videos and logged the proportion of time the children oriented toward the signal of interest. Furthermore, a special software program was used to estimate the speech transmission index (STI) for each situation derived from processing the primary signal of interest through a directional and omnidirectional polar response measured from a hearing aid positioned on KEMAR.

Ching and colleagues (2009) found that children looked in the direction of the primary talker 40% of the time overall. In situations in which two adults conversed while the children played at the side, the subjects only oriented toward the primary talker 20% of the time. They also reported that directional amplification resulted in a 3 dB improvement in the STI when the signal of interest arrived from the front and a 2.8 dB detriment when the signal of interest arrived from behind or from the sides of the user, which when considered collectively, essentially results in no overall net gain or detriment from directional use. In spite of the fact that children did not consistently orient toward the signal of interest and that directional amplification was detrimental when children did not do so, Ching et al. (2009) concluded that hearing aids with directional amplification are "not detrimental and have much potential for benefits in real life. The benefits may be enhanced by fitting directionality early and by counseling caregivers on ways to maximize benefits in everyday situations." At least partially as an outcome of the Ching et al. (2009) study, the Australian Hearing Services program recommends use of automatic directional hearing aids for infants and young children.

Dillon (2012) presents several reasons for the Australian Hearing Services program's support for automatic, adaptive directional use for infants. First, he notes that young children with hearing loss are the population that is most in need of an improvement in the SNR to understand speech in noise, a fact that may be especially critical as children attempt to access intelligible speech as a model for speech and language development. Second, Dillon theorizes that it is likely that children with hearing loss will notice the improvement in SNR afforded by directional amplifi-

cation, and as a result, they will be even more inclined to face the signal of interest. Also, he noted that it is possible to counsel adult caregivers to consistently orient toward the child when speaking with the child. Further, Dillon noted that automatic, adaptive directional hearing aids likely are quite effective in determining which mode enhances access to intelligible speech in the environment. Additionally, Dillon notes that the WDRC present in hearing aids will partially overcome the attenuation of the directional microphone by offering more gain to the reduced signal. Finally, Dillon notes that directional hearing aids only provide a small amount of attenuation to sounds in the rear hemisphere in real-world situations, because reverberation inherent in most real-world environments limits the directivity of a directional hearing aid.

In the end, there is no conclusive evidence that indicates the impact (good or bad) that directional amplification has on a young child's speech, language, and auditory skill development. There is also definitely no consensus amongst professionals as to whether directional amplification should be recommended for infants and young children. Although the Australian Hearing Services program recommends automatic directional hearing aids for children, there are other evidence-based organizations that do not recommend directional amplification for young children (Bagatto, Scollie, Hyde, & Seewald, 2010). The AAA Clinical Practice Guideline on Pediatric Amplification (2013) notes that full-time directional processing is not recommended, but it does state that the audiologist may consider automatic, adaptive directional aids for children. It further states that the audiologist is responsible for understanding the parameters underlying the automatic, adaptive switching as well as the counseling of the family regarding directional use.

The authors of this text contend that more research is needed to fully justify the use of automatic, adaptive directional amplification for infants and young children. This research should explore the auditory, speech, and language development of children using omnidirectional and directional amplification, and should also evaluate the effect of switching parameters on children's development and on children's consistent access to speech and environmental sounds. The authors also contend that omnidirectional amplification is likely most appropriate for infants and toddlers, because of their dependence on incidental listening to develop speech and language as well as their tendency to orient away from the primary talker in an environment. Automatic, adaptive directional amplification should be considered for school-aged children (i.e., 5 years old and up), but the audiologist should conduct periodic hearing aid assessments to objectively ensure that the directional technology is functioning appropriately (see Chapter 6 for examples). Also, it is the audiologist's responsibility to understand the environments in which the child communicates and counsel the family and child on the proper use of directional amplification. Ideally, a formal or informal assessment (i.e., standardized questionnaires, communication diary) should be administered to ensure at the very least that the directional microphone is not causing any deleterious effects. Finally, it should be reiterated that a remote microphone wireless transmission system (e.g., personal digital modulation [DM] radio frequency [RF] system, personal frequency modulated [FM] system) should be recommended for use in noisy/reverberant situations or when the signal of interest originates a great distance from the child. Most modern hearing aids will switch to omnidirectional mode when a child uses a personal remote microphone wireless RF system. In the future, it is likely that many hearing aids will feature three A/D converters to allow for simultaneous use of directional and remote microphone wireless RF technology.

Extended Bandwidth Technology

As previously discussed, children require adequate audibility through at least 9000 Hz in order to optimize speech recognition, particularly when the talker is a female or another child (Stelmachowicz et al., 2002).

It is generally considered best practice to attempt to provide audibility for speech sounds through at least 9000 Hz when fitting hearing aids for infants and young children (AAA Clinical Practice Guideline on Pediatric Amplification, 2013). Unfortunately, as of the writing of this text, the in situ bandwidth of most contemporary hearing aids does not extend much beyond 6000 Hz. Manufacturers have attempted to extend the bandwidth of modern hearing aid receivers and processors and have marketed some new products as "extended bandwidth" devices with a reported bandwidth up to 10,000 Hz. Unfortunately, audibility beyond 6000 Hz is still challenging when a hearing aid is worn on the ear because of limits in available gain before feedback as well as the roll-off that occurs as sound travels through the acoustic plumbing of a BTE earmold.

The clinician should keep several considerations in mind in regards to the bandwidth of a hearing aid. First, the reported bandwidth of a hearing aid may not be indicative of the bandwidth of the device when it is worn on the ear. Clinicians should remember that the reported bandwidth is often based on ANSI (or IEC) standards for hearing aid assessment, which state that the hearing aid's frequency response is calculated by determining the point at which the low- and high-frequency end of the response drops 20 dB below the high-frequency-average full-on gain with the volume control set at the reference test gain position. This measurement is made with the hearing aid output directed to a 2cc coupler. These conditions, including the frequency response, the gain and volume control setting of the hearing aid, and the fact that the measurement is made in a coupler rather than on the ear, are quite disparate from what exists when the hearing aid is used on the child's ear in real life. As a result, one would expect the in situ frequency response to be different from the value published from the standard-based electroacoustic assessment.

Furthermore, some manufacturers may report the bandwidth in relation to the sampling rate of the analog-to-digital converter. The clinician should recall that the Nyquist theorem states that the sampling rate of a

DSP device should be at least twice as much as the highest frequency the device intends to capture and present to the user. For example, if one wishes to provide a frequency response extending to 9000 Hz, then the sampling rate must be at least 18000 Hz. In some instances, manufacturers have reported that the hearing aid possesses a bandwidth of 10000 Hz, because the sampling rate of the DSP is 20000 Hz. A closer inspection of the specification sheet indicated that the frequency response (as defined by the ANSI S3.22 standard) extended to approximately 7000 Hz. As such, clinicians must be aware of the information being presented to describe the hearing aid bandwidth, and clinicians should also conduct in situ electroacoustic measures to evaluate the bandwidth of the aid relative to a child's thresholds when the aid is worn on the ear.

Frequency Lowering Technology

Because of the aforementioned challenges of providing sufficient audibility through 9000 Hz when a hearing aid is worn on a child's ear, manufacturers have introduced frequency lowering technology, which moves high-frequency sounds to a lower frequency range at which sufficient audibility is more likely to be achieved. There are a number of different methods used to achieve frequency lowering including nonlinear frequency compression (NLFC), linear frequency transposition (LFT), and spectral envelope warping. At the time of this writing, there are no published studies showing one method to be inferior to the inferiors. However, there are several studies that show that NLFC and LFT can be beneficial for children with high-frequency hearing loss. Glista et al. (2009) evaluated detection of high-frequency speech sounds and speech recognition for a group of 11 children with sloping, severe high-frequency hearing loss. They found that use of NLFC provided improvements in speech recognition and in the detection of high-frequency speech sounds. Likewise, Auriemmo et al.

(2009b) reported that use of LFT provided an improvement in the recognition of low-level speech in quiet for 11 children with sloping, severe-to-profound high-frequency hearing loss. It should be noted, however, that aural rehabilitation was also provided for the children participating in the Auriemmo study, so it is impossible to unequivocally determine whether their improvement was attributed to the LFT, the therapy, or both.

Wolfe and colleagues (2010, 2011, submitted a, submitted b) have evaluated NLFC for a group of children with mild and moderate high-frequency hearing loss and also showed benefit from the use of NLFC. Specifically, Wolfe et al. (2010) evaluated speech recognition in quiet and in noise as well as detection of high-frequency sounds in a group of 15 children who had moderate high-frequency hearing loss and used hearing aids with NLFC. As a group, use of NLFC resulted in better speech recognition in quiet and better detection of high-frequency sounds with no change in speech recognition in noise when compared with the NLFC disabled condition. Wolfe et al. (2011) evaluated the performance of these 15 children again after they had used NLFC for a consecutive 6-month period and showed continued improvement in speech recognition in quiet as well as better performance in noise with NLFC compared with the NLFC disabled condition. Wolfe and colleagues concluded that an extended period of NLFC use was required for children to acclimate to the frequency-compressed signal and fully realize the potential benefits of NLFC. Furthermore, Wolfe et al. (submitted a) showed improvements in the production of the children's own speech after 6 consecutive months of NLFC use.

Finally, Wolfe and colleagues (submitted b) also compared speech recognition in quiet and in noise as well as detection of high-frequency sounds for children who had mild high-frequency hearing loss and who used hearing aids with extended bandwidth technology and NLFC technology. They reported no differences in speech recognition in noise and also in monosyllabic word recognition in quiet. However, the children did have better recognition of high-frequency phonemes in on-sense syllables with the use of NLFC as well as better detection of high-frequency sounds (8000 Hz warble tones, the phoneme /s/, etc.). Wolfe et al. (submitted b) concluded that NLFC provides better access to low-level high-frequency speech sounds with no apparent detriment in performance of children with mild high-frequency hearing loss when compared with performance with extended bandwidth technology.

It is imperative to note that each of the aforementioned studies employed detailed protocols to ensure that the frequency-lowering strategies were appropriately fitted to meet the individual needs of each subject. This is a critical step in the use of frequency-lowering technology with children, as the default parameters may not always be optimal. It is also important to note that the researchers took care to make certain that the least possible amount of frequency-lowering was used for each subject so as not to overly distort high-frequency phonemes. Objective and behavioral measures were used to verify that frequency-lowering parameters were optimized for the subjects. The AAA Clinical Practice Guideline on Pediatric Amplification (2013) supports the use of frequency-lowering technology when audibility of high-frequency sounds cannot be provided via conventional amplification. The AAA Clinical Practice Guideline on Pediatric Amplification (2013) also indicates that clinicians should conduct verification to ensure that the minimal amount of frequency-lowering is applied for each child in order to restore access to intelligible, high-frequency speech sounds.

Binaural Signal Processing

Several manufacturers have introduced hearing aids that feature binaural audio signal processing. The implementation of binaural processing is quite varied. In one application, binaural processing allows the hearing aid wearer to hear a telephone signal on both ears simultaneously when the telephone receiver is held next to one hearing aid. It is likely that this type of application would offer no degradation in performance and may very well improve a child's performance on the telephone.

Binaural audio processing has also been used to expand the potential effectiveness of directional amplification. Specifically, the input from the directional microphone system of each ear is combined to enable more specific beamforming. There are not published studies that determine whether this feature is suitable for children. Additionally, some manufacturers have attempted to use binaural audio processing to preserve interaural cues to support better localization and speech recognition in noise. Once again, there are no data to indicate the suitability of using this technology with children.

Direct Auditory Input/ Telecoil/Wireless Streaming

Remote microphone hearing assistance technology should be considered for all children with hearing aids. A remote microphone personal radio frequency (RF) personal system is composed of a microphone and transmitting unit and a personal RF receiver that is coupled to the child's hearing aids. Remote microphone personal RF systems represent the best technology option to improve speech recognition in difficult listening situations (Boothroyd & Iglehart, 1998; Hawkins, 1984). Detailed information pertaining to these systems will be provided in a later section in this chapter. It is, however, prudent to state now that all hearing aids fitted for infants and young children should be equipped with a direct auditory input (DAI) port to allow for the connection of a personal RF receiver to the child's hearing aids. Additionally, it may be used to connect a child's hearing aids to handheld electronic devices via a special adapter (obtained from the hearing aid manufacturer) and audio cable.

A telecoil should also be included in hearing aids fitted for children. The telecoil may be used to improve access to hearing aid telecoil compatible telephones and also to induction loop systems. There is a paucity of studies examining telephone performance of children with hearing loss. Clinicians should consider the availability of telecoil use once the child is old enough to manually switch between a regular and telephone program (i.e., 8 to 9 years old). Younger children may inadvertently activate the telecoil in everyday situations and detect noise and distortion from stray electromagnetic signals such as fluorescent lights, monitors, and so on.

A recent trend in hearing aids is the advent of wireless "streaming" devices. Wireless streaming typically refers to the RF transmission on the 2.4 gigahertz RF bandwidth of a signal of interest that is captured by a remote wireless microphone or other accessory that is directly coupled to a personal audio device. These devices typically incorporate a transmitter to "stream" a signal of interest (e.g., mobile telephone signal, television audio, signal from a remote micro-

phone, etc.) to the child's hearing aid. Some manufacturers have chosen to stream the signal of interest to an interface device that the user wears around her neck (Figure 12–6), whereas other manufacturers have opted to stream directly to a small antenna built into the hearing aid (Figure 12–7). Although these hearing assistance technologies may prove to be beneficial in helping children hear better in difficult listening situations, there are no published studies to determine the benefits and limitations of these devices.

Prescriptive Methods for Selection of Real Ear Aided Gain and Maximum Output for Children Using Hearing Aids

Selecting the appropriate real ear aided gain and maximum output of a child's hearing aid is quite possibly the most important part of

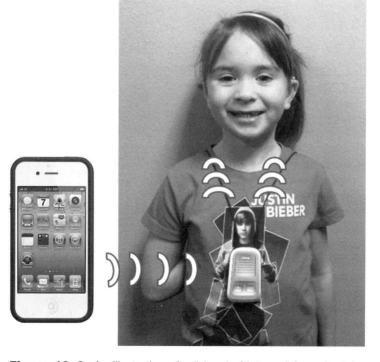

Figure 12–6. An illustration of a "signal of interest" from the telephone being sent to a streamer that then communicates wirelessly with hearing aids.

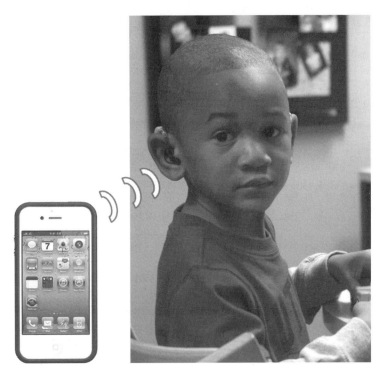

Figure 12–7. An illustration in which a "signal of interest" from the telephone is wirelessly transmitted directly to the hearing aids without an interface.

selecting the optimal amplification for a child with hearing loss. Hearing aid manufacturers offer proprietary hearing aid gain and output prescriptions, and surveys suggest that many audiologists are likely to use these manufacturer-specific prescriptions when fitting hearing aids for adults (Kochkin, 2011). However, it is not appropriate to use proprietary prescriptive approaches to select gain and output for hearing aids fitted to children. As explicitly stated in the AAA Clinical Practice Guideline on Pediatric Amplification (2013), prescriptive methods that are supported by "independent pediatric-focused and pediatric-validated prescriptive targets, normative data, and fitting methods that take into account the unique developmental needs of children should be used for pediatric hearing aid verification (and gain/output selection) instead of a manufacturer's proprietary prescriptive approach." Of course, the clinician should not only use an independent,

evidence-based prescriptive method to select gain and output for a pediatric hearing aid fitting, but electroacoustic assessment (in the form of real ear probe microphone measures or simulated real ear probe microphone measures in a 2cc coupler) of the gain and output present at the eardrum of the child should also be performed to ensure the desired gain and output has actually been provided for the individual child being fitted by the clinician.

The Desired Sensation Level m[i/o] v5.0 (DSL v 5.0) and National Acoustic Laboratories-Non-linear 2 (NAL-NL2) prescriptive fitting methods are the only methods that have been developed for fitting hearing aids for children and also meet the aforementioned criteria for selecting hearing aid gain and output for children as defined by the AAA Clinical Practice Guideline on Pediatric Amplification (2013). The DSL v5.0 and NAL-NL2 methods are each described in the following paragraphs.

DSL m[i/o] v5.0

The Desired Sensation Level (DSL) prescriptive method was first released as a software-based system for clinical use in 1991. The original version of DSL was developed for use with linear hearing aids. The objectives of DSL were to provide an amplified speech signal that was audible to the child across the entire speech frequency range and also comfortable for speech and environmental sounds (Seewald, Ross, & Spiro, 1985; Seewald, Stelmachowicz, & Ross, 1987; Ross & Seewald, 1988). The DSL prescription aimed to place average conversational level speech at a sensational level that would maximize speech recognition while also providing acceptable comfort. The prescribed gain levels to achieve this goal were based on studies that examined speech recognition as a function of sensation level as well as speech sensation levels that corresponded to preferred

listening levels (see Seewald, Moodie, Scollie, & Bagatto, 2005 for a review). Additionally, audiometric threshold-based maximum output targets were also calculated on the basis of loudness discomfort levels (LDL) estimated from Pascoe's (1978) research on uncomfortable loudness levels of persons with hearing loss. The maximum output target values were positioned one standard deviation below the mean LDL values from the Pascoe (1978) study in order to provide a safe and conservative estimate of maximum output for children.

The original DSL was a unique and trend-setting prescriptive method in a number of ways. First, the audiometric thresholds and target values were all converted to sound pressure level (SPL) and displayed in the form of an "SPL-o-gram" (Figure 12–8). As a result, the display naturally facilitated the habilitative/rehabilitative process by allowing for a direct comparison between the

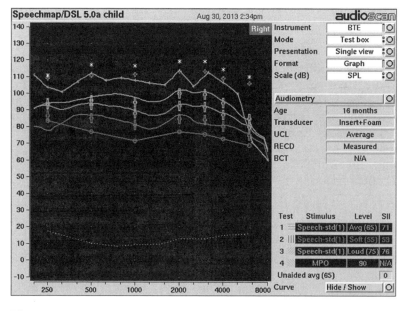

Figure 12–8. An illustration of an SPL-o-gram for a 16-month-old child. Thresholds are plotted in dB SPL at the eardrum (*solid line with circles*). The simulated real ear output of the hearing aid is also plotted in dB SPL at the eardrum for a calibrated, recorded speech passage presented at 55, 65, and 75 dB SPL and also for a 90 dB SPL swept pure tone. Desired Sensation Level version 5.0 (DSL v 5.0) prescriptive targets for children are indicated by the cross symbols.

unaided and aided speech spectrum to the hearing aid wearer's audiometric threshold. This allowed clinicians to easily determine what parts of the speech spectrum are audible for the child, and it provided a relatively simple method to explain the outcome and benefits of amplification to the child's family and interventionists.

Another pioneering feature of the original DSL prescriptive method was the incorporation of an individually specific acoustic measurement to allow for the transformation of audiometric data to dB SPL for plotting in the SPL-o-gram. In particular, the original DSL method introduced the concept of using the real-ear-to-coupler difference (RECD) to improve the accuracy of determining threshold in dB SPL at the eardrum and also to allow for estimation of in situ real ear hearing aid gain and output via measurements made in a 2cc coupler. The DSL method allowed the clinician to use measured or age-specific RECD values in the fitting process. The RECD and its use in the hearing aid selection and fitting of hearing aids is discussed in greater detail in the proceeding section that addresses hearing aid verification.

In 1995, a new version of DSL was introduced to allow for the selection and electroacoustic verification of nonlinear (e.g., wide dynamic range—WDRC) hearing aids. This revised version of DSL was referred to as DSL input/output v4.1 (DSL i/o) and used loudness and speech recognition sensation level data to acoustically map a wide range of inputs (20–90 dB SPL) into the wearer's residual dynamic range. Although it has been suggested that DSL i/o attempts to normalize loudness at each frequency (i.e., it attempts to present amplified sound so that the hearing aid user perceives the sound at the same loudness as a person with normal hearing), the developers of DSL i/o contend that frequency-specific loudness normalization was never a goal. Instead, the primary goal was to make the entire range of speech inputs audible to the hearing aid wearer while avoiding loudness discomfort (Seewald & Scollie, 1999). Subsequent research, however, has shown that DSL i/o users did

report that the overall loudness of speech was normalized within 5 dB across subjects (Jenstad et al., 2000). Research has also shown that DSL i/o provides significant improvement in speech recognition for children with hearing loss (Jenstad et al., 1999).

In 2005, the DSL multistage [input/output] v 5.0 was introduced (DSL v 5.0). The DSL v 5.0 method possessed numerous changes that simplified the process of fitting hearing aids for children and also allowed the clinician to verify the fitting of new hearing aid technology including multiple channel devices as well as a variety of different types of signal processing. Of note, the developers intended for DSL v 5.0 to provide a comprehensive fitting method to assist in the selection and verification of hearing aid gain and output for both children and adults (Bagatto et al., 2005). As with its predecessor, the primary goals of the DSL v 5.0 method was to amplify a range of speech levels to the optimal sensation level across as broad of a frequency as possible to optimize audibility for speech while ensuring comfort for speech and environmental sounds. The DSL i/o algorithm served as the foundation for DSL v 5.0. Specific updates in the DSL v 5.0 platform included:

1. An update of acoustic transforms including the revision of age-specific RECD values and the inclusion of average RECD values that change on a monthly basis through the first 60 months of the child's life. Average RECD measures in the original DSL were segmented into 12 to 24-month age ranges.

2. The DSL v 5.0 fitting method was enhanced to include a protocol for using ABR thresholds to estimate behavioral audiometric thresholds and prescriptive targets. Specifically, correction factors were developed based on David Stapells and colleagues (1995) work to allow for an estimation of audiometric threshold (dB eHL) from ABR thresholds (dB nHL).

3. Unique DSL targets were provided for children and adults with acquired hearing. The extensive research conducted with each group resulted in a slight change

to pediatric targets as compared with the targets provided in DSL 4.1. Additionally, adult gain targets were significantly lower in level than pediatric targets.

4. DSL targets were provided for quiet and noisy environments.

5. DSL v 5.0 included evidence-based calculations to account for verification of multiple-channel devices and hearing aids with multiple-stage processing (i.e., expansion, linear, WDRC, and compression limiting).

The development of DSL v 5.0 was predicated upon the findings of numerous studies with children and adults that determined preferred listening levels of each population as well as establishing that speech recognition was satisfactory when each group (children and adults) used hearing aids programmed to DSL v5.0 targets (Scollie et al., 2005). Subsequent studies have shown that use of DSL v 5.0 allows for satisfactory speech recognition performance in children with hearing loss as well as normalized overall loudness for conversational speech (Scollie et al., 2010).

NAL-NL2

The original National Acoustic Laboratories of Australia (NAL) prescriptive method was first published in 1976 (Byrne & Tonisson, 1976). The primary goal of the NAL approach was to maximize speech recognition while approximating the user's preferred loudness. Loudness is balanced in ⅓-octave bands across the speech frequency range as it has been suggested that equalizing loudness across the frequency range maximizes speech intelligibility (Dillon, 2012).

The NAL developers have conducted extensive research to evaluate the efficacy of NAL, and as a result, the original NAL method has undergone several iterations over the life of the procedure. For instance, it was shown that equal loudness across the spectrum was not achieved for all degrees and configurations of hearing loss (especially precipitously sloping hearing losses), so the NAL-Revised (NAL-R) method was intro-

duced with an updated algorithm that more effectively equalized loudness across the frequency range for a variety of degrees and configurations of hearing loss (Byrne, 1986).

A subsequent round of research indicated that persons with severe-to-profound hearing loss preferred more low-frequency and less high-frequency gain than provided by NAL-R, so the NAL developers introduced the NAL-Revised, Profound (NAL-RP) procedure in the early 1990s (Byrne, Parkinson, & Newall, 1990, 1991). The development of the NAL-RP method was based on measured speech recognition and subjective preferences of sound quality and intelligibility of speech (Byrne et al., 1990, 1991). Follow-up studies suggested that the preferred overall gain and response slope of children with hearing loss was similar to what was prescribed by NAL-RP (Ching, Newall, & Wigney, 1997; Snik, van den Borne, Brokx, & Hoekstra, 1995).

In response to the widespread use of hearing aids with WDRC, NAL introduced the NAL-Nonlinear 1 (NAL-NL1) fitting method in the late 1990s. Once again, the primary objective of NAL-NL1 was to optimize speech intelligibility of the hearing wearer (Dillon, 1999). Two different psychoacoustic models were used to develop NAL-NL1 fitting targets. First, a modified version of the Speech Intelligibility Index (SII) was used to predict speech intelligibility for a given gain prescription. Also, a model designed to estimate loudness as a function of sensation level was used to predict aided loudness associated with a given gain prescription. Both of these models along with 52 audiograms covering a wide range of degrees and configurations of hearing loss were fed to a computer program that sought to compare all of the possible gain combinations in ⅓-octave bands across the aided frequency range to determine the prescribed gain response that maximized speech intelligibility without exceeding normal loudness. The optimal frequency/gain response for each audiogram was determined for speech ranging in 10 dB steps from 40 to 90 dB SPL. Next, from the prescribed frequency responses for the six different speech input levels and 52 audiograms, a formula was derived so that frequency-specific gain could be prescribed for any audiogram a clinician may enter into the NAL-NL1 fitting software. Like the DSL v 5.0 method, the maximum output targets are predicted from hearing thresholds based on studies of loudness discomfort levels associated with different levels of hearing loss. Although the design of NAL-NL1 was predicated on the objective of maximizing speech intelligibility, research has suggested that individual frequency bands are equally loud across the speech frequency range. It should also be noted that the gain/frequency response NAL-NL1 prescribed for average conversational level speech is remarkably similar to the gain NAL-RP prescribed for average conversational level inputs. Finally, a unique feature of the NAL-NL1 method is the fact that the modified SII takes into account hearing-impaired persons' reduced ability to extract speech information from a high-level signal. This phenomenon has been referred to as desensitization, and results in a reduction in prescribed gain in frequency regions with severe-to-profound hearing loss, particularly when it occurs in the high frequencies.

The NAL group conducted extensive studies to examine the merits and limitations of the NAL-NL1 method, and in 2006, they introduced an updated method known as NAL-NL2 (Dillon, 2006; Dillon & Keidser, 2013). NAL-NL2 featured several changes designed to improve speech intelligibility and subjective preference based on their evaluations of NAL-NL1. For instance, a different model of loudness (Moore & Glasberg, 2004) was used to estimate whether the overall loudness for speech did not exceed normal loudness for the given input level. Also, the gain prescribed for mid- (average conversational level speech) and low-level (e.g., soft) speech for pediatric hearing aid wearers was increased, and males were prescribed slightly greater gain than females. Furthermore, the SII model was further revised to account for a hearing impaired person's reduced ability to extract meaningful information from high-level speech (i.e., desensitization, level distortion factor, etc.). Additionally, less gain was

prescribed for binaural fittings to account for binaural summation. There is a paucity of published studies comparing outcomes obtained between use of the NAL-NL1 and NAL-NL2 methods.

Finally, it should be noted that the NAL-NL1 and NAL-NL2 methods possess a number of components that are intended to facilitate a simple and straightforward pediatric fitting. As with the DSL method, average age-specific RECD values are available to allow for the determination of adult equivalent hearing thresholds (to be explained in a later section in this chapter) as well as to allow for accurate estimation of real ear aided output via electroacoustic measurement in a 2cc coupler. Furthermore, the NAL prescriptive method has historically prescribed user gain in the form of insertion gain. However, real ear aided responses are recommended for use with children similar to the approach used in the DSL method.

Comparison of DSL and NAL for Use in Children

Unfortunately, because of the time required to conduct well-designed studies and publish the results in peer-reviewed literature, there is a scarcity of published research describing comparison of potential differences in children's performance obtained between the use of the DSL v 5.0 and NAL-NL2 methods. The DSL and NAL groups did conduct a multiple-center study examining performance and subjective preference for a group of children who used hearing aids programmed to both the DSL v 4.1 and NAL-NL1 methods (Ching, Scollie, Dillon, & Seewald, 2010; Scollie et al., 2010). Forty-eight school-aged children with moderate-to-moderately severe hearing loss participated in the study, in which hearing aids were fitted to the DSL v 4.1 and NAL-NL1 targets in a 2cc coupler with the use of measured RECDs. Subjects wore the hearing aids for 8 weeks programmed to the DSL v 4.1, for 8 weeks programmed to NAL-NL1, and for a final 8-week period in which they were given two programs and asked to switch between the DSL and NAL programs to determine whether a subjective preference existed in the real world. The order in which DSL and NAL were used was counterbalanced across subjects, and the subjects and examiners were both blinded as to what prescriptive method they were using. Approximately one-half of the subjects lived in Australia (where NAL was developed, so they had used hearing aids programmed to the NAL method prior to inclusion in the study) while the other half were from Canada (where DSL was developed), so they had previous experience with DSL prior to the study.

Coupler verification indicated that the DSL v 4.1 method resulted in more gain for low- and mid-level inputs than NAL-NL1. Interestingly, Canadian subjects tended to express a preference for DSL v 4.1, while Australian subjects tended to prefer the NAL-NL1 method. This finding is presumably attributed to the previous experience each group had with the two different methods. There were no differences in measured speech recognition obtained with use of the different methods, and subjects typically performed quite well on measures of nonsense syllable identification with use of each method. However, subjects tended to express a preference for DSL v 4.1 when listening to speech in quiet, particularly when it was low in level or arrived from behind the listener. In contrast, children tended to prefer NAL-NL1 when listening to high-level speech and when listening to speech in noise.

Partially as a consequence of the results of this study, DSL v 5.0 prescribes slightly less gain than DSL v 4.1, and it also provides a "noise target" that provides lower real ear aided gain for use in noisy situations. Likewise, the NAL-NL2 provides greater approximately 5 to 8 dB of gain for children for mid- and low-level speech inputs, respectively.

As a result of the recent revisions to DSL v 5.0 and NAL-NL2, the two prescriptive gain formula, which albeit are not identical, are more similar to one another than their predecessors were (i.e., DSL i/o and NAL-NL1). Because the most recent versions of each of these fitting methods have only been clinically available for a few years, there are no published studies examining performance differences that may arise from use of the two methods. However, the NAL group is conducting a longitudinal study to comprehensively evaluate speech, language, auditory, academic, and social emotional outcomes of a large group of children with hearing loss in Australia. As part of this study, they are examining outcomes for children fitted with the DSL v 5.0 and NAL-NL2 methods. According to Dillon and Keidser (2013), preliminary results suggest no difference in speech and language outcomes between the children using the two different prescriptive methods.

Changes in Ear Canal Acoustics That Affect Results (SPL to HL transform)—ABR Correction—RECD Affecting Results—SPL-o-gram

The physical properties of the external ear and middle ear influence the SPL of audiometric test stimuli that reach the eardrum. These properties also influence the SPL at the eardrum for amplified sound delivered from a hearing aid. In the ideal world, it would be desirable to measure the exact sound pressure level of audiologic test signals (or the sound delivered from a hearing aid) as they reach the eardrum. It is, however, impractical to place a probe tube in the external ear canal to directly measure the sound pressure level of ABR and audiometric test signals as they arrive at eardrum.

Instead, individualized transformation factors may be used to calculate the level of audiometric test signals at the eardrum in dB SPL. Audiologic test signals are calibrated in acoustic couplers. An acoustic coupler is a cavity that provides a controlled environment to make repeatable sound level measurements and is designed to mimic the size (volume) of the adult ear canal past the point at which an eartip/earmold terminates in the ear canal as well as the equivalent volume of the eardrum and middle ear (i.e., the effect that the eardrum and residual volume of the middle ear space have on the SPL of sounds arriving at the eardrum). Insert earphones are also calibrated in 2cc couplers. The human ear is not equally sensitive to sound across the standard audiometric frequency range of 250 to 8000 Hz. If the standard audiogram was displayed in dB SPL, the level corresponding to "normal hearing" would vary as a function of frequency, which would be potentially difficult for patients and other health care providers to interpret. Of course, to address this potential confusion, audiometric test signals are calibrated in 0 dB HL, which corresponds to the level at which a typical young adult is able to just detect a pure tone (or other audiologic test signal) at a given frequency.

Let's say that an audiogram for an "average young adult with normal hearing" is obtained using ER-3A insert earphones. Because this patient is an "average young adult with normal hearing," all of her thresholds are obtained at 0 dB HL. Then, let's say that the insert earphones were coupled to a 2cc coupler (insert earphones are actually calibrated in a 2cc coupler), and the SPL is measured in the 2cc coupler for each test frequency at 0 dB SPL. The level that we would measure would vary as a function of frequency and is referred to as the reference equivalent threshold in sound pressure level (RETSPL). RETSPLs refer to the SPLs measured in an acoustic coupler that are equal to the average hearing thresholds of ontologically normal young adults. Figure 12–9 provides the RETSPL for audiometric test frequencies when measuring with ER-3A insert earphones coupled to an HA-2 2cc coupler. When the audiometer is set to 0 dB HL for a 2000 Hz pure tone presented via insert earphones, the level measured in an HA-2 2cc coupler would be 3 dB SPL. If the audiometer attenuator was changed to 70 dB HL, then the level measured in the HA-2 2cc coupler would be 73 dB SPL.

Unfortunately, acoustic couplers do not provide a perfect approximation of the adult external and middle ear and how sound pressure level develops at the eardrum (Dillon, 2012). As such, sound pressure level measured at the eardrum for the "average young adult with normal hearing" is different from what is measured in a HA-2 2cc coupler. The real-ear-to-coupler difference (RECD) is the difference in SPL measured at the eardrum compared with the SPL measured in a coupler for the same sound. Figure 12–10 provides an illustration of a measured RECD of an adult hearing aid wearer relative to the RECD of an average adult. As shown, the RECD varies as a function of frequency and is typically positive because the SPL measured at the eardrum is typically higher than what is measured in a HA-2 2cc coupler. It should be noted that it is quite simple to measure the RECD with most clinical hearing aid analyzers. Typically, an insert earphone is used to deliver a broadband stimulus to a 2cc coupler, and the measured SPL is stored in the computer. Then, the insert earphone is coupled to a foam eartip or earmold, and the same signal is delivered to the external ear. A probe microphone system is used to measure the SPL that develops at the eardrum from the presentation of the broadband signal, and the difference between the two measures is

Frequency (Hz)	250	500	1000	2000	3000	4000	6000	8000
RETSPL (dB) Insert Earphones – 2 cc HA-2 Coupler	14	5.5	0	3	3.5	5.5	2	0

Figure 12–9. RETSPL.

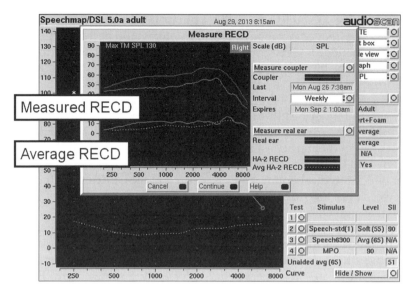

Figure 12–10. An illustration of a real-ear-to-coupler difference response (RECD) measured from an adult hearing aid wearer. This RECD is higher than the average value (*dotted line*).

used to calculate the RECD. Figure 12–11 provides an illustration of the measurement of the RECD measurement.

To determine the SPL at the eardrum for audiologic test stimuli delivered via insert earphones, one can simply add the RECD and RETSPL values to the audiometric dial reading (in dB HL).

Equation 12–2:
   SPL at Eardrum (measured with insert earphones) = Audiometric Threshold (dB HL) + 2cc coupler RETSPL + RECD

So, let's assume a typical adult patient has an audiometric threshold of 70 dB HL at 2000 Hz when measured with an insert earphone. The SPL measured at the eardrum would be:

Equation 12–3:
   80.5 dB SPL = 70 dB HL + 3 dB + 7.5 dB

The SPL that develops at an infant's eardrum for a given audiometric dial level (dB HL) is typically much higher than what would be measured at the eardrum of a typical adult. Boyle's law indicates that the SPL

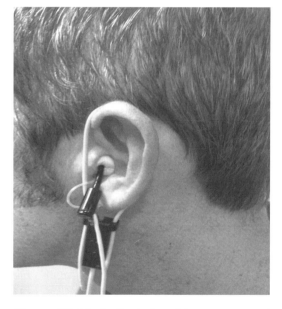

Figure 12–11. An illustration of the measurement of the real-ear-to-coupler difference (RECD).

that is measured in a cavity is inversely proportional to the size of the cavity. Obviously, infants have smaller external ear canals than adults, so the residual volume between the end of a transducer tip (or hearing aid earmold) is significantly smaller than what would exist for an adult. Also, the smaller size of the middle ear cavity influences the SPL that develops at the eardrum as do differences that exist between the physical properties of the ear canal walls, the eardrum, and middle mechanics in general. Because of these differences, the RECD is typically higher for infants and young children than adults. Table 12–3 provides average RECD values for infants and young children.

Let's assume that we use visual reinforcement audiometry with insert earphones and obtain a 2000 Hz pure-tone threshold of 70 dB HL for a 7-month old infant. Then, we measure the RECD for this infant and obtain an RECD of 16 dB at 2000 Hz. The threshold in dB SPL at the eardrum for this infant would be:

Equation 12–4:
$$90 \text{ dB SPL} =$$
$$70 \text{ dB HL} + 3 \text{ db RETSPL} + 17 \text{ dB RECD}$$

This example provides a compelling illustration of the fact that the eardrum SPL at a given audiometric dial level (in dB HL) for an infant or young child is typically higher than what would exist for an adult with a threshold at the same audiometric dial level. This is an important point for at least two reasons. First, as an infant grows, and his ear gets larger and his external and middle ear mechanics change, the RECD will typically decrease. As a result, even if the infant's hearing sensitivity does not change, a higher audiometric dial level will be required to reach the infants threshold. To explain, let's refer back to the previous example provided in Equation 12–4 in which 90 dB SPL was required at the eardrum for detection of a 2000 Hz pure tone. Let's say that the infant was evaluated again at 3 years of age and an RECD of 7 dB was measured at 2000 Hz. As a result, a higher audiometric dial level is now required to reach a level of 90 dB SPL at the ear drum.

Equation 12–5:
$$90 \text{ dB SPL} =$$
$$80 \text{ dB HL} + 3 \text{ dB RETSPL} + 7 \text{ db RECD}$$

At first glance, it may appear as though the child has suffered a 10 dB shift in hearing sensitivity, when in reality, a developmentally related change in external and middle ear acoustics is responsible for the increase in audiometric dial level required to reach threshold.

Table 12–3. RECD Average Values in Infants and Young Children Measured with an Immittance Tip

Age (in months)	Frequency (Hz)								
	250	500	750	1000	1500	2000	3000	4000	6000
1	3	8	9	12	15	15	16	20	23
6	3	7	9	11	12	13	14	17	20
12	3	6	8	10	10	11	11	15	17
24	3	5	7	9	9	10	10	14	15
36	3	5	7	9	8	9	9	13	14
60	3	5	7	9	7	8	8	13	13
> 60	3	4	6	8	7	7	8	13	13

Note how RECD values change most in the mid to high frequencies and are more stable across the age ranges in the lower frequencies.

Based on DSL v5.0. Measurements retrieved from the AudioScan Verifit system (Bagatto et al., 2005).

This dilemma may be addressed in two ways. As already stated, the audiogram may be displayed in dB SPL (SPL-o-gram), so that the clinician may monitor threshold in dB SPL at the eardrum over time. Again, this method lends itself to being quite favorable in the audiology habilitative/rehabilitative process, because the thresholds and hearing aid output are both displayed in dB SPL, so it is quite straightforward to ascertain whether unaided and aided signals are audible for the hearing aid wearer.

Alternatively, the NAL group has proposed a term referred to as "equivalent adult hearing level (HL)" as a strategy to monitor a young child's hearing sensitivity over time. The equivalent adult hearing level is determined by adding the difference between the child's RECD and the average adult RECD to the audiometric dial level reading. To explain, we return to the example provided in Equation 4. This child had an RECD of 17 dB, which is 9.5 dB higher than the average adult RECD at 2000 Hz. Adding this 9.5 dB difference to the 70 dB HL dial reading provides an adult equivalent hearing level of 79.5 dB HL, which closely corresponds to the audiometric threshold measured when the child matured to 3 years of age.

Another reason that it is important to take into account the higher RECD of infants and young children is the fact that we must possess an accurate measure of threshold to specify the gain and output we should select for the child's hearing aids. In the preceding example, it is appropriate to prescribe gain and output for the 7-month child on the basis of a threshold of 90 dB SPL at the eardrum or an adult equivalent hearing level of 80 dB HL. If neither correction were made, then the audiologist would have calculated gain and output on the basis of a 70 dB HL hearing loss.

Of course, the smaller ear canal and unique physical properties of the infant's external and middle ear also influence the SPL that develops at the eardrum for a hearing aid fitting. Specifically, for a given coupler gain setting, the SPL measured at the eardrum of an infant will typically be significantly higher than the SPL measured at an adult's eardrum. For that reason, the RECD is used to provide a more accurate representation of a child's hearing thresholds and also of the gain and output that should be provided by the hearing aid. Additional information pertaining to the RECD and use of the RECD in the hearing aid fitting process is provided in the next section of this chapter, which covers hearing aid verification for children.

VERIFICATION TO ENSURE HEARING TECHNOLOGY IS APPROPRIATE FOR THE PEDIATRIC WEARER

Once the device and the desired features gain/output have been selected, the hearing aid must be appropriately fitted for the child. Fitting a hearing aid is a process with the main goal of optimizing audibility for a child. As part of the process, the hearing aid output and features must be verified to ensure that the hearing aid is, in fact, functioning in the expected and desired manner. For our purposes, verification is defined as measures that audiologists conduct to ensure that hearing aid goals have been met (Johnson & Danhauer, 2002). Validation is another important aspect of the hearing aid fitting process and is defined as the perception of hearing aid performance and benefit from the perspective of the hearing aid wearer or family members as indicated by responses provided on questionnaires or other subjective metrics (Johnson & Danhauer, 2002). Validation of hearing aid performance and benefit for children is discussed later in this chapter.

Research has indicated that verification is critical to ensure hearing aids are fitted appropriately for both children and adults. Studies have shown that simulated gain/output provided by the hearing aid software programming is often higher than that obtained with probe microphone measures

(Campos, Mondelli, & Ferrari, 2011). Another study reported that 64% of the "first fits" from the hearing aid manufacturer failed to come within +/− 10 dB of the target gain for at least one frequency (Aahz & Moore, 2007). Considering these studies, the AAA Clinical Practice Guideline on Pediatric Amplification (2013) strongly recommends that audiologists should conduct real ear measures to ensure that hearing aid output is set to match targets determined from independently developed prescriptive formulas such as DSL or NAL. Furthermore, as mentioned elsewhere, the AAA Clinical Practice Guideline on Pediatric Amplification (2013) states that evidence-based methods such as DSL and NAL, should be used for pediatric hearing aid verification, rather than relying upon a manufacturer's proprietary prescription that is not standardized nor evidence-based for children, and therefore, inappropriate for young hearing aid users.

Prior to verification, the hearing aid's feedback suppression system should be tested and activated to allow the clinician a better idea of how much gain is available before feedback will occur (AAA Clinical Practice Guideline on Pediatric Amplification, 2013). Additionally, conducting the feedback test may be necessary to enable the active feedback cancellation system of some hearing aids. Also, conducting the acoustic feedback test typically results in optimization of the active feedback cancellation system.

The AAA Clinical Practice Guideline on Pediatric Amplification recognizes two methods by which hearing aids may be electroacoustically verified for children: (1) real-ear aided response (REAR) measures via "in situ" probe microphone measurement, and (2) simulated ear-ear probe microphone measures conducted in a 2cc hearing aid coupler. Real-ear probe microphone measures are completed while the hearing aid resides in the child's ear. Simulated real ear measures are made in a 2cc coupler inside the "test box" of a hearing aid analyzer and are completed in conjunction with a measured or average real-ear-to-coupler-difference (RECD) measure. In

situ measurements are the most ideal as they reflect the acoustic influence that the child's earmold has on the REAR. In particular, in situ measures are especially helpful with a highly vented earmold and when earmold tubing is longer than 35 mm (AAA Clinical Practice Guideline on Pediatric Amplification, 2013; McCreery, 2013a). In situ measures also take into account the effect of a reverse horn that is often unintentionally present in small earmolds of children. However, the accuracy of in situ measures is adversely affected when a child will not hold still or cannot hold his or her head in a steady position for the several minutes that are required to complete real ear measures. In such cases, simulated probe microphone measures are preferred (AAA Clinical Practice Guideline on Pediatric Amplification, 2013; McCreery, 2013b). One important point is worth noting at this time. As previously mentioned, the threshold in dB SPL at the eardrum is influenced by an individual's RECD. As such, the RECD should be measured when conducting both simulated and in situ probe microphone measures. The gold standard electroacoustic verification protocol includes in situ real ear probe microphone measures in conjunction with a measured RECD.

One of the most important components of the verification process, especially when children are involved, is the measurement of the real-ear to coupler difference (RECD; Moodie, Seewald, & Sinclair, 1994). The clinical importance of measurement of the RECD was discussed in the preceding section of the hearing aid section. Every attempt should be made to obtain RECD measurements, but these values can be predicted based on age-specific averages whenever it is not possible to measure the response (Baggato, Scollie, Seewald, Moodie, & Hoover, 2002). However, Bagatto and colleagues have demonstrated that the experienced pediatric audiologist is able to successfully measure the RECD in the vast majority of cases.

If the RECD is not accounted for (via measurement or estimated with age-specific average values), then there is a great risk for overamplification (by as much as 20 dB). The greatest change in RECD values occurs in the first 10 to 12 months of life, especially at 4000 Hz. As the child ages, the ear canal volume increases, resulting in a decrease in RECD values (Bagatto et al., 2002; Bingham, Jenstad, & Shahnaz, 2009). Regular measurements of RECDs are needed as earmolds are remade so that the hearing aids can be fit appropriately to target as the child ages. Again, as previously mentioned, the ideal practice is to measure RECD for both ears, but in cases in which a child is resistant to the measure and external and middle ear function is deemed to be essentially symmetrical and normal (no middle ear dysfunction, tympanic membrane perforation, or PE tubes), then it is reasonable to apply the RECD measured in one ear to the contralateral ear. In such cases, previous research has indicated that interaural RECD differences are typically +/− 2 dB (Munro & Howlin, 2010). It is not acceptable to apply RECD measures across ears when external and middle ear abnormalities or asymmetries exist. Middle ear abnormalities tend to have a fairly predictable impact on the RECD. Tympanic membrane perforations and PE tubes are likely to result in a large reduction in the RECD at 500 Hz and below (Martin, Munro, & Lam, 2001). In contrast, negative middle ear pressure (e.g., > 200 daPa) is likely to increase the RECD at 500 Hz and below, while middle ear effusion is likely to result in a fairly substantial increase in the RECD throughout the frequency range.

In addition to the fact that children have much smaller ear canal volumes than adults, between-subject RECD variability is substantial for both custom earmolds and acoustic immittance tips (Baggato et al., 2002; Munro, 2004). Bagatto and colleagues (2002) reported that RECD measurements can vary greatly between children, especially in the low (300 Hz) and high (4000 Hz) frequencies where the poorest repeatability was noted. Specifically, they found that individual differences can vary by as much as 36 dB. These findings are consistent with other studies (Sinclair et al., 1996; Munro, 2004). The aforementioned values underscore the importance of obtaining measured RECD values rather than relying on age-specific averages. It should be noted that slit leaks (gaps between the earmold and external ear which may be accentuated by the presence of the probe tube) can result in a reduction of RECD values in the low frequencies (de Jonge, 1996). The reader is directed to the recommendations below for making accurate RECD measurements (Baggato et al., 2002; McCreery, 2013b).

There are varying opinions about what type of transducer tip (insert earphone foam tip or the child's personal earmolds) should be used to make RECD measurements. Many researchers have suggested that the same coupling method (foam tip or custom earmold) should be used to measure hearing thresholds and obtain RECDs (Gustafson, Pittman, & Fanning, 2013). However, some hearing aid analyzer manufacturers suggest that it is more accurate to measure the RECD using the insert earphone ear tip, and subsequently, they recommend that regardless of the transducer tip used for audiologic assessment. Furthermore, some real-ear hearing aid analyzers allow for the audiologist to specify the coupling method used for threshold measures (Gustafson et al., 2013; Scollie et al., 2011). It is important that the pediatric audiologist understands the protocol for which the hearing aid analyzer has been designed. The AAA Clinical Practice Guideline on Pediatric Amplification (2013) suggests that differences in RECD values measured with transducer tips (earmold versus foam tip) are slight when the ear is very small (i.e., infant ear) and when filtered earhooks are used.

Young children, who are initially fitted within the first several weeks to months of life, often need new earmolds weekly or biweekly, especially when the hearing loss is severe to profound. Ideally, experts have suggested that the RECD is measured every time a new earmold is fitted (Bagatto et al., 2005; Ching & Britton, 2008). At the very least, the RECD should be measured following each audiologic assessment and at least every month during the first 6 months of life (as earmolds are changed frequently during that time). For older children (6 months to 7 years old), RECDs should be measured every time the earmold is changed and after every audiologic assessment (audiologic assessment is recommended every 3 months).

Tips for Successful RECD Measurements

■ Use of lubricant on the probe tube to help reduce slit leaks and the associated reduction that occurs in the RECD at 500 Hz and below

  ■ In such cases where slit leaks cannot be resolved, using measured RECD from 750 Hz and above and applying average adjusted RECD values at 250 and 500 Hz is a reasonable alternative (Bagatto et al., 2002). The following values can be inserted when using an acoustic immittance tip: 250 Hz = 2.4 dB and 500 Hz = 4.3 dB. When an earmold is used for coupling, 3.2 dB and 6.1 dB can be substituted at 250 and 500 Hz, respectively.

  ■ The tip of the probe tube should be placed within 5 mm of the eardrum. When the distance between the tip of the probe tube and the eardrum exceeds 5 mm, standing waves can result in inaccurate RECD measures at 6000 Hz or below (which will manifest as a sharp reduction or notch in the RECD response at or below 6000 Hz). Ideally, the "notch" or roll-off in the RECD will reside beyond 6000 Hz. To achieve this, Tharpe and colleagues (2001) recommended using a constant insertion depth method, where the probe tip was placed so that it extended 4 mm beyond the end of the foam insert, making the probe tube approximately 5 mm from the tympanic membrane (with a 15-mm infant ear canal length).

  ■ Another method to guide in proper placement and insertion depth of the probe tube is to place a "marker" at a specified distance from the tip of the probe tube and then insert the probe tube in the ear canal until the marker is placed in the intertragal notch. The

distance the marker is placed from the tip of the probe tube is based on age-specific average estimates of ear canal length. For instance, the distance from the inter-tragal notch to the eardrum of the average adult is about 35 mm. Positioning the marker 30 mm from the tip of the probe tube and then placing the marker at the intertragal notch results in the probe tube tip to be positioned approximately 5 mm from the eardrum. The following insertion depths are recommended based on age:

  ■ 0–12 months = 15 mm
  ■ 1–5 years = 20 mm
  ■ 5–12 years = 25 mm
  ■ 12 years and older = 30 mm

■ Insert the tip (i.e., insert earphone/immittance tip/earmold such that it is flush with the opening of the ear canal). If using a foam insert tip, make sure the insert has fully expanded in the ear before making the measurement. If the eartip or earmold is not deeply inserted, or if a foam eartip has not yet expanded after being compressed, then the RECD will possess significant roll-off at 500 Hz and below. The astute clinician should aim to place the lateral surface of the insert earphone eartip at the aperture of the external auditory meatus for both audiologic and RECD measures to promote uniformity across measures (Bagatto, Seewald, Scollie, & Tharpe, 2006).

■ Use the average RECD as a guide. If the measured RECD is grossly different (i.e., greater than 10 dB), especially at specific frequencies, the clinician should ensure that measurement error is not responsible for the large deviation from age-specific averages (McCreery, 2013b). In some cases, the child's ear may simply be different from the typical ear resulting in an individual RECD that differs from the average value, but the clinician should confirm that a substantial difference is not attributed to an invalid measure.

■ The acoustic impact of a large vents or open fitting cannot be accurately captured with simulated probe microphone measures, and consequently, in situ real ear measures should be completed in these cases (McCreery, 2013b).

Real Ear Probe Microphone Measurements

Regardless of measurement method (e.g., in situ or simulated), the clinician should measure the REAR at signal levels consistent with soft, average, and loud level speech. The REAR signal used should accurately represent the frequency, intensity, and temporal aspects of speech (AAA Clinical Practice Guideline on Pediatric Amplification, 2013). For some hearing aid analyzers, calibrated recorded speech passages with the same long-term average speech spectrum as typical speech are used as the test signal. Other systems may employ test signals that are not real speech passages but do possess the same temporal and spectral characteristics of "average speech" (e.g., ICRA Signal). Contemporary hearing aid systems often allow for the measurement of hearing aid output to a live speech signal. Although this feature can be useful to demonstrate the benefits and limitations to a child's family members by asking them to speak at a typical level and observe the audibility of their voice, the clinician should not use live speech signals as a primary tool to program and verify a child's hearing aids

The objective of real ear measures is quite simple. The hearing aid output to the soft, average, and high-level calibrated speech or speech-like signals should match (+/− 3 dB) the generic prescriptive target (DSL v5.0 or NAL-NL2; see Figure 12–8). The audiologist's task is to adjust hearing aid gain and compression parameters to achieve such a match. Furthermore, the maximum power output (MPO) should be measured to a high-level (85 to 90 dB SPL) swept pure tone, and the audiologist should ensure that the hearing aid does not exceed maximum output targets.

The audiologist should also seek to verify the function of advanced hearing aid features. When conducting real ear verification on hearing aids possessing frequency-lowering technology, the audiologist should initially disable the frequency-lowering processing and attempt to fit the hearing aid as closely to target as possible without frequency compression/transposition. This allows the clinician to evaluate the full bandwidth of the hearing aid and to determine whether there is insufficient audibility for high-frequency speech sounds. The goal should be to match target out to 6000 Hz and provide as wide of a bandwidth as possible. If adequate audibility cannot be provided through 8000 Hz, then the audiologist should consider enabling frequency-lowering technology.

There is no clear consensus regarding a real ear method to verify the function of frequency-lowering technology. Glista et al. (2009) and Wolfe et al. (2010) described the use of a verification signal specifically designed for use of frequency-lowering technology. Specifically, the calibrated speech signal of the Audioscan Verifit hearing aid analyzer was low-pass filtered by 30 dB with a cutoff frequency of 1000 Hz except for a ⅓-octave band centered around 6300 Hz (e.g., Speech6300). Wolfe et al. (2010) evaluated hearing aid output to the standard calibrated speech signal and to the Speech6300 signal both with and without nonlinear frequency compression (NLFC). They suggested a goal of providing audibility of the Speech6300 signal at an input level of 55 dB SPL for children with mild-to-moderate high-frequency hearing loss, and a goal of providing audibility of the Speech6300 at an input level of 65 dB SPL for children with severe high-frequency hearing loss. Wolfe and colleagues (2010) were typically unable to meet these goals without NLFC but generally were able to achieve these objectives with the use of NLFC.

In cases of severe-to-profound high-frequency hearing loss in which audibility is insufficient in the 2000–3000 Hz range, the clinician may have to select relatively aggressive frequency-lowering parameters to facilitate audibility of the phoneme /s/ or the Speech6300 signal. When frequency-lowering technology is overly aggressive, the user may begin to experience difficulty distinguishing between different high-frequency phonemes. For instance, the /s/ and /sh/ may become indistinguishable. Scollie (2012) provides excellent guidance to determine appropriate frequency-lowering settings. Specifically, she measured hearing aid output to recorded /sh/ and /s/ phonemes, and suggested that the output to the /s/ phoneme approximately 5 dB above threshold (5 dB SL). Additionally, Scollie (2012) suggested that the output for the /s/ and /sh/ should be separated by at least 200 Hz, with an ideal separation of at least 500 Hz (Scollie, 2012).

Although Scollie described measurement to recorded /sh/ and /s/ phonemes, it is also feasible to measure real ear output to /s/ and /sh/ presented via live speech (i.e., live speech mapping; Glista & Scollie, 2009). Regardless of the stimulus the clinician uses, he or she should follow up real ear assessment with a biologic listening check of the hearing aid to ensure that the aided output is free of distortion and excessive noise, and also ensure that a distinct difference can be heard between the /sh/ and /s/ phonemes (i.e., the /s/ phoneme should not sound like /sh/ or possess substantial lisping/lateralization; Scollie, 2012).

If additional features such as directional microphones and digital noise reduction are activated, they also should be verified. The AAA Clinical Practice Guideline on Pediatric Amplification (2013) recommends that both automatic and program specific settings should be verified. Each verification system has ways to complete this, and the reader is directed to his or her specific system to learn how to conduct these measurements. McCreery (2008) also offers excellent suggestions for verification of advanced hearing aid features employed for pediatric hearing aid fittings. There is, however, no consensus at this time in regards to how most advanced features should be verified for use in children (AAA Clinical Practice Guideline on Pediatric Amplification, 2013).

SII/SHARP

Beyond the electroacoustic verification of hearing aid output relative to generic prescriptive targets (NAL or DSL), the audiolo-

gist may wish to incorporate other verification tools including the Speech Intelligibility Index (SII) or the Situational Hearing Aid Response Profile (SHARP), which was recently updated in 2013 to allow transfer of an .XML file directly from the Verifit REM systems (Boys Town National Research Hospital, 2013).

The SII is a standardized tool developed by the American National Standards Institute (1997) that can be used to evaluate the audibility of speech at various input levels (Hornsby, 2004; McCreery, 2013c). For adults, the SII can be used to predict speech recognition scores based on the proportion of the signal that is audible to the recipient, the level of the input signal, and the degree of the recipient's hearing loss. For greater hearing losses, the SII takes into account a level distortion factor that assumes that the impaired ear will be less proficient at processing an audible signal. In other words, the provision of audibility is predicted to result in a lesser extent of benefit in regards to an improvement in speech recognition for more severe hearing losses relative to mild-to-moderate hearing losses.

It is important to note, however, that predictions of speech recognition based on the proportion of the speech signal that is audible are based on adult data and are not appropriate for predicting speech recognition in children. For instance, Gustafson and Pittman (2011) showed that performance on sentence perception improved with increased bandwidth for a group of children even though SII values remained similar with the extension of the aided bandwidth.

Recently, the Marlene Bagatto and colleagues at the University of Western Ontario (UWO) developed the Pediatric Audiological Monitoring Protocol (PedAMP), which includes normative values for the SII to use as a guide to determine if a child's SII is in the range expected for his or her degree of hearing loss (Bagatto, Moodie, Malandrino, et al., 2011). Research has shown that there is a positive correlation between SII and receptive vocabulary outcomes of children with hearing loss. Specifically, a study completed by Stiles and colleagues (2012) suggested higher receptive vocabulary skills in children with an aided SII of 65 (or 0.65) or better. In the

PedAMP protocol, Bagatto and colleagues (2011) incorporate the SII measurement along with other measurements of audibility and hearing aid validation (e.g., questionnaires) to provide a comprehensive battery of validation measures. The PedAMP is discussed in greater detail later in this chapter. See Figure 12–12 for the SII normative chart. Finally, it should be noted that the SII does not take into account the potential improvement in audibility provided by frequency-lowering amplification, and there is currently no consensus as to how the SII should be used as a validation tool for hearing aids with frequency-lowering technology.

The SHARP program provides a calculation of the "Aided Audibility Index" (AAI), which is similar to the SII measurement and may also be used as a tool helpful for determining audibility in various listening conditions. The AAI is designed to represent the proportion of the speech signal that is above the listener's threshold and uses verification data to predict the input/output function in $1/3$ octave bands. As the name suggests, the SHARP addresses situational responses, including audibility for different speakers (male, female, child) different locations/environments (classroom, home, distance, head location), and even explores the extent of audibility of the speech signal when a caregiver is speaking while the child is being cradled or held on his or her lap (Boys Town National Research Hospital, 2013). Currently, the researchers responsible for the SHARP development are working on ways to calculate the AAI/SII for frequency lowering and are also developing ways to predict speech recognition for children on the basis of the AAI/aided SII score (personal communication with Ryan McCreery, 2013).

The SII and SHARP values can also be used as counseling tools to help professionals working with children with hearing loss and their families to better understand how the child is able to hear in various environ-

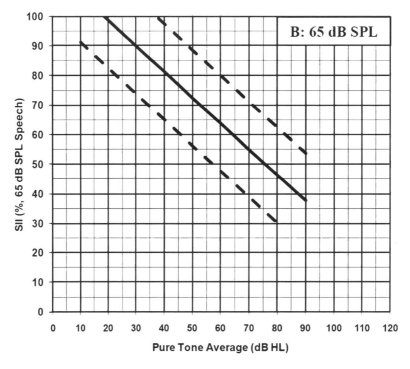

Figure 12–12. PedAMP aided SII normative values for 65 dB SPL signal. PedAMP = Pediatric Amplification Monitoring Protocol.

ments (in distance, background noise, and reverberation) with and without amplification. It will also help those around the child better understand how a child can monitor his or her speech production (auditory feedback loop) and may be used as justification in a request of an FM/DM system for use in a classroom setting where the environment is less than optimal for hearing speech clearly (AAA Clinical Practice Guideline on Pediatric Amplification, 2013).

Cortical Auditory Evoked Potentials

Although real ear probe microphone measures (and the SII/SHARP) are excellent objective verification tools, it is also essential to collect measures that evaluate how the child behaviorally responds to aided signals. For very young children and/or those with developmental delays, these types of behavioral measures may be hard to obtain. Cortical auditory evoked potentials (CAEPs) objectively measure cortical responses evoked by speech sounds at the level of the auditory cortex, thus providing information about the audibility of sounds, especially speech sounds (Golding et al., 2007; Purdy et al., 2004). Furthermore, CAEPs can also be used to evaluate the maturity of the auditory system (Sharma et al., 2005). It has been well-established that young children who are not identified with hearing loss and/or do not receive adequate auditory stimulation at a very early age are at risk for speech and language delays or abnormalities (Sharma et al., 2005; Yoshinaga-Itano et al., 1998). The early ages (0–3) are when the central auditory pathways are maximally plastic (Kral, Hartmann, Tillein, Held, & Klinke, 2002; Sharma et al., 2002). This is also the age when it can be most difficult to obtain behavioral information regarding auditory benefit with hearing aids. Therefore, the measurement of CAEPs may harbor potential as a valuable tool in situations when there is uncertainty in regards to hearing thresholds (i.e., in cases of ANSD) and when children cannot participate in speech perception testing. Researchers have shown that this testing can be completed both with and without amplification (Golding et al., 2007; Sharma et al., 2005). It should be noted that the child must be calm, awake, and quiet in order for CAEP measures to be successfully acquired. Numerous studies have also shown that the CAEP can be used to show that a hearing aid is providing sufficient audibility for various speech sounds presented at an average conversational level (Golding et al., 2007), and it can be used as a biomarker of maturation of the auditory nervous system (Sharma et al., 2002, 2005). Additional research is needed to facilitate clinical implementation of the CAEP.

Aided Testing

Additional behavioral measures may also be used to aid the clinician in the verification process. These behavioral measures include, but are not limited to, aided threshold and aided speech recognition assessment. It is important to note that these measures should not be done in place of real ear measures, but rather should serve as a supplement to verification completed via real ear probe microphone measures.

Aided threshold testing allows for a determination of the lowest-level sound a child can detect while wearing hearing aids. This information is not available from real ear probe microphone measures. Aided threshold assessment is sometimes erroneously referred to as functional gain testing. In reality, the two are not synonymous. Aided threshold testing simply involves the measurement of the lowest-level sound a child responds to when aided, while functional gain testing is a determination of the difference between unaided and aided sound field thresholds. The limitations of functional gain testing are well documented (McCreery, 2013d). The primary limitation is the fact that for a hearing aid with WDRC, the gain provided for low-level warble tones or narrowband noise presented during functional gain testing is unlikely to be representative of the gain the hearing aid provides for speech-level inputs. As such, functional gain assessment (a comparison between unaided and aided sound field thresholds) is not recommended.

However, the audiologist should consider measuring aided sound field thresholds in young children who can attend to the task for this testing to be completed. Again, the aided threshold is the only measure that indicates the lowest level sound a child can detect. Ideally, aided thresholds should not exceed 25 dB HL, so that the child has adequate access to low-level speech and environmental sounds. When aided thresholds are elevated, the audiologist should consider increasing the hearing aid gain for low-level sounds and/or replacing the earmold to provide additional gain (via a better fit, a deeper canal, a horn, etc.). It is imperative to emphasize that any hearing aid adjustments should be verified by real ear measures and a listening check. The audiologist must confirm that prescriptive targets are not significantly exceeded and that the hearing aid sound quality is not poor (i.e., excessive internal noise).

Of course, it should also be noted that there are cases when aided threshold testing is one of the only verification options. Such examples include children who are using cochlear implants or BAHA devices. In these instances and also in the case of verification of air-conduction hearing aids, aided threshold testing should be corroborated with aided speech recognition assessment when possible.

Aided Speech Perception Testing

For children under the age of 2 years old, aided speech perception testing is often difficult to successfully complete (Stelmachowicz, 2004), and testing is often limited to assessment of speech detection. This is also the case for children with developmental delays or other complex factors (difficult to test, English as a second language users, or medically complex). For children around 2.5 to 3 years of age (language age), the likelihood of successfully evaluating speech recognition sub-

stantially improves. There are a variety of options for assessing speech perception at different ages and stages of development. For a full list of currently available test materials, the reader is directed to Advanced Bionic's resource entitled " Test Reference for Cochlear Implants" available at: http://www.advancedbionics.com/content/dam/ab/Global/en_ce/documents/libraries/AssessmentTools/Test%20Reference%20for%20Cochlear%20Implants.pdf

Although the aforementioned resource is provided by a cochlear implant manufacturer, it includes a number of speech recognition materials that are appropriate for use with children with hearing aids. Also, see Table 12–4 for a chart of available and recommended speech perception tests for children. Not included in the list is a newer speech perception tool: (1) the University of Western Ontario (UWO) Plurals Test (Glista & Scollie, 2012), which was designed to assess the child's ability to detect plurality (hear word-final fricatives /s/ and /z/) to better understand if /s/ is audible with frequency lowering or extended bandwidth hearing aids (the UWO Plurals Test may be obtained from the Phonak Hearing Aid Company), and (2) The Phrases in Noise Test (PINT; Schafer & Thibodeau, 2006). The PITN test is attractive for use with young children because it is the first available speech in noise test that is designed for young children (under 5 years of age), is resistant to ceiling and floor effects, and uses multisource noise that is often found in typical classrooms (Schafer & Thibodeau, 2006; Schafer et al., 2012; Schafer et al., 2012). It is particularly useful in determining what classroom supports a child might need including preferential seating, possible directional microphone settings, and hearing assistive technology (i.e., RF or FM systems; Schafer et al., 2012).

When possible, aided speech recognition should be assessed with recorded speech materials, rather than monitored live voice (MLV). However, some young children (2 to 3 years old) may be reluctant to participate when recorded materials are used, and in such cases, the audiologist may have to rely on the

Table 12–4. Speech Perception Tests for Children

Test Name	Open/Closed Set	Test Stimuli	Evaluation Method	Age Range
Northwestern University Children's Perception of Speech (NU-CHIPS)	Four picture Closed set	Phonetically similar monosyllable words	Picture pointing task Chance performance = 25%	2.5–5 years
Word Identification Picture Intelligibility (WIPI)	Six picture Closed set	Phonetically similar monosyllable words	Picture pointing task Chance performance = 16.7%	3–5 years
Early Speech Perception (ESP) Test (updated in 2012)	Four item Closed set	Pictures and objects representing: Detection Pattern perception Spondees Monosyllabic words	Picture pointing/object pointing task Chance performance = 25%	~ 2 yrs + for low standard version; ~ 6 yrs for standard version
Phrases in Noise Test (PINT)	Pseudo open set; Speech in noise testing using four-classroom noise	The child acts out the speech stimuli (i.e., touch his nose)	Child acts out the command Estimates child's speech in noise threshold at the 50% correct level (similar to the BKB-SIN); Not confounded by articulation errors	2–5 years of age (as soon as a child can act out the speech stimuli)
Multisyllabic Lexical Neighborhood Test (MLNT)	Open set	"low frequency occurring words from dense lexical neighborhoods"	Repeat words Can score based on words correct and/or phonemes correct	3–5 years
Lexical Neighborhood Test (LNT)	Open set	Lexically "easy" and "hard" word lists (25 words) "high-frequency occurring words from sparse neighborhoods"	Repeat words	3–5 years

continues

Table 12–4. *continued*

Test Name	Open/Closed Set	Test Stimuli	Evaluation Method	Age Range
Phonetically Balanced Kindergarten (PBK) Words	Open set	Phonetically balanced monosyllabic kindergarten level words	Repeat words and score based on number of phonemes and number of words correct	4–6 years
University of Western Ontario (UWO) Plurals Test (distributed by Phonak)	Closed set (2 picture choice)	Multisyllabic words differing between singular and plural (/-s/ and /-z/) forms	Child chooses between singular and plural form of the word by pointing to the corresponding picture	~ 6 years of age (once a child knows the difference between singular and plural)
HINT Sentences for Children (HINT-C)	Open set sentences	Sentences with background babble (can also be presented in quiet)	Scored based on number of words repeated correctly in the sentence	7 years +
Consonant-Nucleus-Consonant (CNC) Words	Open set words	Monosyllabic words with equal phonemic distribution across lists	Repeat words; can score phonemes correct and/or words correct	7 years +
Bamford-Kowal-Bench Speech-in-Noise Test (BKB-SIN)	Open set sentences	Sentences with background babble	Repeat words in sentence. Scored to determine speech to noise ratio loss (SNR loss)	7 years +

Source: Data adapted from the Advanced Bionics Test Reference for Cochlear Implants, http://www.advancedbionics.com/content/dam/ab/Global/en_ce/documents/libraries/AssessmentTools/Test%20Reference%20for%20Cochlear%20Implants.pdf

use of MLV presentation. The clinician should keep in mind that MLV test results should not be compared across conditions in which the examiner was not the same. Also, MLV test results are heavily dependent on the examiner's effort to articulate the test stimuli. As such, variations in speaker articulation from one test condition to another (e.g., unaided versus aided) may hinder interpretation of differences that are obtained. Finally, performance on MLV tests is usually significantly better than performance on measure with recorded materials. In Roeser and Clark's (2008) study, 72% of the studied population had significantly different results between testing conducted with MLV versus recorded test materials with differences as great as 80 percentage points.

Speech recognition testing should be completed in each monaurally aided (with the opposite ear plugged) and in the binaural condition. Although the binaural condition is most representative of how a child listens in the real world, it is also important to determine how each ear performs independently. Assessment of aided speech recognition may need to be completed over multiple test sessions to obtain reliable results for each monaural condition as well as the binaural condition.

Speech recognition should be assessed at a presentation level consistent with average conversational level speech (45 dB HL/60 dBA) and also at a presentation level consistent with soft speech (35 dB HL/50 dBA; Madell, 2008). The authors suggest evaluating speech recognition in each monaural condition and the binaural condition at an average conversational level and at a soft conversational level in the binaural condition. Speech recognition testing in noise should also be evaluated. The authors recommend evaluating speech recognition in noise at a +5 dB SNR with the speech signal of interest presented at 60 dB HL/75 dBA). The higher presentation level for speech in noise assessment is recommended because it is similar to speech levels that are typically encountered in realistic situations. The SNR may be adjusted if the child encounters ceiling or floor effects at the 5 dB SNR. Also, the clinician may consider the use of a test with an adaptive SNR. Some clinicians may question the need to evaluate speech recognition in noise for children. The clinician should keep in mind the fact that research suggests that infants and young children (under the age of 4) spend as much as one quarter of their day in noisy environments (Jones & Launer, 2010). It is imperative to understand how children understand speech in these situations, so appropriate management and support may be provided.

PRACTICAL ISSUES TO ENSURE REAL-WORLD SUCCESS

Hearing Aid Orientation

Regardless of whether the audiologist is able to perfectly program a hearing aid to meet a child's needs, the child will be at risk for not benefitting from amplification if his or her family does not understand how to properly use and maintain the hearing aids. As such, it is critical for the audiologist to provide a thorough hearing aid orientation for the child's caregivers. Often, a hearing aid orientation is considered to be a one-time event, but for parents who are likely overwhelmed by the diagnosis and the hearing aid fitting itself, it is likely much more effective for the orientation to exist as a dynamic process that meets the child's and family's needs at each age and stage of development.

Because caregivers will often be overwhelmed with emotion on the day their child is initially fitted with hearing aids, the initial orientation should focus only on the most vital aspects of proper hearing aid use. The authors recommend discussing proper insertion/removal (with a demonstration and an opportunity for the caregivers to practice), changing the battery, and a wear schedule (eyes open, ears on). Retention will also quickly become an issue as the child grows and becomes more active.

Continued counseling regarding care and maintenance should be completed across several visits and should also be incorporated into therapy sessions with auditory-verbal therapists, speech therapists, and deaf educators so that the family receives the information redundantly. Additional parts of the hearing aid orientation include cleaning the device (checking earmolds, microphones, and tone hooks for debris), storing the hearing aids, daily listening checks, battery issues, and troubleshooting.

For young children, it is especially imperative that the parents understand the importance of daily listening checks (in which the caregiver listens to the hearing aids with a stethoscope) and also understand the relationship between acoustic feedback and the physical fit of the earmold. The importance of regular earmold impressions should be stressed to these parents in order to promote hearing aids that properly fit the child's ears. For older children, daily listening checks should be composed of a stethoscope listening check and also should include a quick completion of the Ling 6-Sound Test (Ling, 2002) in which the child repeats the six sounds that are spoken by a caregiver (/ah/, /oo/, /ee/, /m/, /s/, /sh/). Ideally, a child should be able to detect and discriminate all six Ling sounds from 6 feet (typical distance for conversation between 2 people) and from 9 feet (typical distance for conversation between more than 2 people).

When ordering the child's hearing aids, a pediatric care kit can be requested through the manufacturer and can be used to guide hearing aid orientation. A comprehensive hearing aid care kit typically includes a dehumidifier, battery tester, earmold blower, wax loop, earmold lubricant, listening stethoscope, retaining clip(s), and double-sided tape.

For older children, whether they are receiving upgraded technology or are using features that have recently been activated, a thorough orientation should be completed with the child and the parents. This includes, but is not limited to operation of the volume control, program/memory switch/button,

and use of the telephone. Anecdotally, many children use the speakerphone or take their hearing aids out and increase the volume on the handset while using the telephone. In those cases, they often do not understand how to hold the telephone so that it is properly oriented to the hearing aid microphones or telecoil. With improved binaural hearing technology that allows wireless streaming of the telephone signal to both ears, it is imperative that audiologists counsel the patient and family on how to facilitate telephone use. They may also benefit from practice while in the office so that any potential issues can be addressed before they become a problem or result in dissatisfaction with phone use with hearing aids.

Incorporating other hearing assistive technologies (HATs), such as wireless devices can improve hearing aid performance and satisfaction for older children. The reader is referred to other sections in this chapter that specifically address HAT devices.

Eyes Open, Ears On: Wear Time

As audiologists who recognize the importance of early amplification to maximize language learning (Sininger, Doyle, & Moore, 1999; Yoshinaga-Itano et al., 1998), we are eager to fit hearing aids closely after diagnosis. Our goal is for full-time hearing aid use to begin immediately after fitting. However, a data-logging study suggests average hearing aid use for children under age 19 was 5.5 hours per day and for infants and young children, average wear time was just under 5 hours per day (consider the amount of time spent sleeping in the early years; Jones & Launer, 2010). Additionally, around 40%, of 5,000 pediatric hearing aid users participating in a pediatric data-logging study wore their hearing aids for 4 hours or less per day (Jones & Launer, 2010).

Consistent and appropriate hearing aid use is essential to support speech and language development, but there are barriers to device use and it is important that audiologists are prepared to help guide families through this part of the process. Immediately following fitting, full-time hearing aid use should be facilitated to the greatest extent possible. "Eyes open, ears on" is a philosophy that is easy for parents to remember. It is not uncommon for infants to have only 4 to 6 hours of wear time because a good deal of the first few months of an infant's life is spent sleeping. Wear time should increase as the child ages and is awake more throughout the day, but the child is also more likely to begin making attempts to remove his or her hearing aids to use as a "chew toy" or for attention getting purposes. For many children, expectations should be established quickly where they know that hearing aids are expected to stay on. At this point in time, it is important for the audiologist to provide good counsel to the family to promote hearing aid retention and full-time use. This counsel may simply involve words of encouragement but should also include strategies to facilitate retention including bonnets/aviator caps, wig tape, retention cords, and so on. The audiologist should be certain to discuss the association between full-time hearing aid use and spoken language development, so that the family has an appreciation for the importance of effective early intervention.

It is also important that the audiologist acknowledges that full-time hearing aid use is not without difficulty, but that establishing full-time use will improve with time. To get a better idea about how each family is adjusting to hearing aid use in different situations and to develop rapport and support of the family, McCreery (2013a) suggests asking questions such as, "When do you feel like your child is most successful with keeping the hearing aids on?" and "What situations are more difficult to keep the hearing aids on?" In a study conducted by Moeller and colleagues (2009), parents identified five main concerns for wear time: safety issues, device loss or damage, retention problems, inclement weather (wind and/or rain), or high noise levels (movie theatres or parades).

Wear time increased when the parents could be close to the child, but challenging situations such as riding in the car (inability to communicate due to reverberation and distance), participating in outdoor play, and engaging in family outings made consistent use more of a barrier. The use of data-logging can also help the audiologist further inquire into what types of environment the child is in and can also be used as a counseling tool for families. McCreery (2013a) recommends presenting data-logging as a way to monitor the function and effectiveness of the hearing aids. Although validity of data-logging has not yet been determined, it can also help with accountability for some families.

Helping parents establish expectations and routines regarding hearing aid use will facilitate consistent hearing aid use as early as possible (Moeller et al., 2009). For children with slight to mild hearing loss, there is not always a obvious difference in a young child's performance with and without hearing aids. Moeller and colleagues (2009) recommended using hearing loss simulations, rather than audiology terms to convey the significance of varying degrees of hearing loss to support hearing aid use.

Remote microphone technologies might also help support hearing aid use and communicative contact with an active toddler who might be exerting his or her independence. This will also address some safety concerns in the car and on outings when a parent can remain in contact with the child despite a less than ideal environment/distance (Thibodeau & Schafer, 2002).

Device Use in Older Children

As children get older, hearing aid use may decrease for cosmetic reasons. Children with disabilities (including hearing loss) are two to three times as likely to experience bullying as compared with children with typical development (PACER, 2012). Bullying and peer pressure may contribute to a child's decision to refrain from hearing aid use. Experts have suggested that older children with hearing loss are often ill-prepared to respond appropriately to bullying and peer pressure, especially if they lack the language, social skills, and self-confidence needed to handle these difficult situations (English et al., 2013). It is important that the child's caregiver and audiologist attempt to maintain an ongoing and constructive dialogue with the child in order to explore the child's social-emotional reaction to his or her hearing loss. Resources like those available from Stop Bullying.gov may help parents, teachers, and hearing health care providers be more effective in addressing bullying (http://www.StopBullying.gov), and the Parent Advocacy Coalition for Education Rights (PACER) center also provides resources to help with IEP and 504 plans that address bullying. Pediatric and educational audiologists should consider recommending goals to help a child with hearing loss learn appropriate social skills such as sharing, taking turns, thinking through actions, and other social pragmatic considerations. It may be necessary to include additional program modifications into the IEP including use of social stories and the provision of in-service trainings for staff and peers to help them better understand hearing loss and hearing technology (English et al., 2013). Hands and Voices (http://www.handsandvoices.org) is also an organization that supports children with hearing loss and can provide additional resources to help with school transitions and concerns.

The Ida Institute has also developed materials that are designed to facilitate hearing aid use at all ages and stages. For younger children, in particular, the My World tool can allow the child to role-play and act out specific situations where they struggle to hear or are feeling bullied. This tool uses open-ended questions/queries to assist an audiologist and other providers in understanding how a child feels in the home, classroom, and outdoor areas. The My World tool includes manipulatives to explore the social-emotional aspects of hearing loss, a documentation form, and a listening guide to help facilitate these conversations. The My World Tool includes three components: (1) Choosing the environment/being curious, (2) Understanding successes and challenges while identifying strategies (for better communication), and (3) Documenting decisions and strategies (http://idainstitute.com/myworld). My World tool resources may be found at http://www.idainstitute.com/myworld

Management and Follow-Up Care

Once the hearing aids have been fitted and the family has received an effective initial orientation, follow-up appointments should be scheduled. Children who are newly fitted with hearing aids should be scheduled to return within 1 week, so the clinician may evaluate the integrity of the earmold fit and also provide further counsel to the family regarding proper hearing aid use. The child should also begin periodic (e.g., weekly) sessions with an Auditory-verbal therapist or other early interventionist who specializes in language development of children with hearing loss. Following the initial checkup, infants should return weekly until 3 to 4 months of age for ear/impressions/earmold fittings and at least monthly after that until 12 months of age.

These authors recommended that children return for audiological monitoring and a hearing aid check every 3 months until the child is 7 years of age and every 6 months thereafter. At those appointments, a biologic listening check, electroacoustic analysis via real ear probe microphone assessment should be completed following the assessment of unaided air-conduction thresholds (and bone-conduction if changes to air conduction are noted). Aided speech recognition testing should also be completed. Aided threshold testing should also be completed as time allows. The follow-up schedule can be adapted as needed if the child cannot attend to assessment tasks for extended periods of time or has developmental delays or other disabilities that affect testing.

Mentoring and Working with Families

Studies examining the needs of families of children with hearing loss have identified several common themes including: (1) the need for parent-to-parent connection, (2) redundancy of information, and (3) multiple education formats (Moeller et al., 2009). Mentor programs and parent/child programs have been shown to be very helpful. Parent/child programs can start with a baby group (for children under 18 months) in which a group of parents of infants with hearing loss periodically meet with facilitators (e.g., pediatric audiologist and Auditory-Verbal therapist) to discuss the issues the families are currently facing as well as strategies for addressing challenges. Additionally, the program at which the authors work has created a parent-toddler group (18–36 months of age), which provides an opportunity for parents of toddlers to meet one another and receive guidance and support in a group setting. These types of programs serve as a helpful resource for families and provide great opportunity for audiologists, speech language pathologists, deaf educators, and parents to share strategies and tips to help the child transition through different stages and to overcome obstacles commonly encountered during these stages.

Additionally, parents and families have expressed a strong desire to connect with other parents going through the same process. Financial concerns are also an issue for families to obtain hearing aids and/or FM/DM systems. Establishing information regarding sources of financial aid in your area and at the state level will be very helpful for families. Financial support can be obtained through AG Bell Association (http://listeningandspokenlanguage.org/), The HIKE (Hearing Impaired Kids Endowment) Fund (http://www.thehikefund.org/), Lions Club (http://www.lionsclubs.org), SERTOMA clubs (http://www.sertoma.org/), and other smaller groups. Audiologists play a crucial role in helping the family obtain funding for such programs by writing letters on their behalf and helping the family navigate the process.

Hearing Assistance Technology

Hearing aid signal processing and technology have improved dramatically over the past two decades. However, children are still likely to encounter difficulty when listening in adverse environments. Pediatric audiologists should support the child and family in identifying hearing assistance technology that will allow the child to overcome even the most significant barriers and challenges hearing loss may impose in the child's daily living situations. Hearing assistance technology refers to a varied array of technologies that have been developed to enhance reception of auditory signals by way of amplification, visual input, or vibrotactile stimulation (Thibodeau, 2004).

The most effective means to improve speech recognition in noisy and reverberant environments and for signals originating from a great distance (e.g., several feet away) is through the use of remote microphone wireless personal RF systems. These systems are composed of a microphone and transmitting unit that captures and transmits a signal of interest via RF transmission to a personal RF receiver that is directly coupled to the DAI port of a child's hearing aid. Research has shown that these systems typically provide a 5 to 20 dB improvement in the SNR (Boothroyd & Iglehart; 1998; Hawkins, 1984).

Historically, these systems have used a frequency modulated (FM) signal to transmit the signal of interest to the RF receiver. So what exactly are FM radio waves? Amplitude modulated (AM) and FM radio waves both incorporate a carrier frequency to transmit to radio signal. For instance, in modern day commercial radio, the carrier frequency is a high-frequency electromagnetic wave created by oscillating a high voltage electrical signal through the transmitting antenna creating a carrier wave that possesses the same frequency as the oscillating signal used to produce the electromagnetic wave. Figure 12–13A provides an illustration of a "signal of interest." In FM transmission, the desired signal is modulated in the frequency domain and overlaid on a sinusoidal high-frequency carrier wave. The frequency on your car's radio dial corresponds to the carrier frequency. By contrast, AM signals are modulated in the amplitude domain before being overlaid on the carrier wave. The radio carrier wave is shown in Figure 12–13B. The carrier wave is amplitude modulated by the signal of interest, which is shown in Figure 12–13C. Figure 12–13D provides an example in which the carrier wave is frequency modulated by the signal of interest.

In both types of transmission, the receiving device (i.e., your antenna and car radio) captures and demodulates the transmitted signal, in effect separating the desired signal (such as music) from the carrier. While a full discussion of the difference between AM and FM transmission is beyond the scope of this article, it is useful to note a few of the reasons that FM is a more desirable transmission method for HAT. First, FM signals have better sound quality than AM signals due to a wider available bandwidth. The FCC has protected higher frequency ranges for FM transmission, providing wide bandwidth for transmission and the potential to use multiple FM channels. Second, FM signals are less prone to interference than are AM signals (consider the difference in quality and the amount of static audible on your car radio's AM and FM stations). Finally, because FM waves are broadcast at a higher carrier frequency than AM waves, FM waves are less able to pass through physical barriers. This means that FM signals are less prone to "leaking" from one room to another compared with AM signals (because FM signals are typically broadcast at higher carrier frequencies)—but certainly not immune to this problem, which is discussed later.

Digital Radio Frequency Transmission

The previous section discusses analog radio transmission. So what is digital radio? How are

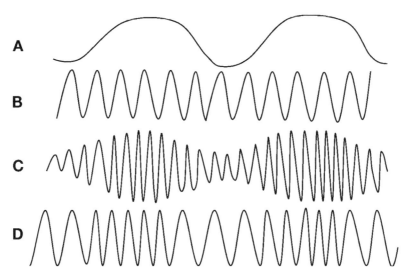

Figure 12–13. A. An illustration of a "signal of interest." **B.** An illustration of a radio carrier wave. **C.** An illustration of the radio carrier wave transmitting the signal of interest via amplitude modulation. **D.** An illustration of the radio carrier wave transmitting the signal of interest via frequency modulation.

zeroes and ones transmitted on radio waves? Is it magic? Not quite, but it does require a quick review of the basics to elucidate.

Digital Signal Processing

Analog signals are converted to digital signals through sampling of the original signal of interest. Figure 12–14 shows an example of an analog signal that is sampled at different points in time. The amplitude of the signal at these points is coded through processes called discretization and quantization into bits, a contraction of the words binary and digits. This refers to the fact that a "bit" of digital information is represented as one of two digits, 0 or 1. For example, let's say that we would like to code the signal in Figure 12–14 with a 3-bit system. The relevant amplitude range of the signal of interest is divided into 8 values (2 options: zero or one, for classification across three opportunities to classify the signal = $2^3 = 8$). First, the digitizer determines whether the amplitude of the signal falls within the top or bottom half of the relevant range of amplitudes. If it falls within the top half, a "1" is assigned, and if it falls within the bottom half, a "0" is assigned. Then, the top and bottom halves are further divided into halves, and a "1" or "0" is assigned based on which half the signal resides. Finally, those halves are further divided, and a "1" or "0" is assigned based on where the signal resides.

A digitized signal can be reconverted to an analog signal through a process called digital-to-analog conversion. Basically, the aforementioned process occurs in reverse. The benefits of digital signal processing are well-established. Most importantly, in hearing technology applications, digital processing allows for more complex and precise analysis and manipulation of a signal of interest relative to analog processing.

Digital RF

So, now can we get to the part about how a radio signal can be digitized? Sure, and there are actually several ways to accomplish this

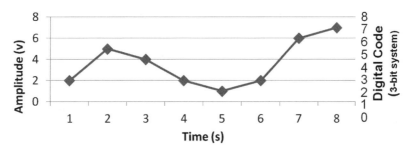

Time	Digital Code	Fours	Twos	Ones
1	2	0	1	0
2	5	1	0	1
3	4	1	0	0
4	2	0	1	0
5	1	0	0	1
6	2	0	1	0
7	6	1	1	0
8	7	1	1	1

Figure 12–14. An illustration of an analog signal sampled at different points in time and converted to a digital code.

goal. Figure 12–15 provides an illustration of one type of approach called Amplitude Shift Keying (ASK), which is utilized to accomplish digital RF transmission. Just as with an AM and FM radio, a carrier frequency is used to deliver the signal of interest. However, the carrier frequency is modulated between "on" and "off" states by a binary digital code. When the system must code a "1," the carrier frequency is transmitted at specified amplitude. Conversely, when the system must code a "0," the carrier frequency is temporarily "muted." In other words, the digital code described above may be transmitted through pulsing the carrier frequency in an "on and off manner" as shown in Figure 12–15.

Gaussian Frequency Shift Keying (GFSK) is another approach utilized to accomplish digital RF transmission. With GFSK, a binary one is represented by a positive frequency deviation imposed on the carrier frequency and a binary zero by a negative frequency deviation imposed on the carrier frequency (Figure 12–16). A potential advantage of GFSK over ASK is less susceptibility to noise/interference for the GFSK approach. Although frequency shift keying does require a wider bandwidth than ASK, the Gaussian filter used in GFSK smoothes the frequency deviation in order to minimize the necessary RF bandwidth.

In most contemporary digital RF systems, the carrier frequency is much higher than that used in AM and FM radio applications. In Bluetooth technology and the system described in this article, the carrier frequency is 2.4 gigahertz (GHz; 2.4 billion Hz). The user must "pair together" the transmitter and the receiver. Once this occurs, they "work together" with one another based on a single agreed-upon protocol. In fact, the name "Bluetooth" refers to the nickname of a tenth-century Scandanavian King, Harald I, famous for uniting warring Danish tribes into one kingdom (supposedly King Harald's teeth were stained blue by blueberries). During transmission, the first segment of the information that is transmitted is used to ensure that the receiver is communicating with the appropriate transmitter. Once this is established, the rest of the digital code may be used to transmit the signal via a GFSK approach.

Because many commercial devices feature digital RF transmission (e.g., Bluetooth, hearing technology, home appliances, etc.),

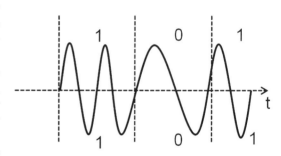

Figure 12–16. An illustration of digital radio frequency transmission via Gaussian Frequency Shift Keying.

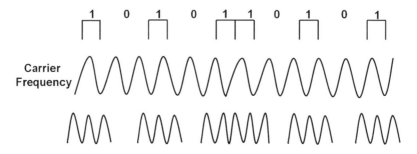

Figure 12–15. An illustration of digital radio frequency transmission via amplitude shift keying.

the carrier frequency continually "hops" from one carrier frequency (each is one Megahertz wide) to another 800 times or more per second. This "channel hopping" dramatically reduces the potential for interference between devices in close proximity to one another. Additionally, many systems will identify channels in which interference may exist and avoid those channels during the roving process.

Theoretical Advantages of Digital RF

The advantages of digital RF are plentiful. First, by means of control data that are broadcast along the digitized audio signal, the analysis and manipulation of the transmitted signal is much more precise and sophisticated compared with what is possible with analog systems. As a result, it may be possible to be more effective in enhancing the speech signal of interest and reducing background noise. Second, every educational audiologist is fully aware that interference may occur when two children with personal FM systems use their devices within the same building. Interference may manifest in the form of static noise, or one child may hear the voice of the other child's teacher rather than that of her own teacher. With a digital RF system such as Roger, many systems can coexist in each other's vicinity without interference. Each Roger system broadcasts audio packets repeatedly at different RF frequencies. If the first packet is lost, the second will be heard. If that one is lost, a third one may be heard, and so on. The creation of networks and subnetworks is easy, and channel planning or channel allocation is not required. Third, digital RF allows for transmission of a wider bandwidth of the signal of interest. This may be very important considering recent research indicating the importance of information above 6000 Hz for children with hearing loss (Pittman, 2008; Stelmachowicz et al., 2002, Wolfe et al., 2010).

Indeed, recent research has indicated that digital personal RF systems have the potential to improve speech recognition in noise compared with performance with personal FM systems. Thibodeau (2012) reported that a group of 10 pediatric and adult hearing aid wearers received a 35 percentage point improvement in speech recognition in high-level noise when using a digital personal RF system (e.g., the Phonak Roger system) when compared with their performance with the previous generation personal FM system. Likewise, Wolfe and colleagues (in press) showed a similar improvement in noise with digital personal RF technology for a group of cochlear implant users.

Adaptive RF Personal Systems

Traditionally, personal FM systems have been fixed-gain systems, which means the strength of the signal from the FM receiver to the hearing aid is fixed at a predetermined value. An American Speech-Language Hearing Association ASHA clinical practice guideline (2002) suggested that the output of the speech signal delivered from the FM system should be 10 dB higher than the output of the same speech signal at 65 dB SPL delivered to the microphone of the hearing aid. This was referred to as a 10 dB FM advantage and was recognized to be a compromise for what the user might prefer across the broad range of acoustical environments encountered from day to day. For example, Lewis and Eiten (2004) showed that FM users preferred a small FM advantage when listening in quiet environments, but a very favorable advantage (+24 dB) when listening in high-level noise environments. The 10 dB FM advantage was suggested as a setting that would be acceptable (but probably not ideal) across all environments.

Adaptive RF technology (also known as Dynamic FM/digital RF) seeks to overcome the need to strike a compromise. Adaptive RF systems provide no gain from the RF receiver when there is no signal of interest present (i.e., speech) from the RF transmitter. When a signal of interest is present in a quiet environment, the RF gain is set to 10 dB. The gain from the RF receiver is adaptively increased once the ambient noise level at the RF microphone exceeds 57 dB SPL to a maximum RF setting of +24 dB at an ambient noise level of approximately 80 dB SPL. Research has shown that adaptive RF technology provides substantial improvement in speech recognition in noise when compared with fixed-gain RF systems (Thibodeau, 2010; Wolfe et al., 2009).

Clinicians should consider personal RF systems for children with hearing loss of all ages. It is imperative that the clinician instruct the child's caregivers on the proper use of personal RF systems, including how and when to best use the technology. It is also imperative that the clinician conduct objective and subjective verification and validation measures to ensure that the personal RF system is fitted properly and is providing adequate benefit for the child. Verification and validation of personal RF systems is beyond the scope of this chapter. However, the interested reader is referred to the American Academy of Audiology's clinical practice guidelines on Remote Microphone Technology for detailed information regarding the selection, fitting, verification, and validation of these systems: http://www.audiology.org/resources/documentlibrary/Pages/Hearing AssistanceTechnologies.aspx

Additional Hearing Assistance Technology

Hearing assistance technology (HAT) includes far more than just remote microphone personal RF systems. Other examples of HAT include amplified telephone handsets, captioned telephones, vibrating alarm clocks, doorbell strobe lights, induction neckloop systems, and so on. Again, a detailed discussion of HAT is beyond the scope of this chapter. However, it is the audiologist's responsibility to equip a pediatric hearing aid wearer with the technology she needs to foster independence and facilitate full inclusion in home, social, occupational, athletic, and educational environments. The individual needs of the child and family must be considered while determining the most appropriate recommendations for HAT.

VALIDATION TO ENSURE THE PEDIATRIC HEARING AID WEARER IS MEETING AGE-APPROPRIATE GOALS AND EXPECTATIONS

Validation of hearing aid benefit is another critical component of the pediatric amplification process. Validation refers to the perception of hearing aid performance and benefit from the perspective of the hearing aid wearer or family members as indicated by responses provided on questionnaires or other subjective metrics. Diligent monitoring of hearing aid benefit and performance is imperative, and materials to assist in the validation process have recently been developed (Bagatto, Moodie, Seewald, Bartlett, & Scollie, 2011).

For very young children, behavioral verification of pediatric amplification is limited. Often, auditory skills questionnaires, parental report, and speech/language assessments take the place of measures such as aided speech recognition. Even for older children who can participate in behavioral verification measures, it is still necessary for audiologists and interventionists to administer other validation measures to ensure a child is achieving age-appropriate auditory, speech, and language skills (Ching et al., 1994, 1999, 20005a, 2005b).

There are a multitude of subjective measures including questionnaires and checklists available to monitor progress of children with and without hearing aids. Ideally, these measures should be normative based, with high levels of validity, feasibility, and utility. In an increasingly busy clinic setting, these measures must be time-efficient and effective in identifying the child's strengths and needs, and determine whether progress is adequate. Historically, many of these questionnaires and measures were limited in their ability to quantify the effectiveness of amplification for children ranging in age from infancy through school-age, with mild to profound hearing losses, and these tests often did not possess normative values to use for comparison between children with normal hearing and those with hearing loss (Ching & Hill, 2007).

Bagatto and colleagues (2011) conducted a critical review of subjective outcome evaluation tools designed for children 0–6 years of age that were questionnaire/interview-based and were designed to evaluate auditory related outcomes of children with hearing aids. Bagatto and colleagues (2011) sought to identify measures that a clinical audiologist could easily administer to a parent/caregiver at a clinic visit. Following a systematic grading and review of 12 different tools, Bagatto and colleagues (2011) determined that the LittlEARS Auditory Questionnaire (Tsiakpini et al., 2004) and the Parents' Evaluation of Aural/Oral Performance of Children (PEACH) Rating Scale (Ching & Hill, 2005a) received high grades in areas including conceptual clarity, normative data, retest validity, discriminant validity, convergent validity, ecological validity, responsiveness, and availability in other languages. They were also deemed to be clinically feasible as outcome evaluation tools for infants and young children. In addition, the two selected measures are available in multiple languages and have normative values based on normal hearing peers for most languages: The LittlEARS is available in 19 languages whereas the PEACH Diary is available in six different languages (Bagatto, Moodie, Malandrino, et al., 2011; Bagatto, Moodie, Seewald, Bartlett, & Scollie, 2011). For these reasons, the authors recommend using the LittlEARS and PEACH Rating Scale for subjective measures of progress along with the PedAMP protocol for verification purposes. Both of these programs are discussed below. The interested reader can review the other available scales at http://www.advancedbionics.com/content/dam/ab/Global/en_ce/documents/libraries/AssessmentTools/Test%20Reference%20for%20Cochlear%20Implants.pdf

The LittlEARs Auditory Questionnaire (Coninx et al., 2009; Tsiakpini et al., 2004) is composed of 35 items to assess auditory development, including expressive and receptive language development, in children with a hearing age in the 0–24 month range, although it can be used up to 48 months of age. Therefore, it is used to determine the development of auditory skills that are seen in the first 2 years of life. The questionnaire was developed with a yes/no format, and all items are listed in age-dependent order. The score is calculated by determining the number of "yes" answers, and results can be plotted on a score sheet to determine the child's progress and whether he or she is meeting expected progress (Figure 12–17) using normative values, set in 1 month age categories (Coninx et al., 2009). That same study by Coninx and colleagues (2009) revealed a strong correlation between the age of the child and overall LittlEARs score, and it also established that the LittlEARS possesses good internal consistency and predictive accuracy. The LittlEARS can also be used for children who have developmental delays by way of an adapted score sheet that maintains the original normative trajectory and cutoff scores but modifies the age range so that it can be plotted beyond 24 months of age (chronological age). The modified score sheet has been included as part of the UWO PedAMP protocol. When the child's performance reaches ceiling levels (score of 27 or better), regardless of age, the child's performance should then be evaluated with the PEACH rating scale (Ching & Hill, 2005a), which has more appropriate items for older children.

The PEACH was developed to solicit parents' observations in order to measure functional performance in everyday life for children with hearing loss regardless of age or duration of hearing aid experience. There are two versions: the PEACH Diary (Ching & Hill, 2005b, 2007) and the PEACH rating scale (Ching & Hill, 2005a). When the PEACH diary is administered, the parents are asked to use the PEACH booklet to document observations about their child's auditory behaviors (13 scenarios) over a 1-week period. Then, the clinician (audiologist, speech language pathologist, or deaf educator) will interview the parents and probe for more information and then assign a score (5-point scale with ratings of 0–4) based on the parents' observations

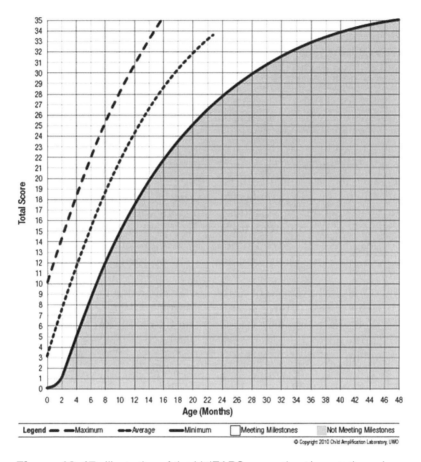

Figure 12–17. Illustration of the LittlEARS score sheet/ normative values chart.

and examples. Scores are assigned based on observed behaviors and number of examples given in response to a specific auditory behavior (Ching & Hill, 2005b). The following ratings are assigned: 0 = never or no examples given, 1 = 25% of the time (seldom) with one to two examples given, 2 = 50% of the time (sometimes) with three to four examples, 3 = 75% of the time (often) with five to six examples, 4 = greater than 75% of the time (always) with more than six examples provided (Ching & Hill, 2005b; 2007). A more time-efficient alternative is the PEACH rating scale that is designed to probe 11 different areas related to auditory behaviors including alertness/detection of environmental sounds, and listening in quiet and in noise. Originally, normative values were only available for the

PEACH diary, but a recent study by Bagatto and Scollie (2013) added to the evidence base for the PEACH, revealing that normative values established for the PEACH diary are valid for use with the PEACH rating scale (Figure 12–18). There is also a TEACH that is the teacher equivalent to the PEACH. In a study conducted by Ching, Hill, and Dillon (2008), the PEACH diary and the TEACH were effective in identifying what hearing aid settings allowed the child to perform most optimally and often these school-aged children preferred those hearing aid settings in a paired-comparison, lending further validity to the subjective outcome measure. The interested reader is referred to (Bagatto, Moodie, Malandrino, et al., 2011) for additional information in the PedAMP protocol.

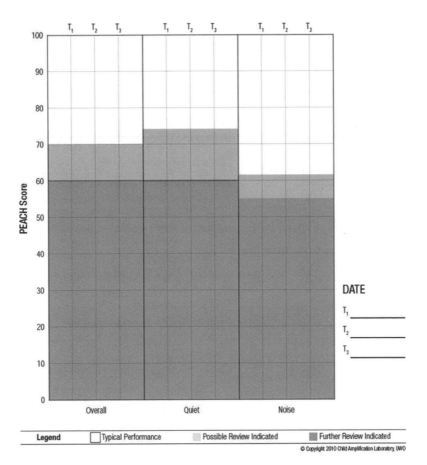

Figure 12–18. Illustration of the score sheet/normative values for the Parents' Evaluation of Aural/Oral Performance of Children's (PEACH) questionnaire.

Monitoring Speech/Language Evaluations/Staffing

In addition to questionnaires used to evaluate auditory development for the purposes of hearing aid validation, it is imperative that a speech-language pathologist administers annual assessments of speech and language development. Ideally, a child with hearing loss should possess age-appropriate speech and language abilities (as indicated by their performance on standardized, norm-referenced measures of speech and language development), and the child should achieve 1 year of speech and language progress for every chronological year. Of course, extenuating circumstances beyond the hearing loss (e.g., neurological/cognitive disabilities) may hinder the progress a child achieves. It is helpful to evaluate a child's nonverbal IQ, to determine whether cognitive disabilities may serve as an obstacle to speech and language development. In such a case, a child's age-referenced speech and language standard scores should be at least as high as the child's nonverbal IQ standard score.

The pediatric audiologist cannot be certain that his or her intervention is successful without an understanding of the child's functional language progress. As such, it is essential for pediatric audiologists to maintain an open and ongoing dialogue with the child's speech-language pathologist in order to possess an understanding of the child's speech and language aptitude. Modifications of audiological intervention are necessary for children making insufficient progress.

Ideally, a team of professionals (pediatric audiologist, Auditory-Verbal therapist/speech-language pathologist, otologist, social worker, teacher, etc.) will coordinate services with the child and family to ensure the child makes satisfactory performance. If an interdisciplinary hearing health care team determines that additional disabilities or factors (e.g., cognition, developmental disabilities/delays, a lack of family support, socioeconomic challenges, etc.) are affecting a child's progress, then the team should seek additional resources and/or referrals to appropriate specialists to provide the intervention the child needs. Examples of additional referrals commonly needed for children with hearing loss include, but are not limited to, vision assessment, genetic assessment, occupational and physical therapy, psychology, and/or social work services. Ultimately, each child should be served as a person rather than as a hearing impairment.

CONCLUSION

In conclusion, the selection, fitting, verification, and validation of hearing aids in children is a dynamic process that that should be supported by evidence-based principles but should also be individualized to meet the unique needs of each child and family. Implementing the protocols and procedures as discussed in this chapter should assist the new and seasoned audiologists in ensuring that each child meets his or her full potential. With the amazing hearing technology and services that are available today, audiologists should strive to provide unlimited opportunities for children with hearing loss.

REFERENCES

Aahz, H., & Moore, B. (2007). The value of routine real ear measurement of the gain of digital hearing aids. *Journal of the American Academy of Audiology, 18,* 653–664. Retrieved from http://audiology.org/resources/journal/

American Academy of Audiology Task Force on Pediatric Amplification. (2013). *American Academy of Audiology clinical practice guideline on pediatric amplification.* Retrieved from http://www.audiology.org/resources/documentlibrary/Documents/PediatricAmplificationGuidelines.pdf

American National Standard Institute. (1997). *American National Standard methods for the calculation of the speech intelligibility index.* New York, NY: Author. Retrieved from http://www.ansi.org

American Speech-Language Hearing Association. (2002). *Guidelines for fitting and monitoring FM systems.* Retrieved from http://www.asha.org/policy/GL2002-00010.htm

American Speech-Language Hearing Association. (2004). *Guidelines for the audiologic assessment of children from birth to 5 years of age.* Retrieved from http://www.asha.org/docs/html/gl2004-00002.html

American Speech-Language Hearing Association Working Group on Classroom Acoustics. (2005). *Acoustics in educational settings: Position statement.* Retrieved from http://www.asha.org/policy/PS2005-00028.htm

Arndt, S., Aschendorff, A., Laszig, R., Beck, R., Schild, C., Kroeger, S., . . . Wesarg, T. (2011). Comparison of pseudobinaural hearing to real binaural hearing rehabilitation after cochlear implantation in patients with unilateral deafness and tinnitus. *Otology and Neurotology, 32,* 39–47.

Auriemmo, J., Kuk, F., Lau, C., Dornan, B. K., Sweeton, S., Marshall, S., & Stenger, P. (2009a). Efficacy of an adaptive directional microphone and noise reduction system for school-aged children. *Journal of Educational Audiology, 15,* 15–27.

Auriemmo, J., Kuk, F., Lau, C., Marshall, S., Thiele, N., Pikora, M., Quick, D., & Stenger, P. (2009b). Effect of linear frequency transposition on speech recognition and production of school-aged children. *Journal of the American Academy of Audiology, 20,* 289–305.

Bagatto, M. P., & Moodie, S. (2007). *Learning the art to apply the science: Common questions related to pediatric hearing instrument fitting.* Audiology Online. Retrieved from http://www.audiologyonline.com/articles/learning-art-to-apply-science-933

Bagatto, M. P., Moodie, S., Scollie, S., Seewald, R., Moodie, S., . . . Liu, K. P. (2005). Clinical protocols for hearing instrument fitting in the Desired Sensation Level Method. *Trends in Amplification, 9,* 199–226.

Bagatto, M. P., Moodie, S. T., Malandrino, A. C., Richert, F. M., Clench, D. A., & Scollie, S. D. (2011). The University of Western Ontario audiological monitoring protocol (UWO PedAMP). *Trends in Amplification, 15*(1), 57–76.

Bagatto, M. P., Moodie, S. T., Seewald, R. C., Bartlett, D. J., & Scollie, S. D. (2011). A critical review of audiological outcome measures for infants and children. *Trends in Amplification, 15*(1), 23–33.

Bagatto, M. P., & Scollie, S. D. (2013). Validation of the Parents' Evaluation of Aural/Oral Performance of Children (PEACH) rating scale. *Journal of American Academy of Audiology, 24*(2), 121–125. doi:10.3766/jaaa.24.2.5

Bagatto, M. P., Scollie, S. D., Hyde, M., & Seewald, R. (2010). Protocol for the provision of amplification within the Ontario infant hearing program. *International Journal of Audiology, 49,* S70–S79.

Bagatto, M. P., Scollie, S. D., Seewald, R. C., Moodie, K. S., & Hoover, B. M. (2002). Real-ear-to-coupler difference predictions as a function of age for two coupling procedures. *Journal of American Academy of Audiology, 13,* 407–415.

Bagatto, M. P., Seewald, R. C., Scollie, S. D., & Tharpe, A. M. (2006). Evaluation of a probe-tube insertion technique for measuring real-ear-to-coupler difference (RECD) in young infants. *Journal of American Academy of Audiology, 17*(8), 573–581.

Baguley, D. M. (2010). Cochlear implants in single-sided deafness and tinnitus. *Seminars in Hearing, 31,* 410–413.

Bentler, R. (2005). Effectiveness of directional microphones and noise reduction schemes in hearing aids: A systematic review of the evidence. *Journal of the American Academy of Audiology, 16,* 473–484.

Berlin, C. I., Hood, L. J., Morlet, T., Wilensky, D., Li, L., Mattingly, K. R., . . . Frisch, S. A. (2009). Multi-site diagnosis and management of 260 patients with Auditory Neuropathy/Dys-synchrony (Auditory Neuropathy Spectrum Disorder). *International Journal of Audiology, 49,* 30–43.

Bess, F., Dodd-Murphy, J., & Parker, R. (1998). Children with minimal sensorineural hearing loss: Prevalence, educational performance, and functional status. *Ear and Hearing, 19,* 339–354.

Bess, F., & Tharpe, A. M. (1984). Unilateral hearing impairment in children. *Pediatrics, 74,* 206–216.

Bess, F., Tharpe, A. M., & Gibler, A. (1986). Auditory performance of children with unilateral sensorineural hearing loss. *Ear and Hearing,* 20–26.

Bingham, K., Jenstad, L. M., & Shahnaz, N. (2009). Longitudinal changes in real-ear to coupler difference measurements in infants. *Journal of American Academy of Audiology, 20,* 558–568.

Boothroyd, A. (1997). Auditory development of the hearing child. *Scandinavian Audiology Supplement, 46,* 9–16.

Boothroyd, A., & Iglehart, F. (1998). Experiments with classroom FM amplification. *Ear and Hearing, 19,* 202–217.

Bourland-Hicks, C., & Tharpe, A. M. (2002). Listening effort and fatigue in school-age children with and without hearing loss. *Journal of Speech, Language, and Hearing Research, 45,* 573–584.

Boymans, M., & Dreschler, W. A. (2000). Field trials using a digital hearing aid with active noise reduction and dual-microphone directionality. *Audiology, 39,* 260–268.

Boys Town National Research Hospital. (2013). *The situational hearing aid response profile (SHARP) version 7.* Retrieved from http://audres.org/rc/sharp/

British Columbia Early Hearing Program. (2008). *Diagnostic audiology protocol* [pdf document]. Retrieved from http://www.phsa.ca/NR/rdonlyres/06D79FEB-D187-43E9-91E4-8C09959F38D8/40115/aDAAGProtocols1.pdf

Buchman, C. A., Roush, P. A., Teagle, H. F. B., Brown, C. J., Zdanski, C. J., & Grose, J. H. (2006). Auditory neuropathy characteristics in children with cochlear nerve deficiency. *Ear and Hearing, 27,* 399–408.

Buechner, A., Brendel, M., Lesinki-schiedat, A., Wenzel, G., Frohne-Buechner, C., Jaeger, B., & Lenarz, T. (2010). Cochlear implantation in unilateral deaf subjects associated with ipsilateral tinnitus. *Otology and Neurotology, 31,* 1381–1385.

Byrne, D. (1986). Effects of frequency response characteristics on speech discrimination and perceived intelligibility and pleasantness of speech for hearing-impaired listeners. *Journal of the Acoustical Society of America, 80,* 494–504.

Byrne, D., Parkinson, A., & Newall, P. (1990). Hearing aid gain and frequency response requirements for the severely/profoundly hearing impaired. *Ear and Hearing, 11,* 40–49.

Byrne, D., Parkinson, A., & Newall, P. (1991). Modified hearing aid selection procedures for severe-profound hearing losses. In G. A. Studebaker, F. H. Bess, & L. Beck (Eds.), *The Vanderbilt Hearing Aid Report II* (pp. 295–300). Parkton, MD: York Press.

Byrne, D., & Tonisson, W. (1976). Selecting the gain of hearing aids for persons with sensorineural hearing impairments. *Scandinavian Audiology, 5,* 51–59.

Campos, P. D., Mondelli, M. F., & Ferrari, D. V. (2011). Comparison: Real ear and simulated insertion gain. *Brazilian Journal of Otorhinolaryngology, 77*(5), 555–558.

Ching, T. Y., & Britton, L. (2008). Repeatability of real-ear-to-coupler differences measured by an acoustic method for determining probe tube insertion depth. *The Australian and New Zealand Journal of Audiology, 30*(2), 91–98.

Ching, T. Y., & Hill, M. (2005a). *The Parents' Evaluation of Aural/Oral Performance of Children (PEACH) Rating Scale.* Chatswood, New South Wales, Australia: Australian Hearing. Retrieved from http://www.outcomes.nal.gov.au/LOCHI%20assessments.html

Ching, T. Y., & Hill, M. (2005b). *The Parents' Evaluation of Aural/Oral Performance of Children (PEACH) Diary.* Chatswood, New South Wales, Australia: Australian Hearing. Retrieved from http://www.nal.gov.au/outcome-measures_tab_peach.html

Ching T. Y., & Hill, M. (2007). The Parents' Evaluation of Aural/Oral Performance of Children (PEACH) scale: Normative data. *Journal of American Academy of Audiology 18*(3), 220–235. Retrieved from http://www.audiology.org/resources/journal/Pages/default.aspx

Ching, T. Y., Hill, M., Birtles, G., & Beecham, L. (1999). Clinical use of paired comparisons to evaluate hearing aid fitting of severely/profoundly hearing impaired children. *Australian and New Zealand Journal of Audiology, 21*(2), 51–63. Retrieved from http://www.audiology.asn.au/anzja.htm

Ching, T. Y., Hill, M., & Dillon, H. (2008). Effect of variations in hearing-aid frequency response on real-life functional performance of children with severe or profound hearing loss. *International Journal of Audiology, 47*, 461–475. doi:10.1080/14992020802116128

Ching, T. Y., Newall, P., & Wigney, D. (1994). Audio-visual and auditory paired comparison judgements by severely and profoundly hearing impaired children: Reliability and frequency response preferences. *Australian Journal of Audiology, 16*(2), 99–106. Retrieved from http://www.audiology.asn.au/anzja.htm

Ching, T. Y., Newall, P., & Wigney, D. (1997). Comparison of severely and profoundly hearing-impaired children's amplification preference with the NAL-RP and the DSL 3.0 prescriptions. *Scandinavian Audiology, 26*, 219–222.

Ching, T. Y., O'Brien, A., Dillon, H., Chalupper, J., Hartley, L., Hartley, D., . . . Hain, J. (2009). Directional effects on infants and young children in real life: Implications for amplification. *Journal of Speech, Language, and Hearing Research, 52*, 1241–1254.

Ching, T. Y., Scollie, S. D., Dillon, H., & Seewald, R. (2010). A cross-over, double-blind comparison of the NAL-NL1 and the DSL v4.1 prescriptions for children with mild to moderately severe hearing loss. *International Journal of Audiology, 49*, S4–S15.

Cole, E. B., & Flexer, C. (2007). *Children with hearing loss: Developing listening and talking: Birth to six.* San Diego, CA: Plural.

Coninx, F., Weichbold, V., Tsiakpini, L., Autrique, E., Bescond, G., Chereches, L., . . . Brachmaier, J. (2009). Validation of the LittleEARS Auditory Questionnaire in children with normal hearing. *International Journal of Pediatric Otorhinolaryngology, 73*(12), 1761–1768. doi:10.1016/j.ijporl.2009.09.036

Crandell, C. C. (1993). Speech recognition in noise by children with minimal degrees of sensorineural hearing loss. *Ear and Hearing, 14*, 210–216.

Davis, J. M., Elfenbein, J., Schum, R., & Bentler, R. A. (1986). Effects of mild and moderate hearing impairments on language, educational, and psychosocial behavior of children. *Journal of Speech and Hearing Disorders, 51*, 53–62.

Dillon, H. (1999). NAL-NL1: A new prescriptive fitting procedure for non-linear hearing aids. *The Hearing Journal, 52*(4), 10–16.

Dillon, H. (2006). What's new from NAL in hearing aid prescriptions? *The Hearing Journal, 59*(10), 10–16.

Dillon, H. (2012). *Hearing aids* (2nd ed.). Turramurra, Australia: Boomerang Press.

Dillon, H., & Keidser, G. (2013). *Siemens Expert Series: NAL-NL2—Principles, background data, and comparison to other procedures.* Audiology Online. Retrieved from http://www.audiologyonline.com/articles/siemens-expert-series-nal-nl2-11355

Elfenbein, J. L., Hardin-Jones, M. A., & Davis, J. (1994). Oral communication skills of children who are hard of hearing, *Journal of Speech, Language, and Hearing Research, 37*, 216–226.

English, K., Grimes, A., Yoshinaga-Itano, C., Squires, M., DeConde Johnson, C., Flexer, C., & Madell, C. (2013, April). *Bullying, children with hearing loss, and the role of pediatric audiologists.* Presentation conducted at the meeting of the American Academy of Audiology, Anaheim, CA.

Gibson, W. P., & Sanli, H. (2007). Auditory neuropathy: An update. *Ear and Hearing, 28*(Suppl. 2), S102–S106.

Glista, D., & Scollie, S. (2009). Modified verification approaches for frequency lowering devices. *Audiology Online.* Retrieved from http://www.audiologyonline.com/articles/article_detail.asp?article_id=2301

Glista, D., & Scollie, S. (2012). Development and evaluation of an English language measure of detection of word-final plurality markers: The university of western ontario plurals test. *American Journal of Audiology, 21*, 76–81. doi:10.1044/1059-0889(2012/11-0036)

Glista, D., Scollie, S., Bagatto, M., Seewald, R., Parsa, V., & Johnson, A. (2009). Evaluation of nonlinear frequency compression: Clinical outcomes. *International Journal of Audiology, 48*, 632–644.

Golding, M., Pearce, W., Seymour, J., Cooper, A., Ching, T., & Dillon, H. (2007). The relationship between obligatory cortical auditory evoked potentials (CAEPs) and functional measures in young infants. *Journal of American Academy of Audiology, 18*(2), 117–125.

Gravel, J. (2000). Audiologic assessment for the fitting of hearing instruments: Big challenges from tiny ears. In R. C. Seewald (Ed.), *A sound foundation through early amplification: Proceedings of an international conference* (pp. 33–46). Stafa, Switzerland: Phonak AG.

Gravel, J. S., Fausel, N., Liskow, C., & Chobot, J. (1999). Children's speech recognition in noise using omnidirectional and dual-microphone hearing aid technology. *Ear and Hearing, 20*, 1–11.

Gustafson, S. J., & Pittman, A. L. (2011). Sentence perception in listening conditions having similar speech intelligibility indices. *International Journal of Audiology, 50*(1), 34–40.

Gustafson, S. J., Pittman, A., & Fanning, R. (2013). Effects of tubing length and coupling method on hearing threshold and real-ear to coupler difference measures. *American Journal of Audiology, 22,* 190–199. doi:10.1044/1059-0889(2012/12-0046

Hakansson, B., Tjellstrom, A., & Rosenhall, U. (1984). Hearing thresholds with direct bone conduction versus conventional bone conduction. *Scandinavian Audiology, 13,* 3–13.

Hall, J. W., III, & Swanepoel, D. W. (2010). *Objective assessment of hearing.* San Diego, CA: Plural.

Hawkins, D. B. (1984). Comparisons of speech recognition in noise by mildly-to-moderately hearing-impaired children using hearing aids and FM systems. *Journal of Speech and Hearing Disorders, 49,* 409–418.

Hawkins, D. B., & Naidoo, S. V. (1993). Comparison of sound quality and clarity with asymmetrical peak clipping and output limiting compression. *Journal of the American Academy of Audiology, 4,* 221–228.

Hol, M. K., Snik, A. F., Mylanus, E. A., & Cremers, C. W. (2005). Longterm results of bone-anchored hearing aid recipients who had previously used air-conduction hearing aids. *Archives of Otolaryngology-Head and Neck Surgery, 131,* 321–325.

Hornsby, B. W. Y. (2004). The speech intelligibility index: What is it and what's it good for? *The Hearing Journal, 57*(10), 10–17.

International Electrotechnical Commission. (2013). *Tamperproof solutions for children under age 36 months.* Retrieved from http://www.ansi.org/

Jenstad, L., Pumford, J., Seewald, R., & Cornelisse, L. (2000). Comparison of linear gain and WDRC hearing aid circuits II: Aided loudness measures. *Ear and Hearing, 21,* 32–44.

Jenstad, L., Seewald, R., Cornelisse, L., & Shantz, J. (1999). Comparison of linear gain and WDRC hearing aid circuits: Aided speech perception measures. *Ear and Hearing, 21,* 32–44.

John, M. S., Brown, D. K., Muir, P. J., & Picton, T. W. (2004). Recording auditory steady-state responses in young infants. *Ear and Hearing, 25,* 539–553.

Johnson, C. E., & Danhauer, J. L. (2002). *Handbook of outcomes measurement in audiology.* Clifton Park, NY: Thomson Delmar Learning.

Johnson, E. E., Ricketts, T. A., & Hornsby, B. W. (2007). The effect of digital phase cancellation feedback reduction systems on amplified sound quality. *Journal of the American Academy of Audiology, 18,* 404–416.

Johnstone, P. M., & Robertson, V. S. (2010). Earmold considerations for optimal spatial hearing in children with unilateral hearing loss. In R. C. Seewald & J. M. Bamford (Eds.), *A sound foundation through early amplification: Proceedings of the Fifth International Conference.* Phonak AG, Stafa, Switzerland.

Joint Committee on Infant Hearing. (2007). Year 2007 position statement: Principles and guidelines for early hearing detection and intervention programs. *Pediatrics, 120,* 898–921.

Jones, C., & Launer, S. (2010). *Pediatric fittings in 2010: The sound foundations cuper project. A sound foundation through early amplification.* Retrieved from http://www.phonakpro.com/us/b2b/en/events/proceedings/soundfoundation_chicago 2010.html

Kawell, M., Kopun, J., & Stelmachowicz, P. (1988). Loudness discomfort levels in children. *Ear and Hearing, 9,* 133–136.

Kochkin, S. (2011). MarkeTrak VIII: Reducing patient visits through verification and validation. *Hearing Review, 18*(6), 10–12.

Kral, A., Hartmann, R., Tillein, J., Held, S., & Klinke, R. (2002). Hearing after congenital deafness: Central auditory plasticity and sensory deprivation. *Cerebral Cortex, 12*(8), 797–807.

Kuk, F., Keenan, D., & Lau, C. C. (2005). Vent configurations on subjective and objective occlusion effect. *Journal of the American Academy of Audiology, 16,* 747–762.

Lewis, D., & Eiten, L. (2004). Assessment of advanced hearing instrument and FM technology. In D. A. Fabry & C. DeConde Johnson (Eds.), *ACCESS: Achieving clear communication employing sound solutions—2003. Proceedings of the First International FM Conference* (pp. 167–174). Safta, Switzerland: Phonak AG.

Ling, D. (2002). *Speech and the hearing-impaired child* (2nd ed.) Washington, DC: A.G. Bell Association for the Deaf and Hard of Hearing.

Madell, J. (2008). Evaluation of speech perception in infants and children. In J. R. Madell & C. Flexer (Eds.), *Pediatric audiology: Diagnosis, technology, and management* (pp. 89–105). New York, NY: Thieme Medical.

Martin, H. C., Munro, K. J., & Lam, M. C. (2001). Perforation of the tympanic membrane and its effect on the real-ear-to-coupler difference acoustic transform function. *British Journal of Audiology, 35*(4), 259–264.

McCreery, R. (2008). Pediatric hearing aid verification: Innovative trends. *Audiology Online.* Retrieved from www.audiologyonline.com/articles

McCreery, R. (2010). Small ears, BIG decisions. *Hearing Journal, 63*(70), 10–17.

McCreery, R. (2013a). Building blocks: Asking the right questions about hearing aid use in children. *The Hearing Journal, 66*(6), 16–18.

McCreery, R. (2013b) Building blocks: RECD is a reasonable alternative to real-ear verification. *The Hearing Journal, 66*(7), 13–14.

McCreery, R. (2013c). Building blocks: Speech intelligibility index: No magic number, but a reasonable solution. *The Hearing Journal, 66*(4), 8–10.

McCreery, R. (2013d). Building blocks: The trouble with functional gain in verifying pediatric hearing aids. *The Hearing Journal, 66*(3), 14–16.

McKay, S., Gravel, J. S., & Tharpe, A. M. (2008). Amplification considerations for children with minimal or mild bilateral hearing loss and unilateral hearing loss. *Trends in Amplification, 12,* 43–54.

Microsonic Earmold Laboratories. (2006). *Custom earmold manual* (8th ed.). Retrieved from http://store

.microsonic-inc.com/manual/earmolds_manual 2.pdf

Moeller, M. P., Hoover, B., Peterson, B., & Stelmachowicz, P. (2009). Consistency of hearing aid use in infants with early-identified hearing loss. *American Journal of Audiology, 18*, 14–23.

Moodie, K. S., Seewald, R. C., & Sinclair, S. T. (1994). Procedure for predicting real-ear hearing aid performance in young children. *American Journal of Audiology, 3*, 23–31.

Moore, B. C., & Glasberg, B. R. (2004). A revised model of loudness perception applied to cochlear hearing loss. *Hearing Research, 188*, 70–88.

Mueller, H. G., Weber, J., & Hornsby, B. W. Y. (2006). The effects of digital noise reduction on the acceptance of background noise. *Trends in Amplification, 10*, 83–94.

Munro, K. J. (2004). *Update on RECD measures in children. A sound foundation through early amplification.* Retrieved from https://www.phonakpro.com/content/dam/phonak/b2b/C_M_tools/Library/Pediatric/Features/en/Update_in_RECD_measures_in_children.pdf.

Munro, K. J., & Howlin, E. M. (2010). Comparison of real-ear to coupler difference values in the right and left ear of hearing aid users. *Ear and Hearing, 31*(1), 146–150.

Mylanus, E. A., van der Pouw, K. C., Snik, A. F., & Cremers, C. W. (1998). Intraindividual comparison of the bone-anchored hearing aid and air-conduction hearing aids. *Archives of Otolaryngology-Head and Neck Surgery, 124*(3), 271–276.

Newborn Hearing Screening Programme. (2010). *Guidance for auditory brain stem response testing in babies* [pdf document]. Retrieved from http://hearing.screening.nhs.uk/audiologyprotocols

Nozza, R. J. (1988). Auditory deficit in infants with otitis media: More than a "mild" hearing loss. In D. Lim, C. Bluestone, J. Klein, & J. Nelson (Eds.), *Recent advances in otitis media: Proceedings of the fourth international symposium* (pp. 376–379). Toronto, Canada: BC Decker.

Oyler, R. (1988). Unilateral hearing loss: Demographics and educational impact. *Language, Speech, Hearing Services in Schools, 19*, 201–210.

Parent Advocacy Coalition for Education Rights (PACER). (2012). *Bullying and harassment of students with disabilities: Top 10 facts parents educators and students need to know.* Retrieved from http://www.pacer.org/publications/bullypdf/BP-18.pdf

Pascoe, D. P. (1978). An approach to hearing aid selection. *Hear Instruments, 29*, 12–16, 36.

Pearce, W., Golding, M., & Dillon, H. (2007). Cortical auditory evoked potentials in the assessment of auditory neuropathy: Two case studies. *Journal of the American Academy of Audiology, 18*, 380–390.

The Pediatric Working Group. (1996). *Amplification for infants and children with hearing loss.* Nashville, TN: Vanderbilt Bill Wilkerson Press.

Phonak Professional website. (n.d.). *IEC standards for tamperproof solution.* Retrieved from http://phonakpro.com

Pittman, A. L. (2008). Short-term word learning rate in children with normal hearing and children with hearing loss in limited and extended high-frequency bandwidths. *Journal of Speech, Language, and Hearing Research, 51*, 785–797.

Pittman, A. (2011). Children's performance in complex listening conditions: Effects of hearing loss and digital noise reduction. *Journal of Speech, Language, and Hearing Research, 54*, 1224–1239.

Ponton, C. W., Eggermont, J. J., Kwong, B., & Don, M. (2000). Maturation of human central auditory system activity: Evidence from multi-channel evoked potentials. *Clinical Neurophysiology, 111*, 220–236.

Preves, D. A., Sammeth, C. A., & Wynne, M. K. (1999). Field trail evaluations of a switched directional/omnidirectional in-the-ear hearing instrument. *Journal of the American Academy of Audiology, 10*, 273–284.

Punch, J. F. (1988). CROS revisited. *ASHA, 30*, 35–37.

Purdy, S. C., Katsch, R., Dillon, H., Storey, L., Sharma, M., & Agung, K. (2004). *Aided cortical auditory evoked potentials for hearing instrument evaluation in infants. A sound foundation through early amplification.* Retrieved from https://www.phonakpro.com/

Rance, G. (2005). Auditory neuropathy/dys-synchrony and its perceptual consequences. *Trends in Amplification, 9*, 1–43.

Rance, G. (2008). *Auditory steady-state response: Generation, recording, and clinical application.* San Diego, CA: Plural.

Ricketts, T. A., & Galster, J. (2008). Head angle and elevation in classroom environments: Implications for amplification. *Journal of Speech, Language, and Hearing Research, 51*, 516–525.

Ricketts, T.A., Galster, J., & Tharpe, A.M. (2007). Directional benefit in simulated classroom environments. *American Journal of Audiology, 16*, 130–144.

Ricketts, T. A., & Hornsby, B. W. (2003). Distance and reverberation effects on directional benefit. *Ear and Hearing, 24*, 472–484.

Ricketts, T., & Hornsby, B. (2005). Sound quality measures for speech in noise through a commercial hearing aid implementing digital noise reduction. *Journal of the American Academy of Audiology, 16*, 270–277.

Roeser, R., & Clark, J. (2008). Live voice speech recognition audiometry: Stop the madness. *Audiology Today, 20*(1), 32–33.

Ross, M., & Giolas, T. G. (1971). Effects of three classroom listening conditions on speech intelligibility. *American Annals of the Deaf, 117*, 580–584.

Ross, M., & Seewald, R. C. (1988). Hearing aid selection and evaluation with young children. In F. H. Bess (Ed.), *Hearing impairment in children* (pp. 190–213). Timonium, MD: York Press.

Roush, P., Frymark, T., Venediktov, R., & Wang, B. (2011). Audiologic management of auditory neuropathy spectrum disorder in children: A systematic review of the literature. *American Journal of Audiology, 20,* 159–170.

Ruscetta, M., Arjmand, E., & Pratt, S. (2005). Speech recognition abilities in noise for children with severe-to-profound unilateral hearing impairment. *International Journal of Pediatric Otorhinolaryngology, 69,* 771–779.

Sanders, D. (1965). Noise conditions in normal school classrooms. *Exceptional Child, 31,* 344–353.

Sarampalis, A., Kalluri, S., Edwards, B., & Hafter, E. (2009). Objective measures of listening effort: Effects of background noise and noise reduction. *Journal of Speech, Language, and Hearing Research, 52,* 1230–1240.

Schafer, E. C., Beeler, S., Ramos, H., Morais, M., Monzingo, J., & Algier, K. (2012). Developmental effects and spatial hearing in young children with normal-hearing sensitivity. *Ear and Hearing, 33*(6), e32–43.

Schafer, E. C., & Thibodeau, L. (2006). Speech recognition in noise in children with cochlear implants while listening in bilateral, bimodal, and FM-system arrangements. *American Journal of Audiology, 15,* 114–126.

Schafer, E. C., Wolfe, J., Algier, K., Morais, M., Price, S., Monzingo, J., . . . Ramos, H. (2012). Spatial hearing in noise of young children with cochlear implants and hearing aids. *Journal of Educational Audiology, 18,* 38–51.

Scollie, S. D. (2012, December). *Frequency lowering hearing aids: New techniques for fitting.* Presented at Advances in Audiology, Las Vegas, NV. Retrieved from http://www.phonakpro.com/content/dam/phonak/gc_hq/b2b/en/events/2012/dec_las_vegas/Proceedings/Tuesday/Scollie_S_Frequency_lowering_hearing_aids_New_techniques_for_fitting.pdf

Scollie, S., Bagatto, M., Moodie, S., & Crukley, J. (2011). Accuracy and reliability of a real-ear-to-coupler difference measurement procedure implemented with a behind-the ear hearing aid. *Journal of the American Academy of Audiology, 22,* 612–622. doi:10.3766/jaaa.22.9.6

Scollie, S. D., Ching, T. Y. C., Seewald R. C., Dillon, H., Britton, L., Steinberg, J., & King, K. (2010). Children's speech perception and loudness ratings when fitted with hearing aids using the DSL v4.1 and NAL-NL1 prescriptions. *International Journal of Audiology, 49*(Suppl. 1), S26–34.

Scollie, S., Seewald, R., Cornelisse, L., Moodie, S., Bagatto, M., . . . Pumford, J. (2005). The desired sensation level multistage input/output algorithm. *Trends in Amplification, 9,* 159–197.

Seewald, R. C., Moodie, S., Scollie, S., & Bagatto, M. (2005). The DSL method for pediatric hearing instrument fitting: Historical perspective and current issues. *Trends in Amplification, 9,* 145–157.

Seewald, R. C., Moodie, K. S., Sinclair, S. T., . . . Scollie, S. D. (1999). Predictive validity of a procedure for pediatric hearing aid fitting. *American Journal of Audiology, 8,* 143–152.

Seewald, R. C., Ross, M., & Spiro, M. K. (1985). Selecting amplification characteristics for young hearing-impaired children. *Ear and Hearing, 6,* 48–53.

Seewald, R. C., & Scollie, S. D. (1999). Infants are not average adults: Implications for audiometric testing. *The Hearing Journal, 52*(10), 64–72.

Seewald, R., Stelmachowicz, P. G., & Ross, M. (1987). Selecting and verifying hearing aid performance characteristics for young children. *Journal of the Academy of Rehabilitative Audiology, 20,* 25–38.

Sharma, A., Cardon, G., Henion, K., & Roland, P. (2011). Cortical maturation and behavioral outcomes in children with auditory neuropathy spectrum disorder. *International Journal of Audiology, 50,* 98–106.

Sharma, A., Dorman, M., & Spahr, A. (2002). A sensitive period for the development of the central auditory system in children with cochlear implants: Implications for age of implantation. *Ear and Hearing, 23,* 532–539.

Sharma, A., Martin, K., Roland, P., Bauer, P., Sweeney, M. H., Gilley, P., & Dorman, M. (2005). P1 latency as a biomarker for central auditory development in children with hearing impairment. *Journal of American Academy of Audiology, 16*(8), 564–573.

Sinclair, S. T., Beauchaine, K. L., Moodie, K. S., Feigin, J. A., Seewald, R. C., & Stelmachowicz, P. G. (1996). Repeatability of a real-ear-to coupler difference measurement as a function of age. *American Journal of Audiology, 5,* 52–56.

Sininger, Y. S., Doyle, K. J., & Moore, J. K. (1999). The case for early identification of hearing loss in children: Auditory system development, experimental auditory deprivation, and development of speech perception and hearing. *Pediatric Clinics of North America, 46*(1), 1–14.

Snik, A. F., Mylannus, E. A., Proops, D. W., Wolfaardt, J. F., Hodgetts, W. E., Somers, T., . . . Tjellström, A. (2005). Consensus statements on BAHA system: Where do we stand at present? *The Annals of Otology, Rhinology, and Laryngology, 195,* 1–12.

Snik, A. F., van den Borne, P., Brokx, J. P., & Hoekstra, C. (1995). Hearing aid fitting in profoundly-impaired children: Comparison of prescription rules. *Scandinavian Audiology, 24,* 225–230.

Stapells, D. R. (2000). Threshold estimation by the tone-evoked auditory brainstem response: A literature meta-analysis. *Journal of Speech-Language Pathology and Audiology, 24,* 74–83.

Stapells, D. (2011). Frequency-specific threshold assessment in young infants using the transient ABR and the brain stem ASSR. In R. Seewald & A. M. Tharpe (Eds.), *Comprehensive handbook of pediatric audiology.* San Diego, CA: Plural.

Stapells, D. R., Gravel, J. A., & Martin, B. A. (1995). Thresholds for auditory brain stem responses to tone in notched noise from infants and young children with normal hearing or sensorineural hearing loss. *Ear and Hearing, 16,* 361–371.

Stelmachowicz, P. G. (2004). *Pediatric amplification: Past, present and future. A sound foundation through early amplification.* Retrieved from https://www.phonakpro.com/com/b2b/en/events/proceedings/pediatric_conference_chicago_2004.html

Stelmachowicz, P., Lewis, D., Hoover, B., . . . (2010). Effects of digital noise reduction on speech perception for children with hearing loss. *Ear and Hearing, 31,* 345–355.

Stelmachowicz, P. G., Pittman, A. L., Hoover, B. M., & Lewis, D. E. (2002). Aided perception of /s/ and /z/ by hearing-impaired children. *Ear and Hearing, 23*(4), 316–324.

Stiles, D. J., Bentler, R. A., & McGregor, K. K. (2012). The speech intelligibility index and the pure-tone average as predictors of lexical ability in children fit with hearing aids. *Journal of Speech, Language, and Hearing Research, 55,* 764–778.

Tharpe, A. M. (2007). Unilateral hearing loss in children: A mountain or a molehill? *Hearing Journal, 60*(7), 10–16.

Tharpe, A. M. (2008). Unilateral and mild bilateral hearing loss in children: Past and current perspectives. *Trends in Amplification, 12,* 7–15.

Tharpe, A. M., Sladen, D., Huta, H. M., & Rothpletz, A. M. (2001). Practical considerations of real-ear-to-coupler difference measures in infants. *American Journal of Audiology, 10,* 41–49.

Thibodeau, L. (2004). Hearing assistance technology (HAT) can optimize communication. *Hearing Journal, 57*(11), 11.

Thibodeau, L. (2010). Benefits of adaptive FM systems on speech recognition in noise for listeners who use hearing aids. *American Journal of Audiology, 19*(1), 36–45.

Thibodeau, L. (2012). *Results with devices that utilize DM technology.* Oral presentation at the Phonak Advances in Audiology conference, Las Vegas, NV.

Thibodeau, L. M., & Schafer, E. (2002). Issues to consider regarding the use of FM systems with infants with hearing loss. *Perspectives on Hearing and Hearing Disorders in Childhood, 12,* 18–21.

Tsiakpini, L., Weichbold, V., Kuehn-Inacker, H., Coninx, F., D'Haese, P., & Almadin, S. (2004). *LittlEARS auditory questionnaire.* Innsbruck, Austria: MED-EL.

Valente, M., Fabry, D. A., & Potts, L. G. (1995). Recognition of speech in noise with hearing aids using dual microphones. *Journal of the American Academy of Audiology, 6,* 440–449.

Valente, M., Sweetow, R., Potts, L., & Bingea, B. (1999). Digital versus analog signal processing: Effect of directional microphone. *Journal of the American Academy of Audiology, 10,* 133–150.

Walden, B. E., Surr, R. K., Cord, M. T., Edwards, B., & Olson, L. (2000). Comparison of benefits provided by different hearing-aid technologies. *Journal of the American Academy of Audiology, 11,* 540–560.

Widen, J. (1993). Adding objectivity to infant behavioral audiometry. *Ear and Hearing, 14,* 49–57.

Wolfe, J., Hudson, M., Caraway, T., John, A., Schafer, E., Hannah, L., & Smith, J. (submitted a). Effects of non-linear frequency compression on speech and language aptitude of children with moderate hearing loss.

Wolfe, J., John, A., Schafer, E., Hudson, M., Boretzki, M., Scollie, S., . . . Neumann, S. (submitted b). Evaluation of wideband frequency responses and non-linear frequency compression for children with mild hearing loss.

Wolfe, J., John, A., Schafer, E., Nyffeler, M., Boretzki, M., Caraway, T. (2010). Evaluation of nonlinear frequency compression for school-age children with moderate to moderately severe hearing loss. *Journal of the American Academy of Audiology, 21,* 618–628.

Wolfe, J., John, A., Schafer, E., Nyffeler, M., Boretzki, M., . . . Hudson, M. (2011). Long-term effects of non-linear frequency compression for children with moderate hearing loss. *International Journal of Audiology, 50,* 396–404.

Wolfe, J., Morais, M., Schafer, E. C., Mills, E., John, A., Hudson, M., . . . Lianos, L. (in press). Evaluation of speech recognition of cochlear implant recipients using a personal digital adaptive radio frequency system. *Journal of the American Academy of Audiology.*

Wolfe, J., Schafer, E. C., Heldner, B., Mülder, H., Ward, E., & Vincent, B. (2009). Evaluation of speech recognition in noise with cochlear implants and dynamic FM. *Journal of the American Academy of Audiology, 20,* 409–421.

Woods, W. S., Van Tasell, D. J., Rickert, M. E., & Trine, T. D. (2006). SII and fit-to-target analysis of compression system performance as a function of number of compression channels. *International Journal of Audiology, 45,* 630–644.

Yoshinaga-Itano, C., Sedey, A. L., Coulter, D. K., & Mehl, A. L. (1998). The language of early- and later-identified children with hearing loss. *Pediatrics, 102,* 1161–1171.

CHAPTER 13

Principles and Clinical Utility of Hearing Aid Fitting Formulas

PHILLIP T. MCCANDLESS

FIG6 (1994)
Independent Hearing Aid Fitting Forum (IHAFF)
Desired Sensation Level (DSL[i/o] v.5.0)
NAL Nonlinear Version 2 (NAL-NL2)

COMPARISON OF TWO FITTING RATIONALES

SUMMARY AND CONCLUSION

REVIEW QUESTIONS

REFERENCES

ENDNOTE

INTRODUCTION

The purpose of hearing aid prescriptive formulas is to estimate electroacoustic amplification requirements for individuals with hearing loss. The need for such prescriptions arise from the belief that different acoustic features are necessary for each individual to hear optimally. To that end, all modern fitting methodologies are considered to be successful to some degree, as all specify at least *some* corrective gain to the ear. While it is true that simply providing amplification will lessen hearing impairment, an arbitrary amount may not always prove to be satisfactory. To provide a satisfactory fitting, a hearing aid must amplify sufficiently to maximize speech recognition at a wide range of inputs, provide comparatively normal loudness, provide good overall sound quality, and do this in an instrument that is both physically and acoustically comfortable.

The trivial application of important electroacoustic features may result in less than optimum speech understanding, poor tolerance of sound in aversive noise environments, and increased returns of hearing aids due to overall user dissatisfaction. Without the benefit of rational and valid scientific methods applied to the fitting process, each patient functions as a unique experiment with variable and unpredictable outcomes.

Although some patient dissatisfaction will persist no matter what fitting method is used, there is wisdom in implementing at least one of the many proven procedures to better estimate the final fitting requirements of the individual, and to verify the outcome via reliable methods such as real ear measurement (REM) or other appropriate means.

Low utilization of REM techniques or other verification methods remains commonplace despite the abundance of advanced fitting and verification software available from manufacturers and hearing aid research laboratories (Kochkin et al., 2010; Mueller & Picou, 2010). It is widely accepted that REM should be used in the fitting process, but when it is used, an appropriate amplification goal should be first selected, or else one cannot say whether the patient is fit adequately to any standard other than providing some arbitrary amount of gain.

Not yet developed, the optimum fitting method would seek to specify all salient electroacoustic parameters required to restore all dynamic acoustic properties lost through cochlear and conductive causes. Such an optimum formula assumes a hearing aid is available and capable of compensating for all the necessary amplification properties such as one that would restore reduced frequency and temporal discrimination of the impaired ear. It is evident from recent user satisfaction studies and modest industry-side return rates that the technology has not yet fully achieved that goal (Kochkin, 2003). Wide Dynamic Range Compression (WDRC), adaptive speech processing, noise reduction schemes, directional microphones, multichannel, expansion, and complex compression circuitry available in nearly all programmable and digital instruments promise to improve hearing through various technical schemes. However, variability introduced through advanced amplification technologies and individual variables preclude simple pencil and paper gain calculations and now rely heavily on proprietary computer software for implementation. Despite these technical hurdles, there has been a certain impetus for developing the optimum formula that will sufficiently address all variables contained in the new nonlinear technologies. Most of the linear approaches and some earlier nonlinear approaches have fallen out of clinical use, but understanding the origins of the simple linear formulas is useful in understanding the rationales of the modern fitting strategies as we move forward.

FOUNDATIONS OF MODERN HEARING AID FITTING

Early fitting methods can be classified into three general categories: comparative approaches, prescriptive approaches, and combination prescriptive-comparative approaches (McCandless, 1995). Approaches, including the DSL[i/o] and NAL-NL2, described later in this chapter are evidence-based prescriptive approaches and have been derived from a body of theoretical electroacoustic and psychoacoustic assumptions combined with data from a large population of successful hearing aid users. Comparative approaches recommend that the optimum hearing instrument is ultimately chosen from a number of "appropriate" models, each judged by measures of speech intelligibility and subjective quality estimates made by the patient.

Conversely, the majority of early prescriptive approaches derive optimum fitting recommendations based on individual threshold and/or loudness scaling procedures with little regard to formal speech intelligibility tests or subjective ratings. Most prescriptive approaches *predict* optimum electroacoustic parameters from the audiometric threshold data alone, while other approaches claim that between-subject differences are significant enough to warrant *direct* loudness scaling measurements be obtained from each individual. The advocates of the various predictive approaches make the assumption that errors in the final calculations for any individual can be corrected for in the clinic by "tweaking" the frequency response or simply by adjusting the volume control. It is apparent that this is an approach that has been quite successful, as most manufacturers deliver hearing aids to the dispenser preprogrammed with a preselected prescriptive rationale from threshold-based algorithms largely because of the difficulties associated with incorporating individual loudness data for each instrument. That is not to say that manufacturers use threshold data exclusively, as some may incorporate measures of MCL or UCL, or they may fine-tune the instrument by incorporating speech data through various proprietary optimization protocols.

EARLY COMPARATIVE APPROACHES

Formal fitting recommendations emerged as early as the late 1920s and 1930s, as can be seen in the works of West (1937) as well as various other U.S. Patents through the decade. In 1946, Carhart developed the popular "comparative fitting approach" that ranks or prioritizes hearing aids from a limited number of models without regard to response gain, maximum output, or other electroacoustic parameters. Still in widespread clinical use (Strom, 2006), the comparative approach selects the "best" hearing aid from a number of appropriate "candidate" hearing aids that would produce best aided speech reception thresholds, most comfortable levels, and discrimination scores measured in quiet and in noise. Some comparative approaches allowed little more than the subjective impression from the user to be applied toward the final selection.

Several problems have been identified with comparative approaches. First, they were considered by some to be too time consuming for practical use, and the final acoustic parameters are not identified with any particular set of electroacoustic parameters that have been demonstrated to contribute to improved performance (McCandless, 1995). Second, poor reliability and to some extent poor validity of word recognition used in the comparative method have been identified (Shore, Bilger, & Hirsch, 1960; Resnick & Becker, 1963). Another drawback is that the final response characteristics may or may not resemble the optimum prescription for the ear, and the comparative method is used with little regard to scientific rationale. Harris (1976) also pointed out that the hearing aids used in comparisons provided no significant measurable differences among various hearing aids. As a result, hearing aids were often chosen by very small differences in actual performance without regard to electroacoustic characteristics. It is interesting to note that the utility of the comparative method was limited, in part by the need to stop the test to change instruments. This tested the auditory memory of the individual between relatively long breaks in the evaluation process.

The advancement of real-time hearing aid tuning capabilities of nearly all modern digital hearing aids has ironically made the comparative method more practical. Today, memory effects are not as much a factor in the selection process as programs may be switched instantaneously from one or more settings during the fitting process. Rapid comparisons of speech intelligibility, loudness discomfort, directionality, and other features can be selected by comparative judgments on the fly. The fast-switch comparative method is not a true prescriptive method in that the hearing aid characteristics cannot be selected and tuned *a-priori* via objective audiometric measures obtained from the audiogram, but may be more useful in fine tuning the individual hearing aid after setting initial programming selections from a preselected prescriptive method.

EARLY PRESCRIPTIVE APPROACHES

Linear Amplification Approaches

West (1937) was the first to describe a prescriptive formula, shortly followed by Watson and Knudsen (1940) that popularized the "audiogram mirror-fitting" technique. This technique essentially provided gain to the ear that "mirrored" the magnitude of loss seen in the audiogram. The rationale simply states that the greatest amount of gain should be delivered to the regions of greatest loss. While at first glance the mirrored-audiogram approach seems logical, the approach has been criticized, as it tended to overamplify at higher sound inputs. This reason for overamplification has been related to the nature of loudness perception contours that tend to normalize at suprathreshold levels (Ross, 1978).

The evolution of the early prescriptive fitting strategies was advanced in 1942 by Lybarger to include the first ½ gain rule; a mathematical scaling factor of 0.5 of the Hearing Loss (0.5 * HL) that was applied against the magnitude of threshold loss at each frequency. For example, a hearing loss of 60 dB at 2000 Hz would receive 30 dB of gain in the hearing aid. Whether it was intentional or not, this ½ gain approach had the positive effect of limiting the overamplification seen in the "mirror-fitting" approach, while having a negative effect of providing too little amplification at low levels or with distant conversation. This was not entirely the fault of the procedure; rather it is an unfortunate characteristic of all linear amplifiers and their inability to accommodate the nonlinear recruitment requirements unique to the impaired ear. However, this ½ gain rule applied to linear hearing aids struck what turned out to be an effective compromise between the undesirable effects relating to overamplification at high inputs and poor audibility at low levels. Interestingly, all subsequent traditional linear approaches utilize some mathematical variation of the ½ gain rule, ranging between ⅓ to ⅔ gain according to the specific fitting rationale and frequency of interest.

Fitting Nonlinear Hearing Loss with Linear Amplification

In Figure 13–1, the 45-degree diagonal line represents the loudness growth function of a normal "reference" ear at 2 kHz. The exponential curved line on the left represents the loudness growth function of a hypothetical

50 dB sensorineural hearing loss. The amount of ideal gain that is required to restore the loudness function of this hypothetical impaired ear is the vertical distance between the curved line (hearing loss) and the diagonal reference line of the normal ear to the right. It can be seen from this graph that the amount of gain required to restore a normal loudness function to this 50 dB hearing loss is not constant. In fact, theoretically, one would need exactly 50 dB insertion gain at 0 dB inputs, and diminishing to 0 dB at 100 dB inputs. The gain requirements to properly restore this hearing loss change as a function of input level, meaning that the amplification requirements at this 2 kHz example are not linear. The three parallel lines that bisect the curved line of the impaired ear illustrate the difficulty in fitting linear hearing aids

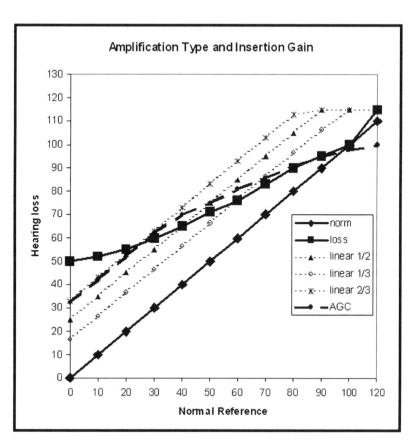

Figure 13–1. The amount of gain required to restore a normal loudness function to this 50-dB hearing loss is not constant.

to a nonlinear hearing loss. At inputs below 40–50dB, the ½ gain linear amplifier provides adequate compensation. This amount of gain at 50 dB inputs would be adequate for typical speech conversation at distances of approximately 6 feet. But at input levels below 40 dB, the gain is probably too little for complete speech perception, and softer environmental sounds are not amplified adequately. At input levels above 40 dB, the gain becomes too high with linear amplification, providing too much gain in noisy environments. What is interesting to note here is that the ⅔ gain can be seen to overamplify over the curved line of the impaired ear more than underamplifies, whereas the ⅓ gain curve illustrates the opposite, where it tends to underamplify sound to the ear.

Figure 13–2 is a "normalized" curve derived from the data in Figure 13–1. The graph shown here is illustrative of the amount of amplification error, or devia-

tion from desired gain depending on linear amplification amount. Also shown here is the error of the wide dynamic range compression (WDRC) amplifier, illustrating the improved accommodation of loudness correction over linear designs.

While the development of prescriptive formulas was in motion, Davis et al. (1946) took another route suggesting that optimum response gain did not seem to be related to patterns that could be seen in the individual's audiometric threshold. The "Harvard Report" emerged from these data suggesting that the frequency response of a hearing aid cannot be prescribed for any individual. The Harvard Report recommended that a flat or gradually rising "6 dB per octave" high pass response characteristic would be sufficient and would satisfy the amplification requirements for most subjects. Some modifications of that 6-dB rule recommendation were implemented at later dates to accommodate the calibration

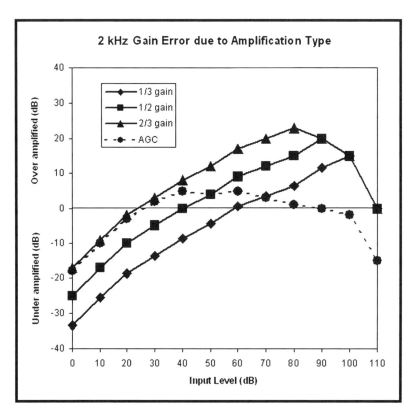

Figure 13–2. Normalized curve derived from data in Figure 13–1.

differences between real-ear and hearing aid coupler data.

The Harvard Report suggested that the "one-size-fits all" approach would satisfy most hearing aid candidates without the need for formal calculations. The Harvard-style of hearing aid fitting lasted for a period extending many years, probably due to its simplicity, and relative success for fitting the "generic" mild to moderate sloping hearing loss.

It was not until the late 1970s and 1980s that prescriptive fitting formulas derived from the audiogram regained widespread acceptance. Among the most popular formulas are the Prescription of Gain and Output, or POGO (McCandless & Lyregaard, 1983), the National Acoustic Laboratories' NAL and the revised version known as NAL-R (Byrne & Dillon 1986), Berger's method (Berger, Hagberg, & Rane, 1977), and Byrne and Tonisson (1976). As stated earlier, these formulas were best suited to the previous state-of-the-art linear broadband instruments utilizing abrupt peak clipping or compression limiting.

These traditional prescriptive formulas (POGO, NAL, Berger, etc.) were elegant in their simplicity, requiring only a pen and paper, addition, subtraction, multiplication, or division skills to derive desired hearing aid characteristics at the time of fitting. These formulas, while still in limited use today, are not particularly well suited to modern digital nonlinear devices that utilize wide dynamic range compression or other advanced processing schemes. Most traditional linear approaches provided individual gain and maximum output sound pressure levels estimated from little more than easily obtainable audiometric thresholds or MCL and UCL measures.

Prescription of Gain and Output (POGO)

McCandless and Lyregaard (1983) developed a prescriptive fitting strategy that provided gain and maximum power output (MPO) recommendations for mild-to-severe sensorineural hearing losses. Still in wide use today as applied to linear amplified hearing aids, POGO has the advantage of being one of the simplest linear formulas to implement clinically. The POGO gain recommendations are derived primarily from the audiometric threshold, similar to Lybarger's approach (Lybarger, 1944). Maximum output recommendations are made from beginning loudness discomfort thresholds obtained from the patient using pure tones or narrowband noise. As in the Lybarger approach, POGO applies a mathematical scaling factor of $0.5 * HL$ to the magnitude of threshold loss at each audiometric frequency to derive recommended gain. They proposed a slight reduction in low frequency gain values (-10 and -5 dB at 250 and 500 Hz, respectively) to optimize speech intelligibility in noise due to the undesirable effects of the upward spread of masking (Table 13–1). Other factors such as speech intelligibility and overall pleasantness were important factors considered in the initial design of the procedure.

In addition, POGO was designed to: (1) avoid the relative complexity and time demands of the comparative approaches, (2) be easily implemented, and (3) be accurate for a large number of users based on routine audiometric threshold data. It was designed to provide a complete, comprehensive method of selection, implementation, and verification for losses of cochlear and conductive origin with proper and easily applied computational corrections. POGO provides recommendations for hearing aid selection using 2cc coupler data provided by the manufacturer.

The authors of POGO claim that, although ideal gain may be calculated from threshold values alone, the actual gain prescription does, more often than not, shift speech and other sounds correctly into the patients' MCL range. Small corrections to the volume control alter the intensity of these sounds to meet the patients' MCL requirements.

Suggested verification of the POGO is through the use of insertion gain measurements obtained at the eardrum using *in situ or REM* probe tube measurements. It is interesting to note that POGO also includes

Table 13–1. POGO Procedures for Insertion Gain

Frequency (Hz)	Formula
250	(½ * HL) – 10 dB
500	(½ * HL) – 5 dB
1000	½ * HL
2000	½ * HL
3000	½ * HL
4000	½ * HL

POGO Procedure for Determining Maximum Power Output:

$$MPO = \frac{(UCL\ 500\ Hz) + (UCL\ 1000\ Hz) + (UCL\ 2000\ Hz)}{3}$$

general, but not specific, recommendations, for reserve gain when the formula is used to choose an appropriate fitting circuit from published manufacturer data. POGO accommodates binaural fittings by allowing the user to adjust gain through use of the volume control, rather than specifying *a priori* compensation values. This is because of the potentially wide variations in loudness discomfort that are reported among patients. Calculation of gain and maximum output of POGO is shown in Table 13–1. Maximum output is calculated by determining the *beginning* threshold of discomfort using an ascending approach at 500, 1K, and 2k Hz tones.

It might be useful to mention here that contrary to popular belief, the often-used POGO II procedure (Schwartz, Lyregaard, & Lundh, 1988) is not a subsequent release to McCandless and Lyregaard's original POGO formula, nor do the original authors claim any title to the subsequent POGO II formulation. It is, however, based largely on the same ½ gain formulation of the POGO for mild-to-moderate hearing loss, with additional gain specifications for severe or greater hearing loss. POGO II argued that the original POGO did not provide enough speech audibility with severe losses, so additional gain was added to POGO II values above 65 dB. The POGO II formula that was designed to modify POGO is shown in Table 13–2.

Table 13–2. POGO II Formula

For thresholds above 65 dB HL:

(½ HTL – C*) + (½ [HTL – 65])

*C = 10 dB at 250 Hz
       5 dB at 500 Hz
       0 dB at all other frequencies

NAL

Among the most popular and easily implemented formula for linear amplification is the National Acoustic Laboratories (NAL) procedure (Byrne & Dillon, 1986). Unlike POGO that based its assumptions on restoring more natural loudness function to the impaired ear, the NAL and its subsequent procedure the NAL-R, employs a rationale that attempts to set all bands of the critical speech frequencies to a "preferred listening level." In doing so, this approach hopes to maximize audibility and speech intelligibility (Table 13–3 shows the NAL calculation). The NAL applies frequency-specific recommendations based on the long-term average speech spectrum, whereas POGO and other linear prescriptive formulations assume a flat response characteristic. The NAL utilizes mathematic scaling corrections slightly different than the straightforward ½ gain rule used in the Lybarger and POGO approaches, yet the earlier NAL procedure is simple enough to incorporate manually without the need for computer software. 2cc and ear simulator corrections were also made available to assist in preselecting hearing aids from published manufacturer matrices. The NAL shares a similar low-frequency attenuation rationale with POGO and many other linear formulas

Table 13–3. Revised NAL Procedure

Step 1. Calculate X where:

  $X = 0.05 (H500 + H1000 + H2000)$

Step 2. Calculate gain at each frequency:

  $G\,250 = X + 0.31\,H\,250 - 17$

  $G\,500 = X + 0.31\,H\,500 - 8$

  $G\,750 = X + 0.31\,H\,750 - 3$

  $G\,1000 = X + 0.31\,H\,1000 + 1$

  $G\,1500 = X + 0.31\,H\,1500 + 1$

  $G\,2000 = X + 0.31\,H\,2000 - 1$

  $G\,3000 = X + 0.31\,H\,3000 - 2$

  $G\,4000 = X + 0.31\,H\,4000 - 2$

  $G\,6000 = X + 0.31\,H\,6000 - 2$

Where:

  G is the required gain at the specified frequency.

  H is the hearing threshold level obtained from the audiogram.

---

to optimize speech information delivered to the ear. The NAL procedure also supplies a formula for correction to a 2cc coupler, so that an appropriate hearing aid may be chosen from published data.

Berger Method

Another popular, linear approach appropriate for linear gain amplification is the Berger prescriptive method initially described in 1976 and again in 1979 by Berger, Hagberg, and Rane. It was updated in 1988. The formula shown in Table 13–4 is relatively simple to implement, yet like the NAL-R, it is derived from a series of comparatively sophisticated rationales based on several key acoustic conditions and observations of normal speech intensities. A key assumption in the Berger approach is that speech is presented at an average sound pressure level of 55 to 70 dB. The desired gain to amplify these levels of speech, therefore, would require amplification of slightly more than ½ the magnitude of the audiometric threshold loss. The Berger approach contends that the most important frequency spectrum relating to speech intelligibility is contained from 2 to 4 kHz. The speech spectrum reveals these high frequencies also have the lowest energy, making amplification in these regions most critical. The contribution of speech discrimination declines after approximately 4 kHz; therefore, these frequencies are not emphasized.

Table 13–4. Berger Procedure for Calculating Full-On 2cc Gain

	Formula	
Frequency (Hz)	*BTE*	*ITE*
500	$(HL_{500}/2.0) + 10$	$(HL_{500}/2.0) + 10$
1000	$(HL_{1000}/1.6) + 10$	$(HL_{1000}/1.6) + 10$
2000	$(HL_{2000}/1.5) + 12$	$(HL_{2000}/1.5) + 10$
3000	$(HL_{3000}/1.6) + 13$	$(HL_{3000}/1.7) + 10$
4000	$(HL_{4000}/1.9) + 10$	$(HL_{4000}/1.9) + 10$
6000	$(HL_{6000}/2.0) + 10$	$(HL_{6000}/1.9) + 10$

Below 500 Hz, voiced vowels and voiced consonants produce a significant amount of low-frequency energy, yet contribute relatively little to overall speech intelligibility. Therefore, frequencies below 500 are also deemphasized in the Berger approach.

Maximum gain is specified in the final recommendations rather than the typical operating or use gain. This is because the operating gain is usually variable according to individual preference and particular listening situations. As such, the maximum gain is set according to the formula: maximum gain = operating gain + reserve gain ± correction factors for BTE versus ITE microphone settings.

For conductive losses, an additional ⅕ gain factor is added to the operating and maximum gain values. Saturation sound pressure levels (SSPL) and binaural correction are also suggested but are not discussed in this text.

Byrne and Tonisson

The Byrne and Tonisson (1976) rationale is based on maximizing speech intelligibility by presenting all of the frequency components of speech presented to the impaired ear at equal loudness levels. To implement this prescriptive method, tables were used to indicate the relationship between the audiometric threshold levels and the user's recommended gain at various critical frequencies. Other modifications of this procedure used MCLs and LDLs of speech to specify the recommended gain at various frequency regions (Byrne & Murray, 1985).

Other Linear Prescriptions

There are several other less well-known linear prescriptive approaches including those from Libby (1985, 1986), utilizing the ½ gain rule for mild to moderate losses and a ⅔ gain rule for more severe losses. Another is by Keller (1973) who derived estimates of the MCL's from essentially bisecting the threshold and

UCL levels. Nearly all of the previously mentioned prescriptive methods incorporate some recommendations for setting the maximum output level, accounting for different coupler types, BTE and ITE hearing aid types, and some recommendations for correcting conductive hearing loss. The reader is encouraged to consult the original literature located in the bibliography for more in-depth specifications on any of these rationales.

THEORETICAL LIMITATIONS OF LINEAR AMPLIFICATION APPROACHES

The traditional formulas described in this chapter are characterized by the single-gain specifications that most often predict insertion or coupler gain values directly from the audiometric threshold data or from direct measurement of the MCLs or UCLs. Gain recommendations are based on rationales derived from unique perspectives, each having distinct outcomes and characteristic response patterns. An exemplary patient is shown in Figure 13–3 as a 65-year-old English speaking male with an acquired bilateral high frequency sensorineural hearing loss. His audiogram is used as a reference by which all prescriptive formulations are compared in this chapter.

Figure 13–4 illustrates the three prescriptive gain recommendations from Berger, POGO, and NAL. There are comparatively large differences between the three in terms of slope and overall gain; however, similarities do exist as all linear formulas provide enough gain sufficient to optimize speech presented at speaker-listener distances of approximately 3 to 6 feet. Notable differences in the high frequency gain are evident between the NAL and Berger methods especially at 2 and 4 kHz. However, there is minimal disagreement among the various methods below 2 kHz. The downside of linear aids and single gain recommendations of course, is that while they do provide adequate amplifica-

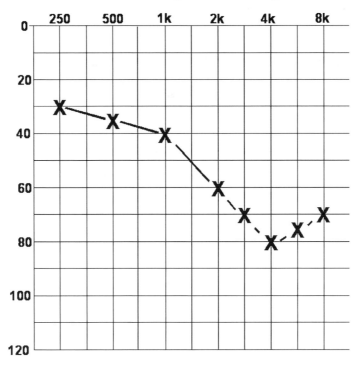

Figure 13–3. Audiogram example. 65-year-old male with acquired hearing loss.

tion in limited conversational situations, they continue to overamplify louder environmental and speech inputs, while underamplifying softer speech signals.

MODERN APPROACHES

Nonlinear Prescriptive Approaches

The current noncomparative fitting rationales are designed to work with the new line of hearing aid amplification that has evolved in the past decade. Current compression-class circuitry in modern hearing aids is capable of providing this nonlinear ampli-

fication characteristic to the ear, which is a clear advantage over linear aids of the past. As shown above, WDRC compression circuitry is capable of "compressing" the wide dynamic range of sound pressures into the relatively narrow range that is required be the impaired ear. Just how much range to be compressed and at what frequencies are to be affected are the main focus of the new nonlinear prescriptive approaches. Most fascinating is that these new formulas presume that you can achieve correct loudness growth and frequency response compensation for a variety of individuals from little more than the audiometric threshold data to work from. The new fitting rationales, therefore, require not only a single gain specification at a single input level, but now provide the specification of different gains at low, mid, and high inputs.

Linear Formulas

Prescription examples

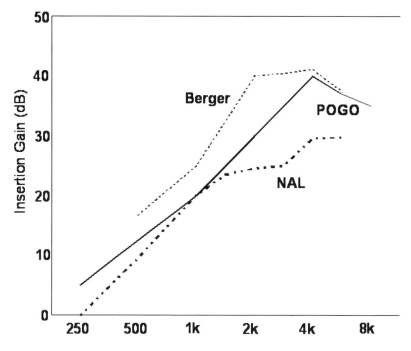

Figure 13–4. Comparison of linear prescriptive formulas.

The following summaries are illustrative of formulas used in modern WDRC instruments. Like their linear counterparts, the nonlinear prescriptions are based on unique rationales and procedures that result in differences in the ultimate fitting.

FIG6 (1994)

Among the first of the nonlinear prescriptive formulas to emerge was by Killion and Fikret-Pasa (1993) and provided calculations for three categories of hearing loss and the amount of gain that would satisfy the loudness compensation for those losses. Figure 6 of that article was an illustration of the gain required to achieve those goals, thus, the origin of the FIG6 procedure. The gain recommendations are calculated from audiometric threshold data derived from loudness-growth data published by several

research sources (Hellman & Meiselman, 1993; Lipmann, Braida, & Durlach, 1981; Lyregaard, 1988) and can be applied, as with the linear prescriptions, with little more than a pen and paper at hand, or is available as a computer program. Like other modern nonlinear formulas, FIG6 calculates the gain on a frequency-by-frequency basis for each of the three different input levels (40, 65, and 90 dB), and an example of the recommendations is shown in Figure 13–5. This formula is generally useful for hearing losses up to 60 dB with very little need for amplification at higher inputs. Generally, FIG6 is not recommended for losses over 70 dB HL.

FIG6—Gain for <40 dB Inputs

The FIG6 formula originates gain recommendations for soft speech inputs from the observation that portions of quiet conversational speech are as low as 20 dB HL (Muel-

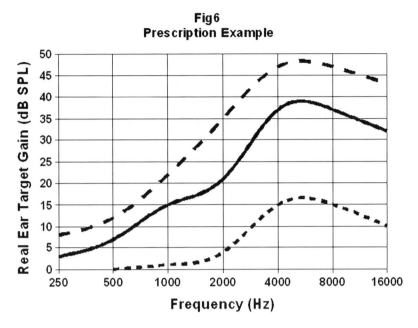

Fig 6
Prescription Example

Figure 13–5. Insertion gain targets response curves at three input levels for audiogram shown in Figure 13–3.

ler & Killion, 1992). Mueller and Killion's count-the-dot audiogram for calculating the articulation index suggests that, if the aided threshold does not provide enough amplification to include speech frequencies at 20 dB, then some of the speech cues will be missed. Gain that restores hearing below 20 dB HL is considered to be excessive because the room noise, as well as hearing aid noise, may mask out lower speech cues. Therefore, the formula is designed to correct hearing to 20 dB, no more and no less. Thus, the formula for 40 dB inputs and lower becomes: $G40 = HL - 20$.

FIG6—Gain for 65 dB SPL (Conversational Speech)

Pascoe (1988) studied the mean MCLs found in subjects with normal, mild, moderate, and severe hearing losses. He found that the mean MCL for normal listeners was 65 dB HL, 77 dB for mild loss, 90 dB for moderate losses, and so forth. Using the mean MCL data for each level of hearing loss, one may target the amount of gain necessary to transfer conversational speech into Pascoe's predicted MCL

levels. The gain formula appropriate for conversational speech inputs is: $G65 = (mean MCL [re HL]) - 65$.

For example, gain at 65 dB for a hearing impaired listener with a 40 dB HL loss would require, 77 dB – 65 dB or 12 dB of gain for a mild 40 dB hearing loss.

FIG6—Gain for 95 dB Inputs

FIG6 prescribes gain based on loudness-growth work reported by Lyregaard (1988) and Lippman et al. (1981). FIG6 assumes that mild losses typically demonstrate complete loudness recruitment at high sound levels, and thus do not need amplification with high inputs. However, as the amount of hearing loss increases into the moderate ranges and above, the amount of required amplification increases only slightly.

Data for two frequency bands are generated in the software package showing the target insertion gain for low, medium, and high input levels. While the FIG6 procedure specifies REIG targets, it also provides 2cc coupler recommendations in tabular and graph form for ITE, BTE, ITC, and deep CIC instruments. In doing this, an appropriate hearing aid may be easily selected from the manufacturers' published data specifications. One feature of the software is that it specifies compression ratios for the independent low- and high-frequency channels found on many of the current two-channel instruments.

Independent Hearing Aid Fitting Forum

The Independent Hearing Aid Fitting Forum (IHAFF) was created by a select forum of researchers, manufacturers, and engineers to reach a consensus for a standardized and comprehensive hearing aid fitting protocol for linear and nonlinear hearing aids. The rationale for the IHAFF is based on the restoration of normal loudness perception across a wide frequency range. Cox (1995) states that the goal underlying the IHAFF procedure is that, "amplification should normalize the relationship between the environmental sounds and loudness perception. This means that a sound that appears to be soft to a normal-hearing listener should be audible but soft, after amplification, to the hearing aid wearer." The same loudness scaling criteria are applied to medium and loud environmental sounds as well. The IHAFF procedure differs from the NAL-NL1 and FIG6 in that gain recommendations are made according to direct loudness scaling measurements obtained from each listener, instead of predicted gain recommendations predicted from the audiometric thresholds.

The implementation of the IHAFF includes direct measures of loudness scaling estimations using 500 and 3000 Hz warble tone stimuli. A computer program, having the acronym Visualization of Input/Output Locator Algorithm (VIOLA) assists in categorization of the loudness estimations at 500 and 3000 Hz. These loudness categories are shown in Table 13–5 of Cox (1995; Cox, Alexander, Taylor, & Gray, 1997). Using these data of loudness scaling, the VIOLA program aligns the categories into a meaningful loud-

Table 13–5. Categories of Loudness Used in the Contour Test

7. Uncomfortably loud
6. Loud, but okay
5. Comfortable, but slightly loud
4. Comfortable
3. Comfortable, but slightly soft
2. Soft
1. Very soft

Source: Reprinted with permission from "Using Loudness Data for Hearing Aid Selection," by R. M. Cox, 1995. *Hearing Journal*, *47*(2), 39–42.

ness prescription for the hearing aid, so that soft sounds are perceived as soft, and loud sounds are perceived as loud, approaching but not exceeding the user's LDLs. The procedure uses audiometric pure tone-threshold data, combined with the loudness scaling data, to derive three input level recommended targets for entry into the nonlinear hearing aid. The software program also assists in setting gain, compression thresholds, and output characteristics. Verification procedures are also available on the software. Provisions are also included to predict gain characteristics for those unable to participate in loudness-scaling tasks.

The IHAFF approach is one of the few procedures that relies strongly on direct loudness measures from the patient. The time-factor has been a major point of criticism, as some suggest that it takes a considerably longer time to implement than other procedures. Although this method may prove to be more accurate for any given patient, the time needed to implement may discourage clinical use.

Desired Sensation Level

The earliest version of the Desired Sensation Level (DSL) relied on look-up tables that specified target sensation levels for amplified speech for various hearing degrees and slopes of hearing loss. It was based on data that are associated with demonstrated comfortable listening levels for various hearing levels (Kamm, Dirks, & Mickey, 1978; Pascoe, 1978). The principal of the DSL strategy was in normalizing loudness, so that sounds for a hearing-impaired person would sound on the same level on which it would be perceived by a normal listener. The most recent version of the DSL modifies that approach to make accommodations for a number of variables in order to optimize speech information aid account for limitations of hearing aids in noise; also included are recommendations for establishing maximum output levels to maintain user comfort. The pencil and paper look-up tables of the early DSL, considered to be too simplistic and cumbersome for practical use, has since evolved in later versions to accommodate nonlinear hearing aids.

The DSL came to be known as the first comprehensive, commercially available software-driven hearing aid fitting protocol optimized for the fitting of children (Cornelisse, Seewald, & Jamieson, 1995; Seewald, 1994; Seewald, Ross, & Spiro, 1985). Cornelisse et al. (1995) stated that it was the goal of the DSL to develop a threshold-based formula that would specify ideal electroacoustic parameters for a wide range of inputs, regardless of the unique hearing device characteristics, as is the stated goal of nearly all other modern fitting prescriptions.

The DSL m[i/o] v5.0 (m stands for multilevel family of targets, i/o stands for input/output) is the latest version that takes into consideration the need to fit the very young patient due to the improved early hearing loss identification methods. Long gone are the days of pen and paper calculations to derive the fitting recommendations; rather the DSL m[i/o] relies on proprietary software to generate the recommendations. This limits access to the software, as it is available commercially or through manufacturer's programming software. However, the program is quite comprehensive in its recommendations and scope. Version 5 has been enhanced beyond infant and children specifications to include a family of targets such as one that

accounts for lower gain requirements in adults who have acquired hearing loss (Scollie et al., 2005). The reason for incorporating the family of targets based on age and etiology is from empirical evidence found from a large database of varied users who suggested that more than one choice is needed depending on the individual. There are significant differences in electrophysiologic requirements between adults and children that warrant fine-tuning of prescriptions based on average group data. Version 5.0 includes the principal goals of: (1) avoidance of excessive loudness, (2) the maximization of the number of acoustic cues contained in conversational speech, (3) support for early intervention programs, (4) optimization protocols for compression circuitry, (5) account for differences in congenital versus acquired hearing loss in children and adults, and (6) making accommodations for comfortable listening in both noisy and quiet environments.

One of the hallmarks of the DSL procedure recognized among hearing aid professionals is recognized as the SPLogram. For years, it has been incorporated into manufacturer's fitting and verification equipment to provide a graphical display of the appropriate ear canal SPL or gain target verification, usually used in conjunction with the real-ear analysis. An example of one such SPLogram shown in Figure 13–6 contains the unaided auditory thresholds, *predicted* thresholds of discomfort and what lies in between as the useable auditory area between 250 Hz and 6 KHz. Within the useable auditory area, targets for maximum output power and conversational speech range targets for soft, medium, and loud conversation are plotted, and are easily compared at a glance.

There is an important distinction from other prescriptive formulas that bears mentioning at this point. The DSL prescription uses complex speech input instead of puretone stimuli in its recommendations. It is argued that the use of dynamic speech stimuli is more representative of real-life conditions under which a hearing aid must operate, and, therefore, the amount of "true" gain of a hearing aid produces not only by the steady-state

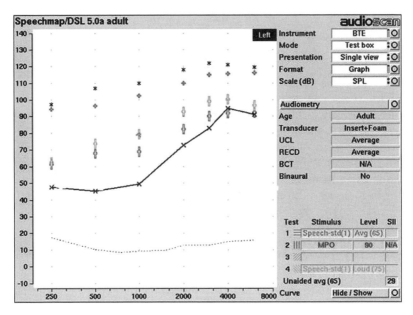

Figure 13–6. *Speechmap* showing DSLm[i/o] 5.0 real-ear targets for an exemplary subject. The dashed line on the lower portion of the graph indicates Minimum Audible Pressure for normal-hearing individuals. The connected line is the hearing loss of one exemplary individual converted to SPL. Top asterisk line show the maximum recommended output levels of the hearing aid and the crosses indicate target levels for low, mid, and high input levels. Up to a 3 dB compensation should be subtracted for a binaural fitting. Note: The inputs for this display are shown using complex speech input signal and is not directly comparable with other prescriptive methods that use pure tones as inputs (see text). *Speechmap* and Audioscan are registered trademarks of Etymonic Design Inc. Used with permission.

levels of gain and compression thresholds, but is also determined in part by the temporal attack and release characteristics of the digital processing circuitry.

The new DSL m[i/o] 5.0 also claims advances in specifying input-output functions by determining knee points, expansion rates, expansion, and compression ratios for various hearing losses. DSL 5.0 has the ability to take into account the number of compression channels and group them, so that targets for each channel can be determined for hearing aids that have numerous independent processing channels.

DSL 5.0 also recognizes that speech is highly variable by nature and has numerous peaks that, if not properly managed, can easily exceed the patient's uncomfortable loudness levels. The updated protocol rec-

ognizes that the peaks typically exceed the long-term average speech levels by 10 to 12 dB (known as the crest factor), and hearing aids can faithfully reproduce these peaks often into uncomfortable levels, so a variable called the Broadband Output Limiting Threshold (BOLT) is calculated against the long-term speech average response to lower the response on the SPLogram to make sure the speech peaks remain at levels that are not objectionable (Figure 13–7).

Advanced data inputs are allowed in the software for the calculation of real-ear-to-coupler-difference (RECD), real-ear-unaided-gain (REUG), and real-ear-to-dial-differences (REDD). There are many other subtleties and rationales to the DSL m[i/o] implementation that exceed the space limitations of this chapter, so the reader is urged to seek out further

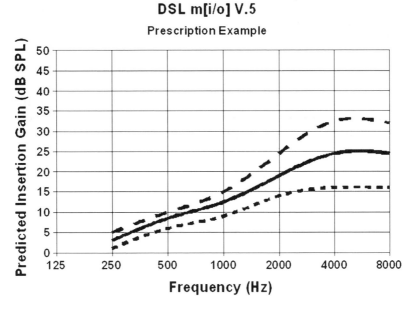

Figure 13–7. A prescription for the patient shown in Figure 13–3.

information from the University of Western Ontario's National Centre for Audiology web site or an Internet search for DSL[i/o] hearing aid fitting procedure.

NAL Nonlinear Version 2 (NAL-NL2)

The NAL-NL2 is the latest iteration of several prescriptive formulas useful for prescribing gain in modern nonlinear amplification devices. As in the DSL and other modern prescriptive formulae, it is not a simple pen and paper formula; rather it is a computer-driven prescription procedure that generates multi input compression level frequency response recommendations mainly from the audiogram data alone. The goal of the NAL-NL2 is similar, but not identical to the previous NAL-NL1, in that it strives to maximize speech intelligibility for any level above the compression threshold, while keeping overall loudness at or below that of normal listeners (Keidser & Dillon, 2009).

For those already familiar with the NAL-NL1, the NL2 differs from its prede-cessor in that the most recent version adds or subtracts gain-response, compression, or other electroacoustic parameters values to the basic formula based on the patient's age, gender, experience level, native language type, severity of loss, and other individual characteristics. Due to the complexity involved with these added criteria and assumptions, the NAL-NL2 procedure requires a "neural network-based" computer software program to arrive at an appropriate fitting recommendation, and no longer can be calculated with simple pencil and paper as in the original linear-based NAL.

The previous nonlinear NAL-NL1 version used portions of the Speech Intelligibility Index (SII) and loudness models from Moore and Glasberg (1983) and applied them to 52 different audiograms from which an optimized formula was derived. The results of this fitting approach provided gain recommendations that made the loudness of speech bands approximately equal across a wide range of frequencies. However, the basic underlying assumptions and rationales used to formulate the NAL-NL1 were questioned in the formulation of the NAL-NL2 to find out if they could be further improved. It was asked whether the appropriateness of recommending equal loudness relationships across frequencies of hearing impaired was better than recommending a loudness relationship that was referenced to loudness judgment functions of normal listeners (Dillon, 1999; Dillon, Flax, Ching, Keidser, & Brewer, 2009) The results suggest that the NAL-NL2 should, in fact, maintain much of the loudness corrections used in the NAL-NL1 procedure with a number of slight modifications that is in accordance with their internal assumptions and research.

Another assumption in the latest NAL version of the prescription stems from the understanding that not all hearing losses result in the same speech understanding or clarity, even if speech is amplified adequately (Dillon, Flax, Ching, Keidser, & Brewer, 2009). They found, on average, as hearing loss becomes worse in terms of both degree and slope, the speech cues that can be extracted from the acoustic signal may become more distorted. This means that as hearing loss becomes more severe, less information is extracted from the speech signal, even if it is above threshold, may be less than optimum. Therefore, this degradation of speech understanding in more severe hearing losses and especially in the presence of noise must be accounted for in the amplification recommendation.

Additional assumptions incorporated into the most recent NAL-NL2 fitting formula considers everything in the fitting chain, from the transducer used in testing, to the type of venting used in the fitting and subject variables. The assumptions based on subject variations include previous experience of the user, age, gender, binaural and monaural fitting, type of hearing loss, etiology, coupler calibration differences, and many other factors. It is difficult to describe the actual differences between the current and previous versions, but in general, the current version provides:

1. Less gain provided in adults than was originally prescribed by the NAL-NL1.

2. Males prefer slightly more gain than females.
3. With moderate or severe losses, old users preferred more gain than new users.
4. The compression ratio is increased slightly for mild to moderate loss.
5. Gain is reduced 2 to 6 dB for binaural fittings greatest reduction at high input levels.
6. More gain for children at low input levels, less gain at high inputs for adults.
7. Variation in gain specifications for acquired versus congenital hearing loss.
8. Frequency-dependent gain differences in native language (tonal versus nontonal language).
9. Recommendations for compression speed (attack and release times).

A fitting example using the NAL-NL2 is provided in Figure 13–8. Unlike other fitting procedures, we included the data that would adjust for a 65-year-old English-speaking male with a bilateral acquired high-frequency sensorineural hearing loss shown in the audiogram of Figure 13–3. For those interested in learning more about this procedure, the reader is referred to Australia's National Acoustics Laboratory's Internet website at http://www.nal.gov.au for more information.

COMPARISON OF TWO FITTING RATIONALES

It is necessary to have a fitting protocol that approximates as closely as possible the true fitting requirement that the hearing-impaired ear needs and one that the subject finds satisfactory. However, because of the highly complex imbedded rationales, patient databases, stimulus type used in the analysis (tones versus narrow band noise), and other assumptions buried within the computer software, it is difficult to quantify the differences among the new generation prescriptions. It is a lot like comparing apples with oranges on some scale, but the good news is that Johnson and

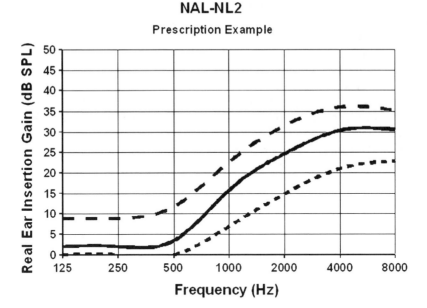

Figure 13–8. The NAL-NL2 prescription for the audiogram shown in Figure 13–1. Fitting data provided courtesy of National Acoustics Laboratory, Australia.

Dillon (2011) have done just that for two of the most common prescription formulas; the NAL-NL2 and the DSL m[i/o], and the reader is encouraged to refer to the original articles for more details.

SUMMARY AND CONCLUSION

Ever since the introduction of a commercially available carbon hearing aid developed in 1902 by Hutchinson, there have been valiant efforts to derive a fitting formula that best compensates for the type and magnitude of a given hearing impairment. There have been a number of attempts to develop appropriate fitting formulas, most of which were based on predicting specific gain functions based on threshold data for discrete frequencies. Most, if not all, of the early fitting rationales attempted to compensate for hearing loss using linear amplifiers. It was not until the

introduction of nonlinear hearing aid systems that new or modified formulas were introduced to include the advantages offered by these nonlinear instruments. Regardless of the fitting procedure, it is safe to say that all provide at least some, if not a great deal, of benefit to the user. Fitting formulas are largely insensitive to the presenting pathology contributing to the loss, the survivability, and distribution of the hair cell population of the cochlea, and central neural pathways contributing to the conduction and ultimate central processing of environmental sounds. These factors cannot be controlled for in any single fitting formula, as all fitting recommendations are based on average data, and one single approach may not be appropriate for all individuals. It is not the intent of this chapter to differentiate—or to imply the best formula— but only to educate the reader on the background, rationale, and differences among the most popular fitting strategies. The question of what is the appropriate fitting procedure has been raised many times in the past, and is no less a valid question for modern formulas.

The rationale underlying any fitting formula is to improve signal audibility and word recognition, and to provide corrective loudness compensation to the impaired ear. The "ideal" prosthetic device is designed to minimize the impact of an impairment by making it as inconsequential and unnoticed as possible. That "ideal" hearing aid fitting requires a target be identified and met for each and every individual in so far as possible from the audiogram as the primary data source. What is interesting to note, is that despite the large amount of research that has been applied to deriving the "ideal target," differences in prescriptive recommendations persist, and the choice of which one is "best" is still a matter of clinical choice and to what rationales and foundations that each formula makes most sense. In the final analysis, as new and more complex signal processing hearing aids are developed, and as we understand more of the behavior of impaired auditory systems, fitting methods will be developed to embrace these new and challenging contributions.

REVIEW QUESTIONS

1. What arguments have some made against the use of the "comparative method" of hearing aid fitting?
   a. It is too time consuming.
   b. It has poor reliability.
   c. It uses too many audiometric frequencies in the calculation of functional gain and output maximums.
   d. B and C
   e. A and B

2. The problem with the "mirrored-audiogram" approach is that it:
   a. Undercompensates hearing by providing too little gain.
   b. Overcompensates hearing by providing too much gain.
   c. Reflects too many sounds from the ear.
   d. None of the above.

3. Which linear approaches reported in the article rely solely on audiometric threshold data to arrive at appropriate gain recommendations?
   a. POGO and NAL-R
   b. Berger and NAL-R
   c. POGO, NAL-R, and Berger
   d. None of the above.

4. The limitations of linear formulas are seen as:
   a. They specify gain recommendations at only one input level.
   b. They specify gain recommendations at only three (soft, medium, and loud) input levels.
   c. A and B
   d. None of the above.

5. An appropriately fit linear hearing aid better satisfies the loudness requirements of the impaired ear at all input intensities.
   a. True
   b. False

6. The NAL-NL1 is a complex predictive formula that optimizes speech intelligibility within the constraints of loudness perception for soft, medium, and loud inputs.
   a. True
   b. False

7. The FIG6 procedure routinely amplifies speech so that sound is audible below 20 dB HL.
   a. True
   b. False

8. The early version of the DSL was optimized for prescribing electroacoustic hearing aid parameters to children.
   a. True
   b. False

9. Most nonlinear fitting recommendations appropriate for the use in modern WDRC instruments specify gain for inputs of approximately:

a. 20, 40, and 60 dB
b. 20, 40, and 90 dB
c. 40, 65, and 90 dB
d. 20, 75, and 85 dB

10. Linear formulas assume that loudness accommodation is made with inputs of approximately 60 dB SPL. This sound pressure translates into a typical speaker-listener limitations ranging from ___ feet.
a. 1 to 3
b. 3 to 6
c. 5 to 12
d. 8 to 32

REFERENCES

Berger, K., Hagberg, E., & Rane, R. (1977). *Prescription of hearing aids: Rationale, procedures, and results.* Kent, OH: Herald.

Byrne, D., & Dillon, H. (1986). The National Acoustic Laboratories' (NAL) new procedure for selecting the gain and frequency response of a hearing aid. *Ear and Hearing, 7*(4), 257–265.

Byrne, D., & Murray, N. (1985). Relationships of HTL's, MCL's, LDL's and psychoacoustic tuning curves to the optimal frequency response characteristics of hearing aids. *The Australian Journal of Audiology, 7*(1), 7–16.

Byrne, D., & Tonisson, W. (1976). Selecting the gain of hearing aids for persons with sensorineural hearing impairments. *Scandinavian Audiology, 5,* 51–59.

Cornelisse, L. E., Seewald, R. C., & Jamieson, D. G. (1995). The input output formula: A theoretical approach to the fitting of personal amplification devices. *Journal of the Acoustical Society of America, 97,* 1854–1864.

Cox, R. M. (1995). Using loudness data for hearing aid selection: The IHAFF approach. *The Hearing Journal, 47*(2), 10, 39–42.

Cox, R. M., Alexander, G. C., Taylor, I. M., & Gray, G. A. (1997). The contour test of loudness perception. *Ear and Hearing, 18,* 388–400.

Davis, H., Hudgins, C. V., Marquis, R. J., Nichols, R. H., Peterson, G. E., Ross, D. A., & Stevens, S. S. (1946). The selection of hearing aids. *Laryngoscope, 56,* 85–115, 135–163.

Dillon, H. (1999). NAL-NL1: A new procedure for fitting non-linear hearing aids. *Hearing Journal, 52*(4), 10–16.

Dillon, H., Flax, M., Ching, T., Keidser, G., & Brewer, S. (2009). The NAL-NL2 Prescription Procedure. *National Acoustic Laboratories, Research & Development Report 2008/2009,* 41–45.

Harris, J. D. (1976). Introduction to hearing aids: Current developments and concepts. In M. Rubin (Ed.), *Hearing aids* (pp. 3–6). Baltimore, MD: University Park Press.

Hellman, R. P., & Meiselman, C. H. (1993). Rate of loudness growth of pure tones in normal and impaired hearing. *Journal of the Acoustical Society of America, 2,* 966–975.

Johnson, E., & Dillon, H. (2011). A comparison for gain in adults from generic hearing aid prescriptive methods: Impacts on predicted loudness, frequency bandwidth, and speech intelligibility. *Journal of the American Academy of Audiology, 22,* 441–459.

Kamm, C., Dirks, D., & Mickey, M. R. (1978). Effect of sensorineural hearing loss on loudness discomfort level and most comfortable loudness judgments. *Journal of Speech and Hearing Research, 21,* 668–681.

Keidser, G., & Dillon, H. (2009). The NAL-NL2 prescription: Background, derivation and how it differs from the NAL-NL1. *Audiology Online Continuing Education Course.*

Keller, F. (1973). *Technische Hilfe bei der Rehabilitation Horgeschadigter.* Schildele Verlag, Neuburgweier.

Killion, M. C., & Fikret-Pasa, S. (1993). The three types of sensorineural hearing loss: Loudness and intelligibility considerations. *Hearing Journal, 46*(11), 31–34.

Kochkin, S. (2003). MarkeTrak VI: On the issue of value: Hearing aid benefit, price, satisfaction, and repurchase rates. *Hearing Review, 10*(2), 12–29.

Kochkin, S., Beck, D. L., Christensen, L. A., Compton-Conley, C., Fligor, B. J., Kricos, P. B., . . . Turner, R. G. (2010). Marketrak VIII: The impact of the hearing healthcare professional on hearing aid user success. *The Hearing Review, 17*(4), 12–34.

Libby, R. (1985). State of the art hearing aid selection procedures. *Hearing Instruments, 36*(1).

Libby, R. (1986). The 1/3–2/3 insertion gain hearing aid selection guide. *Hearing Instruments, 37*(3).

Lipmann, P., Braida, L., & Durlach, N. (1981). Study of multichannel amplitude compression and linear amplification for persons with sensorineural hearing loss. *Journal of the Acoustical Society of America, 69*(2), 524–534.

Lybarger, S. F. (1944). *Method of fitting hearing aids.* United States Patent Application No. 543,278. Filed July 3, 1944.

Lyregaard, P. (1988). POGO and the theory behind. In J. Jensen (Ed.), *Hearing aid fitting: Proceedings of the 13th Danavox Symposium* (pp. 92–94). Copenhagen, Denmark: GN Danavox.

McCandless, G. A. (1995). Hearing aid formulae and their application. In R. E. Sandlin (Ed.), *Handbook of hearing aid amplification. Volume 1: Theoretical and technical considerations* (pp. 221–238). San Diego, CA: Singular.

McCandless G., & Lyregaard, P. (1983). Prescription of gain and output (POGO) for hearing aids. *Hearing Instruments, 34,* 16–21.

Moore, B. C., & Glasberg, B. R. (1983). Suggested formulae for calculating auditory-filter bandwidths and excitation patterns. *Journal of the Acoustical Society of America, 74,* 750.

Mueller, H. G., & Killion, M. C. (1992). An easy method for calculating the Articulation Index. *Hearing Journal, 46*(9), 14–17.

Mueller, H. G. & Picou, E. M. (2010). Survey examines popularity of real-ear probe-microphone measures. *Hearing Journal,63*(5).

Pascoe, D. P. (1978). An approach to hearing aid selection. *Hearing Instruments, 29*(6), 12–16, 36.

Pascoe, D. P. (1988). Clinical measurements of the auditory dynamic range and their relation to formulas for hearing aid gain. In J. Jensen (Ed.), *Hearing aid fitting: Proceedings of the 13th Danavox symposium* (pp. 81–94). Copenhagen, Denmark: GN Danavox.

Resnick, D., & Becker, M. (1963). Hearing aid evaluation: A new approach. *Asha, 5,* 596–699.

Ross, M. (1978). Hearing aid evaluation. In J. Katz (Ed.), *Handbook of clinical audiology* (2nd ed., pp. 524–549). Baltimore, MD: Williams and Wilkins.

Schwartz, D., Lyregaard, P., & Lundh, P. (1988). Hearing aid selection for severe to profound hearing loss. *Hearing Journal, 41,* 13–17.

Scollie, S., Seewald, R., Cornelisse, L., Moodie S., Bagatto, M., Laurnagaray, D., Beaulac, S., & Pumford, J. (2005). The desired sensation level multistage input/output algorithm. *Trends in Amplification, 9*(4), 159–197.

Seewald, R. C. (1994). Fitting children with the DSL method. *Hearing Journal, 47*(9), 10, 48–51.

Seewald, R. C., Ross, M., & Spiro, M. (1985). Selecting amplification characteristics for young hearing impaired children. *Ear and Hearing, 6,* 48–53.

Shore, I., Bilger, R. D., & Hirsch, I. J. (1960). Hearing aid evaluation: Reliability of repeated measurements. *Journal of Speech and Hearing Disorders, 25,* 152–170.

Strom, K. (2006). The HR 2006 Dispenser Survey. *Hearing Review, 13*(6), 16–39.

Watson, N., & Knudsen, V. (1940). Selective amplification in hearing aids. *Journal of the Acoustical Society of America, 11,* 406–419.

West, R., Kennedy, L., & Carr, A. (1937). *The rehabilitation of speech* (p. 9). New York, NY: Harper Brothers.

ENDNOTE

In my practice, I have found that the results of specifying gain based on speech stimuli is that the target recommendations are on the order of 10 to 15 dB lower than the gain found in formulas that assume pure tone inputs. This makes comparing the gain recommendations of the DSL with previous linear formulas difficult, if not impossible due to differences in stimulus type. Therefore, one cannot easily compare the target gain recommendations of Berger, Pascoe, POGO or linear NAL in Figure 13–2 with modern versions that use more sophisticated stimuli. However, technical support at Etymonic Design Inc (Audioscan), makers of the AudioScan hearing aid analyzers, has informed me that pure-tone recommendations for the DSL m[i/o] v. 5.0 are for those interested in more advanced research.

CHAPTER 14

Real Ear Measures

GEORGE FRYE

OUTLINE

WHAT DOES THIS CHAPTER COVER?

The chapter starts off with a set of definitions of terms used in real ear measures. It then covers the reason for doing real ear measures and the basics of the operation. Gain and SPL-based targets are discussed, as well as the importance of the audiogram. General instructions for setting up and performing real ear measures are covered, but many of the details of the button presses and mouse clicks needed for individual instruments are not covered. Those actions are dependent on the manufacturer of the individual real ear test equipment.

The annex lists more detailed explorations of subjects as probe microphones, sound field speaker placement, test signals, spectra, and analysis methods. It ends with a list of manufacturers of real ear test equipment and their Internet site addresses.

Hopefully what is covered is a description of the processes and the foundation of the many different ways in which real ear tests can be made so that some clarity is found.

DEFINITIONS OF TERMS

Terms used in this chapter include:

REAR   Real Ear (RE) aided response-in sound pressure level

REUR   RE unaided response-in sound pressure level

REUG   RE unaided gain-in dB of gain

REAG   RE aided gain-in dB of gain

REIG   RE Insertion gain = REAG minus REUG—the gain you get over and above unaided

RESR   RE saturation response-in sound pressure level

Gain   Gain in dB

SPL   Sound pressure level in dB; not the same as Gain or HL

HL   Hearing threshold level in dB

REDD   Real ear to dial difference

RECD   Real ear to coupler difference

TM   Tympanic membrane, or eardrum

UCL   Uncomfortable listening level in dB HL or dB SPL

FFT   Fast Fourier Transform, a method of spectral analysis

ANSI   American National Standards Institute

RMS   Root Mean Square; the amplitude of the signal; a linear, rather than a dB value

NAL   The National Acoustics Laboratory of Australia

DSL   The desired sensation level program from the University of Western Ontario, Canada

dB   10 times the log to the base 10 of a power ratio; 20 times log base 10 of a linear ratio

BAHA   Bone-anchored hearing aid

Notes

A response (REAR, REUR . . .) typically includes a complete spectrum of sound or set of frequency amplitude points and is plotted in dB of Sound pressure level (dB SPL). Gain (REUG, REAG, REIG) on the other hand, while also in dB, indicates the gains at each of these frequencies, or in other words, output in dB minus input in dB. Insertion gain (REIG) is a derived figure, and as noted above, calculated from two responses or gain graphs. Of course, SPL is related to a fixed sound level (20 micropascals), whereas HL (or HTL) is related to the threshold of hearing for an individual as compared against what is considered to be a normal hearing sensitivity; it is given in dB HL.

It is important to recognize these terms and how they are used. A more complete description is given in the standard ANSI S3.46-1997 (R2007). These terms are often seen used incorrectly; REAR, for instance, has been used when REAG was appropriate. A message is better understood when terminology is used correctly.

The term "Real ear measurements" means a measurement as done on a real ear, not some artificial device. It is done to get a better idea of the acoustic performance of a hearing aid mounted on the "real ear." The accuracy of the measurement depends on the skill and experience of the operator.

The FFT is an efficient form of the Discrete Fourier Transform (DFT).

UNAIDED EAR GAIN (REUG)

The typical unaided adult ear has an internal resonance around 2.7 kHz with an amplitude of about 16 dB, which raises the amplitude of sounds coming to the ear by that amount. Frequencies above the resonance also get picked up, but not by as much. The unaided ear thus exhibits gain in that frequency range. See Figure 14–1.

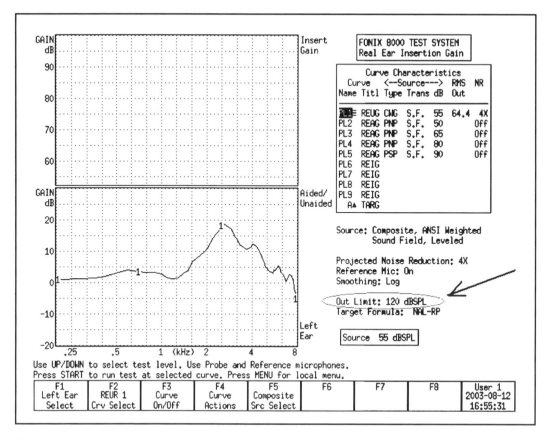

Figure 14–1. Output limit and unaided gain graph (REUG).

INSERTION GAIN (REIG)

The fact of gain in an unaided ear has given meaning to the use of "insertion gain," which is the amount of gain that a hearing aid gives an ear over and above that of the unaided condition. Insertion gain is measured by taking two gain or SPL curves of the aided and unaided conditions, and subtracting the unaided curve from the aided. This test can also be used in other ways. One is in the measure of the gain obtained from a CROS aid; the other is the determination of the amount of gain received by a directional aid.

WHY REAL EAR? IS IT REALLY NECESSARY?

Is real ear really necessary? This question is a valid one. Many hearing professionals do not use the real ear approach when fitting hearing aids. But could the real ear measurement approach allow them to be more confident of their fittings and help their patients hear better?

The world is an interesting place. We humans have inhabited it for many thousands of years. But only in the past few years have we made significant progress in understanding how it works. How has this rapid advance been possible? A simple answer is that we have stopped taking things for granted. We now observe and measure. From these actions, we theorize and make modifications to the way we do things to try to correct problems.

The author has worked as a design engineer for 50 years and has noticed these simple truths:

There is no such thing as magic.

Things may not work as intended. Instead,

They work the way they should, given the circumstances.

It is up to the professional to determine why they work as they do.

Success is rarely achieved on the first try.

Fitting an individual with a hearing aid is basically a design job. Each hearing loss is an individual case. Each requires a somewhat different approach. The proper fitting of a hearing correction must be thought of as a design job. Complicating this picture is that the hearing aid may not behave as intended. It is up to the hearing professional to learn what is happening and make changes if necessary. The real ear measure is a fairly efficient way to determine hearing aid operation on an individual.

Performing real ear measurements is like shining a light into a dark place to see what is there. Is it absolutely necessary? No, but in the dark, it is easier to stumble.

HOW LONG SHOULD A REAL EAR MEASURE TAKE?

Assuming that the professional has thought out the process and performed a few measures, the real ear analysis should take no more than 5 to 10 minutes on a single ear. Of course,

practice makes perfect, and a real ear measure is no exception to this rule. Time may stretch out if significant problems are found that are not easily solved. In a case like this, the real ear measure may be a significant time saver because it can show up unforeseen problems.

THE BASIC REAL EAR MEASURE

How is the real ear measurement accomplished? In abbreviated terms, a sound known in amplitude and spectra is presented to the person wearing the hearing aid to be tested. The sound coming to the patient is usually picked up and analyzed by use of a reference microphone located near the tested ear, and the sound from the hearing aid picked up by the use of a small thin silicone rubber probe tube placed within the ear and which is terminated in a second externally located microphone. The analyzer compares the incoming to the amplified sounds and displays the results on a screen.

Questions as to whether the aid is acting in an appropriate manner are answered by reference to targets that are placed on the screen along with the measurement graphs. The targets are guidance graphs generated by a special program and derived from the patient's audiogram, the sound levels presented to the ear and the spectrum of the test signal. Target generation is discussed later in the chapter.

An office is the typical location for a real ear measurement; it is also a location that is typical of the environment in which the patient may normally find himself.

OUTPUT LIMITING

To prevent overamplifying the aided patient while making hearing aid programming adjustments, most analyzer manufacturers provide a way to stop a test if the sound at the TM gets too loud. The sound level loudness is monitored by the probe microphone. When it goes beyond a preset level, the test is interrupted and a message is provided.

Each manufacturer, and probably each analyzer design, is a bit different. But the maximum amplitude setting can usually be found in a prominent menu. See Figure 14–1 for one location. It may also be displayed on the screen during a test. Normally, adjustment of the hearing aid output is needed to correct the loudness problem. If the analyzer is set to a level that is deemed incorrect, then use the manufacturer's menu system to set the allowable amplitude to a proper level.

MEASUREMENT METHODS

To complicate things, there are two methods of approaching the real ear measurement: Gain and SPL. The gain method is more straightforward because it reduces the problems created by the spectral differences in broadband test signals and the ways in which these signals are analyzed. The gain approach is used in the NAL formulae. NAL has gone through at least three iterations of gain target formula generation as hearing aids have changed and as NAL has collected more patient data. The present version is labeled NAL/NL2.

Initially, real ear measures were confined to the use of pure or warbled tone signals. With this form of signal, all types of analysis tools will give the same answers if properly calibrated. Those that come to mind are the sound level meter (used with C scale weighting), the Fast Fourier (FFT) analyzer, and the fractional octave band analyzer (usually ⅓ octave). The amplitude of a pure or warble tone should read the same with any one of these tools. Also, when the real ear approach was first introduced, the only hearing amplification device available was the linear circuit, combined with the use of automatic gain control (AGC).

Hearing Aids— Unpredictable Operation

A further problem the professional is faced with today is that modern digital hearing aids often do not use predictable, linear processing. If a pure tone or any steady signal is presented to a modern hearing aid, it thinks of it as noise or feedback and turns the gain down. This fact means that it is not possible to use pure-tone or steady-state amplitude signals in real ear testing. Modulated broadband signals, including speech, must be used.

Gain and Insertion Gain Measures

Starting with gain, concepts may be easier. When people have a history of hearing well much of their life, they become accustomed to sound without a hearing aid. As mentioned above, the unaided ear has a 16 dB resonance at around 2.7 kHz. If you amplify sound with a hearing aid, especially one that uses an earmold that plugs the ear, then the hearing aid has to restore that resonance to sound natural. This fact is where the term insertion gain comes. A first step in the real ear gain measure is to determine the unaided gain or response curve (REUG or REUR). (See Figure 14–1 again.) The next step is to measure the amplified gain or response curve (REAG or REAR) and then subtract the unaided curve. The result is the aid's insertion gain. It is the curve of the gain that the aid gives the patient over and above the unaided condition. See Figure 14–2. In this display, the measured graphs are kept separate from the calculated, insertion gain graph and fitting target.

The insertion gain can also be calculated by using a "normal" unaided gain curve. This approach works if the patient physically has a nearly "normal" ear. The "normal" or "average" ear response is available in most real ear systems. But some people, however, have short ear canals with higher frequency resonances, and some have big canals with lower

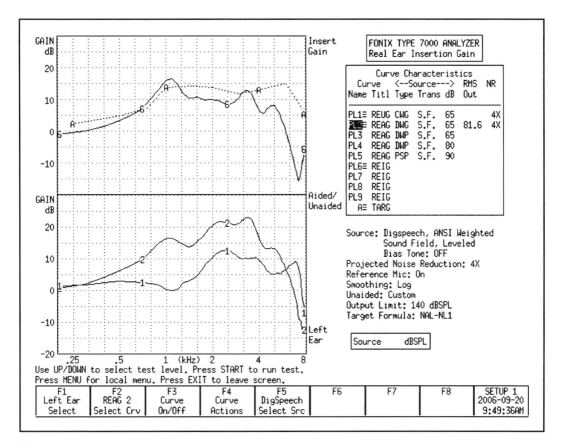

Figure 14–2. Unaided gain, aided gain, and insertion gain.

resonances. Some canals have hard walls with higher amplitude resonances, and so on. If the professional is set up to do real ear measures, it is a relatively quick and simple job to run the unaided gain test (REUG) first.

The generation of gain targets by the NAL and other programs is typically based on the insertion gain principle.

SPL Measures

SPL measures allow the presentation of targets representing the UCL and the HL as well as the amplification curves for different signal levels. As long as the targets are presented correctly, taking into account the spectrum of the test signal and the method of analysis used, there should be no problem getting an accurate result.

It is also possible to measure the unaided SPL curve, as it allows the professional to see just how much output is obtained from the hearing aid over and above the unaided condition.

SPL measures can also be used with targets generated by the NAL system, which is based on gain, rather than SPL, by the use of mathematical conversions, using the spectral and analysis factors mentioned above. The analyzer system may make this conversion.

Targets

Targets are generated by the use of a formula such as one of the NAL programs, or one of the University of Western Ontario's Desired Sensation Level (DSL) programs. The latter are often recommended for the younger hearing impaired population, although the NAL system also accommodates this class of patient. The formulae use the patient's audiogram, obtained in a number of ways. They also modify the target based on:

Signal level

Signal spectra

Audiogram method

Bone audiogram values

Patient age

One or both ears amplified

Unaided ear gain

Real ear measurement setup

Hearing aid internal structure, including compression channels and knee-points.

Some of the formulae are set as delivered (default setting) to accommodate the average hearing loss, but can be changed to reflect special cases. These formulae are usually available on real ear analyzers. For more specific detail on the target formulae, see the chapter in this book devoted to the subject.

Gain Versus SPL

Targets from the NAL formulae are based on gain, because SPL analysis of broadband signals can get complicated by factors such as the analysis method and the spectrum of the signal. When gain is used to determine amplifier frequency band performance, these spectral and analysis SPL differences mathematically cancel out. The use of gain is not ideal, however, when trying to determine if the sound output is too loud or too soft. Determination of SPL is needed to answer these questions.

SPL-Based Targets

The DSL program is based on SPL rather than gain for the reason that it was primarily intended for fitting hearing aids on very

young patients. The hearing of these persons has to be treated as fragile, easily damaged by too much power. They are not able to directly tell us that the sound is just too loud, or that they can't hear it. The DSL program has also been expanded to allow it to also cover a wider range of the hearing impaired population.

SPL-Based Speech Analysis Targets

A popular fitting tool uses the analysis of either real speech or a recorded speech signals. This analysis is generally in the form of the SPL pattern of the averaged amplitudes, maximums and minimums of each frequency band in the speech spectrum. The target for one of these systems is the audiogram itself, converted to SPL. In a real speech SPL display, a term called the speech banana has been used to define the SPL pattern. When amplified speech is analyzed over a period of time, the averaged SPL pattern ideally should lie above the SPL target audiogram, indicating that the amplified speech will be audible to the person wearing this hearing aid. Sometimes an additional figure of merit known as the speech intelligibility index (SSI) is added to the display.

The SSI is generated by use of a formula in the standard ANSI S3.5-1997 (R2007). See Figure 14–3* for a roadmap that describes one manufacturer's display of the amplified speech banana.

SPL analysis is also possible using modulated synthetic signals. If the signal exactly repeats and is locked with the analysis system, often a very fast real ear answer can be obtained as compared with the use of a random noise or speech signal. The spectrum for a random signal is only developed by an averaging process over a period of time, after enough information is collected to form a smooth response.

A number of discussions have taken place as to which type of signal is preferable. One point of view has the person's "significant other" talking to the aided person during the real ear test. If audibility can be shown in this situation, then the aided person has a better chance of being able to understand what is being said.

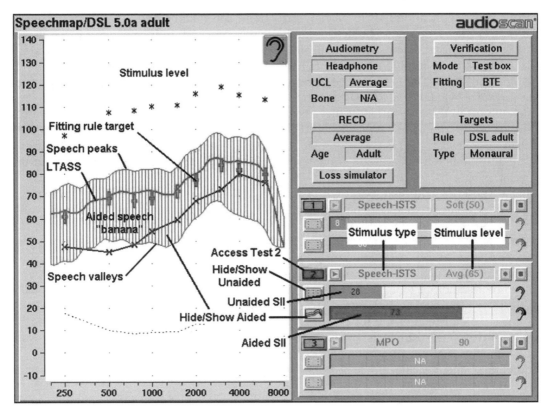

Figure 14–3. Display of SPL analysis of moderate amplitude speech. *Speechmap is a registered trademark of Audioscan. Photo courtesy of Audioscan.

UCL Target

This SPL target is derived (Pascoe, 1988) from either the measured or predicted UCL for an individual. The predicted UCL for each frequency band is based on the audiogram. A favorite set of hearing threshold-based target SPLs are from a study done by Pascoe[1] that was published in 1988.

The Audiogram and the REDD

How good is the audiogram? Some people who question the hearing aid responses supplied by the manufacturer also question the accuracy of the audiogram. Because it is the basis for the development of the fitting target, the audiogram has to be accurate if the target is to mean anything. The audiometer is calibrated by use of a system that assumes that everyone's ear mechanics are "normal";

individual physical variations are not taken into account. The resultant audiogram thus can contain errors that can be as much as 5 to 10 dB. Fortunately, most adults have ears that come close to fitting a normal profile, and the audiogram can be used as taken.

But the audiogram can be questioned when testing very young members of the population. Normal earphones and insert receivers are not designed to fit small heads and ears. A special measurement to determine the real ear to dial difference (REDD) may thus be in order. The REDD is typically written out in the form of a frequency table that maps the differences between the audiometer's dial reading and the actual sound pressure at the tympanic membrane. To determine the REDD, a test tone is presented to the ear at a moderate sound level, such as 70 dB HL, and a probe tube microphone is used to measure the actual SPL. This measure can be done with audiometric head worn transducers or with sound field. Once the REDD table is established, then the professional can be more confident of the obtained hearing threshold. The NAL or DSL formulae also are able to take the REDD audiogram into account in the generation of the target. Pure or warble tones are typically used to obtain the REDD.

Equipment manufacturers often have special programs for the measure of the REDD. The instructions supplied with each individual analyzer need to be followed. Some manufacturers provide audiometric testing as well as the hearing aid analyzer function and allow complete automatic capture of the REDD. These programs can also provide another tool, the RECD, at the same time. The RECD is mentioned later in this chapter. Much of the time, however, the capture of the REDD is a frequency-by-frequency manual operation since the audiometer and hearing aid analyzers are separate instruments.

Setting Up for the Real Ear Measurement

What has to be done to set up an office for real ear testing? Hopefully the suggestions listed below will give the reader an idea of how to proceed.

Acoustic Environment

What is the ideal acoustic environment for a real ear test? Few professionals have the luxury of an anechoic chamber. And, it could be argued, people who wear hearing aids live in regular rooms and offices, not ideal testing facilities. The testing should, therefore, be done in a similar environment. This argument is not necessarily true, as good data is more important than a pleasant environment, but specialized rooms are sometimes not affordable or available.

Before a real ear measurement is attempted, the area where the fitting is to occur must be prepared. Modern real ear equipment can take care of a variety of acoustic environmental problems, but a place that is relatively free of them is a good place to start. What are acoustic problems? The two biggest are reflections and noise. Things reflect sound. All kinds of things. Keep the test area as free of objects as possible. Sound bounces off of objects and interferes with the measurement. The operator has to be considered as an object, too. Stay clear of the area around the ear when making a measurement.

Keep the measurement in as large a room as possible and avoid hard surfaced walls. A thick rug on the floor helps. Also, if the office is small, hanging rugs or ornamental carpets on the walls can heap deaden sound reflections. Special foam wedges are also available and lend a professional acoustic look (even if they are not perfect sound dead eners). Ceilings can be treated with acoustic tiles. Don't locate the patient too close to a wall.

Quiet Needed

Because it is not possible to obtain a good audiogram in a noisy environment, quiet is also needed for real ear measurements.

Placement of Patient and Sound Field Speaker

Real ear measures are done with one, or sometimes two, sound field speakers. Some professionals like to place a single speaker in front of the seated patient, up to less than a meter away from the test ear. Others use a closer spacing of up to one foot, or about 30 centimeters, and off to one side, aimed at the ear. The speaker can be at the same level as, or slightly elevated above the ear.

Use a smaller sized speaker. A good rule of thumb is the smaller, the better. Large speaker enclosures work better at lower frequencies, but real ear tests are done at frequencies where small enclosures work well. And the speaker itself is a re-reflector of sound.

Figures 14–4 and 14–5 show the responses of real ear tests run from patient/speaker spacing of one meter and 30 cm, respectively. The closer spacing test was also done with

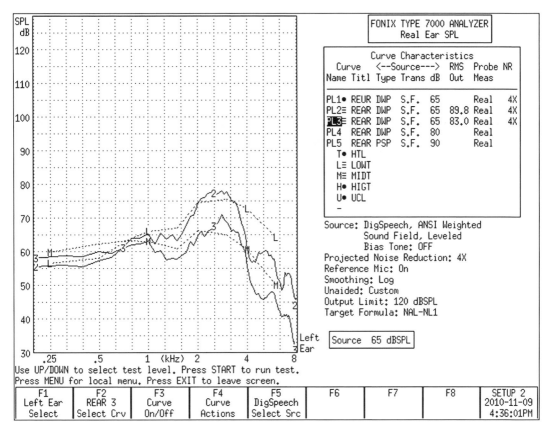

Figure 14–4. Real ear tests using 1 meter spacing, 0 degree azimuth speaker with ANSI and ICRA spectra.

the speaker directed at the test ear instead of directly in front of the patient. Two spectra were used in each of the tests. The upper and lower curves were done with ANSI and ICRA weighting, respectively, at amplitude of 65 dB SPL. (These spectra are defined in the annex at the end of the chapter. See the section labeled Test signals and spectra.) The test results from the two speaker positions are similar, with the closer spacing looking a bit cleaner. The illustration shows that it is possible to perform repeatable real ear tests in a variety of setups. The NAL target program has inputs for the two speaker locations used. FFT analysis.

Probe and Reference Microphones

Probe systems include both probe and a reference microphones for each ear. The probe is used to measure the sound close to the TM of the ear. The reference is often used to monitor and sometimes control the sound level presented to the test ear. It is placed near the ear, but not in the immediate vicinity of the outer ear canal. A popular location is immediately below the ear. Another location is directly above the ear.

Computer and/or Real Ear Instruments

The equipment required to perform the real ear measurement varies from one manufacturer to the other. The simplest at the moment requires only a USB connection to the computer on which the test program is loaded. In this system, a self-powered speaker is driven from a connector located in the small USB module that looks a lot like a computer

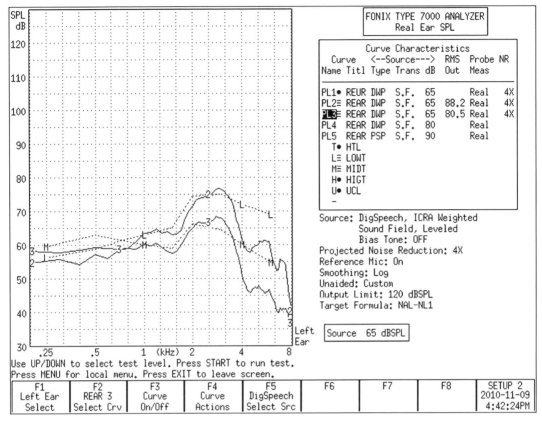

Figure 14–5. Real ear tests using 30 cm spacing, 45 degree azimuth speaker with ANSI and ICRA spectra.

"thumb drive." The more complicated units provide a separate module to which the speaker and probes are connected. A computer may or may not be used with this system. A listing of manufacturers of real ear equipment is given in the chapter annex.

General Arrangement—Wires and Cables

Try to set up the equipment to avoid, as much as possible, entanglement with the wires that connect the speaker and probe microphones with the electronics. Some equipment manufacturers have external modules to bring the real ear electronics closer to the patient and thus to reduce the wiring problem. Another uses a wireless approach to the probe microphone system, which can help reduce the clutter. Of course, this introduces the problem of supplying power to the remote devices.

Performing a Real Ear Measurement

1. **Select the test method.** Select the measurement method and signal, as discussed above, or as outlined in the specification/instruction manual of the equipment manufacturer. Import the audiogram and establish the amplification target curves.

2. **Calibrate the probe system.** Some systems require calibration of the probe system as the first step. This is best done before the patient is readied for testing. Calibration typically consists of placing the tip of the probe next to the

sound inlet of the reference microphone and then holding this assembly in front of and moderately close to the sound field speaker. The calibration system, when activated, will present a signal to the microphone pair and record the differences between the two, using the response of the reference as the comparison standard (Figure 14–6).

Some systems do not require calibration, but this test can still be performed as a check.

3. **Seat the patient.** Assuming that the patient has already been examined physically and audiometrically, and that an appropriate hearing aid has been selected and prepared for compensating the hearing loss, the real ear test can then be performed. Remember cerumen; it can easily plug the probe microphone tube.

Before placing the hearing aid(s) on the patient, seat him or her comfortably with the sound field speaker in position.

4. **Insert the probe.** Always use a new probe tube for each patient. Place and insert the probe(s) into the ear(s). Look in the Annex for hints on various ways in which the probe can be inserted and positioned within the ear for best results.

5. **Level the sound field.** Some systems require that the frequency and amplitude response of the acoustic system is leveled before testing is done. The leveling is done at a moderate, not loud, sound intensity. This function should be done before hearing aids are fit to the patient.

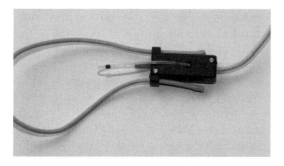

Figure 14–6. Setup of probe microphone set for calibration. Photo courtesy of Audioscan.

Systems that require calibration may not require leveling.

6. **Run an unaided response (REUG, REUR).** With the probe in place, run an unaided response, noting the curve and equipment operation.

7. **Place the hearing aid on the ear to be tested.** Fit the hearing aid on the ear, keeping the probe properly positioned. While fitting the hearing aid, make sure that the probe and reference microphones remain in position.

8. **Run a moderate level aided response (REAR, REAG).** Run a response at a moderate sound level, such as 65 dB SPL. Sound at this level should be satisfactorily amplified, and the gain or SPL response curve should match the target. Look for sharp peaks in the response curve and correct them if possible by making adjustments to the acoustic system and hearing aid programming. Large peaks in the response can be an indication of an impending or even active oscillation.

9. **Run a low level response test.** If satisfied with performance at the moderate sound level, then lower the test signal level to 50 or 55 dB SPL and run a low level test. Again, the target for low amplitudes should be reached. If environmental noise is present, it may be more difficult to make tests at this level.

10. **Check that the UCL target is not exceeded (RESR).** If possible, switch the test signal to a series of short pure-tone impulses and run a quick SPL response test to insure that the UCL target is not exceeded. The hearing aid's response to these quick tone presentations allow UCL testing, but with the patient subjected to as little discomfort as possible.

11. **Document the results of the real ear fitting.** As a last step, record the results of the tests just run. If problems arise in the future, this record may prove to be valuable. It may also be advantageous to run a test using a sound chamber and coupler. This test allows future verification of the hearing instrument without the patient being needed as a part of the process.

RECD

The real ear to coupler difference is a useful tool for the verification of amplification properties of hearing aids before they are placed on the patient's ear. The RECD is especially useful for children, especially those with short attention spans.

Measurement of the RECD

Test equipment manufacturers often have developed programs for the measurement of the RECD. In general, however, the procedure goes as follows:

1. Using a transducer device, such an insert earphone coupled with the hearing aid analyzer, present a signal to the test ear. The signal can be a set of pure tones or a broadband signal. If an insert earphone is used with a foam seal, the seal may be punctured with a device like a knitting needle, then threading the probe through the hole (Figure 14–7).
2. Record the frequency response sound levels in the ear with the use of the probe microphone.
3. Repeat the step 1, but this time use a 2cc coupler using the same drive signals as

was used in step 1. With some analyzers, the microphone may be the one normally used with coupler measurements.
4. Develop the RECD table, listing the differences in dB between the two environments as a function of frequency.

The 2cc coupler response of the insert transducer may already exist as a table in the manufacturer's analyzer. If this is the case, then step 3 of the above procedure is not necessary.

A number of analyzer manufacturers have hearing aid fitting procedures, complete with target curves, using the RECD with the analyzer's test chamber and 2cc coupler. The analysis and performance verification of the hearing aid in this way is done off-patient.

As a final precautionary step, the real ear verification with probe microphone and sound field speaker can then be done on the patient.

Real ear and RECD coupler test data should be stored in the patient's file for future reference.

TESTING CROS AND BICROS AIDS

Some people have one "bad" ear. They typically have a problem hearing sounds directed to their "bad" ear because of the head baffle (shadow) effect. The principle purpose of the CROS aid is to allow the wearer to hear those sounds better by placing a microphone on the bad ear and routing its signal to an amplifier located on the good ear. In the best of worlds, a limited amount of gain is required. If the good ear has a hearing impairment, then more gain from a BICROS may be required.

The question of how much gain is required to overcome the head shadow effect is nicely answered with real ear analysis. In the setup for this analysis, the reference and probe microphones must be placed on opposite ears. The probe is inserted into the aided, good ear, and the reference microphone is placed close to the bad ear. Sound is directed

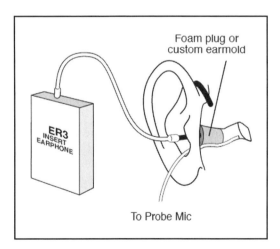

Figure 14–7. RECD setup.

to and equalized at the bad ear. The amplified sound is presented by the CROS amplifier to the good ear and analyzed there.

If the patient physically has a "normal" ear, the normal unaided response can be used as a gain comparison. Using the analyzer's insertion gain mode, level the system with the sound directed directly at the dead ear and away from the good ear. Select the use of a normal unaided response for the analyzer. Then place the CROS aid system on the ears and run an insertion gain response. If the good ear has close to normal hearing, adjustment of the amplification to give a flat insertion gain curve should satisfy the patient's needs for contralateral amplification.

If the patient has a hearing loss, then the BICROS form is needed, and an audiogram related fitting target should be established. Use of a speaker location directly in front of the patient may be a better approach in this case, using the test procedure for a normal target. The reference microphone would still be located next to the dead ear. For an insertion gain approach, measure the unaided response (aid off of the ear) first and then the aided response, the analyzer doing the math to build the insertion gain curve, which is then used to match the target.

Unfortunately, most real ear systems locate the two microphones in a single package that cannot be broken apart and separated. Some manufacturers, however, build dual probe microphone sets that allow signal routing for the correct CROS microphone configuration. Both probe systems are placed on the ears and then the systems allow the reference microphone from one set and the probe microphone of the other set to be used at the same time for the CROS measurement. Follow the manufacturer's instructions for CROS aid analysis.

THE OCCLUSION EFFECT

This effect may be called the hearing aid sales killer. Especially for a patient with a substantial hearing loss, the sound of one's own voice

changes substantially when the aided ear is plugged with an occluding earmold. The problem arises from the patient's own voice vibrating the soft tissue in the outer part of the ear canal. With the ear normally open, this sound disperses to the outside. Plugging the ear traps it inside so that it is heard. "My voice sounds like I'm in a barrel."

Fitting an aid with a substantial vent allows the sound to escape, reducing the occlusion effect. How much? That question can be answered with a simple real ear test. The patient is his own sound generator in this test. Before aiding the ear, place the probe tube in the ear canal to be aided. Set the test for unaided gain in insertion gain mode. Choose a wideband gain measurement mode. With the sound turned off, have the patient say the vowel sound "eee" continuously and measure the spectrum and amplitude of the sound in the unaided ear.

Now set the system to measure aided gain. Place the aid on the ear and repeat the test, leaving the aid and the sound turned off. The resultant insertion gain curve will indicate the increase in the sound in the ear canal caused by the occlusion effect.

Sometimes a change in the phase of the amplified sound can nullify the occlusion effect. This may be tried with the aid turned on. It can be easily seen if the amplified sound adds to the unaided occlusion effect. Flipping the amplified phase by reversing the receiver drive may help to lower the occlusion effect.

People find open-fit aids are easier to adapt to because the occlusion effect is smaller. The sound produced by one's own voice leaks out through the almost open canal.

Sometimes it is impossible to reduce the occlusion effect in a patient with a severe hearing loss. In a case like this, the patient will have to have patience and wear the aid for an extended period of time. Eventually the patient will accept the amplified sound as normal, but it will take a period of several weeks, wearing the aid constantly. The brain will take time to adjust, but it will. If the effect can be minimized "up front," it makes the unaided/aided transition a lot easier.

BODY WORN AIDS

Testing body worn aids is complicated somewhat by the off of the ear location of the body worn microphone. The basic setup, however, for real ear testing is still valid. One exception may be to make the elevation of the sound field speaker a bit lower, so that the body worn microphone is addressed at about the same amount as the ear mounted reference microphone; an elevation of somewhere between the ear and the position of the body aid, maintaining a distance of one foot or so from the patient, is suggested. The reference and probe microphones are still used and positioned as for a normal real ear test. Some manufacturers make special provisions in the gain and SPL targets for body aids.

BAHA AIDS

Bone-conduction aids are not good real ear test candidates. The basic problem is that the output of the anchored bone vibrator is not a sound wave that can be detected by an air conduction microphone. The sound going to the ear can be detected by the reference microphone, but the sound from the vibrator goes into the skull, bypassing the air conduction path.

Testing of the BAHA has to be done with the use of an artificial mastoid, but even here, manufacturers of hearing aid analyzers have not supplied a relatively inexpensive mastoid device for this class of hearing aid. An obvious problem is that use of an artificial mastoid is more equivalent to a sound box/coupler test, anyway. Perhaps this lack of verification equipment will be overcome in the future.

ANNEX

Probe Microphones

While there are a number of variations in the equipment supplied by the different manufacturers to make real ear measures, a few items have become standardized. With few exceptions, the 3-inch long, 1-mm diameter silicone rubber probe tube is used. This tube is typically terminated at an external electret condenser microphone. The microphone housing is usually hung from and located under the tested ear with an adjustment system provided to allow ear size variations. Again see Figure 14–6. Another system uses a different type of ear hanger and positions the reference microphone over the ear and the probe under the ear, with a height adjuster (Figure 14–8).

Small diameter tubes increasingly attenuate sound as a function of increasing frequency. Sound waves also bounce back and forth in the tube. The response of a probe tube microphone is thus not flat and needs to be corrected for use in a measuring instru-

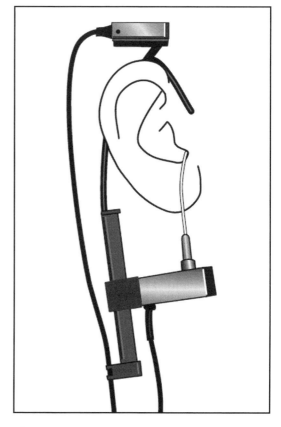

Figure 14–8. Probe microphone set with reference microphone. Located above test ear.

ment. Most systems require a calibration of the microphone set prior to a measurement. This procedure is described above in step 2 of the section "Performing a Real Ear Measurement." Other systems use an acoustic damping system and an equalizer that is built into the probe electronics, so that the calibration step is unnecessary.

Insertion of the Probe Tube Microphone

To get a good idea of the patient's real ear sound level, the input end of the probe tube needs to be located close to the TM. The operator should avoid locating the probe tube inlet too close to the output sound port of the hearing aid because the actual sound intensity presented to the TM may then be substantially less than indicated. How to go about locating the probe tube end in the proper position? Three methods are described below:

1. **The Earmold Method.** If the hearing aid uses an earmold, it can be used as a guide for setting the position of the probe tube. Lay down the earmold next to the tube, making the tube extend about 5 to 7 mm beyond its end. Mark the tube with some means where it passes the outside surface of the earmold. Probe tubes are supplied with sliding markers or a marking pen for this purpose. Moderately sized vents can be used as probe tube channels. Most earmolds are not fit tightly into the ear. There is usually, therefore, little problem in passing the probe tube past the earmold in the ear. There are, of course, exceptions. In a worst case, a 1-mm diameter hole for the probe tube can be drilled in the earmold, whose hole can then be plugged after testing is complete (Figure 14–9).
2. **The 6–7 kHz Dropout Method.** Another method of locating the end of the tube close to the TM is to apply a broadband test signal while sliding the probe into the open ear until a 6 to 7 kHz notch appears in the frequency response. Then slide the tube into the ear enough to reduce the size of the notch. Mark the tube at the point

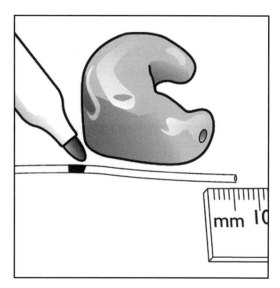

Figure 14–9. Marking the probe tube.

where it passes the ear's tragal notch, so that it can be repositioned again if needed.
3. **The "Ouch" Method.** There is another method that is used by some professionals. Slide the tube into the ear until the patient says "ouch!" and then pull it back out 2 to 3 mm. The "ouch" is an indication that the TM has been touched. It is pretty sensitive. Care must be taken in this approach so that the patient's comfort is not compromised.

Use the ear's tragal notch as a gage for insertion of the probe tube. When the tube has been positioned, it can be held in position by the application of a small length of surgical tape on the ear lobe.

Caution Note

Always use a new probe tube for each patient. Do not be in the position of being accused of providing the accidental transmission of some form of disease.

Cerumen

Probes are easily clogged with earwax. Waxy ears cannot be tested until they are cleared of cerumen. Use of an otoscope is advised before real ear testing or hearing aid fitting to avoid cerumen problems. If a tube is clogged with cerumen, it is very difficult to clean and/or use.

A Tip on Probe Insertion

Sometimes hair in the ear can make it difficult to insert the highly flexible, small diameter probe tube. However, tubes can be inserted easily into most ears by spinning the tube with the two fingers holding it as it is guided into the ear.

The Reference Microphone

Some manufacturers use this microphone to control the level and frequency response of the signal being used for the real ear analysis. Others use it to set the amplitude and response of the signal in an initial step and then as a monitor to determine the gain of the amplification system or as a way to ascertain the amplitude of the incoming signal.

For some systems, this microphone provides a standard response against which the probe microphone is compared in an initial calibration step. This step is not required in some other systems. But all systems can be checked by holding the tip of the probe microphone close to the opening of the reference microphone and running a gain response. A smooth flat line with close to a zero gain should be seen.

Open-Fit Hearing Aids

The reference and the probe microphones form a pair in most real ear measurements. With the open-fit aid, however, it is advisable to do what is necessary to calibrate the system as a preliminary step, including the equalization of the sound field. Then use the analyzer menu tools to remove the influence of the reference microphone from the measurement. The reason is that the open-fit hearing aid injects a good deal of amplification signal into the external environment, which signal can be picked up by the reference microphone and cause a measurement error. Disabling the reference microphone in the measurement system makes it necessary to more closely control the physical positions of the people and equipment in the measurement's acoustic environment.

Patient/Sound Field Speaker Placement

The traditional location of the patient with respect to a sound field speaker has been directly in front of the speaker (0 degrees azimuth) and one meter distant. This position was established years ago for sound field audiometry. It is significant that the traditional signal then used was either narrow band noise or warble tone. The reason that pure tone was not used was that because of acoustic reflections in the environment, the signal amplitude with pure tones was not dependable at that distance. This setup was also carried over and used for real ear testing.

The author examined some of the early real ear test results and wondered if some of the resulting curves were the result of the response of the hearing aid or of other factors in the environment. A series of tests were then carried out which determined that a cleaner response could be obtained if the distance between speaker and patient were reduced to ⅓ meter, and if the speaker were moved around to more directly point at the ear being tested. In 1987, Killion and Revit verified and improved upon this setup, suggesting an azimuth of 45 degrees, a close speaker spacing and a slight elevation of the speaker with respect to the test ear. With these changes, either pure tones or broadband composite signals could be used successfully. The closer spacing has the disadvantage that the absolute SPL of the drive signal is more sensitive to speaker distance changes. On the other hand, the reduction of response errors from acoustic reflections made the sensitivity increase worth it. The author notes that several manufacturers now suggest a somewhat closer spacing than one meter.

The placement of the reference microphone is also a factor in setting the speaker azimuth angle. This device is used by many systems to control the sound source. And it is typically hung from the ear, thus positioned a short distance from the patient's neck. With the reference microphone in this position, a side speaker position will cause a high frequency signal dropout. The speaker should, therefore, be located directly in front of the patient.

To use a side speaker location, place the reference microphone over the ear, which is close to the acoustic center of the head. Keeping the microphone next the head's surface reduces the artifact mentioned in the above paragraph.

Positioning the speaker directly in front of the patient has obvious advantages for those who wish to use systems with probe microphones placed in both ears because it is not necessary to reposition the speaker when switching the test ear. On the other hand, it is possible to get the benefits of the side speaker location by having the patient rotate his head to the side being tested, "listening to the speaker." Mounting the speaker on a wall bracket with a swing arm can also be helpful.

Test Signals and Spectra

Random Noise Versus Deterministic Signals

Signals fall into these two different categories. The spectra of random noise signals are only predictable in the long term; taking a look at the spectral characteristics of such a signal by only looking at a short period of time yields unpredictable results. An example of a noise signal is the sound generated by an FM radio tuned between stations. Speech can also be classified as a noise signal because it is constantly and almost randomly varying in amplitude and frequency content.

A deterministic signal, on the other hand, is constant and stable with a defined repetition period, each of which contains the complete spectral signature. If this kind of signal is synchronized to the analysis system, a very quick analysis of spectrum of the amplified output of a device can be obtained. A pure tone is an example of a deterministic signal. Another example is the broadband composite signal used by some manufacturers, which consists of a number of pure tones added together.

Signals and Hearing Aid Operation

A number of different signals have been used for real ear analysis. It has been argued that real speech signals are the best, because that is what the hearing aids are meant to amplify. And the modern digital algorithms used in hearing aids sometimes make it difficult to use conventional test methods and deterministic signals.

Although warbled pure tones were originally used, the deterministic broadband composite signal was used in some early real ear tests. A mathematical device called a FFT was used to extract the frequency amplitude information, with the result available in a fraction of a second. The advantage was that the real ear test could then be made interactively, with changes made to the hearing aid program resulting in the immediate observation of changes to its spectral output. These deterministic signals were steady state, and remained constant while the test was running.

However, as digital versions of hearing aids were introduced, one of the first attempts to program the aid to reduce the effects of noise in the environment was to look at the amplified frequency bands. If one or more of the bands were steady state, then the signal in that band was obviously noise, and the gain was reduced. Thus, it became more difficult to test this hearing aid, either in a sound box or on the real ear.

One answer was to continue to use the composite signal, but to introduce time modulations, turning the signal on and off at intervals that approximated speech. Most of the new hearing aid circuits were happy with this compromise. One term for this modulation was "digital speech."

As time went on, more and more "interesting" hearing aid algorithms were introduced, making the testing of these products also more "interesting." Fortunately, most of these products can still be tested with synthetic signals by the introduction of more interesting forms of "digital speech."

It is still true that actual speech is a signal that hearing aids are designed to amplify, and it is argued, therefore, that speech is the ideal test signal. However, using speech as a test signal does take some time, as a clean response is only obtained after waiting for an average to build up. Synthetic forms of repeating signals, on the other hand, can be analyzed quickly, and interactive adjustments can be made to hearing aids by way of the hearing aid's programming systems, allowing a quick resolution to a problem response.

When all is said and done, speech is the gold standard for hearing aid testing. If a person can't understand his spouse's sweet voice, then the aid is not doing its job.

Spectra

As mentioned above, there is an almost infinite variety of spectral shapes that can be used in broadband test signals. A few have been recognized as standard. All of these can be generated in either noise or deterministic formats. A listing:

    Flat

    Pink

    ANSI

    ICRA

    LTASS

White

This signal has a flat spectrum when analyzed by an FFT system.

Pink

The pink spectrum falls at the rate of 3 dB per octave as frequency rises when analyzed by a

FFT system. So why use that? When analyzed by a fractional octave band analyzer, such as a ⅓-octave bandwidth analyzer, the pink spectrum appears to be constant versus frequency. The ear behaves a lot like a fractional octave bandwidth filter system.

ANSI

The ANSI spectrum is defined in the ANSI standard S3.42–1992 (R2007) and is moderately flat to 900 Hz, where it is down 3 dB, then falls at a rate approaching 6 dB per octave as the frequency increases (FFT analysis). It was once used for the testing of hearing aids in the Veterans Administration program. It represents a spectral compromise; speech has a faster falloff in high frequencies than the ANSI, but has high frequency dynamics that do not follow this faster falloff.

ICRA

This is a signal spectrum generated by the International Collegium of Rehabilitative Audiology and has been made available by Widex (1996). In its original form, it has a relatively constant amplitude to the frequency of 500 Hz, and then falls at the rate of 9 dB per octave above that (FFT analysis). It represents a somewhat different compromise to the generation of a standardized speech test signal. It has been available as a noise and also as a speech-like signal generated using modified speech segments. Later versions contain several different spectra variations corresponding to raised voice, loud voice, female talker, and others.

LTASS

The long-term average speech spectrum, as mentioned above. Two references to this spectrum are the Cox and Moore study published in 1988, and the international effort led by the National Acoustics Laboratory of Australia and published by Byrne et al. (1994). That study employed the efforts of at least 17 well-known auditory researchers around the world to collect male and female speech samples of 12 languages with digital recorders. The formats in both studies are presented in ⅓-octave analysis spectra. Both spectra are very similar to each other.

Test Signal Equalization

The acoustic signals for real ear testing are provided by sound field speakers. The frequency response and sensitivity of these devices are not exactly predictable. A speaker may sound "great," but that is not sufficient for audiometric or hearing aid testing. Every individual speaker system adds its own coloration to the sound. One of the jobs of the analysis system is to remove the effects of this coloration by modifying the test signal, so that its amplitude and spectrum is correct at the physical point where the test takes place.

One Frequency at a Time

For analysis systems that use pure tones, the coloration adjustment has been done either by the use of a controlling monitor (reference) microphone or the preadjustment of the signal level before the measurement is attempted. The preadjustment technique can also be used for the construction of the deterministic composite signals described above. The level of each frequency in the composite is corrected in amplitude, and then the corrected composite is used in the test.

Spectral Modification of Stored Random Signals

Unfortunately, preadjustment doesn't work when a signal has a random nature, like a noise or a speech signal. Sometimes, if a "random" signal has been digitally recorded, and its image stored, the corrections necessary to correct the response of the system can be built into a modified form of the prerecorded "random" signal before it is used. Then when the corrected version of the signal is used, the amplitude and spectrum can be made to be correct at the test point.

Real-Time Spectral Equalization

Another method is to apply real-time equalization filters to the test signal on its way to the output amplifier. Thus any desired signal, random or deterministic, can be used for testing. No matter what is sent to the analysis sound system, it arrives at the test point the way the operator intended. Real-time equalization has been done in various different ways for a number of years.

Broadband Analysis Methods

The Sound Level Meter

First, there is the sound level meter. In basic form, it consists of a calibrated microphone/amplifier followed by an RMS detector circuit. It typically has a broadband response and reads out the RMS SPL of the signal it is measuring. All frequencies are equally included in the measurement. To use one for hearing aid analysis with a pure tone, set the level of input with the sound level meter, and then with the hearing aid in place and turned on, make a measurement of the hearing aid output using a microphone coupler. Use "c" or flat spectral weighting if possible. Very straightforward, although it is a little hard to make a real ear measurement with one. Also, pure tones are not amplified well by modern hearing aids.

The FFT Audio Analyzer

This device uses a calibrated microphone with analog to digital converter that creates a set of digital samples of the amplitudes of a signal as a series of points in time. The output is thus a set of numbers that represent the amplitudes of the collected samples. The samples set is then routed to a mathematical FFT algorithm, which calculates the signal's frequency content. The lowest, or base, frequency analyzed is equal to the inverse of the sample set's period. The highest frequency passed to the system and analyzed must be lower than one half of the sampling rate. The FFT calculation is usually based on a set of samples, the number of which is a power of 2. In other words, the set has to have 16, 32, 64, 128, 256 or . . . samples. It is an efficient way of doing a Discrete Fourier Transform (DFT), which can be done on a set containing any number of samples. Analyzed frequencies may consist of integer multiples of the lowest possible analyzed frequency.

As mentioned above, the FFT frequency analysis yields a flat amplitude response to a signal with a white noise spectrum. The FFT analysis of pink noise yields a downward slope of 3 dB per octave with increasing frequency.

Fractional Octave Band Audio Analyzer

Like FFT analyzers, fractional octave band audio analyzers use calibrated microphones for sound pick up. They include the ⅓ octave band analyzers used extensively in analysis of speech sounds for hearing. This device displays information on the frequency content of signals in bands, the widths of which are proportional to the frequency analyzed. Originally, these analyzers used analog inductance/capacitance/resistance elements in the filtering process. The operation of this class of filter system is covered in the standard ANSI/ASA S1.11–2004 (R2009).

As mentioned above, the fractional octave band analyzer will show white noise to be increasing in amplitude at the rate of 3 dB per octave for increasing frequency. Pink noise has been used to provide a flat spectral output for this type of analyzer. Fractional octave filters are used for acoustic analysis because they are more closely related to human hearing function than the FFT.

Several techniques have evolved to implement fractional octave band filters, even including the use of the FFT sampling and analysis process listed above. Thus it is possible to use a system that can switch back and forth between FFT and fractional octave band analysis by the use of mathematical operations.

Dual Probe Systems

Some real ear analyzers provide two probe/reference microphone sets. The analyzers are equipped with selection systems to allow the operator to select the ear to be tested. Typically, only one ear is tested at a time. An exception to this rule is the CROS test, where for some analyzers the probe microphone of one set is used on the good ear, and the reference microphone of the other set is used on the opposite ear. Actually, only one ear is again tested, but both microphone sets are used. On some analyzers, the two microphones of a single set can be separated for use in the CROS test.

The sound field speaker in a dual probe system may, for convenience, be located centrally to equally address the two ears, or may be moved from one side to the other to address the ear being tested.

Directional Hearing Aids

Is a hearing aid programmed to be directional? A directional verification test can be done on a real ear system by one of several methods. One method is use the insertion gain approach, where two curves are run, the result being the difference between the two. Make two aided tests, one with the sound field speaker positioned for maximum sensitivity and the other with the speaker positioned behind, or at the programmed system null. The first test would be done using the "unaided" part of the insertion gain program, and the second as the "aided" test. The difference curve, normally labeled as the insertion gain response, shows how much the aid attenuates sound coming from the reverse direction.

This test can be quite useful, as some supposedly directional aids may be operating in an undesirable way. Also, if the aid is a modern one, with automatic switching of the directional function, then it may be wise to program the special automatic features off. Sometimes a directional pattern can be seen using the newer forms of digital speech.

At the time of this writing, most manufacturers do not actually test the directionality characteristics of their products. Instead, they rely on a measure of the sensitivity and phase output difference of the two microphones of the hearing aid when it is placed in a certain position in a test chamber. Unfortunately, at least two factors can make this factory measurement invalid. The first is that the two microphones may be wired in backwards. The second is that the outputs of the two microphones may be shorted together. There may be others. Tests on actual products have shown that "directional" aids may actually be more sensitive to sound from behind the patient, or that the hearing aid is not directional at all. Sometimes aids that have been in service for a period of time can lose their directional programming. Verification can be useful.

Manufacturers of Real Ear Equipment

This listing of manufacturers was taken by internet search. Manufacturers are listed alphabetically and are included with internet addresses.

AudioScan (http://www.audioscan.com)

Frye Electronics (http://www.frye.com)

Interacoustics (http://www.interacoustics -us.com)

MedRx (http://www.medrx-usa.com)

Otometrics (http://www.otometrics.com)

Real Ear Systems (http://www.audit data.com/fitting-systems/primus/ real-ear-measurement/)

REFERENCES

Byrne, D., Dillon, H., Tran, K., Arlinger, S., Wilbraham, K., Cox, R., . . . & Ludvigsen, C. (1994). An international comparison of long-term average speech spectra. *Journal of the Acoustical Society of America, 96,* 2108.

Cox, R. M., & Moore, J. N. (1988). Composite speech spectrum for hearing aid gain prescriptions. *Journal of Speech and Hearing Research, 31,* 102–107.

Killion, M. C., & Revit, L. J. (1987). Insertion gain repeatability versus loudspeaker location: You want me to put my loudspeaker W H E R E? *Ear and Hearing, 8.5,* 68–73.

Pascoe, D. P. (1988). Clinical measurements of the auditory dynamic range and their relation to formulas for hearing aid again. In J. Jensen (Ed.), *Hearing aid fitting: Theoretical and practical views* (pp. 129–154). Copenhagen: Stougaard.

Widex. (1996). *ICRA speech shaped noise compact disk* (Personal correspondence).

CHAPTER 15

Making Hearing Aid Fitting Decisions

ROBERT L. MARTIN

INTRODUCTION

Audiologists are conducting fewer in-office measurements of hearing aids. Most practitioners rely on the manufacturers' fitting formula to generate an initial "first fit." There are times when the patient rejects the hearing aid. It is difficult to determine if the problem is related to the hearing aid settings, a defective component of the hearing aid, or the patient's expectations.

Many dispensing offices do not utilize in-office measuring equipment. This is unfortunate. In many instances, the patient's complaints can be resolved more efficiently when appropriate measures are done. This chapter discusses the advantages obtained when one employs hearing aid test systems.

Hearing aid test systems measure the acoustical properties of hearing aids in a sound chamber (a test box) and in the real ear. If the test-box is used, a hearing aid is placed in a sound chamber, input signals are presented, and the amplification is evaluated. When tests are done on the real ear, a probe microphone is positioned properly in the ear, input signals are presented, and the sound is evaluated. This current chapter takes a slightly different approach and focuses on the clinical use of test-box and real-ear information in the decision-making process.

The clinician receives information about the patient's hearing aid performance from many different sources: the patient, the family, the initial audiometric evaluation, and so on. This information must be studied and integrated before it is used to solve hearing aid user's problems (Revit, 1997). The focus of the audiologist and hearing aid specialist should be on the whole person, not just the ears, hearing loss, and hearing aids. It is imperative to treat each patient as an individual and to talk to them about their health, life, and the problems they are facing (Byrne, 1996; Staab, 1985; Valla, & Sweetow, 2000).

We need to understand the patient's fears. For example, some patients hate feedback; others are afraid of complex electrical systems. We especially need to understand the patient's dexterity, memory capacity, mechanical aptitude, and special needs. Some patients look forward to the use of remote controls and Bluetooth interconnections. Other patients are terrified by the idea of using these technologies.

The inclusion of electroacoustical measurements, hereafter called "tests," is part of the verification process (Frye, 1998; Hosford-Dunn & Huch, 2000; Kasten, Lotterman, & Revoile, 1967). When we conduct these measurements, we demonstrate our professional interest to the patient. We show the patient we are dedicated to achieving a successful fitting. These tests help confirm adequate amplification and are useful in documenting the proper regulation of output to comfortable levels.

The clinician's goal is to improve the quality of hearing aid fittings. This task is difficult! Hearing aid adjustments and the number of possible hearing aid settings increase exponentially each year. Years ago hearing aids were single channel amplifiers. The goal concerned gain, output, AGC settings, and high- and low-frequency tone controls. Now the practitioner is forced to consider hundreds, perhaps thousands of possible settings.

The era of adjusting a hearing aid with a small screwdriver is ending. We are in the digital era and all aspects of the amplification are controlled by software. Adjustments are made using a computer and a digital interface system called a Hi-Pro box. The manufacturer-specific software used to program the hearing aids needs to be updated several times each year.

The modern hearing aid is a small computer. Most new hearing aids have computer-based algorithms running behind the amplification process. These algorithms: reduce feedback, adjust the amount of amplification when the background noise level is significant, extend the frequency response, and keep track of the amount of time the patient is in various background-noise listening environments (Siemens 2010a, technical reference). Most of these algorithms impact the quality of the test-box measurements (Frye, 2010). The reader is advised to consult the owners' manual and the manufacture regarding the special techniques needed to obtain reliable data.

The hearing aid programming software provides "estimated" performance curves of the amplified sound (Frye, 1998). One might question if we need to do additional tests in a test box or real ear to evaluate the amplified sound. In this author's opinion, as well as that of many professional academies, additional measurements are an absolute necessity. It is common to see huge differences between the "estimated" curves and the curves measured on a hearing aid test system.

Hearing aid measurements must accurately measure both the *quality* and *quantity* of the amplified sound. When an assessment of sound quality is needed, various measures of distortion can be made: harmonic inter modulation and frequency (Frye, 1998). Studies of sound quantity include: gain, bandwidth, input-output tests, and other measurements. Some hearing aid tests, such as real ear target studies, check both quality and quantity issues.

THE DECISION-MAKING PROCESS

Patients wearing new hearing aids return to the office for follow-up visits and report problems that must be resolved quickly to avoid having the hearing aids returned for credit.

To remedy these issues, a substantial amount of information is needed. This includes:

- Audiometric studies. (Referred to below to as "thresholds").
- The patient's description of the problem. (The "Problem").
- The family report.
- Data logged in the hearing aid showing the duration and type of noises encountered.
- Watching the patient adjust the volume controls to verify proper use-gain.
- Test-box and real ear measurements ("Test-box").
- Sound field studies.

Decisions are made by listening carefully to the patient's definition of the problem, then gathering and analyzing pertinent information. The following case studies of fictitious patients are used to illustrate the decision-making process.

Case Study #1

"The hearing aids are too noisy and word understanding is poor when away from home." This case study introduces the decision-making process.

Custom instruments are ordered for the patient following the traditional audiometric evaluation. The patient has a mild-to-moderate, sensorineural hearing loss. Thresholds are the same in both ears, see Table 15–1.

Table 15–1. Judy

Frequency	Threshold	Use-Gain	Background Noise	% of Speech Information
250 Hz	35 dB	+16	High	8%
500 Hz	45 dB	+18	Med High	14%
1000 Hz	50 dB	+20	Medium	22%
2000 Hz	60 dB	+20	Low	33%
4000 Hz	70 dB	+10	Very Low	23%

After wearing the new hearing aids for a week, the patient returns to the office and says, "I cannot stand to wear these hearing aids, they are too noisy. I cannot understand what my husband/wife is saying when we are out . . . and that is the reason I purchased the aids."

This case represents numerous complaints that hard-of-hearing people who have difficulty hearing and understanding words in typical background noise listening situations. They hear a substantial amount of sound, but they don't understand enough words to carry on a comfortable conversation.

The problem is evaluated in two parts: data gathering and data analysis. The data collected includes: thresholds, description of the problem, and use-gain values. These values are compared with typical noise levels and the speech information values.

The first task is to determine how much amplification is active when the hearing aids are adjusted to the most comfortable listening levels. These values (this amount of amplification) are called *use-gain levels.*

After adjusting the volume controls to a comfortable level, we put the hearing aids in a test-box and run a series of tests. We can do standard frequency response measurements, or RECD tests (Real Ear Coupler Difference) that estimate real ear use-gain (Frye & Martin, 2008). We can also obtain this information with sound field tests (Walker, 2000) or with real ear measurements.

Data Analysis

We then compare thresholds and use-gain values to typical background noise levels and speech information values (discussion below). See Table 15–1.

The world is very noisy. Patients are exposed to increasing levels of irritating background noise. But, they are not aware of this noise until they get hearing aids. Unless we exercise high degrees of skill during the hearing aid fitting process, the patient will be unexpectedly and unwillingly thrown back into the natural world of irritating noise when they wear their new hearing aids. The

complaint, "Too much noise" is one of the main reasons hearing aids are returned for credit (Kochkin, 2003).

We can minimize the patient's exposure to background noise by understanding the frequency distribution of typical noise; then cautiously controlling the amount of amplification within these frequencies. Most background noise is low frequency in nature because it is easy to make something vibrate a few hundred of times a second and difficult to make anything vibrate thousands of time per second (Bernstein, 1966).

Active patients spend time at church/synagogue, shopping, at restaurants, and in meetings. In these environments, the human voice is a primary noise source. The spectrum and level of the human voice has been discussed in earlier literature (Martin, 1985). The shape of typical background noise (discussed below) is similar to the spectrum of the human voice. Higher energy is observed in the lower frequencies.

The relative terms "High" and "Low" are used for teaching purposes only. The actual frequency distribution and associated intensity levels will depend on the distance between speaker and listener, gender, amount of effort used during speaking, and many other factors. The terms "High . . . " are approximations used, so the reader can better "see" the factors needed in the decision-making process. This information is used to create hearing conditions that are more comfortable for the patient.

Observe the 16 and 18 decibels of gain at 250 and 500 Hz. This zone of amplification is dominating Judy's hearing from a loudness point of view. The octave bands at 250 and 500 Hz have high natural noise levels in comparison with the octave bands at 2000 and 4000 Hz.

When Judy is not wearing hearing aids, she judges typical background noise as "soft" or "comfortable." With hearing aids adjusted to provide the use-gain values shown in Table 15–1, Judy perceives the background noise sound as "loud and irritating."

The use-gain settings in Table 15–1 were obtained in a quiet listening environment.

When Judy is around background noise, she adjusts the volume of her hearing aids down to the point where she is comfortable. Unfortunately, this reduction eliminates most of the helpful amplification in the higher octave bands. The higher frequencies provide 78% of the speech energy cues needed for word understanding (American National Standards Institute, 1969). We discuss this topic in the next section.

Table 15–2 is an analysis of the gain in the lower frequencies. The patient's unaided hearing is not significantly impaired in this zone. The fitting has substantial amplification and the use-gain versus noise level study suggests "bass overload" (i.e., overamplification in the lower frequencies). We test this conclusion by having the patient listen to an environmental noise recording set to 75 dB. If the patient judges this sound as "noisy or irritating," our conclusion of "bass overload" is confirmed.

In addition, we compare the current hearing aid settings to a similar setting with a 15 dB gain reduction in the lower frequencies. When this comparison is made, Judy reports a strong preference for a reduction in the lower frequencies.

Judy's problem had two parts: the perceived noise level is too high and word understanding is poor. The data comparison in Table 15–2 studied the fitting from the perceived "background noise" point of view. We next consider the "word understanding" part of the problem.

Speech Intelligibility

The term "speech intelligibility" implies the ability to differentiate between words, for example, "shoe" sounds like "shoe," not "blue." Amplified sound can facilitate the patient's ability to hear the difference between similar speech sounds (e.g., "ch" and "sh"). Sounds are clear if they are easily identifiable, intelligible. The enhancement or improvement of this ability is one of the primary goals of most hearing aid fittings (Purdy, 1999a, 1999b).

Perceptual sharpness can be improved by providing quality, clear amplification, free of distortion. Word recognition is usually easy, and background noise does not interfere when the proper amount of amplification is provided in each zone. Ideally word recognition is done with precision and ease. The speech sounds are separated from each other.

Clear hearing means the patient perceives completely and clearly the words the speaker is saying. If a spoken word has five syllables, the listener picks up every syllable precisely and the way the speaker produced them.

The softer higher pitched speech sounds are more important to word understanding than the louder lower pitched speech sounds. The amount of information in speech contained in the octave bands has been studied extensively. A National Standard (1969) exists showing the relative amount of information in each octave band. In the American National Standards Institute standard, these values are presented as weighting factors. The author converted the weighting factors to an easier to understand format (percentages):

8% @ 250 Hz

14% @ 500 Hz

22% @ 1000 Hz

33% @ 2000 Hz

23% @ 4000 Hz

Table 15–3 shows the use-gain, typical noise level, and speech information (intelligibility) values in the higher frequencies for Judy. This side-by-side comparison shows mild (inadequate) amplification in the higher frequencies. Increasing the gain by 10 to 20 dB gives the patient a substantial increase in speech information, and because typical

Table 15–2. Judy: Low Frequency

	250	500 Hz
Threshold	60	70 dB
Use-Gain	+16	+18 dB
Background Noise	High	Med High

Table 15–3. Judy: High Frequency

	2000	4000 Hz
Threshold	60	70 dB
Use-Gain	+20	+10 dB
Background Noise	Low	Very low
Speech Intelligibility	33%	23%

background noise levels are low in this zone, adding substantial gain to the higher frequencies will not markedly increase the patient's exposure to background noise. The patient will be comfortable in most listening situations. The exceptions are cases of high-frequency noises (e.g., children crying, etc.). In these cases, the AGC (Automatic Gain Control) settings need to be carefully selected to reduce the surges in noise.

Case Study #2

This is a complex case that deals with an in-depth use of the data-gathering, data-analysis process.

The patient, Samuel, has a moderate, flat, sensory neural hearing loss shown in Table 15–4. Impressions are made, and hearing aids are ordered. When the hearing aids are received from the manufacturer, they have been preprogrammed for the patient's hearing loss. When Samuel adjusts the instruments to a comfortable level, the use-gain settings shown in Table 15–4 are obtained.

Samuel is being fitted with a flat frequency response: low knee-points (50 dB) and high ratios (2.25 to 1.0) provide considerable compression. The patient is initially happy with the hearing aids when they are worn in the office.

After wearing the hearing aids for a week, the patient expresses frustration: "If I turn the hearing aids up to hear, all the sound drives me crazy. If I turn them down to a comfortable level, I don't hear well at all. They work fine when I watch TV, but I can-

not wear them to Lion's club, church, or out to lunch."

Our initial analysis compares use-gain settings with typical noise levels and speech information values. Once again, it appears that there is substantial amplification in the zones where typical noise levels are elevated and moderate, and limited amplification in the zones where noise levels are much lower.

We modify the frequency response by reducing gain in the low frequencies by about 10 decibels and increasing gain in the highs by about 10 decibels; the modified use-gain settings are shown in Table 15–5.

After wearing the hearing aids for an additional week, Samuel returns saying, "Well, the hearing aids are better, but I don't like the quality of the sound. They sound very artificial; like I am talking into a microphone."

Our next level of *decision making* address the topic of perceived sound quality and specifies ways to improve "quality." We start with the authors' definition of "quality" amplification.

Perfectly clear hearing aid fittings produce a listening condition much like looking through perfectly clean glass, we are not aware the glass is there. If the amplified sound is excellent—perfectly clear—the hard-of-hearing patient is not aware of listening to amplification. The action of the hearing aids become invisible, and the listener is only aware that they are hearing and understanding what has been said precisely and accurately.

Much of what we know about perceived sound quality comes from the music and recording industry (Bernstein, 1966). For years, musicians have emphasized the importance of a flat frequency response, wideband amplification, complete elimination of all types of distortion, and a wide dynamic range driven by powerful amplifiers. Substantial power is needed so the recording faithfully follows the high "peaks" and deep "valleys" inherent in music. These concepts can be summarized as:

■ Perceived flat frequency response
■ Wideband amplification
■ Elimination of all types of distortion.

Table 15–4. Samuel

Frequency	Threshold	Use-Gain	Background Noise	% of Speech Information
250 Hz	50 dB	+22	High	8%
500 Hz	55 dB	+26	Med High	14%
1000 Hz	60 dB	+28	Medium	22%
2000 Hz	60 dB	+22	Low	33%
4000 Hz	60 dB	+16	Very Low	23%

Table 15–5. Samuel: "Lows" Decreased, "Highs" Increased

Frequency	Threshold	Use-Gain	Background Noise	% of Speech Information
250 Hz	50 dB	+12	High	8%
500 Hz	55 dB	+16	Med High	14%
1000 Hz	60 dB	+36	Medium	22%
2000 Hz	60 dB	+30	Low	33%
4000 Hz	60 dB	+12	Very Low	23%

We need to add to this list:

■ Maintaining the ear's natural resonance (on average, a 16 dB peak at 3000 Hz) if the patient's hearing is sufficiently acute, so they are aware of this peak.

Five additional defects in Samuel's fitting need to be discussed: three can be discerned from the data in Table 15–5; a fourth, feedback, is seen in the fitting software and the real ear data; a fifth is found by studying the compression settings.

First defect: Observe the use-gain values at 1000 and 2000 Hz (see Table 15–5). This fitting has more use-gain at 1000 Hz than 2000 Hz. This is a minor issue but problematic in terms of perceived quality. Remember, we are attempting to create perfectly clear hearing. There is more speech information and less noise in the zone near 2000 Hz than 1000 Hz. Patient's with typical "falling" audiograms, usually need more amplification in the 2000 Hz zone.

Second defect: The human ear has a natural resonance, a peak, near 3000 Hz. If the patient's hearing in this zone is sufficiently acute (good enough so they are aware of this natural enhancement), we must reproduce this resonant peak within the amplified sound; otherwise, the patient will report dissatisfaction with the quality of the sound. In the case of Samuel, we "add the peak" by reducing gain near 1000 Hz and increasing gain near 3000 Hz.

Third defect: Observe the 12 decibels of use-gain in the 4000 Hz zone (see Table 15–5) where the patient's threshold is 60 dB. This amount of amplification is grossly inadequate because this patient has "highly usable hearing" in the higher frequencies. We want to provide amplification in highly functional zones and avoid amplification in "dead" zones.

All practitioners are aware of the degradation of word understanding as hearing loss increases substantially. When thresholds are near "0" dB, most people have perfect word understanding ability. When all thresholds are near 100 dB HTL, most people have very poor word understanding abilities.

The "usable hearing range" was discussed by this author (2004). Table 15–6 shows the estimated amount of speech information available at various hearing levels for the "average" or typical patient. Note how most speech cues (information) remain available through 70 dB hearing level. If the patient's hearing falls within this range (0–70 dB), amplification is typically highly productive. If hearing sensitivity falls below this range, a decreasing amount of speech information is usually available to the listener.

One exception to this 0 to 70 rule of thumb is the zone at 4000 Hz, which processes signals at a higher speed. According to Harvey Dillon (personal correspondence), hearing in the 4000 Hz octave band needs to be 10 dB "better" than hearing in the lower frequencies to be defined as equally "usable." Study the 70 dB HTL line in Table 15–7 and observe the marked reduction in speech information at this point (70 dB and 4000 Hz). Note: The values in Table 15–6 differ from those published earlier (Paper presented by the author at Frye Electronics, August 19, 2004). These values have been modified to present the author's current understanding. Harvey Dillon, PhD in Australia and Carl Asp, PhD at the University of Tennessee, Knoxville, were consulted regarding these values.

Because Samuel's hearing threshold at 4000 Hz is 60 dB, if his hearing follows typical averages, he can use significant amplification in this zone. We improve this hearing aid fitting by adding about 20 dB of gain in the 4000 Hz zone. This additional high frequency gain gives the patient *wideband amplification*, and it provides substantial speech information in a zone that has little natural background noise.

Up to this point, we have adjusted the amount of use-gain for Samuel in the various frequency zones. We continue our efforts to improve the "quality" of the amplified sound

Table 15–6. Speech Information Available at Various Hearing Levels for the "Average" Patient

	250 Hz	500 Hz	1.0k Hz	2.0k Hz	4.0k Hz	8.0k Hz
0	8	14	22	33	23	0
10	8	14	22	33	23	0
20	8	14	22	33	23	0
30	8	14	22	33	23	0
40	8	14	22	33	23	0
50	8	13	21	32	19	0
60	7	12	19	28	14	0
70	6	10	14	22	4	0
80	4	6	8	12	2	0
90	3	4	6	6	1	0
100	1	1	1	2	1	0

Table 15–7. Samuel

Frequency	Threshold	Use-Gain	Background Noise	% of Speech Information
250 Hz	50 dB	+12	High	8%
500 Hz	55 dB	+16	Med High	14%
1000 Hz	60 dB	+28	Medium	22%
2000 Hz	60 dB	+36	Low	33%
4000 Hz	60 dB	+32	Very Low	23%

by studying distortion. In Samuel's case, two types of distortion (frequency and temporal) were degrading the perceived sound quality: a preoscillatory peak in the real ear frequency response curve (frequency distortion) and excessive compression (temporal distortion). These topics are discussed below.

Fourth defect: When a hearing aid fitting operates in or near feedback, the quality of the perceived sound suffers markedly. All practitioners have seen patients wearing hearing aids that are in constant feedback, yet the patient is unaware of the feedback because their hearing is poor in the frequency range where the feedback is occurring. When this happens, AGC circuits and the noise reduction algorithm are activated and useful amplification is reduced. Samuel's hearing aids had a preoscillatory peak in the real ear response curve. We were alerted to this problem by the feedback detection feature in our hearing aid fitting software (Siemens, 2010b). This feature is called the critical gain measurement. It generates two curves: a "feedback" curve and a "use-gain" curve. When these two curves are apart, there is no feedback; when they approach each other or overlap, feedback is indicated at the point of overlap. When the two curves closely approach each other, a condition called "insipient feedback" occurs. In Samuel's case, the feedback was insipient, neither the patient nor the audiologist heard feedback. The "insipient" peaks were easily seen in the real ear tests; these small peaks grow quickly into huge peaks

(and audible feedback) when you place your hand near the ear.

There are many types of distortion that impact the quality of amplified sound. The time delays (attack and release) in the compression circuits in hearing aids can alter the natural relationship between the peaks and valleys in speech. As compression is increased, temporal distortion increases. Some patients are sensitive to high degrees of compression; their perceived sound quality suffers as compression is increased.

Fifth defect: Samuel was asked to listen to the hearing aids under two conditions: AGC deactivated, and AGC adjusted to the initial settings (marked compression). He preferred the quality of the amplified sound without compression. A compromise setting was used: low AGC thresholds, mild AGC ratios. This approach provided sufficient reduction in loudness, so his UCL (Uncomfortable Level or ULL-Uncomfortable Loudness Level) was not exceeded. The quality of perceived sound improved when compression was reduced.

So far in this discussion, we have focused on the patient's primary hearing program, Program 1. Most practitioners call this program the Everyday Program, or the quiet listening situation program. Another program often used with hearing aids is a noise reduction program. There are numerous approaches to modifying a standard hearing aid fitting, so the patient is able to function well in background noise. Most hearing aid fitting protocols recommend activating a secondary microphone and increasing the compression slightly.

The author taught a class for Frye Electronics on this topic in August 2004. The following information was taken from that class. This approach is called the Adverse Listening Protocol. It is used to create and evaluate a hearing aid fitting that provides the patient with as-good-as-possible word understanding in high-level noise listening situations.

Before we discuss the specifics of the protocol, we should overview the most common hearing aid fitting errors that preclude a patient from hearing and understanding speech in the presence of high-level noise. Three errors are egregious. These include:

1. Not evaluating the patient hearing ability in background noise.
2. Overuse of low-frequency amplification.
3. Elimination of speech cues by overuse of compression.

We discuss these topics at length in the next section.

THE ADVERSE LISTENING PROTOCOL

Many patients are very active and spend a great deal of time in restaurants, meetings, airports, and other situations where there is a substantial amount of background noise. The goal of this protocol is to first identify those patients who have adequate hearing-in-noise abilities—people who have the potential to hear and understand words in a high-level competing noise environment—and to create an amplification strategy that works for these people.

The QuickSIN (Quick Signal in Noise) test measures the degree of impairment for hearing in noise. Patients can be sorted into three groups: those who have the capacity to hear well in high-level background noise, those who cannot, and the borderline people who have problems in high-level background noise, but still want to be fitted with hearing aids rather than FM systems.

The steps of the protocol include:

1. Administer the QuickSIN test.
2. Do test-box measurements to determine whether or not the hearing aid is operating in or near saturation (see below).
3. Use a high-level input to load the amplifier and do real rear tests to see if the patient is getting "speech cues" (usable amplification). This simulates wearing the instruments in a high-level noise environment.
4. Measure the real ear gain in the lower frequencies using moderate and high level inputs.
5. Check to see whether or not the output exceeds the patient's UCL (Uncomfortable Level).
6. Do live voice testing to make sure the patient can understand words in high-level noise.

The QuickSIN test presents speech-test signals (sentences) at a variety of SNR, S/N. The test starts with a favorable, easy-to-hear signal (speech in low-level noise), and sequentially increases the background noise in 5 dB steps. According the Mead Killion and the literature supplied with the QuickSIN test, most of the people coming in for their first hearing aid have a 5 dB loss of capacity (i.e., they need a 5 dB improvement in signal-to-noise to hear like normal). The prognosis for these people is excellent. According to Mead Killion, most directional microphone systems can improve the SNR about 5 dB.

When the author administers the QuickSIN test, he records the patient's QuickSIN scores for the +5, +10, and +15 dB signal-to-noise levels. If the patient has poor word understanding at these levels, they are counseled about FM systems.

The second step in the protocol is to determine how "cleanly" the hearing aid is operating when the amplifier is subjected to a substantial "sound load." Intense background noise "loads" all parts of the amplifier system (microphone, amplifier, and receiver). If the "amplifier" is operating near saturation (e.g., a receiver is operating near or above its maximum output capacity), or if the background noise algorithms are working "poorly," the sound quality suffers, and the patient is not able to understand speech.

The test-box can be used to quickly and efficiently determine the presence of harmonic and intermodulation distortion. High-intensity pure tones are used as input for the harmonic distortion test. High-intensity composite noise is used as input for the intermodulation distortion test.

The harmonic distortion test recommended by the author for this adverse listening protocol is made by placing the hearing instrument in the test box set to the use-gain level and presenting a 90 dB pure-tone test sweep. The high intensity of the input signal "pushes" the amplifier system toward an "overload" position (i.e., saturation). This measurement simulates high-level noise situations by placing equivalent "loads" on the hearing aid. A quality fitting should have no significant distortion with an intense input. The amplification should be clean, clear.

Years ago, peak clipping was a common problem with class A amplifiers. Now, the era of digital hearing aids has replaced the analog hearing aids, yet, we continue to see digital hearing aids that distort the signal. When a hearing aid begins to saturate, it cuts off the peaks of the amplified sound. As the amplifier is pushed into full saturation by louder and louder sounds, the degree of peak clipping rapidly increases and the harmonic distortion values exceed 30% to 60%.

Years ago, audiology students were taught to reject hearing aids that have harmonic distortion values greater than 10% on the initial ANSI distortion test. This is helpful for identifying a hearing aid with a broken microphone or broken receiver. It is not a helpful test is evaluating the "clearness" or "cleanness" of the amplified sound as it relates to hearing in the presence of high-level noise. The "soft" input level of the ANSI test provides no information about the amplifier's ability to cleanly handle high-intensity input.

Another test-box measurement that is helpful in evaluating the "quality" of the sound in high-level noise is the intermodulation test. A composite-noise input-signal is used, and a series of increasing-level inputs are presented. The frequency response curve is studied to be sure the curve remains smooth. If the amplifier approaches saturation, the response curve gets ragged or rough. Small amounts (2%–4%) of intermodulation distortion are easily heard (Bernstein, 1966), so the acceptable level of intermodulation distortion is zero.

The third step in this protocol—perhaps the most critical—is to see if the patient is receiving speech cues when the instruments are worn in a high-level noise. High-level noise activates the compression circuits. If the compression settings are too aggressive, the compression circuit can "turn the hearing aid off" from the point of view of the available speech cues.

An example of the "overuse" of compression is illustrated in Figure 15–1. This graphic is the real ear test data for a patient with a moderate sensory neural hearing loss: 35 dB @ 250 Hz; 45 dB @ 500 Hz; 50 dB @ 1000 Hz; 60 dB @ 2000 Hz; 75 dB @ 4000 Hz.

The patient is receiving about 20 dB of usable gain in the mid frequencies when a 70 dB input signal is used (see Figure 15–1). This amount of sound is "loud" enough, so the patient believes the hearing aids are working properly. When the input test signal is increased to 80 dB; the real-ear gain in the higher frequencies drops below 10 dB. This is an inadequate level. Little speech information is available to the patient under this condition.

There are no universally accepted "targets" that may be used in evaluating hearing aid fitting in high level nose situations. However, the author has a "guide," or a "reference" response. It is the hand-behind-the-ear real ear response. The author recommends this curve be used as a least-possible-gain guide for the noise reduction program. Most people agree that they can hear well in high-level noise situations if they simple put their cupped hands behind their ears without hearing aids. The REUR (Real Ear Unaided Response) curve is a "boost" in the higher frequencies; the peak of this curve is about 16 to 18 dB at 3000 Hz. When a person puts their cupped hands behind their unaided ears, an additional 5 to 10 dB is added to the REUR curve.

When the author teaches this concept, he has the class participants talk to each other; then listen with and without cupped hands behinds their ears. Class participants universally agree they hear much better in a noisy room when they cup their hands behind their ears. The hand-behind-the-ear response curve is easily measured. It is reference curve, a real ear guide for the Hearing In Noise program. The term "guide" is used, rather than "target" because this curve does not identify the "best" or maximum response; rather it is used as a professional suggestion that indicates amplification should be more than this amount. The exact quantity is unknown, but the gain that matches this curve is a good starting point.

Figure 15–2 shows the real ear test data for a patient with a severe sensory neural hearing loss: 50 dB @ 250 Hz; 55 dB @ 500 Hz; 70 dB @ 1000 Hz; 70 dB @ 2000 Hz; and 75 dB @ 4000 Hz. In this case, like the previous, there is little usable amplification provided by the patients' hearing aids when the patient is in a high-level noise environment. The noise level activates the AGC circuits and markedly reduces the amplification.

If there is no "usable" amplification in a fitting, there are no available speech cues. The patient is comfortable, and the UCL has not

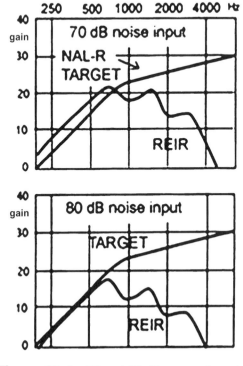

Figure 15–1. 70 and 80 dB composite noise inputs, notice absence of HF speech cues with higher level inputs.

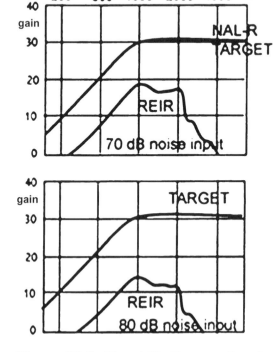

Figure 15–2. 70 and 80 dB composite noise inputs, notice absence of HF speech cues with higher level inputs.

been exceeded; however, the patient has little or no speech information available, so word understanding approximates zero.

When creating a hearing aid program that works well in high-level noise, one needs to know which part of the amplified spectrum is responsible for the perceived "loudness." Let's consider two opposing possibilities: substantial amplification in the lower frequencies, substantial amplification in the higher frequencies. If perceived "loudness" is "coming from" the lower frequencies, the patient will adjust the volume control downward whenever typical ambient noise is high in that zone. The same is not necessarily true for the "highs" (depending on the spectrum of the noise).

The acoustic inherent in human speech is distributed across a wide spectrum. Most of the energy, however, is in the lower frequencies near 250 Hz. When a patient wearing a pair of hearing aids enters a high-level noise environment, we need to know how much amplification they are experiencing in each frequency zone, so we can avoid the typical reaction of having the patient turn the volume control down because they are experiencing too much "loudness." Speech cues can only be preserved if the hearing aids provide usable sound in the adverse listening situation. When patients turn the volume down, they are reducing or eliminating speech cues in all zones.

Technical note: If the practitioner wants to evaluate (study) the delivery of speech information to the patient in a noisy listening situation, real ear or sound field measurements are required. It is not possible to test the instruments in the test box and determine the amount of sound the hearing aids are delivering to the ears. Most hearing aids have vents, and the amount of sound that escapes from the ear is substantial and unpredictable.

Years ago, there were charts in textbooks that attempted to show the amount of amplified sound lost through various sized vents. The advent of real ear tests taught us that these approximations were usually meaningless. Ears differ in shape, hardness, size, and other factors. If you want to accurately determine the use gain, do real ear tests or sound field measurements.

There are two additional parts of the Adverse Listening Protocol: ensure the amplified sound does not exceed the patients UCL (Uncomfortable Level) and do live-voice speech tests to confirm the hearing aid fitting is working well. Measurements regarding the patients' UCLs have been discussed at length in the literature and will not be discussed here.

Conventional hearing tests include the SRT (Speech Reception Threshold) and the Word Understanding test: neither how well the patient will hear in high-level noise environments. When a speech articulation function is generated by doing speech understanding at varying intensity levels, the practitioner can "see" the zone (on the intensity scale) where the patient understands speech. Figure 15–3 shows one such measurement. Note how word understanding is poor (less than 40%) at levels below 70 dB HTL. This patient has a very narrow intensity zone of usable hearing. Also observe that this patient —like many people with severe to profound hearing loss—has decreasing word understanding in the upper levels. Above 80 dB HTL (about 100 dB SPL), this patient's word understanding decreases with increases in intensity. Appropriately fit hearing aids will keep the output below the upper zone where speech understanding deteriorates.

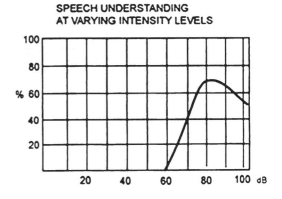

SPEECH UNDERSTANDING AT VARYING INTENSITY LEVELS

Figure 15–3. Word understanding tests show a very narrow range of functional hearing.

Patients with a severely reduced dynamic range of hearing are challenges when fitting hearing aids in adverse listening conditions. The frequency response curve must ideally "fit" the patient's hearing. Excessive amplification in the lower frequency will lead to upward spread of masking. Overuse of AGC (too much compression) will result in the patient receiving few speech cues when the patient experiences high-level noise.

Last, but not least, the practitioner should verify the fitting. Live voice test words can be quickly and efficiently presented to the patient and the patient's responses noted. Substantial background noise (the author uses a 80 composite noise) should be turned on behind the patient, the hearing aids switched to the Noise Reduction Program, and the live voice testing administered. Live voice testing is used, rather than recorded voice, due to time constraints and the number of variables: distance from the patient, hearing aid program selection, and so on.

Most patients have the potential to have high-quality word understanding in the presence of high-level background noise, but this potential is often not realized. Achieving this goal requires substantial work, and the patient must have: the capacity to hear well in noise (as measured by the QuickSIN test and other signal-to-noise types of tests), hearing aids that are operating far from saturation, the availability of substantial speech information with the compression circuits activated, and a sound level that should not exceed the patient's UCL.

REFERENCES

American National Standards Institute. (1969). S3.5. *Methods for the articulation index*. New York, NY: American National Standards Institute.

Bernstein, J. (1966). *Audio systems*. New York, NY: Wiley.

Byrne, D. (1996). Hearing aid selection for the 1990s: Where to? *Journal of the American Academy of the Audiology, 7*, 377–395.

Frye, G. (1998). *Manual for the Fonix FP40 portable hearing aid analyzer*. Tigard, OR: Frye Electronics.

Frye, G. (2010). *Personal communications*. Tigard, OR: Frye Electronics.

Frye, K., & Martin, R. (2008). Real ear measurements. In M. Valente, H. Hosford-Dunn, & S. Roeser (Eds.), *Audiology treatment* (2nd ed.). New York, NY: Thieme Medical.

Hosford-Dunn, H., & Huch, J. (2000). Acceptance, benefit, and satisfaction measures of hearing aid user attitudes. In R. Sandlin (Ed.), *Hearing aid amplification: Technical and clinical considerations* (2nd ed.). San Diego, CA: Singular Thomson Learning.

Kasten, R. N., Lotterman, S. H., & Revoile, S. G. (1967). Variability of gain versus frequency characteristics in hearing aids. *Journal of Speech and Hearing Research, 10*, 377–383.

Kochkin, S. (2003). *MarkeTrak: The U.S. hearing instrument market*. Book of MarkeTrak reprints, published by Knowles Electronics.

Libby, E. R., & Westerman, S. (2000). Principles of acoustic measurement and ear canal resonances. In R. E. Sandlin (Ed.), *Hearing aid amplification* (Vol. 1, pp. 188–190). San Diego, CA: Singular.

Martin, R. L. (1985). Audiometric assessment and interpretation. In R. E. Sandlin (Ed.), *Hearing instrument science and fitting practices*. Livonia, MI: National Institute for Hearing Instruments Studies.

Martin R. L. (2004). Presenting the speech cues audiogram. *The Hearing Journal, 59*(1).

Purdy, J. K. (1999a). Linear fitting prescriptions. *Hearing Review, 6*(2), 42–45.

Purdy, J. K. (1999b). Nonlinear fitting prescriptions. *Hearing Review, 6*(3), 22–30.

Revit, L. (1997). The circle of decibels: Relating the hearing test, to the hearing instrument, to real ear response. *Hearing Review, 4*, 35–38.

Siemens Hearing Instruments. (2010a). *Technical specification sheets for the Motion 700 series hearing aids*.

Siemens Hearing Instruments. (2010b). Connexx 6.4 fitting software including SIFIT 6.4.

Staab, W. J. (1985). *Hearing aid handbook*. Phoenix, AZ: Wayne Staab.

Walker, G. (2000). Technical considerations for sound field audiometry. In R. Sandlin (Ed.), *Hearing aid amplification: Technical and clinical considerations* (2nd ed.). San Diego, CA: Singular Thomson Learning.

Valla, A. F., & Sweetow, R. W. (2000). Psychology of individuals with hearing impairment. In R. Sandlin (Ed.), *Hearing aid amplification: Technical and clinical considerations* (2nd ed.). San Diego, CA: Singular Thomson Learning.

CHAPTER 16

Inventories of Self-Assessment Measurements of Hearing Aid Outcomes

JUDY L. HUCH

Hearing Handicap Scale: HHS
Hearing Measurement Scale: HMS
Hearing Performance Inventory: HPI
McCarthy-Alpiner Scale of Hearing Handicap:
  M-A Scale
Self-Assessment of Communication and the
  Significant Other Assessment of Communication:
  SAC and SOAC

GROUP III: BENEFIT SCALES
Abbreviated Profile of Hearing Aid Benefit: APHAB
Client Oriented Scale of Improvement: COSI
Glasgow Hearing Aid Benefit Profile: GHABP
Hearing Aid Performance Inventory: HAPI
Hearing Functioning Profile: HFP
Profile of Aided Loudness: PAL
Listening and Communication Enhancement (LACE)

GROUP IV: SATISFACTION INVENTORIES
Hearing Aid Users' Questionnaire: HAUQ
Satisfaction with Amplification in Daily Life: SADL
International Outcome Inventory for Hearing Aids
  (IOI-HA)
Office Satisfaction Surveys
Industry Standards

CONCLUSION

REVIEW QUESTIONS

REFERENCES

APPENDIX 16–A. COMMUNICATION SCALE FOR
OLDER ADULTS

APPENDIX 16–B. HEARING HANDICAP INVENTORY
FOR THE ELDERLY-SCREENER

APPENDIX 16–C. HEARING HANDICAP INVENTORY
FOR THE ELDERLY

APPENDIX 16–D. HEARING PERFORMANCE
INVENTORY REVISED

APPENDIX 16–E. ABBREVIATED PROFILE OF
HEARING AID BENEFIT

APPENDIX 16–F. GLASGOW HEARING AID BENEFIT
PROFILE

APPENDIX 16–G. HEARING AID PERFORMANCE
INVENTORY

INTRODUCTION

This chapter reads like books of lists. Its corpus is an inventory and commentary on available structured patient questionnaires that are designed to measure and validate hearing aid outcomes using a variety of separate and possibly related factors. The inventory is not exhaustive, but its length remains impressive. Readers may ask themselves why there are so many instruments and which one is best.

There are many instruments for evaluating program outcomes. There are a number of independent factors that influence different dimensions of hearing aid outcome in complex ways. As Humes (1999, p. 29) commented, "The development of separate measures of performance, benefit, satisfaction, and use reflect the clinical and research communities' belief that these are, in fact, independent aspects of outcome that must be measured separately."

■ Until we understand enough about the multidimensionality of hearing aid outcome factors to develop a "complete" hearing aid outcome instrument, the "best" tool depends on what factor we want to measure.

The following scales and profiles are separated into four overlapping groups, according to application:

■ I: Success Predictors
■ II: Handicap Profiles
■ III: Benefit Scales
■ IV: Satisfaction Inventories

Benefit scales (Group III) are designed for pre- and postintervention administration, with measured difference indicating degree of aided improvement. Items in Group II can also be used after treatment intervention, but their original intent was to profile pretreatment handicap in order to determine appropriate intervention strategies. The Hearing Handicap Inventory for the Elderly (HHIE) is a good example of this. The original intent was to determine the emotional and social effects of a hearing loss on individuals, but many clinicians use it as a pre- and postintervention tool to measure hearing aid benefit. Group IV scales measure satisfaction, which encompasses factors from the other three groups and also surveys that ask about the office environment directly. The latter factor is sometimes overlooked when clinicians evaluate satisfaction. There is another tool that is emerging in the industry that involves cognitive and listening skills but can show benefit. Instead of creating another group for the chapter, the Listening and Communication Enhancement (LACE) is added into Group III, Benefit, as there is a before and after measurement.

GROUP I: SUCCESS PREDICTORS

Since the original writing of this chapter over a decade ago, more research has been in the area of hearing in noise and the success of hearing aid use. This is happening in the booth with specialized testing, rather than inventories in a question/answer format. This is another chapter in of itself, and this chapter is limited to outside the booth so to speak. More information on ANL and other booth procedures may have more of an impact in this author's opinion than question/answer formats.

Expected Consequences of Hearing Aid Ownership (ECHO)

Development

The ECHO was developed by Robyn Cox and Genevieve Alexander in 2000 as a companion with the Satisfaction with Amplification in Daily Life (SADL). The development was to uncover unrealistic concepts an individual would have before hearing aids were fit and determine if there was a correlation between prefitting expectations and postfitting satisfaction.

Description

Similar to SADL, there is a Global Score and four subscales: Positive Effect Service and Cost, Negative Features and Personal Image.

Positive Effect: Includes six items that involves performance and function. Acoustic benefit, sound quality,

and psychological dividends with hearing aid use are examined. Cox and Alexander based this group to be the largest single contributor to satisfaction.

Service and Cost: Three items make up this section. This subscale can be removed if the individual did not purchase the hearing aids themselves.

Negative Features: There are three items in this set that examines hearing aid use. This area highlights the status of items that can take away an overall satisfying fitting.

Personal Image: The final subscale examines self-image and hearing aid stigma. "This area can be highly influential in the decision to try amplification and ultimate satisfaction" (Cox & Alexander, 2000).

The ECHO items are slightly reworded items of the SADL to form a statement of expectation. The SADL question number one, "Compared with using no hearing aid at all, do your hearing aids help you understand the people you speak with most frequently?" The responses are in the form of a 7-point, equally spaced semantic scale, ranging from "Not at all" (A) to "Tremendously" (G). The ECHO question one, "My hearing aids will help me understand the people I speak with most frequently." Continuing the 7-point responses from "Not at all" (A) to "Tremendously" (G).

Application

The ECHO would be given after hearing aid candidacy is determined. The items outside of the norms can be highlighted for counseling not only with the patient, but friends and family as well. Cox and Alexander (2000) point out that friends and family many times have inaccurate perceptions about benefits and problems with hearing aids. They further state it may be beneficial to have the spouse fill out the ECHO as well as to discuss hot spots.

Interpretation and Scoring

The Global score is the mean of the scores for all of the completed items. Subscales are scored separately by averaging the item responses (e.g., if the three scores for Personal Image are 5, 2, and 6 = 14, the score is (6 + 3 + 5/3 = 4.3). The higher the number, the more favorable the expectation is, whether it is on the individual subscale or the global scale.

The authors note, "If the box is checked in item 11 (hears well on the telephone without hearing aids), omit this item even if an answer was also selected from the scale."

The software for scoring can be purchased from the AUSP Software Group at the School Communication Sciences and Disorders at the University of Memphis.

Advantages and Disadvantages

This is a quick inventory to have the patient fill out and score. Donald Schum brought up an interesting point from Cox and Alexander's initial study of the ECHO, as they found the outcome from the SADL was better than the expectation of the ECHO on how the hearing aid fitting process went. His comment was, "Because of the nature of sensorineural hearing loss, we are never going to solve hearing loss totally, but we certainly can create in the patients' mind the sense that they were well taken care of, and they received good care out of the process, whether or not their hearing loss is totally solved" (Schum, 2013). If some of the scores show unrealistic expectations though, counseling prior to fit would be warranted. The counseling should be tailored to the specific area of trouble and not have a global counseling lecture.

Hearing Aid Needs Assessment: HANA

Development

In 1999, Schum developed the HANA as part of a self-report battery that examines the relationship between perceived communication needs/expectations and benefit achieved with new hearing aids. It is a companion scale to the Hearing Aid Performance Inventory (HAPI) and the shortened HAPI (described in section III). The HANA was administered to an unselected group of 82 patients. The HAPI was then administered after the hearing aid fittings to provide information on the relationship between expectations and results for the hearing aid fitting process (Schum, 1992).

Description

The HANA consists of 11 situational questions (Table 16–1) from the HAPI. The questions are grouped into four categories: noise, quiet, no visual cues, and nonspeech. Patients assign three ratings to each question that characterizes their unaided listening needs and hearing aid expectations. Patients who are previous hearing aid users answer the questions from their aided perspective. The ratings for the 11 situations are:

1. How often are you in this type of situation (hardly ever, occasionally, frequently)?
2. How much listening trouble do you have in situations like this one (very little, some, very much)?
3. How much help do you expect the hearing aid to provide (very little, some, very much)?

Application

The HANA is intended for use at the evaluation appointment or when amplification is selected. The patient rates the 11 situations prior to hearing aid fitting.

The follow-up with the HAPI should be 2 to 3 months after fitting to give ample time for the patient to acclimatize to amplification. The HANA results are then compared with the HAPI to determine if prefit expectations match postfit benefit.

Interpretation and Scoring

The situations were scored on a 3-point system, "Hardly Ever" or "Very Little" equal to

Table 16–1. Hearing Aid Needs Assessment Questions

Question	Categories
1. You are one of only a few customers inside your bank and are talking with a teller.	Quiet
2. You are at home reading the paper. Two family members are in another room talking quietly, and you want to listen in on their conversation.	No Visual Cues
3. You are in a quiet conversation with your family doctor in an examination room	Quiet
4. You are driving your car with the windows down and are carrying on a conversation with others riding with you.	Noise
5. You are home in face-to-face conversation with one member of your family.	Quiet
6. You are at church listening to a sermon and sitting in the back pew.	No Visual Cues
7. You are at a large, noisy party and are engaged in conversation with one other person.	Noise
8. You are in your backyard gardening. Your neighbor is using a noisy power lawnmower and yells something to you.	Noise
9. Someone is trying to tell you something in a small quiet room while you have your back turned.	No Visual Cues
10. You are starting to cross a busy street, and a car horn sounds a warning.	Nonspeech
11. You are at home alone listening to your stereo system (instrumental music).	Nonspeech

Source: From Perceived Hearing Aid Benefit in Relation to Perceived Need, by D. J. Schum, 1999, *Journal of the American Academy of Audiology*, 3. Copyright 1999, by American Academy of Audiology. Reprinted with permission.

1 point and "Frequently" or "Very Much" corresponding to 3 points. The higher the score, the more difficulty the patient is reporting. Each category (quiet, no visual cues, etc.) is scored separately.

The scores from the HAPI are inverted to compare them with the HANA, as seen in Figure 16–1. Direct comparisons allow the clinician to evaluate the patient's expectations versus perceived benefit.

Schum (1999) found that most previous users' expectations are more realistic in noisy situations than those of new users. Both groups expected less benefit from amplification in noise than in quieter environments. The HANA can be used as a tool to identify unrealistic user expectations before they experience the situations. For example, if a new user answered the question, "You are driving your car with the windows down and are carrying on a conversation with others riding with you" with the statement, "I expect the hearing aids to help very much," then counseling on SNR in automobiles should be addressed immediately.

Advantages and Disadvantages

Schum (1999) reported that the HANA is a useful tool to evaluate patient expectations of hearing aid benefit. It is likely to be a reliable measure, because its items are derived from the HAPI, which has already been shown to be reliable (Walden, Demorest, & Helper, 1984). Nonetheless, the HANA had been tested only once at the time of writing.

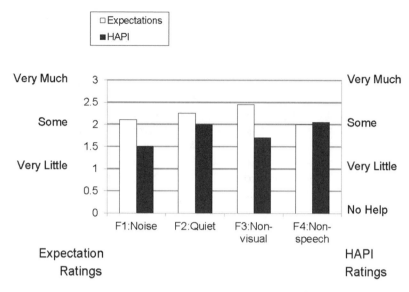

Figure 16–1. Average ratings for the HANA categories for the frequency of similar situations section. Data from Perceived Hearing Aid Benefit in Relation to Perceived Needs, by D. J. Schum, 1999, *Journal of the American Academy of Audiology*, *3*, Figure 2. Copyright 1999, by the American Academy of Audiology. Reprinted with permission.

GROUP II: HANDICAP PROFILES

Communication Profile for the Hearing Impaired: CPHI

Development

The CPHI provides a systematic and comprehensive assessment of a broad range of communication problems (Demorest & Erdman, 1986). It was initially standardized on active duty service members at Walter Reed Army Medical Center. Later normative studies included older and wider ranges of clinical populations (Erdman et al., 1995; Garstecki & Erler, 1996; Hyde, Malizia, Riko, & Storms, 1992, 1996).

The initial item pool was written to be relevant for the general population of individuals with hearing impairment. Two different but equivalent versions of the CPHI allow administration of a short (one form) or long

(two forms) profile without the memory factor confounding results. The items, scales, and subscales of the CPHI have undergone rigorous statistical analyses to ensure their validity and reliability (Demorest & Erdman, 1987).

Description

The CPHI contains 145 items in five areas. For purposes of analysis, the areas are internally divided into 22 "scales." The five areas are described as follows:

The Communication Performance Scales assess ability to give and receive information or carry on a conversation. The authors recognize that individual communication in daily life is influenced by many factors depending on the patient's situations, expectations, and priorities. For this reason, the 18 items are designed to cover various types of situations and listening conditions. In contrast with other profiles developed around the same time (e.g., The Hearing Performance Inventory, HPI), the scales are not designed to provide detailed or specific information of the situation, listener, or speaker.

Through the development of Communication Performance, another area emerged. Communication Importance examines communication problems in different situations. The handicapping effects of a hearing loss may be less severe than if the same degree of difficulty is discovered in situations where communication is determined to be very important or essential (Demorest & Erdman, 1986). The 18 items of the Communication Performance scale have two response scales. The responses relating to importance range from "Not Important" (1) to "Essential" (5).

The Communication Environment Scales, consisting of 31 items, assess the external environmental factors, strategies, and emotional adjustments the patient experiences in everyday life. Because the communication environment is the environment perceived by the patient, the possibility exists that the patient may incorrectly blame the environment and other persons for creating communication problems.

Communication Strategies Scales assess the person's verbal and nonverbal behaviors in 25 different situations. Behaviors are viewed as adaptive or maladaptive depending on their effects on communication. Maladaptive behavior items describe avoidance and other negative behaviors, such as ignoring others, dominating conversations, and avoiding social interaction (Garstecki & Erler, 1996).

Personal Adjustment is composed of eight subscales, which assess the patient's acceptance of and adjustment to hearing loss and reaction to related communication problems. The subscales are as follows:

■ Self-Acceptance: Negative feelings toward the self as a direct consequence of hearing loss.
■ Acceptance of Loss: The patient's ability to admit hearing impairment.
■ Anger: Frustration from hearing loss and inability to communicate effectively.
■ Displacement of Responsibility: Determines whether the patient places blame externally for communication difficulties.

■ Exaggeration of Responsibility: Degree to which the patient blames external factors.
■ Discouragement: General feelings of discouragement or depression associated with communication difficulty or hearing loss.
■ Stress: The patient's reported discomfort, tension, nervousness, or anxiety in reaction to communication difficulties.
■ Withdrawal: The extent to which the patient removes himself or herself from communication situations or experiences feelings of isolation.

The Denial scale is equivalent to the Problem Awareness scale. Its purpose is to identify patients' responses in the Personal Adjustment section that are inordinately positive given that they have a hearing loss. The items were designed to have the majority of the hearing impaired population agree with the statements. Most of the time these questions are qualified by the word "sometimes." The Denial section is not set as a main area, but intertwined in the Personal Adjustment section and given a separate score. The Denial scale reliability is reported to be very good (Demorest & Erdman, 1987).

Application

The CPHI is administered by the paper and pencil method before aural rehabilitation begins to define the patient's hearing profile and help plan appropriate intervention. The questionnaire generally takes less than 40 minutes to complete (Demorest & Erdman, 1987). The response scales range from 1 to 5 on a frequency ("almost never" to "almost always") or agree-disagree continuum.

Interpretation and Scoring

Because there are 25 individual scores on the CPHI, an automated database and scoring system are recommended. Responses can be entered in the computer by the clinician and a profile generated and printed within 2 minutes. Hand scoring is not recommended due to the number of items, and the fact that some questions are reversed. Demorest and Erdman (1990) developed a database system and automated scoring system, which is available for a nominal fee.

When interpreting the scores, a low score may suggest problems in a given area. Ineffective use of verbal communication strategies or a variable (ambient noise), for example, could contribute to communication difficulties. A high score that reflects effective communication may be due to appropriate use of compensatory strategies or indicate that the conditions described are not contributing to communication difficulty.

Advantages and Disadvantages

The scales give a wide range of clinical data that may be useful in creating an intervention plan. Perhaps the biggest advantage of the CPHI is that it is a demonstrably reliable and valid method to profile communication ability of patients with hearing loss.

The length of the CPHI and the cost of purchasing a database for scoring may discourage many offices from using this profile. Although there are norms for military and older populations, it is advisable to develop local norms where individual clients can be more appropriately compared (Demorest &Erdman , 1990). This may be too great a task for most offices to take on.

Communication Scale for Older Adults: CSOA

Development

The CSOA is a self-assessment scale that evaluates the communication strategies and attitudes of independent, older patients (Kaplan, Bally, Brandt, Busacco, & Pray, 1997). It was normed on 135 subjects with a mean age of 75 (60–88 years).

CSOA items were designed to "evaluate positive and negative communication strategies; perceived attitudes and behaviors of family, friends, and others; and interpersonal and emotional factors related to communication" (Kaplan et al., 1997, p. 204). The CSOA

is based on the Hearing Performance Inventory (HPI) and the Communication Profile for the Hearing Impaired (CPHI), both described in this chapter. The CSOA has good internal consistency and high test-retest reliability (Kaplan et al., 1997).

Description

CSOA has two scales: Communication Strategies (41 items) and Communication Attitudes (31 items). The Communication Strategies scale measures actual or perceived communication breakdowns and strategies pertaining to each situation. The strategies may be positive or negative. An example of a positive strategy on this scale is when an individual with hearing loss asks someone to repeat a part of a sentence that he or she missed. Negative strategies include bluffing or avoidance behaviors on the part of the person with hearing loss.

The Communication Attitudes scale evaluates the patient's attitude toward his or her hearing loss and self perceptions as a hearing-impaired individual. It also touches on other people's perceptions of the hearing loss. Positive and negative perceptions of self and others are questioned.

Two response formats are available, a 3-point item response and a 5-point item response. The 3-point scale should be used when a complex format is too difficult for older adults who frequently only use the endpoints of scale responses (Kaplan, Feeley, & Brown, 1978). The 5-point scale is designed for those older adults who desire more choices (Appendix 16–A). On the 3-point scale, the responses are: (1) Almost Always, (2) Sometimes, and (3) Never. If the patient answers "never," he or she receives a score of 3. The higher the score, the more communication difficulty. Some items are answered in reverse, and "Almost Always" is 3.

The two scales are administered by the paper-and-pencil method and can be used independently of each other. The scores are computed separately by using the scale mean, and items that are not answered are not used in the mean score.

Application

The CSOA is used to help set up intervention. It is administered before and after treatment (which may or may not include amplification) to compare the change in communication. The initial COSA is given at the initial appointment and the final at 3 to 6 months postintervention. Aural rehabilitation and communication intervention can be used in situations of normal to mild hearing losses.

Interpretation and Scoring

An individual score on the Communication Strategies scale that exceeds 0.10 indicates benefit on the 3-point scale, and 0.04 or greater indicates benefit on the 5-point scale (Kaplan et al., 1997). For the Communication Attitude scale, a difference of 0.10 on the 3-point scale and of 0.11 on the 5-point indicates benefit (Kaplan et al., 1997).

One recommendation made in the original study is to compare scale results with the patient's case history and audiological testing results. A low score on the attitude scale with reported difficulty in the case history and aidable hearing loss could indicate denial of the hearing loss.

Advantages and Disadvantages

The ability to use a 3- or 5-point response is good when the clinician knows when a patient needs things a bit simpler. Another advantage of this scale is helping with planning intervention. The CSOA can be a tool to help the clinician customize intervention and decide whether amplification should be part of the rehabilitation process. This scale has not had other clinicians conduct test-retest studies on it and can be quite lengthy.

Denver Scales

The following four scales originated from the Denver Scale of Communication Function (Alpiner, Chevrett, Glascoe, Metz, & Olsen, 1974) for purposes of estimating hearing handicap and effects of intervention on adults of different ages, abilities, and living situations.

Denver Scale of Communication Function: DSCF

The DSCF is a 25-item scale that queries adults with hearing impairment on the impact of hearing loss in a variety of experiential areas. The 25 statements are divided into four categories: family, self, social-vocational, and general communication experience. The response scale is a seven-level semantic difference continuum from "agree" (1) to "disagree" (7). It is recommended that patients complete the scale with a 15-minute time limit to encourage first-impression responses.

Schow and Nerbonne (1980) quantified the scores of the DSSF and called it the Quantified Denver Scale (QDS). The scores are graphically represented on a profile form, with no handicap ranging from 0% to 15%, slight hearing handicap scores in the 16% to 30% range, and mild-moderate handicap scores 31% or greater. Degree of handicap increased with degree of hearing impairment based on pure-tone averages.

Denver Scale of Communication Function for Senior Citizens: DSCF-SC

This scale was one of the first designed for confined elderly patients. Zarnoch and Alpiner (1977) modified the original DSCF to allow older individuals to report their communication performance prior to and following rehabilitative intervention.

This scale is administered interview style because self-scoring scales are not always feasible with older confined persons. The questionnaire consists of seven key questions that cover the following topics:

- family
- emotions
- other persons
- general communication
- self-concept

■ group situations
■ rehabilitation

Each question is followed by one "Probe Effect" and one "Exploration Effect" question, which examine the question further. The Probe Effect question isolates specific problem situations. The Exploration Effect determines how applicable the general question is to the individual. This area of the scale serves to eliminate questions that are irrelevant to the patient and, therefore, unnecessary in establishing intervention goals. The responses are "yes" or "no," scored with pluses and minuses. A form for scoring is helpful when interpreting and comparing pre- and postintervention. This scale does not have scoring norms or group comparisons, but postintervention improvement is manifest by more pluses and fewer minuses than in the preintervention interview.

Denver Scale of Communication Function— Modified: DSCF-M

The modified version of the DSCF also was designed for use with older individuals living in retirement homes (Kaplan et al., 1978). DSCF was modified for this population, as follows:

■ All items concerned with vocation were removed.
■ The family category was changed to "peer and family attitudes" because many older people do not live with their families.
■ The "self" and "socialization" categories were combined into one "socialization" category aimed at probing degrees and feelings of participation in social activities.
■ A new category was added for "specific difficult listening situations."

In addition to these changes, an interview technique is used.

The DSCF-M consists of 34 items that are rated on a 5-point "agree" to "disagree" continuum instead of the 7-point scale in the original. Each of the five points is defined for the patient on the form.

Advantages and Disadvantages

These scales offer different versions to cover a wide variety of populations. The scales can be given in either the interview format or the paper-and-pencil method according to clinician preference. When a clinician is setting up intervention, these scales help develop counseling strategies.

Except for the DSCF-M, these scales do not provide norms or group comparisons. Instead, they focus on the individual to provide an analysis of his or her communication performance. The DSCF-M is reliable when using group data, but individual test-retest reliability is highly variable. For that reason, Kaplan et al. (1978) cautioned against using the scale as a pre- or postintervention evaluation tool.

Hearing Handicap Inventory for the Elderly: HHIE

Development

The HHIE was published by Ventry and Weinstein in 1982. The inventory assesses the perceived effects of hearing impairment on the emotional and social adjustment of elderly patients. Although originally the HHIE was designed to assess hearing impairment, it also is a reliable tool for measuring benefit (Newman & Weinstein, 1988). The HHIE has two areas interwoven throughout the profile, the Emotional Scale and the Social Scale. The Emotional Scale estimates the patient's attitudes and emotional responses to his or her hearing loss. The Social Scale measures the perceived effects of hearing loss in a variety of social situations.

Prototype testing was performed on 42 subjects with hearing loss who were over the age of 65. Internal consistency of the total scale was .82; reliability was .93 on the emotional subsection and .83 on the social/situational section (Ventry & Weinstein, 1982). A sensitivity section in the prototype was not included in the final inventory because of poor reliability (.24). The authors selected a 3-point answering scale to simplify the response format for elderly patients.

The items used for the final version were selected on the basis of their strong correlation with pure-tone hearing sensitivity. The HHIE was administered to 100 subjects 65 years and older who had sensorineural hearing loss and no evidence of neurological or psychological problems. Results showed large standard deviations in the total score and both subscales, consistent with the prediction that patients respond differently to their hearing losses (Ventry & Weinstein, 1982). Weinstein, Spitzer, and Ventry (1986) subsequently evaluated reliability and found high test-retest correlations in the scores. They concluded that the HHIE is a highly reliable index of self-perceived hearing handicap in the elderly.

The HHIE-S (Appendix 16–B) is a 10-item version, derived from the HHIE, that serves as a screening tool for profiling emotional and social aspects of hearing handicap. A companion inventory to the HHIE, called the HHIE-SP, is the spouse's version. It is identical to the HHIE except for small working changes in the questions (e.g., "your spouse" instead of "you"). The HHIE-SP supports using the spouse's judgments as an indicator of the outcome of future rehabilitative intervention (Newman & Weinstein, 1988). A study conducted in Japan (Tomioka et al., 2013) found the HHIE-S an effective tool to assess hearing impairment and quality of life in the elderly community.

Description

The HHIE is composed of 25 questions in two subscales, Social (S) and Emotional (E) (Appendix 16–C). All questions are labeled according to the scale to which they pertain. Administration time in the initial study was approximately 10 minutes (Ventry & Weinstein, 1982).

There is a 3-point scale response system, "yes" (4 points), "sometimes" (2 points), "no"/not applicable (0 points). The maximum score is 100, and the minimum is 0.

Application

Self-perceived hearing handicap following a program of rehabilitation can be scruti-nized using the interview format in the initial administration. Newman and Weinstein (1989) recommended that the HHIE be administered initially in a face-to-face interview format to reduce the "not applicable" answers.

If the HHIE is used as a benefit scale, the second application can be completed with the paper-and-pencil method by the patient. When the follow-up survey is given by paper and pencil, the results vary more than if it is given by face to face (Weinstein et al., 1986). If given face to face, there is a 95% confidence interval for detecting a change of 10 points, as opposed to 36 points from the paper-and-pencil administration.

Interpretation and Scoring

The higher the score, the greater the perceived hearing handicap. A "yes" response receives 4 points, "sometimes" receives 2 points, and "no" receives 0 points. Scores for the total scale range from 0 (no perceived handicap) to 100 (significant perceived hearing handicap; Newman & Weinstein, 1989). A percentage change of 18% or greater is a significant change for each subscale when used as a benefit scale. One study reported a significant reduction in perceived emotional and social effects of hearing impairment following 1 year of hearing aid use (Newman & Weinstein, 1988).

Advantages and Disadvantages

This scale is easy for elderly patients to complete. It is straightforward to score and interpret. In addition, its reliability and validity are well-documented for elderly persons with hearing loss. The screening version is a quick way to evaluate a patient's perceived hearing handicap. For these reasons, the HHIE and its variants have been widely used in the profession (Dancer & Gener, 1999).

Hearing Handicap Inventory for Adults: HHIA

Similar to the HHIE, the HHIA (Newman, Weinstein, Jacobson, & Hug, 1990) is a 25-item self-assessment scale composed of emotional and social/situation subscales that is scored in the same manner as the HHIE. This inventory is used to measure hearing handicap, as well as hearing aid benefit.

The HHIA was developed and normed on patients under the age of 65. Two questions differ from the HHIE, one social and one emotional. They focus on the occupational effects of hearing loss. A third item relates to leisure time activities. Table 16–2 shows the HHIE items that were omitted from the HHIA and the new items that were included. The HHIA has high internal reliability and excellent test-retest reliability (Newman, Weinstein, Jacobson, & Hug, 1991). Recently a poster session was presented suggesting the classification of handicap is not inline with the World Health Organization's (WHO) International Classification of Functioning, Disability and Health. (IFC) Because the HHIA was created prior to the classifications, the paper suggests hearing is more socially centered than just focusing on activity limitations (Miller, Zapala, & Heckman, 2010).

Hearing Handicap Scale: HHS

Development

The Hearing Handicap Scale, developed in 1964, was the first self-report questionnaire to assess hearing handicap (High, Fairbanks, & Glorig, 1964). Handicap in the HHS is defined as "any disadvantage in the activities of everyday living which derives from hearing impairment" (High et al., 1964, p. 215). In the original study, 40 items were given to 50 adults with hearing impairment along with a comprehensive audiological exam. The HHS is designed to estimate the effects of hearing loss on communication in various environments.

Description

The HHS has 40 questions on two equivalent forms (A and B) that have 20 questions each. The forms are used in pre- and posttesting. There are four content areas: Speech Perception, Localization, Telephone Communication, and Noise Situations. The 5-point responses range from "Almost Always," "Usually," "Sometimes," "Rarely," to "Almost Never."

Application

The HHS is given in a paper-and-pencil format at the initial appointment. The second form is given after intervention if it is used as a benefit scale.

Interpretation and Scoring

Schow and Tannahill (1977) suggested a categorical method for interpreting HHS results.

Table 16–2. Items Omitted from HHIE and Substituted in HHIA

HHIE	*HHIA*
E. Does a hearing problem cause you to feel "stupid" or "dumb?"	E. Does a hearing problem cause you to feel frustrated when talking to coworkers, clients, or customers?
S. Do you have difficulty hearing when someone speaks in a whisper?	S. Does a hearing problem cause you difficulty in the movies or theater?
S. Does a hearing problem cause you to attend religious services less often than you would like?	S. Does a hearing problem cause you difficulty hearing/understanding coworkers, clients, or customers?

Source: From The Hearing Measure Scale: A Questionnaire for the Assessment of Auditory Disability, by W. G. Noble and G. R. C. Atherley, 1970, *Journal of Auditory Research, 10,* 229–250. Copyright 1970, by Journal of Auditory Research. Reprinted with permission.

Scores of 0% to 20% indicate no hearing handicap, 21% to 40% indicate a slight handicap, 41% to 70% indicate a mild-moderate hearing handicap, and 71% to 100% indicate severe handicap.

Advantages and Disadvantages

The two forms allow pre- and postrehabilitation assessment and can be used as a benefit scale as well (Schow & Tannahill, 1977). The HHS does not assess social or psychological impacts of hearing loss, however.

Hearing Measurement Scale: HMS

Development

The Hearing Measurement Scale (HMS) was published in 1970. It assesses the degree of hearing handicap in patients with noise-induced hearing loss and relates handicap to audiological data (Nobel & Atherley, 1970). Four generations of the scale were tested on men engaged in trades that were noisy enough to cause chronic acoustic trauma.

The final version has 42 items and two identical forms, one for the subject (form A), the other for the subject's nearest relative (form B). Form B is used to check the reliability of the subjects' statements (Noble & Atherley, 1970).

Description

The HMS is a 42-item questionnaire of four sections (Table 16–3) divided into seven subsections:

Sections
1. Speech hearing
2. Hearing handicap
3. Acuity
4. Localization

Subsections
1. Speech hearing
2. Acuity for nonspeech sound
3. Localization
4. Emotional response
5. Speech distortion
6. Tinnitus
7. Personal opinion

The seven subsections were weighted for importance by a panel of judges. The panel consisted of an otolaryngologist, a director of an audiology clinic, a psychologist, and a physician. The latter two were the authors of the HMS. Four main sections were developed grouping the original subsections with the corresponding weighting scale (see Table 16–3).

The authors retested the same individuals 6 months later and found the test-retest scores were reliable over time. A 6-month interval was chosen to minimize noise and

Table 16–3. Hearing Measurement Scale Sample Nonscoring Question

---

5. Do you have difficulty in hearing when shopping or traveling in a car or bus?

| All | Most | Half | Occasionally | Never |

5. Modifier

Is this due to your hearing, due to background noise, or a bit of both?
Circle 1, 2, or 3.

1. Due to hearing
2. Due to noise
3. A bit of both

Source: From The Hearing Measure Scale: A Questionnaire for the Assessment of Auditory Disability, by W. G. Noble and G. R. C. Atherley, 1970, *Journal of Auditory Research,* *10,* 229–250. Copyright 1970, by *Journal of Auditory Research.* Reprinted with permission.

age effects on hearing while ensuring that subjects would not recall the test items.

Most answers are on a 5-point scale ranging from "Always" to "Never." A few questions have answers that are designed specifically for the question (e.g., item 5 in Table 16–4). Several nonscoring questions are included (e.g., the nature of the tinnitus, information about lip-reading ability).

Application

The HMS is given at the initial appointment in paper-and-pencil form to the patient. It is best if used with a comprehensive audiogram in order to estimate expected and perceived handicap.

Interpretation and Scoring

Higher scores correlate with higher perceived handicap. In cases of denial, the perceived handicap does not correspond with the audiogram, and this discrepancy can be used during counseling. If the patient has a 50 dB hearing loss at 2000 Hz and reports no trouble in any situation, for example, denial is most likely present.

Advantages and Disadvantages

This scale is reliable for individuals with noise-induced hearing loss (Noble & Atherley, 1970). The authors are unsure of the validity in other populations. Scoring is not consistent and can be complicated. Not surprisingly, self-assessment of communication difficulties is consistent with audiological findings, but not highly correlated (Noble & Atherley, 1970).

Hearing Performance Inventory: HPI

Development

The HPI is designed to assess a patient's hearing performance in a variety of everyday listening situations to determine areas of communication breakdown (Giolas, Owens, Lamb, & Schuber, 1979). Later the HPI was used as a measure of benefit during and after intervention (Hosford-Dunn & Baxter, 1985; Owens & Fujikawa, 1980).

In the initial prototype, 500 items were narrowed to 289 items, which were administered to 190 patients with mild-to-severe hearing losses. Statistical analysis of these responses narrowed the selection to the 158 items that composed the HPI in its final form. There is also a screening form, HPI-S, which Henoch (1998) found reliable as a quicker form to use in a clinical setting.

Description

The HPI is divided into six sections. These sections address common listening situations that vary according to the speaker(s), communication situations, and noise environments. The six sections are as follows:

Table 16–4. Number of Items and Maximum Possible Scores in Sections Combined According to Subject Matter

Sections	Subject Matter	Number of Items	Maximum Score Possible
1, 5	Speech Hearing	14	96
4, 6, 7	Hearing Handicap	13	74
2	Acuity	8	28
3	Localization	7	28

Source: Reprinted from Newman et al., 1990, with permission.

1. Understanding Speech Section: Patients judge how well they understand people whose voices are loud enough.
2. Intensity Section: Patients report their awareness of a particular sound in various situations (e.g., speech, doorbell, whistle).
3. Auditory Failure Section: Patients respond to how frequently they use particular behaviors in various situations (e.g., asking for repeats).
4. Social Section: Patients respond to selected items from Understanding Speech and Auditory Failure regarding situations in which a group of more than two people are gathered away from any occupational setting.
5. Personal Section: The patients report how they feel about the impairment and how it influences self-esteem and social interaction.
6. Occupational Section: Patients judge certain dimensions within an occupational context.

In 1983, Lamb, Owens, and Schubert revised the HPI to eliminate redundant items and shorten administration (Appendix 16–D). The 90 items are arranged in the same six sections as the original. The shortened form has 43 items, again in the same six sections.

Application

The HPI is administered by the clinician in an interview format in approximately 30 to 40 minutes (HPI-R about 20 minutes) at the initial visit. The 27 occupational items at the end of the profile can be omitted if the respondent is not employed. The spouse can fill an inventory out as well to highlight discrepancies that reflect the patient's denial of a hearing loss. If the HPI is used as a benefit scale, it is readministered face-to-face or in a paper-and-pencil format after intervention.

Interpretation and Scoring

The responses are answered in a 5-point scale. There are several questions in the Personal Section and Auditory Failure Section that are

answered in reverse and need to be flagged before scoring is completed. To score, the numbers are added for all items answered, divided by the number of items answered, and multiplied by 20. (This does not apply to those not answered. They are counted as not attempted.) Scoring inventory can be conducted by individual sections individually as well. Templates have been used, as well as a computer program (Giolas et al., 1979).

Scores range from 20% (least amount of difficulty) to 100% (most difficulty). The more the scores between the spouse and the patient covary, the more likely the patient is realistic about communication difficulties. The greater the disparity of scores, the more likely that there is a lack of acknowledgment on the patient's part (Giolas et al., 1979).

The HPI-R authors found that the global inventory score was difficult to interpret due to poor correlation between audiometric hearing loss and individual patients' adjustment to the hearing loss. Rather, they recommend using individual section scores, with special emphasis on the Understanding Speech and the Intensity sections (Lamb et al., 1983).

Advantages and Disadvantages

An advantage to the HPI and HPI-R are the rigorous development studies with large numbers of subjects, which lead to good statistics and high reliability. The HPI-R inventory is also appropriate for those with profound hearing losses (Owens & Fujikawa, 1980).

At 90 items, it still takes 20 minutes to complete the HPI-R, but it is much shorter than the HPI. Either inventory can be mailed out before the initial visit. The authors of the HPI-R felt that further item reductions would sacrifice the integrity of the inventory (Lamb et al., 1983).

McCarthy-Alpiner Scale of Hearing Handicap: M-A Scale

Development

The McCarthy-Alpiner Scale of Hearing Handicap, developed in 1983, assesses the psychological, social, and vocational effects of hearing loss for an adult (McCarthy & Alpiner, 1983). The M-A Scale also has a parallel scale for a family member. Initially 100 items were given to a pilot group of 100 adults with acquired sensorineural hearing loss. Two weeks later a randomized form of the scale was readministered. Using a criteria of > 0.80 test-retest correlation, 34 items remained.

Sixty additional subjects and family members were given the 34-item scale to determine internal item consistency and correlation between subjects' scores and those of their family members on three subscales (Psychological, Social, and Vocational Effects). Results showed high correlations, high consistency, and good stability for the scales when administered to the subjects and their family members (McCarthy & Alpiner, 1983).

Description

The 34 items are divided into three categories:

■ Psychological
■ Social
■ Vocational Effects

An example question is, "My hearing loss has affected my relationship with my spouse" (McCarthy & Alpiner, 1983, p. 265). Response choices are on a 5-point scale ranging from "Always" to "Never." Audiometric results are also recorded for comparison with the reported perceived handicap.

Application

This scale is given prior to intervention and is used to design a rehabilitation program for the patient family members.

Interpretation and Scoring

Responses are weighted 1 to 5, with maximum handicap assigned a 5. Because the scale includes reversals, negative items are coded "N," and positive items are coded " P. " For "N" items, "Always" is 5 points, and "Never" is 1 point. For "P" items, "Always" is 1 point, and "Never" is 5 points. The higher the score, the greater the perceived handicap reported by the individual.

Attitudes and relationships of family members are compared with those of the patient and used for counseling. Several scenarios can emerge:

1. The patient does not accept, understand, or deal with the hearing problems, whereas the family member is keenly aware of the handicap.
2. The family member does not recognize, understand, or deal with the patient's hearing impairment.
3. The two people fail to agree on the impact of problem areas.
4. A combination of the above exists (McCarthy & Alpiner, 1983).

Advantages and Disadvantages

This scale is used to get family members involved in the patient's rehabilitation process. It is important to target and prioritize areas of counseling, and this scale helps in this area of intervention.

Self-Assessment of Communication and the Significant Other Assessment of Communication: SAC and SOAC

Development

The Self-Assessment of Communication (SAC) and the Significant Other Assessment of Communication (SOAC) are two companion questionnaires developed by Schow and Nerbonne (1982) to screen primary communication difficulty and secondary emotional and social consequences of hearing impairment. The SAC and SOAC represent the nonaudiometric, subjective portion of Schow and Nerbonne's Communication Assess Profile (CAP).

In the initial phase of developing these scales, guidelines were developed through a Task Force. The CAP emerged from these guidelines.

There are two parts of the CAP, audiometric measures and nonaudiometric measures. The nonaudiometric section has two components:

1. Self-Assessment of Communication (SAC)—Personal attitudes of the patient regarding the hearing loss
2. Significant Other Assessment of Communication (SOAC)—Assessment of the hearing loss by a significant other. This component is useful in cases where a patient is either unaware of the extent of the hearing loss or attempts to minimize the severity (Schow & Nerbonne, 1982).

The SAC and the SOAC have high test-retest reliability, 0.80 and 0.90, respectively (Schow & Nerbonne, 1982). Elkayam and English (2003) adapted the SAC for adolescents as this group has not had a specific assessment. They found it to be a reliable tool to use for this age group.

Description

The SAC is a 10-item screening test. Items 1 through 6 estimate communication in different environments. Items 7 and 8 look at the patient's overall feelings about the hearing handicap, and items 9 and 10 assess the patient's perception of other people's impression of the hearing loss. The SOAC contains the same questions, but changes the pronouns in the questions to be appropriate for a family member.

Application

The authors suggested mailing the profiles and instructions prior to the initial appointment in order to save time.

Interpretation and Scoring

The responses are on a 5-point continuum from "Almost Never" (1) to "Practically Always" (5). The corresponding numerical responses are summed for a raw score. The raw score is converted to a percentage by

multiplying by 2, subtracting 20, and multiplying by 1.25. For example, if the raw score is 43, the equation is: $43 \times 2 = 86 - 20 = 66 \times 1.25 = 82.5\%$.

The higher the percentage, the greater perceived hearing handicap of the patient. Percentage differences between the patient's and the family member's scores are taken into account to look for signs of denial on the patient's part.

Clinicians should develop their own norms over time to compare with individual patients (Schow & Nerbonne, 1982).

Advantages and Disadvantages

Using a quantifiable test battery helps set up guidelines for what constitutes normal overall communication functioning, to which individual patient responses can be compared. Even if clinicians do not complete their own norms, this test is quick and easy to administer, whether it is mailed out beforehand or done in the office. Including the SOAC provides another perspective on the hearing impairment, which supports the patient's perceptions or serves as a counseling tool in cases of denial.

GROUP III: BENEFIT SCALES

Abbreviated Profile of Hearing Aid Benefit: APHAB

Development

The Abbreviated Profile of Hearing Aid Benefit, the APHAB, is a third-generation instrument whose precursors are the Profile of Hearing Aid Performance (PHAP) and the Profile of Hearing Aid Benefit (PHAB). All three instruments were developed at the University of Memphis, Hearing Aid Research Laboratory (HARL), by Dr. Robyn Cox and colleagues.

The PHAP was developed to measure hearing handicap in seven dimensions (Cox & Alexander, 1995). The PHAP is scored using three categories of speech communication and one environmental sound category: speech communication under relatively favorable conditions (SA), speech communication under unfavorable conditions that are not due primarily to background noise (SB), speech communication in noise (SC), and perception of environmental sounds (ES). Three of the categories or scales are further divided into subscales as seen in Table 16–5.

The PHAP was expanded to include responses to the items from the point of view of a listener in unaided and aided conditions. The differences between responses for "with my hearing aid" and "without my hearing aid" were compared to measure the user's subjective benefit from hearing aid use. Because it measures benefit as well as handicap, this expanded version of the PHAP was named the Profile of Hearing Aid Benefit (PHAB).

The PHAP and the PHAB both have 66 items and are too long for routine clinical use. As a result, 24 items were extracted from the PHAB and constructed into an Abbreviated PHAB (the APHAB). Item selection for the APHAB began by eliminating three of the PHAB subscales because of ceiling effects, and low internal consistency and test-retest correlations (Cox & Rivera, 1992). The items for the APHAB were then selected based on an analysis of responses to the items in remaining four PHAB subscales: Ease of Communication (EC), Reverberation (RV), Background Noise (BC), and Aversiveness (AV).

Cox and Alexander (1995) established norms for the APHAB by administering it to three study groups that varied in their reported communication difficulties, hearing aid use, and age:

■ Group I: Established wearers of linear hearing aids
■ Group II: Elderly persons with few or no self-assessed hearing problems who do not wear amplification
■ Group III: Young normal hearing listeners

Cox and Alexander (1995) reported good item-total correlation, ranging from .54 to .66, for each of the subscales and also high internal reliability scores (.78 to .87).

Description

The APHAB is a three-page questionnaire with items arranged on the left and two response columns for "without my hearing aid" and "with my hearing aid" answers. The APHAB is composed of 24 items that are scored in four subscales, as described in the previous section and as seen in Appendix 16–E. Each item belongs to one subscale. The items are statements that describe a specific situation (e.g., "I can understand my family at the dinner table."). Patients respond on a 7-point Likert scale by rating the frequency of the time that the statement is true in their experience. The responses range from "Always" (99%) to "Never" (0%).

The complete APHAB questionnaire is reproduced in Appendix 16–E. The APHAB and associated scoring software are available through HARL's website (http://www.ausp.memphis.edu/harl) and are included in software fitting applications from several hearing aid manufacturers (e.g., Starkey PFS and Phonak).

Application

Probably the most common application of the APHAB is to evaluate benefit of new hearing aid fittings (Cox, 1997). In this case, the

Table 16–5. Scales and Respective Subscales for the PHAP

Scales of PHAP	Subscales of PHAP
SA	F T: Familiar Talkers
	EC: Ease of Communication
SB	RV: Reverberation
	RC: Reduced Cues
SC	BN: Background Noise (referred to only)
ES	AV: Aversiveness
	DS: Distortion

recommended procedure is to obtain the patient's "without my hearing aid" responses before the amplification device is fitted, and the "with my hearing aid" responses at least 2 weeks postfitting. The two sections can be completed at the same time, answering the "without my hearing aid" completely before starting "with my hearing aid."

To maximize the validity and reliability of the data, Cox suggested that patients be allowed to see their responses to the "without my hearing aid" portion while they are completing the "with my hearing aid" section. She also suggested encouraging patients to review and even change the responses if they no longer agree with them (Cox, 1997).

The scale can be given in the office at initial appointment and follow-up or mailed out for completion after the fitting. If a patient fills out both "without" and "with" at the same time, instruct them to complete the "without" before starting the "with" column in order to minimize confusion and the possibility that data will be entered into the wrong column.

Patient responses are entered into the computer by the audiologist (see above for information on obtaining the scoring program). The program generates subscale scores and displays them graphically. The patterns of the graphs indicate areas of benefit and communication difficulty; they also help the audiologist determine whether the patient understood the APHAB and provided valid responses. This is because of the different types of items in the profile and the fact that some of them are presented in a reverse scoring paradigm (i.e., where "always" means fewer rather than more problems). As a result, it is likely that most of the response alternatives will be used at least once and the pattern of usage will not be systematic. Patterns that do not vary, suggesting similar responses for all or most items, suggest that the patient does not understand the talk or did not read the instructions carefully.

Interpretation and Scoring

The average unaided score and average aided score is calculated. The Global Score is the mean of the scores for all the items in the EC, RV, and BN subscales. These scores show how frequently clients experience performance problems.

A difference of 22 points between unaided and aided scores is required to be certain of a significant difference between EC, RV, or BN conditions. Globally, the aided scores must exceed unaided scores on all three subscales by at least 10 points to establish true benefit accrues from hearing aid use (Cox, 1997). The AV score has become better understood over time, and with the development of other algorithms for hearing aid technology, there is a change over time with these norms. It is not grouped with the other three subscales for interpretive purposes. Because the AV subscale focuses on perception of environmental sounds, answers on aided statements may give information about the appropriateness of an aid's maximum output level, and some clinicians have reported successfully using the AV scores as a basis for adjusting the SSPL 90 settings on linear type aids (Cox, 1997). Johnson, Cox, and Alexander (2010) collected data from private clinics in 2005 to establish updated normative data that showed the other three subscales have stayed stable, but AV is lower with better technology. See Figure 16–2 for both sets of norms.

Advantages and Disadvantages

The APHAB is widely used due to its brevity and high internal reliability and because its software is readily available and automatically scored. The graphical representation of APHAB provides a quick way for the audiologist to understand the patient's communication needs and the effect of amplification on those needs. The graph is useful for explaining and discussing hearing handicap and aided benefit with a patient. It can also be printed and put in the patient's chart for future reference and comparison of hearing handicap status and aided benefit.

A recurring problem for most Group III questionnaires is that not all of the situationally specific items are relevant to all patients.

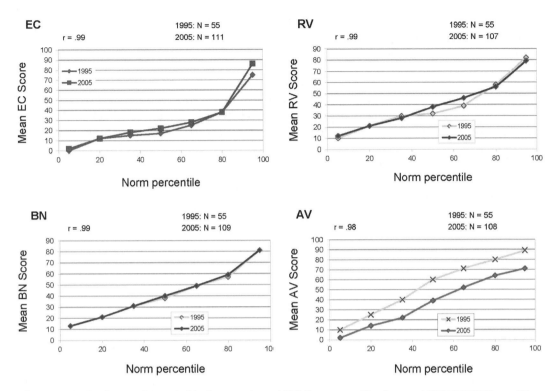

Figure 16–2. Comparison of aided norms from 1995 linear amplification and 2005 WDRC amplification across all four norms of the APHAB. (EC, RV, BN, and AV subscales).

The APHAB suffers from this problem and instructs patients to answer such items by estimating how they might respond, even if they are not likely to experience the situation. The APHAB was normed on patients who wore hearing aids with linear circuitry. The norms were published in a national journal by Johnson et al. (2010) with circuits using WDRC (Wide Dynamic Range Compression) that showed problems understanding amplified speech did not decrease compared with linear, but there were less negative reactions to amplified environmental sounds. An update to the normative data for compression circuits was studied in 2005, but started to be circulated in 2006 during presentations but was not published until 2009 to 2010. Finally, the APHAB may be difficult for some patients to read and understand. Cotugna, Vickery, and Carpenter-Haefele (2005) recommends patient education materials be at a 5th- to 6th-grade level, but the APHAB's reading level is

at or above the 11th-grade level when applying the Flesch-Kincaid readability formula.

As with all of the outcome applications and hearing aid fitting applications, links can be found at the Hearing Aid Research Lab (HARL) at http://www.harlmemphis.org/index.php/clinical-applications/

Client Oriented Scale of Improvement: COSI

Development

The Client Oriented Scale of Improvement (COSI) is an individually constructed statement of the patient's needs and the improvements resulting from the hearing rehabilitation process (Dillon, James, & Ginis, 1997). The COSI was developed by clinicians at the National Acoustic Laboratories (NAL) over several years in the early 1990s. In 1994, audiologists at different facilities were asked to use the COSI and five other outcome measures to estimate the benefits of the aural rehabilitation process and the value of the outcome measures. The audiologists reported a preference of the COSI over the others due to the simplicity, brevity, and the focus on the individual's particular situations (Dillon et al., 1997).

The COSI was normed on 98 Australian adults who were new hearing aid users. In that study, Dillon and colleagues (1997) reported on the scale's reliability, test-retest stability, validity, convenience of use, and capability to improve as well as measure rehabilitation outcomes. The first section of the COSI was completed at the initial appointment. The second section was administered 4 to 7 weeks after the hearing aid fitting and again at a 3-month checkup appointment. Test-retest scores show that the COSI is a reliable scale, with coefficients ranging from 0.73 to 0.84.

Description

In conference with the clinician, the patient identifies up to five situations in which he or she would like to hear better. These situations should be specific; for example, the patient should not state, "I would like to hear better." The audiologist should help narrow this down to something like "I would like to understand conversational speech with a grocery store clerk."

After amplification is fitted, and after the patient has had a reasonable time to adapt to the aids (1 to 3 months), the patient rates how well the fitting has helped in the previously defined listening situations. There are two types of ratings to evaluate the COSI at this time, which are recorded on the same sheet on which the situations were outlined:

1. Relative (degree of change): How much better do you hear in this situation (Worse, No Difference, Slightly Better, Better, Much Better)?
2. Absolute (final ability): How well do you do in this situation? I can hear: Hardly

Ever, Occasionally, Half of the Time, Most of the Time, Almost Always.

Examples of the ratings are: "I hear my grandchildren on the phone" "slightly better," and I hear them "most of the time" or, "I hear the bids when playing bridge" "better," but I still only hear them "Half of the time."

Application

It is best to use the COSI at the initial appointment to individualize the patient's aural rehabilitation. The follow-up can be within the 30-day evaluation time or within a few months of the fitting, depending on acclimatization and other fitting factors.

Interpretation

The final assessment may highlight areas that require further improvement or counseling. Because the rehabilitation process is individualized according to patient needs and desires, the COSI helps clarify expectations, as well as remind the patient and clinician of original fitting goals. The COSI can also help define an endpoint for the fitting process.

Advantages and Disadvantages

This outcome measure is a quick, individualized tool that not only measures outcome, but also helps assess patient needs. For instance, non-hearing aid solutions can emerge from the assessment that solve needs that are not corrected by amplification. The COSI has proven to hold up to the test of time. Most of this information was in the previous edition of this chapter and is still used today. Many manufactures encourage its use by putting the COSI in their programming software.

As with many other hearing aid outcome measures, it is difficult to determine to what extent the patients' answers are related to how much they like their practitioners. The patients may overrate their responses if they admire the audiologist helping them (Dillon et al., 1997). The COSI can be downloaded from NAL (http://www.nal.gov.au/outcome-measures_tab_cosi.shtml).

Glasgow Hearing Aid Benefit Profile: GHABP

Development

The Glasgow Hearing Aid Benefit Profile (GHABP; Gatehouse, 1998) evaluates the effectiveness of rehabilitation services for adults with hearing impairment. It is based on data from the Hearing Disability and Aid Benefit Interview (HDABI; Gatehouse, 1998). The HDABI contained 14 listening situations that were most likely to occur in everyday life. It was given to 943 subjects who were asked seven questions pertaining to each of the 14 listening situations. The seven follow-up questions are as follows:

1. How often does this happen?
2. Without your hearing aid, how much difficulty did you have in this situation?
3. Without your hearing aid, how much does any difficulty worry, annoy, or upset you in this situation?
4. In this situation, what proportion of the time do you wear your hearing aid?
5. In this situation, how much does your hearing aid help you?
6. In this situation with your hearing aid, how much difficulty do you have?
7. For this situation, how satisfied are you with your hearing aid?

After data collection, four of the most common situations were used to develop the GHABP, based on either maximum frequency of occurrence or maximum occurrence of hearing difficulty. Although test-retest reliability is high (0.86), the author suggested that this measure may be inflated because the scale is so short that subjects can recall the answers between test and retest.

Description

The GHABP has six scales:

1. Initial Disability
2. Handicap
3. Reported Hearing Aid Use

4. Reported Benefit
5. Satisfaction
6. Residual Disability

Information on these scales is obtained based on patient's answers to the seven questions of the HDABI, in each of the four specified listening circumstances. There are also up to four additional listening circumstances described by the patient (Appendix 16–F). The GHABP combines the features of both standardized and open ended questioning.

Application

The author's goal is to use this profile during rehabilitation to help the patient and clinician focus on positive and negative aspects of amplification for the individual patient. It is best administered in an interview format.

Three questions are answered (Appendix 16–F) at the visit when the decision to proceed with amplification is made:

1. Does this situation happen in your life? Yes (go to next question) No (stop)
2. How much difficulty do you have in this situation?
3. How much does any difficulty in this situation worry, annoy, or upset you?

Most patients give at least one (and as many as four) other examples in the subject-specified section, as seen in Appendix 16–F and initially answer the two pertinent questions of difficulty (Gatehouse, 1999).

Interpretation

Questions are examined individually, but in each case the higher the number associated with the particular answer, the less difficulty.

Advantages and Disadvantages

The GHABP is a comprehensive profile that does not take much clinical time. This inventory has been used in clinical settings and for research over the past 13 years with success. The Scottish Government has made the

GHABP part of fitting protocol along with Real Ear Measurements (Davis, Evans, Martin, & Orton, 2007).

Hearing Aid Performance Inventory: HAPI

Development

The HAPI is a self-reported scale that measures success with amplification (Walden, Demorest, & Hepler, 1984). The main question asked by the developers was: "Is perceived benefit from amplification relatively consistent across situations or is benefit too situation-specific to be assessed with a single, global criterion measure?" (Walden et al., 1984, p. 49).

The HAPI was normed on 128 experienced hearing aid users (119 males, 9 females) who wore their aids an average of 10.8 hours per day and had a sloping sensorineural hearing loss. Subjects filled out the inventory at an appointment or mailed it and were instructed to answer based on the benefit received from the hearing aids and not based on the difficulty of the situation itself (Walden et al., 1984). Each situation had a "does not apply" option included in the answer format. The latter were not included in the statistical analysis.

The reliability of the HAPI is high (.96), even though there is high intersubject variability. The reliability factor opened the door to shorter versions that were created later. Two different Shortened HAPI scales (both have been referred to as SHAPI) were modified by Schum (1992) and Dillon (1994) to decrease administration time but keep the reliability of the scale.

Description

The HAPI has 64 items organized into four subsections according to listening situations:

1. Noisy situations
2. Quiet situations with the speaker in proximity

3. Situations with reduced signal information
4. Situations with nonspeech stimuli

Common environments such as home and work are represented several times throughout the questionnaire. The items are broad in scope, applying to a variety of listening environments.

The patient chooses from a 5-item scale, as seen in Appendix 16–G, ranging from "Very Helpful" (1) to "Hinders Performance" (5). In contrast with most other profiles, a low score is preferable.

Application

The original intent was to administer the HAPI when intervention is near completion by the paper-and-pencil method.

Interpretation and Scoring

The HAPI and its offspring were designed to report the amplification performance and the success of hearing aid use in daily life as one combined measure. The scores of all items are added together and averaged (leaving out the "not applicable" answers). The closer to "1" the averaged score is, the better the individuals feel they are doing.

Advantages and Disadvantages

Both the HAPI and Shortened HAPIs provide aided scores only. Although the scale is not designed for pre- and postintervention testing, some clinicians use it in this manner even though its reliability is not known for this application.

Because the items apply to a variety of listening environments, the HAPI may not be applicable to some elderly respondents (Newman & Weinstein, 1988). Schum (1992) and Dillon's (1994) Shortened HAPIs target the elderly population for ease of use. These scales do help clinicians reliably determine self-perceived benefit for those individuals who have been using amplification. The shortened forms reduce administration and scoring-time involvement.

Hearing Functioning Profile: HFP

Development

Singer, Healey, and Preece (1997) described The Hearing Functioning Profile (HFP). This profile helps clinicians use rehabilitation tactics over and beyond amplification, such as communication strategies and closed captioning.

The HFP focuses on the psychological and behavioral changes that patients must go through in order to accept amplification. The profile is based on a psychological "transtheoretical approach" in which success and failure are related to "learned helplessness" (Singer et al., 1997). The HFP helps the clinician understand the patient's psychological profile based on learned helplessness and how different factors may influence the patient's function with hearing instruments. The HFP looks at the extent to which a patient is actively working to change his or her behaviors and whether his or her outlook is pessimistic or optimistic. The latter dictates whether an individual is at high risk for failure with amplification on this profile.

Description

The HFP examines three categories that encompass at least 10 hearing situations:

1. Alerting Category: Telephone bell, doorbell, sound (e.g., baby), alarm clock, fire, and a section to add another alerting sound for that particular individual.
2. Listening Category: Television and phone conversation.
3. Communication Category: Planned (one to one), unplanned (one to one), group, and a fourth can be added to fit the needs of the individual.

Application

The HFP was designed for postfitting management, but the authors did not feel it was limited to this intervention stage (Singer et al., 1997). The profile is conducted in an interview format with the clinician asking the patient about situations in each category and recording the responses. Each relevant situation is evaluated in terms of whether a problem is present in aided and unaided listening. If a problem exists, the patient is asked whether it is due to overall hearing, listening angle (e.g., if there is a "dead" ear or monaural fit), competing noise, distance, or visibility. Each situation has room for comments to elaborate on problems. If the patient has amplification, the final limitation that is examined is usage (i.e., is the individual a full-time or part-time user?)

Interpretation and Scoring

The HFP is not scored numerically. Rather, the clinician checks it on the form when a problem area is identified. A comments section is used for elaboration of the problem situation if needed. Evaluating the difficulties that patients report with amplification helps the clinician organize continuing rehabilitation for the patient. Treatment recommendations are based on "S.E.T." categories: Strategies, Environmental Manipulations, and Technology (Singer et al., 1997). Strategies include getting the individual's attention before speaking in an unplanned situation to optimize use of visual cues. Environmental manipulations can be as simple as turning the television down when conversation takes place or waiting for commercial breaks to converse. Technology refers to assistive listening devices of all types.

Advantages and Disadvantages

This profile encompasses many factors that are beneficial to the patient and clinician when searching for hearing solutions beyond amplification. As the authors pointed out, "The use of the Hearing Functioning Profile greatly enhances management of hearing loss. It benefits those fitted with hearing instruments, but should also be considered for individuals who do not use hearing instruments. The Profile forces the hearing health care professional to organize management around the numerous demands on a person in everyday life" (Singer et al., 1997, p. 26).

A few underlying issues are not clear on the form. For example, a limitation to communication is lack of hearing aid use, but daily (hourly) use is not queried on the form. The HFP might be easier to use if more question areas were on the form instead of relying on the clinician to think of unstated items when the profile is given to a patient.

Profile of Aided Loudness: PAL

Development

Mueller and Palmer developed the Profile of Aided Loudness (PAL) in 1998 to determine if loudness restoration is accomplished with amplification. In 1997, 53 subjects were fit binaurally with two-channel programmable CICs. The instruments had the capability of wide dynamic range compression (WDRC) or compression limiting (Mueller & Palmer, 1998). The authors found that the WDRC performance had better ratings for soft speech, but no difference was found in word understanding in noise using the speech perception in noise (SPIN) test. Mueller and Palmer reported a high consistency correlation of .70 or better on the PAL.

The pilot study normed loudness ratings for individuals without a hearing loss on 95 different sounds. This normative data is used when comparing answers of hearing aid users.

Description

There are 12 situations or noises in which the patient rates the loudness and the loudness satisfaction (see Appendix 16–H). The loudness rating uses a 7-point scale as "cannot hear" (0) to "uncomfortably loud" (7). Each loudness (soft, medium, and loud) has four different examples to represent that situation.

The loudness rating is compared with the ratings of the normed (normal hearing)

subjects. The target rating for each item is where 70% of the norm group selected that particular item. The acceptable rating is within ±1 standard deviation from the target, which establishes the loudness profile rating. Thus, soft speech goal is 2, ±1. For medium sounds, such as average speech, the target is 4, ±1.

Application

The original design is for administration after amplification is fit, but the PAL can also be executed prior to hearing aid fitting in order to establish baseline (Mueller & Palmer, 1998). It is not to be completely filled out after fitting to judge prefit as it is difficult to remember some items before hearing aids are fit.

Interpretation and Scoring

There are four possible outcomes:

1. Goal of normal aided loudness perception met, patient is satisfied.
2. Goal of normal aided loudness perception met, patient is dissatisfied.
3. Goal of normal aided loudness perception not met, patient is satisfied.
4. Goal of normal aided loudness perception not met, patient is not satisfied.

Each satisfaction rating is evaluated for each loudness level (soft, medium, and loud). The satisfaction profile is then compared with the loudness profile.

Advantages and Disadvantages

The PAL is easy to administer. It measures a specific component that affects wearer satisfaction and gives insight into the patient's fitting needs for loudness. The PAL does not show norms for satisfaction, but targets items that rate below "okay" or #3 (Taylor & Mueller, 2012). This scale has been used to help in WDRC settings for comfort in individuals. There have been off shoots of the PAL, such as Blamey and Martin (2009) ESQ (Environmental Sounds Questionnaire), which uses the same scaling and nine of the twelve items with some items removed (dryer, sermon, marching band).

Listening and Communication Enhancement (LACE)

Development

Sweetow and Sabes (2006), while at UCSF, developed and subsequently, NeuroTone produced a computerized version of Aural Rehabilitation (AR) and Auditory Training (AT) to help individuals who report difficulty understanding speech in problematic situations, but also to use as a tool alongside with the process of fitting and follow-up with hearing aids for better cognitive processing. With hearing loss, comes sensory deprivation (Arlinger, 2003). Depending on how long the individual takes to be fit with hearing aids, the deterioration may or may not be reversible. As audiology works more closely with other disciplines such as neuroscience, there are more opportunities to help those with hearing loss. There are links between auditory skill improvement with training that works neural plasticity and reorganization cognitively through aural rehabilitation (Hawkins, 2005; Kricos, Holmes, & Doyle, 1992; Montgomery, Walden, Schwartz, & Prosek, 1984; Rubinstein & Boothroyd, 1987; Sweetow & Palmer, 2005). The challenge has been to encourage those in the audiology profession to utilize aural rehabilitation.

LACE is a computerized home-based, interactive program to have the adult hearing impaired listener be engaged in the hearing device fitting process (Sabes & Sweetow, 2007). To build on other AR and APD therapies while increasing listening strategies, increase confidence and acknowledge the cognitive changes that develop during aging. The original LACE was 30-minute sessions, 5 days a week for a period of 4 weeks (Sabes & Sweetow 2007). The versions that are available today through NeroTone and Sycle.net are shorter. Sweetow and Sabes conducted a follow-up study in 2007, and found that for those who scored the worst on the baseline showed the most improvement. This is encouraging that we are targeting help to those who most need it. Song, Skoe, Banai, and Kraus (2011) supported that there was improvement in scores and were still evident after 6 months of the training.

Description

The software program gives tasks that are divided into three main categories: (1) better comprehension of degraded speech, (2) enhancement of cognitive skills, and (3) improvement of communication strategies. Each section has designated tasks for the patient to participate in.

Degraded speech includes speech that is either time-compressed, liken to rapid speech, along with multitalker background babble noise or a single competing speaker. There are multiple choice options of which the patient chooses what they feel is the correct answer of the main signal. With every correct answer, the next sentence will be more difficult, but easier if the answer was incorrect.

The LACE CD Home Edition from NeuroTone is 20 sessions long and will send daily reports to the prescribing professional; with the 20 sessions, they are 30 minutes each and cover a 4-week time period to complete. For those who do not have Internet access, there is a DVD LACE version where the users use a remote control to work through the program. This version has 10 30-minute sessions that covers a 2-week time period. The patient must report their compliance as opposed to the computerized version and is monitored remotely by the professional.

Application

Training is conducted at the patient's MCL, which is determined at the beginning of the exercise. The program can be given to the patient to do at home, or come into the office postfit to work on the office's program for 30 minutes.

Advantages and Disadvantages

The LACE is not designed for those with dementia or poor English language skills (8th-grade reading level). There have been reports of high number of patients dropping out of the training, especially in the 4-week course. Sweetow and Sabes also found that most of the improvement showed in the first 2 weeks. Obtaining patient compliance can be challenging. What our offices experience, as well as reports coming back for us to monitor, like many upgrade glitches, we must be ever vigilant on our own follow-up and ensure reports show in the patients Sycle file.

GROUP IV: SATISFACTION INVENTORIES

Hearing Aid Users' Questionnaire: HAUQ

Development

The Hearing Aid Users' Questionnaire (HAUQ) was developed and reported in Australia in 1988 (Dillon et al., 1997). The HAUQ contains questions that relate to hearing aid use, difficulties, and other satisfaction-related issues. Little information is available on the HAUQ, and it is not widely known in the United States.

Description

This multi-item questionnaire looks at several different areas of hearing aid use. The primary goal is to detect problems that may affect the person's ability to use and benefit from the hearing aid (Dillon, Birtles, & Lovegrove, 1999). Dillon described the questionnaire as:

■ Questions 1 and 2 deal with usage of the hearing aid with the categories in question 2 scaled from 1 to 6.

■ Question 3 deals with benefits, with "not at all" scaled as a 1, "a little" scaled as a 2, and "a lot" scaled as a 3.
■ Question 4 deals with problems, with "no" scaled as 2 and "yes" scaled as 1.
■ Questions 5 to 7 deal with satisfaction, each scaled from 1 to 4. In all cases, the larger the number, the more favorable the outcome.
■ Question 8 attempts to find clients' assessment of whether they have problems that require another appointment.
■ Questions 9 to 11 are open-ended questions to determine what the clients like and dislike are of the services and instruments they have received (Dillon et al., 1999, p. 71).

Application

This questionnaire is given at some point postintervention. Although no information is available on administration, it lends itself to a paper-and-pencil format.

Interpretation and Scoring

This scale is useful when looking at the individual's satisfaction in several practical dimensions, but it is not appropriate to use it to rank patients according to satisfaction (Dillon et al., 1999). Dillon suggested looking at each question individually and using the data to identify those aspects of the hearing aid fitting that are less than satisfactory.

Advantages and Disadvantages

The scale is quick to administer and can be mailed to patients. Use of the HAUQ is primarily used in Australia. It is used by some professionals in Australia and has been reported on in the United States through the *Journal of the American Academy of Audiology.* It is helpful in identifying the needs of individual people, but not if benefit is good or great in a group program (Dillon et al., 1999). It can be downloaded by National Acoustic Laboratories (http://www.nal.gov.au/out come-measures_tab_cosi.shtml).

Satisfaction with Amplification in Daily Life: SADL

Development

The SADL examines the overall outcome of hearing aid fittings from the patient's point of view, using satisfaction rather than benefit as the measure of interest (Cox & Alexander, 1999). As the authors stated, "the focus on benefit as an outcome measure is in danger of becoming too narrow."

The investigator has hearing aid users rank a set of "Importance Factors." Those rankings showed that items of importance clustered into four factors: Benefit and Sound Quality, Physical and Psychological Comfort, Value, and Hearing Aid Stigma. Based on these four factors, a series of proposed satisfaction questions were developed and tested on older hearing aid users. The subjects wore conventional aids, one-half of which were dispensed in a VA setting. The results showed that satisfaction and importance were similar constructs but not identical. For example, a patient might be satisfied with one measure in an Importance Factor (e.g., phone use) but dissatisfied with another measure in the same factor (e.g., hearing in groups). Principal components analysis of the satisfaction data showed that items grouped into five Satisfaction Factors of varying importance to hearing aid users. Ultimately, this analysis and further testing produced a 15-item questionnaire with four subcategories corresponding to four dimensions of satisfaction.

Description

The SADL has 15 items that are scored into four subscales that correspond to these four satisfaction dimensions:

1. Positive Effect consists of 6 items associated with benefit and performance.
2. Service and Cost consists of 3 items that address dispenser services and cost.
3. Negative Features looks at 3 disparate areas of frustration with hearing aid use.
4. Personal Image addresses hearing aid stigma and cosmetics in 3 items. The scale is shown in Appendix 16–I.

The responses are in the form of a 7-point, equally spaced semantic scale, ranging from "Not at all" (A) to "Tremendously" (G).

There is a separate section that includes the experience, use, and hearing difficulty as recorded by the clinician. The SADL form has a back section for describing hearing aid information, which is also filled out by the clinician.

Application

The SADL is filled out by patients after they have become accustomed to their hearing aids. Responses can be compared with interim norms. The administration can be repeated at intervals (e.g., 3 months to 1 year) after the initial administration to track the patient's satisfaction over time.

The SADL requires less than 15 minutes. Some questions are reversed and may confuse a few patients. If a question is not applicable, patients are instructed to leave it unanswered. The scale can also be used to rate the difference in satisfaction between amplification devices.

The subscale scores allow more complete analysis of a patient's satisfaction status. If a patient is reporting global dissatisfaction, there is most likely an underlying cause that would show up in that particular subscale.

Intervention in that area can be applied to improve satisfaction.

Interpretation and Scoring

The Global score is the mean of the scores for all of the completed items. Subscales are scored separately by averaging the item responses (e.g., if the three scores for Service and Cost are 6, 3, and 5 = 14, the score is (6 + 3 + 5/3 = 4.6). The higher the number, the more satisfied the patient is, whether it is on the individual subscale or the global scale.

Cox and Alexander (1999) reported that a critical difference (CD) calculated by test-retest scores, in global scores of 0.9, happens by chance only 10% of the time. Therefore, if the global scores differ by 0.9, there is a significant difference in satisfaction between the responses of one SADL and another for the same patient.

As of this writing, the scale is new and only interim norms from linear fittings are available.

Advantages and Disadvantages

The SADL is short and does not take long to complete (about 10 minutes). It can be mailed to patients or filled out in the clinic. It has found to be quick and an accurate reading of satisfaction for those fit with hearing aids (Humes et al., 2002).

One of the disadvantages of the APHAB that Cox also developed was the high reading level (Abrams & Hnath-Chisolm, in press; the SADL is written at a seventh-grade reading level). Hosford-Dunn and Halpern (2000) duplicated the validity of the SADL giving quick and reliable measured outcomes that are important to hearing aid users. It can be used in conjunction as stated before with the ECHO and compared if the expectations and results worsen or improve. Cox and Alexander (2001) again reinforced the validity of the SADL. Since then, the questionnaire has been translated to Chinese (Cantonese and Mandarin), Danish, Spanish, Portuguese (Brazilian), Swedish, German, and Odia.

The software for scoring can be purchased from the AUSP Software Group at the School Communication Sciences and Disorders at the University of Memphis.

International Outcome Inventory for Hearing Aids (IOI-HA)

Development

Robyn Cox along with Dafydd Stephens and Sophia Kramer (2002) developed the IOI-HA on the tail end of a workshop covering Self-Report Outcome Measures in Audiological Rehabilitation (Cox et al., 2000). The authors intention was to design a brief general measure that could be used easily across disciplines and countries using different languages.

In Cox's original development and presentation at the International Collegium of Rehabilitative Audiology (ICRA) in May of 2001, the original IOI-HA was given to several other professionals to translate. There have been 24 careful translations of the IOI-HA. It was not designed to replace outcome measures that are currently being used but to help with those existing measures when looking into research. It is also a quick way for busy clinics to cover several areas of hearing aid use and satisfaction if nothing else is done.

Description

Originally, the IOI-HA scale consisted of seven questions. An eighth question was added after the Norms were examined in 2002 (Cox et al., 2002) and is not included in the overall score but used to group results for the norm comparisons. The questions cover Use (1), Benefit (2), Residual Activity Limitations (3, 5), Satisfaction (4), Impact to Others (6), and Quality of Life (7).

It is scored on a 5-point scale. Each of the responses are specific to each question.

Application

The patient's responses should be obtained on a return mail format. Given to the patient about the 30-day postfit time frame at an appointment or mailed. A return postage paid envelope is enclosed with a return by date, no later than 6-months postfit.

The eight questions should be filled out by the patient themselves at home or away from the clinic, not by phone or face to face with the clinician.

Interpretation and Scoring

A higher number corresponds to a better outcome. The responses are specific to each question on a 5-point scale. Question one: Think about how much you used your present hearing aid(s) over the last 2 weeks. On an average day, how many hours did you use the hearing aid(s)? Which is answered by the amount of time, None to More than 8 hours per day. Question six "Over the past 2 weeks, with your present hearing aid(s), how much do you think other people were bothered by your hearing difficulties?," where the answers varied from "Very much" to "Not at all."

Advantages and Disadvantages

This is an appropriate questionnaire in large-group collection, spanning different languages. The U.S. Veteran Administration has implemented the IOI-HA in late 2008 to help identify trends in the VA population (Gonzenbach, 2010). The individual VA clinics are encouraged to use other standardized outcome measures in addition to the IOI-HA.

The IOI-HA norms in the United States lean more toward the VA population, which Smith, Noe, and Alexander (2009) showed higher outcomes from the original established norms, possibly because the population or the hearing aid technology was more current. This questionnaire is a fast way to obtain how the patient is doing, and it is used in many countries along with several languages. With the widespread use, the norm pool is the largest that most clinics are able to tap into.

Office Satisfaction Surveys

There are several surveys that relate to the user's overall satisfaction office and service delivery variables. An in-office adaptation of the ASHA survey (Appendix 16–K) can be filled out by patients in the office, or it can be mailed. Another quality-of-service survey by Martin (1997) helps clinicians focus on quality issues in their own practices (see Appendix 16–K). It is important that clinicians remain aware of other services besides hearing aid delivery that influence patients' satis-

faction. A remodeling project in the office, for instance, may interfere with mobility, patient flow, or scheduling. Any of these can reduce a patient's satisfaction with the overall hearing aid fitting process.

Industry Standards

Several surveys used by the hearing aid industry track hearing aid user satisfaction and other statistics. The MarkeTrack uses variations of the Knowles' Satisfaction and Benefit surveys (Kochkin, 1992, 1993, 1995, 2000, 2003, 2005, 2007). It is modified periodically to address changes in hearing aid technology and service delivery. The data are used by some audiologists to compare industry standards to the performance of individual offices or clinics. Some practices use this information to model incentive programs for their clinicians, using measures such as return-for-credit rate to reward employees whose rates are lower than the industry as a whole. *The Hearing Review, The Hearing Journal*, and Better Hearing Institute also publish national hearing aid dispensing trends and statistics.

A term that has come up is "Best Practices" in recent years. When it comes to fitting hearing aids, there has to be more than just the instruments themselves. Audiology has faced many challenges, and one that we need to face is the rise of internet sales. Audiologists will complain about how this is not the proper way to fit amplification, but complaining honestly in this authors opinion doesn't change the public wave. Internet sales are here to stay. One way to keep audiology prudent is putting our best practices where our mouths are, so to speak. Using tools, such as those described in this chapter can help. Using Real Ear, communication strategy hand outs, anything! We will always be crying how we are the best to fit aids, well then do something about it.

In the offices I run, we use COSI, HINT (Hearing In Noise), LACE, RealEar, and hand out communication strategies for both the patient and family members or close friends.

If we are able to bill for AR or separate testing, we take advantage of this, or in the case of private pay do a partial unbundling price structure.

CONCLUSION

An exhaustive list of self-reported measures is beyond the scope of this book and would be incomplete at any time, but there are some "tried and true" that have stood the test of time since the last publication. There are updates on Audiology Online and Hearing-HealthMatters.org periodically on Benefit and Satisfaction updates.

When selecting and using outcome measures, it is important to first ask what factor needs to be measured. Is the goal to predict acceptance, to determine perceived benefit, or to measure satisfaction in one or more dimension? The clinician must evaluate the tools that best measure the desired factor(s). When the appropriate scale or scales are selected, clinicians must apply them consistently in their practices to realize improvement for their patients and their practices. In the long run, the tools only help if we use them.

REVIEW QUESTIONS

1. What is the main procedural difference between the "Benefit" scales and the other three types of profiles?

2. Name the four areas of scales in this chapter.

3. Name two examples for each group.

4. Which scales could be used on an elderly population to help design an aural rehabilitation program? Name two.

5. When would be an appropriate time to give a scale on satisfaction?

REFERENCES

Abrams, H. B., & Hnath-Chisolm, T. (2000, in press). Outcome measures: Audiologic difference.

Alpiner, J., Chevrett, W., Glascoe, O., Metz, M., & Olsen, B. (1974). *The Denver Scale of Communication Function* (Unpublished study.) University of Denver, Colorado.

Arlinger, S. (2003). Negative consequences of uncorrected hearing loss-a review. *International Journal of Audiology, 42*(2), S17–S20.

Blamey, P., & Martin, L. (2009). Loudness and satisfaction ratings for hearing aid users. *Journal of the American Academy of Audiology, 20*(2), 272–282.

Cotugna, N., Vickery, C. E., & Carpenter-Haefele, K. M. (2005). Evaluation of literacy level of patient education pages in health-related journals. *Journal of Community Health, 30*(3), 213–219.

Cox, R. M. (1997). Administration and application of the APHAB. *The Hearing Journal, 50,* 32–48.

Cox, R. M., & Alexander, G. C. (1995). The abbreviated profile of hearing aid benefit. *Ear and Hearing, 16,* 176–186.

Cox, R. M., & Alexander, G. C. (1999). Measuring satisfaction with amplification in daily life: The SADL scale. *Ear and Hearing, 20*(4), 306.

Cox, R. M., & Alexander, G. C. (2000). Expectations about hearing aids and their relationship to fitting outcome. *Journal of the American Academy of Audiology, 11,* 368–382.

Cox, R. M., & Alexander, G. C. (2001). Validation of the SADL questionnaire. *Ear and Hearing, 22*(2), 151–160.

Cox, R. M., & Rivera, I. M. (1992). Predictability and reliability of hearing aid benefit measured using the PHAB. *Journal of the American Academy of Audiology, 3,* 242–254.

Cox, R., Hyde, M., Gatehouse, S., Noble, W., Dillon, H., Bentler, R., . . . & Hallberg, L. (2000). Optimal outcome measures, research priorities, and international cooperation. *Ear and Hearing, 21*(4), 106S–115S.

Cox, R. M., Stephens, D., & Kramer, S. E. (2002). Translations of the international outcome inventory for hearing aids (IOI-HA). *International Journal of Audiology, 202*(41), 3–26.

Dancer, J., & Gener, J. (1999). Survey on the use of adult hearing assessment scales. *The Hearing Review, 6*(1), 35.

Davis, A., Evans, M., Martin, M., & Orton, L. (2007). *Audiology modernisation: Clinical audit of NHS audiology services in Scotland.* MRC Hearing and Communication Group School of Psychological Sciences, University of Manchester.

Demorest, M. E., & Erdman, S. A. (1986). Scale composition and item analysis of the communication profile for the hearing impaired. *Journal of Speech and Hearing Research, 29,* 515–535.

Demorest, M. E., & Erdman, S. A. (1987). Development of the Communication Profile for the Hearing Impaired. *Journal of Speech and Hearing Disorders, 52,* 129–142.

Demorest, M. E., & Erdman, S. A. (1988). Retest stability of the Communication Profile for the Hearing Impaired. *Ear and Hearing, 9,* 237–242.

Demorest, M. E., & Erdman, S. A. (1990). *User's guide to the CPHI database system* (2nd ed.). Simpsonville, MD: CPHI Services.

Dillon, H. (1994). Shortened hearing aid profile inventory for the elderly. *Journal of Australian Audiology, 16,* 37–34.

Dillon, H., Birtles, G., & Lovegrove, R. (1999). Measuring the outcomes of a national rehabilitation program: Normative data for the Client Oriented Scale of Improvement (COSI) and the Hearing Aid User's Questionnaire (HAUQ). *Journal of the American Academy of Audiology, 10,* 67–79.

Dillon, H., James, A., & Ginis, J. (1997). Client Oriented Scale of Improvement (COSI) and its relationship to several other measures of benefit and satisfaction provided by hearing aids. *Journal of the American Academy of Audiology, 8,* 27–43.

Elkayam, J., & English K. (2003). Counseling adolescents with hearing loss with the use of self-assessment/significant other questionnaires. *Journal of the American Academy of Audiology, 14*(9), 485–499.

Erdman, S. A., Demorest, M. B., Wark, D. J., Skinner, M. W., Deming, J., Montano, J. J., & Madory, R. D. (1995). Psychosocial and behavioral adjustment to hearing impairment. *American Speech, Language and Hearing, 37*(10), 107.

Garstecki, D. C., & Erler, S. F. (1996). Older adult performance on the Communication Profile for the Hearing Impaired. *Journal of Speech and Hearing Research, 39,* 28–42.

Gatehouse, S. (1998). *The Glasgow Hearing Aid Benefit Profile: Derivation and validation of a client-centered outcome measure for hearing aid services* (Unpublished study). MRC Institute of Hearing Research (Scottish Section), Glasgow, Scotland.

Gatehouse, S. (1999). The Glasgow Hearing Aid Benefit Profile: Derivation and validation of a client-centered outcome measure for hearing aid services. *Journal of the American Academy of Audiology, 10,* 80–103.

Giolas, T. G., Owens, B., Lamb, S. H., & Schuber, E. E. (1979). Hearing Performance Inventory. *Journal of Speech and Hearing Disorders, 44,* 169–195.

Gonzenbach, S. A. (2010). *Selecting and using an outcome measure.* Presentation at the Joint Defense Veterans Audiology Conference.

Hawkins, D. B. (2005). Effectiveness of counseling-based adult group aural rehabilitation programs: A systematic review of the evidence. *Journal of the American Academy of Audiology, 16*(7), 485–493.

Henoch, M. A. (1998). Evaluation of the Hearing Performance Inventory-Short Form. *Journal of the Academy of Rehabilitative Audiology, 31,* 97–110.

High, W. S., Fairbanks, G., & Glorig, A. (1964). Scale for self-assessment of hearing handicap. *Journal of Speech and Hearing Disorders, 29,* 215–230.

Hosford-Dunn, H., & Baxter, J. H. (1985). Prediction and validation of hearing aid wearer benefit: Preliminary findings. *Hearing Instruments, 36,* 35–41.

Hosford-Dunn H., & Halpern, J. (2000). Clinical application of the Satisfaction with Amplification in Daily Life Scale in private practice I: Statistical, content, and factorial validity. *Journal of the American Academy of Audiology, 11,* 523–539.

Humes, L. E. (1999). Dimensions of hearing aid outcome. *Journal of the American Academy of Audiology, 10,* 26–39.

Humes, L. E., Wilson, D. L., Humes, L., Barlow, N. N., Garner, C. B., & Amos, N. (2002). A comparison of two measures of hearing aid satisfaction in a group of elderly hearing aid wearers. *Ear and Hearing, 23*(5), 422–427.

Hyde, M. L., Malizia, K., Riko, K., & Storms, D. (1992). *Evaluation of a self-assessment inventory for the hearing impaired* (Project Rep. No. 66064122-45). Toronto, Ontario, Canada: Mount Sinai Hospital, The Toronto Hospital, Otologic Function Unit.

Hyde, M. L., Malizia, K., Riko, K., & Storms, D. (1996). *CPHI results in a general clinical population.* Paper presented at the meeting of the Academy of Rehabilitative Audiology, Snowbird, UT.

Johnson, J. A., Cox, R. M., & Alexander, G. C. (2010). Development of APHAB norms for WDRC hearing aids and comparisons with original norms. *Ear and Hearing, 31*(1), 47–55.

Kaplan, H., Bally, S., Brandt, F., Busacco, D., & Pray, J. (1997). Communication Scale for Older Adults (CSOA). *Journal of the American Academy of Audiology, 8,* 203–217.

Kaplan, H., Feeley, J., & Brown, J. (1978). A modified Denver scale: Test-retest reliability. *Journal of the Academy of Rehabilitative Audiology, 11,* 15–32.

Kochkin, S. (1992). MarkeTrak III identifies key factors in determining consumer satisfaction. *The Hearing Journal, 45,* 39–44.

Kochkin, S. (1993). *Customer satisfaction with hearing instruments in the United States.* The Marketing Edge. Washington, DC: Hearing Industries Association.

Kochkin, S. (1995). *Subjective measures of satisfaction and benefit: Establishing norms.* Collaborative Marketing Committee (CMC).

Kochkin, S., (2000). MarkeTrak V: Why are my hearing aids in the drawer: The consumers' perspective. *The Hearing Journal, 53,* 34–42.

Kochkin, S. (2003). Isolating the impact of the volume control on customer satisfaction. *The Hearing Review, 10*(1), 26–35.

Kochkin, S. (2005). MarkeTrak VII: Customer satisfaction with hearing instruments in the digital age. *The Hearing Journal, 58*(9), 30–39.

Kochkin S. (2007). MarkeTrak VII: Obstacles to adult nonuser adoption of hearing aids. *The Hearing Journal, 60*(4), 24–50.

Kricos, P. B., Holmes, A. E., & Doyle, D. A. (1992). Efficacy of a communication training program for hearing-impaired elderly adults. *Journal of the Academy of Rehabilitative Audiology, 25*, 69–80.

Lamb, S. H., Owens, B., & Schubert, E. E. (1983). The revised form of the hearing performance inventory. *Ear and Hearing, 4*, 152–157.

McCarthy, P. A., & Alpiner, J. G. (1983). An assessment scale of hearing handicap for use in family counseling. *Journal of the Academy of Rehabilitative Audiology, 16*, 256–270.

Martin, R. L. (1997). Nuts and bolts; Are you providing quality service? *The Hearing Journal, 8*, 66.

Miller, L., Zapala, D., & Heckman, M. (2010). *Development and validation of new subscales for the hearing handicap inventory for adults and their relationship to WHO ICF constructs.* **AudiologyNow** (Poster session).

Montgomery, A. A., Walden, B. E., Schwartz, D. M., & Prosek, R. A. (1984). Training auditory-visual speech reception in adults with moderate sensorineural hearing loss. *Ear and Hearing, 5*, 30–36.

Mueller, H. G., & Palmer, C. V. (1998). The profile of aided loudness: A new "PAL" for 98. *The Hearing Journal, 51*, 10–19.

Newman, C. W., & Weinstein, B. E. (1988). Test-retest reliability of the Hearing Handicap Inventory for the Elderly using two administration approaches. *Ear and Hearing, 10*, 90–191.

Newman, C. W., & Weinstein, B. E. (1989). The Hearing Handicap Inventory for the Elderly as a measure of hearing aid benefit. *Ear and Hearing, 9*, 81–85.

Newman, C. W., Weinstein, B. E., Jacobson, G. P., & Hug, G. A. (1990). The Hearing Handicap Inventory for Adults: Psychometric adequacy and audiometric correlates. *Ear and Hearing, 11*, 430–433.

Newman, C. W., Weinstein, B. E., Jacobson, G. P., & Hug, G. A. (1991). Test-retest reliability of the Hearing Handicap Inventory for Adults. *Ear and Hearing, 12*, 355–357.

Noble, W. G., & Atherley, G. R. C. (1970). The Hearing Measure Scale: A questionnaire for the assessment of auditory disability. *Journal of Auditory Research, 10*, 229–250.

Owens, E., & Fujikawa, S. (1980). The Hearing Performance Inventory and hearing aid use in profound hearing loss. *Journal of Speech and Hearing Research, 23*, 470–479.

Rubinstein, A., & Boothroyd, A. (1987). The effect of two approaches to auditory training on speech recognition by hearing impaired adults. *Journal of Speech and Hearing Research, 30*, 153–160.

Sabes, H. J., & Sweetow, R. W. (2007). Variables predicting outcomes on listening and communication enhancement (LACE) training. *International Journal of Audiology, 46*(7), 374–383.

Schow, R. L., & Nerbonne, M. A. (1980). Hearing handicap and Denver scales. Applications, categories, interpretation. *Journal of the Academy of Rehabilitative Audiology, 13*, 66–77.

Schow, R. L., & Nerbonne, M. A. (1982). Communication Screening Profile: Use with elderly clients. *Ear and Hearing, 3*, 135–147.

Schow, R., & Tannahill, C. (1977). Hearing handicap scores and categories for subjects with normal and impaired hearing sensitivity. *Journal of the American Auditory Society, 3*, 134–139.

Schum, D. J. (1992). Responses of elderly hearing aid users on the Hearing Aid Performance Inventory. *Journal of the American Academy of Audiology, 3*, 308–314.

Schum, D. J. (1999). Perceived hearing aid benefit in relation to perceived needs. *Journal of the American Academy of Audiology, 10*, 40–45.

Schum, D. J. (2013). *Course #21732. Does the fitting satisfy the patient?* Retrieved from Audiologyonline.com

Singer, J., Healey, J., & Preece, J. (1997). Hearing instruments: A psychologic and behavioral perspective. *High Performance Hearing Solutions, 1*, 23–27.

Smith, S. L., Noe, C. M., & Alexander, G. C. (2009). Evaluation of the international outcome inventory for hearing aids in a veteran sample. *Journal of the American Academy of Audiology, 20*(6), 374–380.

Song, J. H., Skoe, E., Banai, K., & Kraus, N. (2011) Training to improve hearing speech in noise: Biological mechanisms. *Oxford Journals: Cerebral Cortex.* Retrieved from http://cercor.oxfordjournals.org/content/early/2011/07/28/cercor.bhr196.full

Sweetow, R., & Palmer, C. V. (2005). Efficacy of individual auditory training in adults: A systematic review of the evidence. *Journal of the American Academy of Audiology, 16*(7), 494–504.

Sweetow, R., & Sabes, J. H. (2006). The need for and development of an adaptive listening and communication enhancement (LACE) program. *Journal of the American Academy of Audiology, 17*(8), 538–558.

Sweetow, R. W., & Sabes, J. H. (2010). Auditory training and challenges associated with participation and compliance. *Journal of the American Academy of Audiology, 21*(9), 586–593.

Taylor, B., & Mueller, H. G. (2012). Getting aided loudness right: A three step approach. *Audiology Practices, 4*(1), 16–23.

Tomioka, K., Ikeda, H., Hanaie, K., Morikawa, M., Iwamoto, J., Okamoto, N., . . . Kurumatani, N. (2013). The Hearing Handicap Inventory for Elderly-Screening (HHIE-S) versus a single question: Reliability, validity, and relations with quality of life measures in the elderly community, Japan. *Quality Life Research, 22*(5), 1151–1159.

Ventry, I., & Weinstein, B. (1982). The Hearing Handicap Inventory for the Elderly: A new tool. *Ear and Hearing, 3*, 128–134.

Walden, B. E., Demorest, M. E., & Hepler, E. E. (1984). Self-report approach to assessment benefit derived from amplification. *Journal of Speech and Hearing Research, 27,* 49–56.

Weinstein, B., Spitzer J., & Ventry, I. (1986). Test-retest reliability of the Hearing Handicap Inventory for the Elderly. *Ear and Hearing, 7,* 295–299.

Zarnoch, J. M., & Alpiner, J. G. (1977). The Denver scale of communication function for senior citizens living in retirement centers. In *The handbook of adult rehabilitative audiology* (2nd ed.). Baltimore, MD: Williams & Wilkins.

APPENDIX 16–A
· COMMUNICATION SCALE FOR OLDER ADULTS

INSTRUCTIONS: Please read each situation. Decide if the situation is true. **Please respond to each question.**

Communication Strategies

Please read each situation. Decide if the situation is true:

   3-point: (1) Almost always, (2) Sometimes, or (3) Almost never

   5-point: (1) Always, (2) Almost always, (3) Sometimes, (4) Almost never, or (5) Never

Please circle the appropriate answer. PLEASE RESPOND TO EACH QUESTION.

1. You are talking with someone you do not know well. You do not understand. You ask her to repeat.
   (1) Almost always   (2) Sometimes   (3) Almost never
   (1) Always   (2) Almost always   (3) Sometimes   (4) Almost never   (5) Never

2. You are talking with two people. You are not understanding. You change the topic so that you can control the conversation.
   (1) Almost always   (2) Sometimes   (3) Almost never
   (1) Always   (2) Almost always   (3) Sometimes   (4) Almost never   (5) Never

3. You ask a stranger for directions. You understand part of what he says. You tell him the part you understand and ask him to repeat the rest.
   (1) Almost always   (2) Sometimes   (3) Almost never
   (1) Always   (2) Almost always   (3) Sometimes   (4) Almost never   (5) Never

4. A friend introduces you to a new person. You do not understand the person's name. You ask the person to spell her name.
   (1) Almost always   (2) Sometimes   (3) Almost never
   (1) Always   (2) Almost always   (3) Sometimes   (4) Almost never   (5) Never

5. A stranger spells his name for you. You miss the first two letters. You ask him to say each letter and a word starting with that letter (A as in Apple, B as in Boy).
   (1) Almost always   (2) Sometimes   (3) Almost never
   (1) Always   (2) Almost always   (3) Sometimes   (4) Almost never   (5) Never

6. A person tells you his address. You do not understand. You ask him to repeat the street number, one number at a time.
   (1) Almost always   (2) Sometimes   (3) Almost never
   (1) Always   (2) Almost always   (3) Sometimes   (4) Almost never   (5) Never

7. You are talking with one person but are not understanding. You interrupt the person before he finishes to say what you think.
   (1) Almost always   (2) Sometimes   (3) Almost never
   (1) Always   (2) Almost always   (3) Sometimes   (4) Almost never   (5) Never

8. Your friend asks you to buy seven hamburgers. You do not understand how many he wants. You ask him to start counting from zero and stop at the correct number.
(1) Almost always   (2) Sometimes   (3) Almost never
(1) Always   (2) Almost always   (3) Sometimes   (4) Almost never   (5) Never

9. You are at a meeting. The speaker says something you do not understand. You pretend to understand and hope to get the information later.
(1) Almost always   (2) Sometimes   (3) Almost never
(1) Always   (2) Almost always   (3) Sometimes   (4) Almost never   (5) Never

10. Two people are talking. You do not understand the conversation. You ask them to tell you the topic.
(1) Almost always   (2) Sometimes   (3) Almost never
(1) Always   (2) Almost always   (3) Sometimes   (4) Almost never   (5) Never

11. You are talking with one person in a restaurant. His face is in the shadows. You know you could understand better if you changed seats with him. You ask to change seats.
(1) Almost always   (2) Sometimes   (3) Almost never
(1) Always   (2) Almost always   (3) Sometimes   (4) Almost never   (5) Never

12. You are visiting the doctor. He tells you what to do for your illness. You do not understand his speech. You ask him to write.
(1) Almost always   (2) Sometimes   (3) Almost never
(1) Always   (2) Almost always   (3) Sometimes   (4) Almost never   (5) Never

13. You are at a meeting. The speaker does not look at you when he talks. You feel angry but do nothing about it.
(1) Almost always   (2) Sometimes   (3) Almost never
(1) Always   (2) Almost always   (3) Sometimes   (4) Almost never   (5) Never

14. You are at a meeting. You realize you are too far from the speaker to understand him. There are empty seats in the front of the room. You change your seat.
(1) Almost always   (2) Sometimes   (3) Almost never
(1) Always   (2) Almost always   (3) Sometimes   (4) Almost never   (5) Never

15. You are at a meeting. You are the only hard-of-hearing person. You are afraid that you will not understand, but you do not ask for help. You do the best you can.
(1) Almost always   (2) Sometimes   (3) Almost never
(1) Always   (2) Almost always   (3) Sometimes   (4) Almost never   (5) Never

16. You are talking to the dentist. He speaks very fast. You cannot lip-read him. You ask him to slow down.
(1) Almost always   (2) Sometimes   (3) Almost never
(1) Always   (2) Almost always   (3) Sometimes   (4) Almost never   (5) Never

17. You are taking a class. The teacher talks while she writes on the board. You talk to her after class. You explain that you need her to face you in order to speech read.
(1) Almost always   (2) Sometimes   (3) Almost never
(1) Always   (2) Almost always   (3) Sometimes   (4) Almost never   (5) Never

18. A speaker likes to move around the room while she lectures. You have problems reading her lips. You ask her after class to lecture from one place in the room.
    (1) Almost always   (2) Sometimes   (3) Almost never
    (1) Always   (2) Almost always   (3) Sometimes   (4) Almost never   (5) Never

19. You are going to a series of meetings or lectures. You ask the speaker to use slides, pictures, or the overhead projector whenever possible.
    (1) Almost always   (2) Sometimes   (3) Almost never
    (1) Always   (2) Almost always   (3) Sometimes   (4) Almost never   (5) Never

20. You are going to a series of meetings or lectures. You ask the speaker to find a person to take notes for you.
    (1) Almost always   (2) Sometimes   (3) Almost never
     (1) Always (2) Almost always 3) Sometimes (4) Almost never (5) Never

21. You are going to a series of meetings or lectures. You ask for an outline or a reading list.
    (1) Almost always   (2) Sometimes   (3) Almost never
    (1) Always   (2) Almost always   (3) Sometimes   (4) Almost never   (5) Never

22. You are going to a play. You read the play or reviews of the play before you see it.
    (1) Almost always   (2) Sometimes   (3) Almost never
    (1) Always   (2) Almost always   (3) Sometimes   (4) Almost never   (5) Never

23. You are talking with a clerk at the bank. A fire truck goes by. You ask him to stop talking until the noise stops.
    (1) Almost always   (2) Sometimes   (3) Almost never
    (1) Always   (2) Almost always   (3) Sometimes   (4) Almost never   (5) Never

24. You ask a person to repeat because you don't understand. He seems annoyed. You stop asking and pretend to understand.
    (1) Almost always   (2) Sometimes   (3) Almost never
    (1) Always   (2) Almost always   (3) Sometimes   (4) Almost never   (5) Never

25. You ask a stranger for directions to a place. You really want to understand his speech. You ask very specific questions like: "Is this place north or south of here?"
    (1) Almost always   (2) Sometimes   (3) Almost never
    (1) Always   (2) Almost always   (3) Sometimes   (4) Almost never   (5) Never

26. You need to ask directions. You avoid asking a stranger because you think you will have trouble understanding him.
    (1) Almost always   (2) Sometimes   (3) Almost never
    (1) Always   (2) Almost always   (3) Sometimes   (4) Almost never   (5) Never

27. You are at a store. You have trouble hearing the clerk because his voice is soft. You explain you are hearing impaired and ask him to talk louder.
    (1) Almost always   (2) Sometimes   (3) Almost never
    (1) Always   (2) Almost always   (3) Sometimes   (4) Almost never   (5) Never

28. You ask your family or friends to get your attention before they speak to you.
(1) Almost always   (2) Sometimes   (3) Almost never
(1) Always   (2) Almost always   (3) Sometimes   (4) Almost never   (5) Never

29. You are with five or six friends. You miss something important. You ask the person next to you what was said.
(1) Almost always   (2) Sometimes   (3) Almost never
(1) Always   (2) Almost always   (3) Sometimes   (4) Almost never   (5) Never

30. You have trouble understanding a man who is chewing gum. You explain that you need to speech read. You politely ask him to remove the gum when he talks.
(1) Almost always   (2) Sometimes   (3) Almost never
(1) Always   (2) Almost always   (3) Sometimes   (4) Almost never   (5) Never

31. You try to avoid people when you know you will have trouble understanding them.
(1) Almost always   (2) Sometimes   (3) Almost never
(1) Always   (2) Almost always   (3) Sometimes   (4) Almost never   (5) Never

32. You hate to bother other people with your hearing problem, so you pretend to understand.
(1) Almost always   (2) Sometimes   (3) Almost never
(1) Always   (2) Almost always   (3) Sometimes   (4) Almost never   (5) Never

33. You avoid wearing your hearing aid because it makes you feel different.
(1) Almost always   (2) Sometimes   (3) Almost never
(1) Always   (2) Almost always   (3) Sometimes   (4) Almost never   (5) Never

34. You are at a lecture on a subject of great interest. There is a microphone, but the speaker does not use it. You raise your hand and request that the speaker use the microphone.
(1) Almost always   (2) Sometimes   (3) Almost never
(1) Always   (2) Almost always   (3) Sometimes   (4) Almost never   (5) Never

35. You are at a lecture on a subject of great interest. There is a microphone, but it is not set loud enough for you to understand. You leave the meeting angry to complain to someone "in charge."
(1) Almost always   (2) Sometimes   (3) Almost never
(1) Always   (2) Almost always   (3) Sometimes   (4) Almost never   (5) Never

36. You are at a lecture on a subject of great interest. The speaker is talking too fast for you to understand. You leave the lecture because it has become a waste of time.
(1) Almost always   (2) Sometimes   (3) Almost never
(1) Always   (2) Almost always   (3) Sometimes   (4) Almost never   (5) Never

37. You are at a lecture on a subject of great interest. The speaker moves around so much that you have trouble understanding her. You complain to the organizers of the lecture after it is over.
(1) Almost always   (2) Sometimes   (3) Almost never
(1) Always   (2) Almost always   (3) Sometimes   (4) Almost never   (5) Never

38. You are at a holiday dinner. You can't understand the conversation because everyone is talking at once. You promise yourself you will not go back next year.
(1) Almost always   (2) Sometimes   (3) Almost never
(1) Always   (2) Almost always   (3) Sometimes   (4) Almost never   (5) Never

39. You are at a holiday dinner. You can't understand the conversation because everyone is talking at once. You ask for everyone's attention, explain the problem, and ask people to take turns so you can understand.
(1) Almost always   (2) Sometimes   (3) Almost never
(1) Always   (2) Almost always   (3) Sometimes   (4) Almost never   (5) Never

40. You are at a holiday dinner. You can't understand the conversation because everyone is talking at once. You explain the problem to the host so that he can handle the situation.
(1) Almost always   (2) Sometimes   (3) Almost never
(1) Always   (2) Almost always   (3) Sometimes   (4) Almost never   (5) Never

41. You are at a holiday dinner. You can't understand the conversation because everyone is talking at once. However, you don't say anything because you are glad to be at the party.
(1) Almost always   (2) Sometimes   (3) Almost never
(1) Always   (2) Almost always   (3) Sometimes   (4) Almost never   (5) Never

Attitudes

Please read each situation. Decide if the situation is true:

    3-point: (1) Almost always, (2) Sometimes, or (3) Almost never

    5-point: (1) Always, (2) Almost always, (3) Sometimes, (4) Almost never, or (5) Never

Please circle the appropriate answer. **Please respond to each question.**

1. I feel embarrassed when I don't understand someone.
(1) Almost always   (2) Sometimes   (3) Almost never
(1) Always   (2) Almost always   (3) Sometimes   (4) Almost never   (5) Never

2. I get upset when I can't follow a conversation.
(1) Almost always   (2) Sometimes   (3) Almost never
(1) Always   (2) Almost always   (3) Sometimes   (4) Almost never   (5) Never

3. I become angry when people do not speak clearly enough for me to understand.
(1) Almost always   (2) Sometimes   (3) Almost never
(1) Always   (2) Almost always   (3) Sometimes   (4) Almost never   (5) Never

4. I feel stupid when I misunderstand what a person is saying.
(1) Almost always   (2) Sometimes   (3) Almost never
(1) Always   (2) Almost always   (3) Sometimes   (4) Almost never   (5) Never

5. It's hard for me to ask someone to repeat things. I feel embarrassed.
(1) Almost always   (2) Sometimes   (3) Almost never
(1) Always   (2) Almost always   (3) Sometimes   (4) Almost never   (5) Never

6. Most people think I could understand better if I paid more attention.
(1) Almost always (2) Sometimes (3) Almost never
(1) Always (2) Almost always (3) Sometimes (4) Almost never (5) Never

7. I get angry when people speak too softly or too fast.
(1) Almost always (2) Sometimes (3) Almost never
(1) Always (2) Almost always (3) Sometimes (4) Almost never (5) Never

8. Sometimes I can't follow conversations at home. I still feel part of family life.
(1) Almost always (2) Sometimes (3) Almost never
(1) Always (2) Almost always (3) Sometimes (4) Almost never (5) Never

9. I feel frustrated when I try to communicate with people.
(1) Almost always (2) Sometimes (3) Almost never
(1) Always (2) Almost always (3) Sometimes (4) Almost never (5) Never

10. Most people do not understand what it is like to be hard of hearing. This makes me angry.
(1) Almost always (2) Sometimes (3) Almost never
(1) Always (2) Almost always (3) Sometimes (4) Almost never (5) Never

11. I am ashamed of being hearing impaired.
(1) Almost always (2) Sometimes (3) Almost never
(1) Always (2) Almost always (3) Sometimes (4) Almost never (5) Never

12. I get angry when someone speaks with his mouth covered or with his back to me.
(1) Almost always (2) Sometimes (3) Almost never
(1) Always (2) Almost always (3) Sometimes (4) Almost never (5) Never

13. I prefer to be alone most of the time.
(1) Almost always (2) Sometimes (3) Almost never
(1) Always (2) Almost always (3) Sometimes (4) Almost never (5) Never

14. My hearing loss makes me nervous.
(1) Almost always (2) Sometimes (3) Almost never
(1) Always (2) Almost always (3) Sometimes (4) Almost never (5) Never

15. My hearing loss makes me depressed.
(1) Almost always (2) Sometimes (3) Almost never
(1) Always (2) Almost always (3) Sometimes (4) Almost never (5) Never

16. My family does not understand my hearing loss.
(1) Almost always (2) Sometimes (3) Almost never
(1) Always (2) Almost always (3) Sometimes (4) Almost never (5) Never

17. I get annoyed when people shout at me because I have a hearing loss.
(1) Almost always (2) Sometimes (3) Almost never
(1) Always (2) Almost always (3) Sometimes (4) Almost never (5) Never

18. People treat me like a stupid person when I don't understand their speech.
(1) Almost always   (2) Sometimes   (3) Almost never
(1) Always   (2) Almost always   (3) Sometimes   (4) Almost never   (5) Never

19. Hard of hearing and hearing people often have difficulty communicating. It is only the responsibility of the hearing person to improve communication.
(1) Almost always   (2) Sometimes   (3) Almost never
(1) Always   (2) Almost always   (3) Sometimes   (4) Almost never   (5) Never

20. Hard of hearing and hearing people often have difficulty communicating. It is only the responsibility of the hard of hearing person to improve communication.
(1) Almost always   (2) Sometimes   (3) Almost never
(1) Always   (2) Almost always   (3) Sometimes   (4) Almost never   (5) Never

21. Members of my family get annoyed when I have trouble understanding them.
(1) Almost always   (2) Sometimes   (3) Almost never
(1) Always   (2) Almost always   (3) Sometimes   (4) Almost never   (5) Never

22. People who know I have a hearing loss think I can hear when I want to.
(1) Almost always   (2) Sometimes   (3) Almost never
(1) Always   (2) Almost always   (3) Sometimes   (4) Almost never   (5) Never

23. Members of my family leave me out of conversations.
(1) Almost always   (2) Sometimes   (3) Almost never
(1) Always   (2) Almost always   (3) Sometimes   (4) Almost never   (5) Never

24. Hearing aids don't always help people understand speech, but they can help in other ways.
(1) Almost always   (2) Sometimes   (3) Almost never
(1) Always   (2) Almost always   (3) Sometimes   (4) Almost never   (5) Never

25. I feel speech reading is helpful to me.
(1) Almost always   (2) Sometimes   (3) Almost never
(1) Always   (2) Almost always   (3) Sometimes   (4) Almost never   (5) Never

26. Even though people know I have a hearing loss, they don't help me by speaking clearly or repeating.
(1) Almost always   (2) Sometimes   (3) Almost never
(1) Always   (2) Almost always   (3) Sometimes   (4) Almost never   (5) Never

27. My family is willing to make telephone calls for me.
(1) Almost always   (2) Sometimes   (3) Almost never
(1) Always   (2) Almost always   (3) Sometimes   (4) Almost never   (5) Never

28. My family is willing to repeat as often as necessary when I don't understand them.
(1) Almost always   (2) Sometimes   (3) Almost never
(1) Always   (2) Almost always   (3) Sometimes   (4) Almost never   (5) Never

29. People get frustrated when I don't understand what they say.
(1) Almost always   (2) Sometimes   (3) Almost never
(1) Always   (2) Almost always   (3) Sometimes   (4) Almost never   (5) Never

30. Members of my family make it easy for me to speech read them.
   (1) Almost always   (2) Sometimes   (3) Almost never
   (1) Always   (2) Almost always   (3) Sometimes   (4) Almost never   (5) Never

31. Strangers make it easy for me to speech read them.
   (1) Almost always   (2) Sometimes   (3) Almost never
   (1) Always   (2) Almost always   (3) Sometimes   (4) Almost never   (5) Never

Source: Kaplan, H. (1997). Communication Scale for Older Adults. *Journal of the American Academy of Audiology, 8,* 203–217. Copyright 1997 American Academy of Audiology. Reprinted with permission.

APPENDIX 16–B
HEARING HANDICAP INVENTORY FOR
THE ELDERLY—SCREENER

INSTRUCTIONS: The purpose of this questionnaire is to identify the problems your hearing loss may be causing you. Circle Yes, Sometimes, or No for each question. **Do not skip a question if you avoid a situation because of a hearing problem.**

E-1	Does your hearing problem cause you to feel embarrassed when meeting new people?	Yes	Sometimes	No
E-2	Does a hearing problem cause you to feel frustrated when talking to members of your family?	Yes	Sometimes	No
S-1	Do you have difficulty when someone speaks in a whisper?	Yes	Sometimes	No
E-3	Do you feel handicapped by a hearing problem?	Yes	Sometimes	No
S-2	Does a hearing problem cause you to visit friends, relatives, or neighbors less often than you would like?	Yes	Sometimes	No
S-3	Does a hearing problem cause you to attend religious services less often than you would like?	Yes	Sometimes	No
E-4	Does a hearing problem cause you to have arguments with family members?	Yes	Sometimes	No
S-4	Does a hearing problem cause you difficulty when listening to the TV or radio?	Yes	Sometimes	No
E-5	Do you feel that any difficulty with your hearing limits or hampers your personal or social life?	Yes	Sometimes	No
S-5	Does a hearing problem cause you difficulty when in a restaurant with relatives or friends?	Yes	Sometimes	No

Score E:

Score S:

Score T:

Source: Reprinted with permission of Barbara Weinstein.

APPENDIX 16–C
HEARING HANDICAP INVENTORY FOR THE ELDERLY

INSTRUCTIONS: The purpose of this questionnaire is to identify the problems your hearing loss may be causing you. Circle Yes, Sometimes, or No for each question. **Do not skip a question if you avoid a situation because of a hearing problem.**

S-1	Does your hearing problem cause you to use the phone less often than you would like?	Yes	Sometimes	No
E-2	Does your hearing problem cause you to feel embarrassed when meeting new people?	Yes	Sometimes	No
S-3	Does your hearing problem cause you to avoid groups of people?	Yes	Sometimes	No
E-4	Does a hearing problem make you irritable?	Yes	Sometimes	No
E-5	Does a hearing problem cause you to feel frustrated when talking to members of your family?	Yes	Sometimes	No
S-6	Does a hearing problem cause you difficulty when attending a party?	Yes	Sometimes	No
E-7	Does a hearing problem cause you to feel "stupid" or "dumb"?	Yes	Sometimes	No
S-8	Do you have difficulty when someone speaks in a whisper?	Yes	Sometimes	No
E-9	Do you feel handicapped by a hearing problem?	Yes	Sometimes	No
E-10	Does a hearing problem cause you difficulty when visiting friends, relatives, or neighbors?	Yes	Sometimes	No
S-11	Does a hearing problem cause you to attend religious services less often than you would like?	Yes	Sometimes	No
E-12	Does a hearing problem cause you to be nervous?	Yes	Sometimes	No
S-13	Does a hearing problem cause you to visit friends, relatives, or neighbors less often than you would like?	Yes	Sometimes	No
S-14	Does a hearing problem cause you to have arguments with family members?	Yes	Sometimes	No
S-15	Does a hearing problem cause you difficulty when listening to the TV or radio?	Yes	Sometimes	No
S-16	Does a hearing problem cause you to go shopping less often than you would like?	Yes	Sometimes	No

E-17	Does any problem or difficulty with your hearing upset you at all?	Yes	Sometimes	No
E-18	Does a hearing problem cause you to want to be by yourself?	Yes	Sometimes	No
S-19	Does a hearing problem cause you to talk to family members less often than you would like?	Yes	Sometimes	No
E-20	Do you feel that any difficulty with your hearing limits or hampers your personal or social life?	Yes	Sometimes	No
S-21	Does a hearing problem cause you difficulty when in a restaurant with relatives or friends?	Yes	Sometimes	No
E-22	Does a hearing problem cause you to feel depressed?	Yes	Sometimes	No
S-23	Does a hearing problem cause you to listen to TV or radio less often than you would like?	Yes	Sometimes	No
E-24	Does a hearing problem cause you to feel uncomfortable when talking to friends?	Yes	Sometimes	No
E-25	Does a hearing problem cause you to feel left out when you are with a group of people?	Yes	Sometimes	No

Score E:

Score S:

Score T:

Source: Reprinted with permission of Barbara Weinstein.

APPENDIX 16–D
HEARING PERFORMANCE INVENTORY REVISED

We are interested in knowing how your hearing problem has affected your daily living. Below you will find a series of questions that describe a variety of everyday listening situations and ask you to judge how much difficulty you would have hearing in these situations. Once we know which situations cause a person difficulty, we can begin to do something about them. Your answers will be confidential.

The questions cover many different listening situations. Some ask you to judge how well you can understand what people are saying when their voices are loud enough. The term *understand* means hearing the words a person is saying clearly enough to be able to participate in the conversation. Other questions ask whether you can hear enough of a particular sound (doorbell, speech, etc.) to be aware of its presence. Other questions concern occupational, social, or personal situations. Still others ask what you *do* when you miss something that was said.

To answer each question, you are asked to check the phrase that best describes how often you experience the situation being described:

Practically always	(or always)
Frequently	(about three-quarters of the time)
About half the time	
Occasionally	(about a quarter of the time)
Almost never	(or never)

For example, if you can understand what a person is saying on the telephone about 100% of the time, then you should check *practically always*. On the other hand, if you can understand almost nothing of what a person is saying on the telephone, then you should check *almost never*. If you can understand what a person is saying on the telephone about 50% of the time, then you should check *about half the time.*

Your answers to the questions should describe your hearing ability as it is now. If you wear a hearing aid in the situation described, answer the question accordingly. Please check one, and only one, phrase for each question. You should check *Does not apply* only if you have not experienced a particular situation or one similar to it.

There are also questions that appear identical but differ in at least one important detail. Please read each question carefully before checking the appropriate phrase.

We know that all people do not talk alike. Some mumble, others talk too fast, and others talk without moving their lips very much. Please answer the questions according to the way most people talk to you.

If the question does not specify whether the person speaking is male or female, answer according to which gender you have the most difficulty hearing.

1. You are watching your favorite news program on television. Can you understand the news reporter (female) when her voice is loud enough for you?

2. You are reading in a room with music or noise in the background. Can you hear a person calling you from another room?

3. You are with a male friend or family member in a fairly quiet room. Can you understand him when his voice is loud enough for you and you can see his face?

4. Can you hear an airplane in the sky when others around you can hear it?

5. You are watching a drama or movie on television. Can you understand what is being said when the speaker's voice is loud enough for you and there is music in the background?

6. Can you understand what a woman is saying on the telephone when her voice is loud enough for you?

7. You are at a restaurant and you hear only a portion of something the waitress/waiter said. Do you repeat the portion when asking him/her for a repetition?

8. You are with a child (6–10 years old) in a fairly quiet room. Can you understand the child when his/her voice is loud enough for you and you can see his/her face?

9. You are the driver in an automobile with several friends or family members. One or more of the windows are open. Can you understand the passenger behind you when his/her voice is loud enough for you?

10. You are at a restaurant and there is background noise such as music or a crowd of people. Can you understand the waiter/waitress when his/her voice is loud enough for you and you can see his/her face?

11. You are talking with a close friend. When you miss something important that was said, do you immediately adjust your hearing aid to help you hear better?

12. You are with five or six strangers at a gathering of more than 20 people and there is background noise such as music or a crowd of people. One person talks at a time. When you are aware of the subject, can you understand what is being said when the speaker's voice is loud enough for you and you can see his/her face?

13. You are at a play, movie, or are listening to a speech. When you miss something important that was said, do you ask the person with you?

14. You are with a child (6–10 years old) and several people are talking nearby. Can you understand the child when his/her voice is loud enough for you and you can see his/her face?

15. You are playing cards, Monopoly, or some similar game with several people and there is background noise such as music or a crowd of people. Can you understand what a friend or family member is saying to you when his/her voice is loud enough for you and you can see his/her face?

16. Does your hearing problem discourage you from attending lectures?

17. You are talking with five or six friends. When you miss something important that was said, do you ask the person talking to repeat it?

18. You are in an auditorium listening to a lecturer (female) who is using a microphone. Can you understand what she is saying when her voice is loud enough for you and you can see her face?

19. Can you hear water running in another room when others around you can hear it?

20. You are with a friend or family member and you hear only a portion of what was said. Do you repeat that portion before asking him/her for a repetition?

21. You are at a party or gathering of less than 10 people and the room is fairly quiet. Can you understand what a friend or family member is saying to you when his/her voice is loud enough for you, but you cannot see his/her face?

22. Does your hearing problem lower your self confidence?

23. You are in a fairly quiet room with five or six strangers. One person talks at a time. When you are aware of the subject, can you understand what is being said when the speaker's voice is loud enough for you, but you cannot see his/her face?

24. You are with five or six friends or family members at a gathering of more than 20 people and several people are talking nearby. One person talks at a time and the subject of conversation changes from time to time. Can you understand what is being said when the speaker's voice is loud enough for you and you can see his/her face?

25. When an announcement is given over a public address system in a bus station or airport, is it loud enough for you to hear?

26. You are talking with a stranger. When you miss something important that was said, do you ask for it to be repeated?

27. You are talking with a friend or family member. When you miss something important that was said do you pretend you understood?

28. You are at a fairly quiet restaurant. Can you understand the waiter/waitress when his/her voice is loud enough for you and you can see his/her face?

29. You are seated with five or six strangers around a table or in a living room. Often two persons are talking at once and one person frequently interrupts another. When you miss something important that was said, do you pretend you understood?

30. You are playing cards, Monopoly, or some similar game and the room is fairly quiet. The subject of conversation changes from time to time. Can you understand what is being said when the speaker's voice is loud enough for you, but you can his/her face?

31. You are at a party or gathering of less than 10 people and the room is fairly quiet. Can you understand what a friend or family member is saying to you when the speaker's voice is loud enough for you and you can see his/her face?

32. Does your hearing problem discourage you from going to concerts?

33. Do you find that children (6–10 years old) speak loudly enough for you?

34. When an announcement is given over a public address system in a bus station or airport, can you understand what is being said when the speaker's voice is loud enough for you?

35. You are seated with five or six strangers around a table or in a living room. Often two persons are talking at once and one person frequently interrupts another. Can you understand what is being said when the speaker's voice is loud enough for you and you can see his/her face?

36. You are seated with five or six friends around a table or in a living room. Often two persons are talking at once and one person frequently interrupts another. When you miss something that was said, do you ask the person talking to repeat it?

37. You are with a female stranger in a fairly quiet room. Can you understand her when her voice is loud enough for you and you can see her face?

38. You are with a stranger and there is background noise such as music or a crowd of people. Can you understand the person when his/her voice is loud enough for you, but you cannot see his/her face?

39. Does your hearing problem tend to make you impatient?

40. You are talking with five or six strangers. When you miss something important that was said, do you let the person talking know you have a hearing problem?

41. You are at a party or gathering of less than 10 people and several people are talking nearby. Can you understand what a friend or family member (female) is saying to you when her voice is loud enough for you and you can see her face?

42. Does your hearing problem discourage you from going to plays?

43. You are having dinner with five or six friends. When you miss something important that was said, do you ask the person talking to repeat it?

44. You are at a restaurant with a friend or family member and there is background noise such as music or a crowd of people. Can you understand the person when his/her voice is loud enough for you and you can see his/her face?

45. When you have difficulty understanding a person who speaks quite rapidly, do you ask him/her to speak more slowly?

46. You are talking to a woman sitting in a ticket or information booth and it is fairly noisy. She is giving directions or information. Can you understand her when her voice is loud enough for you and you can see her face?

47. You are having dinner with five or six friends. When you miss something important that was said, do you ask the person talking to repeat it?

48. When others are listening to speech on the radio or television, is it loud enough for you?

49. Does your hearing problem discourage you from going to the movies?

50. You are riding in an automobile with several friends or family members. One or more of the windows are open and you are sitting in the front seat. Can you understand the driver when his/her voice is loud enough for you and you can see his/her face?

51. You are at home watching television or listening to the radio. Can you hear the doorbell ring when it is located in the same room?

52. You are in a fairly quiet room talking with five or six strangers. One person talks at a time and the subject of conversation changes from time to time. Can you understand what is being said when the speaker's voice is loud enough for you and you can see his/her face?

53. You are seated with five or six friends or family members around a table or in a living room. Often two persons are talking at once and one person frequently interrupts another. When you miss something important that was said, do you remind the person talking that you have a hearing problem?

54. You are attending a stage play. Can you understand what the actors/actresses are saying when their voices are loud enough for you and you can see their faces?

55. You are with a friend or family member in a fairly quiet room, can you understand him/her when his/her voice is loud enough for you, but you cannot see his/her face?

56. A person is talking to you from a distance of no more than six feet with music or noise in the background. Would you be aware that he/she is talking if you did not see his/her face?

57. You are with five or six friends or family members and there is background noise such as music or a crowd of people. Can you understand what is being said when the speaker's voice is loud enough for you, but you cannot see his/her face?

58. When you have difficulty understanding a person with a pipe, toothpick, or similar object in his/her mouth, do you ask him/her to remove the object?

59. You are the driver in an automobile with several friends or family members. The windows are closed. Can you understand the passenger behind you when his/her voice is loud enough for you?

60. When you have difficulty understanding a person because he is holding his hand in front of his mouth, do you ask him to lower his hand?

61. You are at a party or gathering of more than 20 people and several people are talking nearby. Can you understand what a stranger is saying to you when his voice is loud enough for you and you can see his face?

62. Do you feel that others cannot understand what it is to have a hearing problem?

63. You are at a movie. Can you understand what the actors/actresses are saying when their voices are loud enough for you and you can see their faces?

64. You are talking with five or six strangers. When you miss something important that was said, do you ask the person talking to repeat it?

65. You are at a party or gathering of less than 10 people and several people are talking nearby. Can you understand what a friend or family member (male) is saying to you when his voice is loud enough for you and you can see his face?

66. You are in a fairly quiet room. Can you carry on a conversation with a man in another room if his voice is loud enough for you?

67. You are with a male friend or family member and several people are talking nearby. Can you understand him when his voice is loud enough for you and you can see his face?

68. You are with five or six friends or family members. One person talks at a time. When you miss something important that was said, do you pretend you understood?

69. You are watching a drama or movie on television. Can you understand what is being said when the speaker's voice is loud enough for you and there is no music in the background?

70. You are with five or six friends or family members and there is background noise such as music or a crowd of people. One person talks at a time. When you are aware of the subject, can you understand what is being said when the speaker's voice is loud enough for you, but you cannot see his/her face?

71. You are at a lecture. If you have difficulty hearing what is being said, do you move to a place where you can hear better?

72. Does your hearing problem tend to make you nervous and tense?

73. You are with a female stranger and there is background noise such as traffic, music, or a crowd of people. Can you understand her when her voice is loud enough for you and you can see her face?

74. You are in a quiet place and the person seated on the side of your better ear whispers to you. Can you hear the whisper?

75. You are at a small social gathering. If you have difficulty hearing what is being said, do you move to a place where you can hear better?

Occupational Items

76. You are with a male coworker at work in a fairly quiet room. Can you understand him when his voice is loud enough for you and you can see his face?

77. You are with five or six coworkers at work. One person talks at a time. When you miss something important that was said, do you pretend you understood?

78. Does your hearing problem interfere with helping or instructing others on the job?

79. You are with a female coworker at work and there is background noise such as traffic, music, or a crowd of people. Can you understand her when her voice is loud enough for you and you can see her face?

80. You are with a coworker at work and you hear only a portion of what was said. Do you repeat that portion before asking the speaker for a repetition?

81. You are talking with a coworker at work. When you miss something important that was said, do you ask for it to be repeated?

82. You are talking with your employer (foreman, supervisor, etc.) and several people are nearby. Can you understand him/her when his/her voice is loud enough and you can see his/her face?

83. You are with a female coworker at work in a fairly quiet room. Can you understand her when her voice is loud enough for you and you can see his face?

84. You are talking with a coworker or employer. When you miss something important that was said, do you remind him/her that you have a hearing problem?

85. You are in a fairly quiet room at work with five or six coworkers. One person talks at a time and the subject of conversation changes from time to time. Can you understand what is being said when the speaker's voice is loud enough for you and you can see his/her face?

86. Does your hearing problem interfere with learning the duties of a new job easily?

87. You are seated with five or six coworkers around a table at work. Often two persons are talking at once and one person frequently interrupts another. Can you understand what is being said when the speaker's voice is loud enough and you can see his/her face?

88. You are talking with a coworker at work. When you miss something important that was said, do you pretend you understood?

89. You are with a male coworker at work and there is background noise such as traffic, music, or a crowd of people. Can you understand him when his voice is loud enough for you and you can see his face?

90. You are talking with a coworker at work. When you miss something important that was said, do you immediately adjust your hearing aid to help you hear better?

Source: Reprinted with permission from Stanford H. Lamb, PhD

APPENDIX 16–E
ABBREVIATED PROFILE OF HEARING AID BENEFIT

INSTRUCTIONS: Please circle the answers that come closest to your everyday experience. Notice that each choice includes a percentage. You can use this to help you decide on your answer. For example, if a statement is true about 75% of the time, circle C for that item. If you have not experienced the situation we describe, try to think of a similar situation that you have been in and respond for that situation. If you have no ideas, leave that item blank.

A. Always (99%)

B. Almost Always (87%)

C. Generally (75%)

D. Half-the-time (50%)

E. Occasionally (25%)

F. Seldom (12%)

G. Never (1%)

	Without My Hearing Aid	**With My Hearing Aid**
1. When I am in a crowded grocery store, talking with the cashier, I can follow the conversation.	A B C D E F G	A B C D E F G
2. I miss a lot of information when I'm listening to a lecture.	A B C D E F G	A B C D E F G
3. Unexpected sounds, like a smoke detector or alarm bell, are uncomfortable.	A B C D E F G	A B C D E F G
4. I have difficulty hearing a conversation when I'm with one of my family at home.	A B C D E F G	A B C D E F G
5. I have trouble understanding dialogue in a movie or at the theater.	A B C D E F G	A B C D E F G
6. When I am listening to the news on the car radio, and family members are talking, I have trouble hearing the news.	A B C D E F G	A B C D E F G
7. When I am at the dinner table with several people and am trying to have a conversation with one person, understanding speech is difficult.	A B C D E F G	A B C D E F G
8. Traffic noises are too loud.	A B C D E F G	A B C D E F G
9. When I am talking with someone across a large empty room, I understand the words.	A B C D E F G	A B C D E F G

	Without My Hearing Aid	With My Hearing Aid
10. When I am in a small office, interviewing, or answering questions, I have difficulty following the conversation.	A B C D E F G	A B C D E F G
11. When I am in a theater watching a movie or play, and the people around me are whispering and rustling paper wrappers, I can still make out the dialogue.	A B C D E F G	A B C D E F G
12. When I am having a quiet conversation with a friend, I have difficulty understanding.	A B C D E F G	A B C D E F G
13. The sounds of running water, such as a toilet or shower, are uncomfortably loud.	A B C D E F G	A B C D E F G
14. When a speaker is addressing a small group, and everyone is listening quietly, I have to strain to understand.	A B C D E F G	A B C D E F G
15. When I'm in a quiet conversation with my doctor in an examination room, it is hard to follow the conversation.	A B C D E F G	A B C D E F G
16. I can understand conversations even when several people are talking.	A B C D E F G	A B C D E F G
17. The sounds of construction work are uncomfortably loud.	A B C D E F G	A B C D E F G
18. It's hard for me to understand what is being said at lectures or church services.	A B C D E F G	A B C D E F G
19. I can communicate with others when we are in a crowd.	A B C D E F G	A B C D E F G
20. The sound of a fire engine siren close by is so loud that I need to cover my ears.	A B C D E F G	A B C D E F G
21. I can follow the words of a sermon when listening to a religious service.	A B C D E F G	A B C D E F G
22. The sound of screeching tires is uncomfortably loud.	A B C D E F G	A B C D E F G
23. I have to ask people to repeat themselves in one-on-one conversation in a quiet room.	A B C D E F G	A B C D E F G
24. I have trouble understanding others when an air conditioner or fan is on.	A B C D E F G	A B C D E F G

Source: Reprinted with permission of Robyn L. Cox.

APPENDIX 16–F
GLASGOW HEARING AID BENEFIT PROFILE

Does this situation happen in your life?

0 ____ No   1 ____ Yes

Listening to the television with other family or friends when the volume is adjusted to suit other people.

How much difficulty do you have in this situation?	How much does any difficulty in this situation worry, annoy or upset you?	In this situation, what proportion of the time do you wear your hearing aid?	In this situation, how much does your hearing aid help you?	In this situation, with your hearing aid, how much difficulty do you now have?	For this situation, how satisfied are you with your hearing aid?
0 __ N/A	0 __ N/A	0 __ N/A	0 __ N/A	0 __ N/A	0 __ N/A
1 __ No Difficulty	1 __ Not at all	1 __ Never	1 __ Hgn aid no use	1 __ No difficulty	1 __ Not sat at all
2 __ Only sl difficulty	2 __ Only a little	2 __ about 1/4	2 __ Hng aid some help	2 __ Only slt difficulty	2 __ A little satisfied
3 __ Moder difficulty	3 __ A moder amount	3 __ about 1/2	3 __ Hng aid quite helpful	3 __ Mod diff	3 __ Reasonably
4 __ Great difficulty	4 __ Quite a lot	4 __ about 3/4	4 __ Hng aid is great help	4 __ Great diff	4 __ Very satisfied
5 __ Can't manage	5 __ Very much	5 __ All the time	5 __ Hng is perfect w/ aid	5 __ Can't manage	5 __ Delighted

Source: Reprinted with permission from Stuart Gatehouse.

APPENDIX 16–G
HEARING AID PERFORMANCE INVENTORY

INSTRUCTIONS: We are interested in knowing the extent to which your hearing aid helps you in your daily life. In this questionnaire you are asked to judge the helpfulness of your hearing aid in a variety of listening situations. You are asked to rate the benefit of your hearing aid in each situation and not the difficulty of the situation itself.

To answer each question, check the phrase that best describes how your hearing aid helps you in that situation.

— —Very Helpful

— —Helpful

— —Very Little Help

— —No Help

— —Hinders Performance

There are items that appear similar but differ in at least one important detail. Therefore, read each item carefully before checking the appropriate phrase. We know that all people do not talk alike. Some mumble, others talk too fast, and others talk without moving their lips very much. Please answer the questions according to the way most people talk.

If you have never experienced the situation but can predict your hearing aid performance, respond to the item. A "Does Not Apply" response box is also provided. However, use the response "Does Not Apply" only if you do not know how helpful your hearing aid would be in the given situation.

Items

1. You are sitting alone at home watching the news on TV.

2. You are involved in an intimate conversation with your spouse.

3. You are watching TV and there are distracting noises such as others talking.

4. You are at home engaged in some activity and the telephone rings in another room.

5. You are at home in conversation with a member of your family who is in another room.

6. You are at a crowded outdoor auction bidding on an item.

7. You are listening to a speaker who is talking to a large group and you are seated toward the rear of the room. His back is partially turned as he makes notes on a blackboard.

8. You are starting to cross a busy street and a car horn sounds a warning.

9. You are riding on a crowded bus. You are in conversation with a friend seated next to you and you do not want others to overhear your conversation.

10. You are walking in the downtown section of a large city. There are the usual city noises and you are in conversation with a friend.

11. You are in a large office with the usual noise in the background (e.g., typewriters, air conditioners, fans, etc.). A coworker is telling you the latest gossip from close range in a soft voice.

12. You are riding in the back seat of a taxi. The window is down and the radio is on. The driver strikes up a conversation in a relatively soft voice.

13. You are driving your car and listening to a news broadcast on the radio. You are alone and the windows are closed.

14. You are in a crowded grocery store checkout line and talking with the cashier.

15. You are alone in a small office with the door closed. People are talking quietly outside the door and you want to overhear their conversation.

16. You are at a crowded office picnic talking with a friend.

17. You are at home watching television and the doorbell rings.

18. You are with your family at a noisy amusement park and you are discussing which attraction to go to next.

19. You are taking an evening stroll with a friend through a quiet neighborhood park, there are the usual environmental sounds around (e.g., children playing, dogs barking).

20. You are at home alone listening to your stereo system (instrumental music).

21. You are listening to an orchestra in a large concert hall.

22. You are in whispered conversation with your spouse at an intimate restaurant.

23. You are in the kitchen in conversation with your spouse during the preparation of an evening meal.

24. You are at home in face-to-face conversation with a member of your family.

25. You are shopping at a large busy department store and talking with a salesclerk.

26. You are at church listening to the sermon and sitting in the front pew.

27. You are listening to a speaker who is talking to a large group and you are seated toward the rear of the room. There is an occasional noise in the room (e.g., whispering, rattling papers, etc.).

28. You are having a conversation in your home with a salesman, and there is background noise (e.g., TV, people talking) in the room.

29. You are attending a business meeting where people are seated around a conference table. The boss is talking; everybody is listening quietly.

30. You are at church listening to the sermon and sitting in the back pew.

31. You are talking with a friend outdoors on a windy day.

32. You are driving your car with the windows up and carrying on a conversation with your spouse in the front seat.

33. You are in a small office interviewing for a job.

34. You are ordering food for the family at McDonald's.

35. You are at home reading the paper. Two family members are in another room talking quietly, and you want to listen in on their conversation.

36. You are in a courtroom listening to the various speakers (witness, judge, lawyer).

37. You are talking with a teller at the drive-in window bank.

38. You are in a noisy business office talking with a stranger on the telephone.

39. You are in conversation with someone across a large room (such as an auditorium).

40. You are in conversation with a neighbor across the fence.

41. You are in a crowded reception room waiting for your name to be called.

42. You are in you backyard gardening. Your neighbor is using a noisy power lawnmower and yells something to you.

43. You are listening in a small quiet room to someone who speaks softly.

44. You are on an airplane and the stewardess is requiring a meal selection.

45. You are riding in a crowded bus and are in conversation with a stranger seated next to you.

46. You are alone driving your automobile and the cars around you are pulling to the side of the road. You begin to listen for what you anticipate is an emergency vehicle (fire truck, rescue squad, etc.).

47. Someone is trying to tell you something in a small quiet room while you have your back turned.

48. You are driving with your family and are listening to a news broadcast on the car radio. Your window is down and family members are talking.

49. You are driving your car with the windows down and are carrying on a conversation with others riding with you.

50. You are at an exciting sports activity (baseball, football game, etc.) and talk occasionally with those around you.

51. You are in a large business office talking with a clerk. There is the usual office noise (e.g., typing, talking , etc.).

52. You are in a quiet conversation with your family doctor in an examination room.

53. You are talking to a large group and someone from the back of the audience asks a question in a relatively soft voice. Audience is quiet as they listen to the question.

54. You are walking through a large crowded airport and are in conversation with a friend.

55. You are at a large noisy party and are engaged in conversation with one other person.

56. You are alone in the woods listening to the sounds of nature (e.g., birds, insects, small animals, etc.)

57. You are at the dinner table with your whole family and are in conversation with your spouse.

58. You are attending a business meeting where people are seated around a conference table. The discussion is heated as everyone attempts to make a point. The speakers are frequently interrupted.

59. You are one of only a few customers inside your bank and are talking with a teller.

60. You are at a theater watching a movie. There are occasional noises around you (e.g., whispering, wrappers rustling, etc.).

61. You are alone at home talking with a friend on the telephone.

62. You are downtown in a large city requesting directions from a pedestrian.

63. You are riding in a car with friends. The windows of the car are rolled down. You are in the back seat carrying on a conversation with them.

64. You are driving your car with the windows up and radio off and are carrying on a conversation with your spouse who is in the front seat.

APPENDIX 16–H
PROFILE OF AIDED LOUDNESS (PAL)

Name: _____ Date: _____

Status: _____ Unaided: _____ Previous Hearing Aids: _____

Current Hearing Aids: _____

INSTRUCTIONS: Please rate the following items by both the level of loudness of the sound, and also by the level of satisfaction that you have for that loudness. For example, you might rate a particular sound as "Very Soft." If "Very Soft" is your preferred level for this sound, then you would rate your loudness satisfaction as "Just Right." If on the other hand, you would like the sound to be louder than "Very Soft," then your loudness satisfaction rating might be "Not Too Good" or "Not Good At All." The Loudness Satisfaction rating is not related to how "pleasing" the sound is to you, but rather, the appropriateness of the loudness. Here is an example:

1. The hum of a refrigerator motor:

Loudness Rating		*Loudness Satisfaction*	
0	Cannot Hear	5	Just Right
1	Very Soft	4	Pretty Good
2	Soft	3	Okay
3	Comfortable, But Slightly Soft	2	Not Too Good
4	Comfortable	1	Not Good At All
5	Comfortable, But Slightly Loud		
6	Loud, But Okay		
7	Uncomfortably Loud		

In this example, the hearing aid user rated the loudness level of a refrigerator motor running as "Comfortable, But Slightly Soft" and rated his Loudness Satisfaction for this sound as "Just Right." This satisfaction rating indicates that this person believes that it is appropriate for a refrigerator motor to sound "Comfortable, But Slightly Soft."

Circle the responses that best describe your listening experiences. If you have not experienced one of the sounds listed (or a similar sound), simply leave that question blank.

Profile of Aided Loudness (PAL)

1. An electric razor:

Loudness Rating
0   Cannot Hear
1   Very Soft
2   Soft
3   Comfortable, But Slightly Soft
4   Comfortable
5   Comfortable, But Slightly Loud
6   Loud, But Okay
7   Uncomfortably Loud

Loudness Satisfaction
5   Just Right
4   Pretty Good
3   Okay
2   Not Too Good
1   Not Good At All

2. A door slamming:

Loudness Rating
0   Cannot Hear
1   Very Soft
2   Soft
3   Comfortable, But Slightly Soft
4   Comfortable
5   Comfortable, But Slightly Loud
6   Loud, But Okay
7   Uncomfortably Loud

Loudness Satisfaction
5   Just Right
4   Pretty Good
3   Okay
2   Not Too Good
1   Not Good At All

3. Your own breathing:

Loudness Rating
0   Cannot Hear
1   Very Soft
2   Soft
3   Comfortable, But Slightly Soft
4   Comfortable
5   Comfortable, But Slightly Loud
6   Loud, But Okay
7   Uncomfortably Loud

Loudness Satisfaction
5   Just Right
4   Pretty Good
3   Okay
2   Not Too Good
1   Not Good At All

4. Water boiling on the stove:

Loudness Rating

0 Cannot Hear
1 Very Soft
2 Soft
3 Comfortable, But Slightly Soft
4 Comfortable
5 Comfortable, But Slightly Loud
6 Loud, But Okay
7 Uncomfortably Loud

Loudness Satisfaction

5 Just Right
4 Pretty Good
3 Okay
2 Not Too Good
1 Not Good At All

5. A car's turn signal:

Loudness Rating

0 Cannot Hear
1 Very Soft
2 Soft
3 Comfortable, But Slightly Soft
4 Comfortable
5 Comfortable, But Slightly Loud
6 Loud, But Okay
7 Uncomfortably Loud

Loudness Satisfaction

5 Just Right
4 Pretty Good
3 Okay
2 Not Too Good
1 Not Good At All

6. The religious leader during the sermon:

Loudness Rating

0 Cannot Hear
1 Very Soft
2 Soft
3 Comfortable, But Slightly Soft
4 Comfortable
5 Comfortable, But Slightly Loud
6 Loud, But Okay
7 Uncomfortably Loud

Loudness Satisfaction

5 Just Right
4 Pretty Good
3 Okay
2 Not Too Good
1 Not Good At All

7. The clothes dryer running:

Loudness Rating
0 Cannot Hear
1 Very Soft
2 Soft
3 Comfortable, But Slightly Soft
4 Comfortable
5 Comfortable, But Slightly Loud
6 Loud, But Okay
7 Uncomfortably Loud

Loudness Satisfaction
5 Just Right
4 Pretty Good
3 Okay
2 Not Too Good
1 Not Good At All

8. You chewing soft food:

Loudness Rating
0 Cannot Hear
1 Very Soft
2 Soft
3 Comfortable, But Slightly Soft
4 Comfortable
5 Comfortable, But Slightly Loud
6 Loud, But Okay
7 Uncomfortably Loud

Loudness Satisfaction
5 Just Right
4 Pretty Good
3 Okay
2 Not Too Good
1 Not Good At All

9. Listening to a marching band:

Loudness Rating
0 Cannot Hear
1 Very Soft
2 Soft
3 Comfortable, But Slightly Soft
4 Comfortable
5 Comfortable, But Slightly Loud
6 Loud, But Okay
7 Uncomfortably Loud

Loudness Satisfaction
5 Just Right
4 Pretty Good
3 Okay
2 Not Too Good
1 Not Good At All

10. A barking dog:

Loudness Rating

0 Cannot Hear
1 Very Soft
2 Soft
3 Comfortable, But Slightly Soft
4 Comfortable
5 Comfortable, But Slightly Loud
6 Loud, But Okay
7 Uncomfortably Loud

Loudness Satisfaction

5 Just Right
4 Pretty Good
3 Okay
2 Not Too Good
1 Not Good At All

11. A lawn mower:

Loudness Rating

0 Cannot Hear
1 Very Soft
2 Soft
3 Comfortable, But Slightly Soft
4 Comfortable
5 Comfortable, But Slightly Loud
6 Loud, But Okay
7 Uncomfortably Loud

Loudness Satisfaction

5 Just Right
4 Pretty Good
3 Okay
2 Not Too Good
1 Not Good At All

12. A microwave buzzer sounding:

Loudness Rating

0 Cannot Hear
1 Very Soft
2 Soft
3 Comfortable, But Slightly Soft
4 Comfortable
5 Comfortable, But Slightly Loud
6 Loud, But Okay
7 Uncomfortably Loud

Loudness Satisfaction

5 Just Right
4 Pretty Good
3 Okay
2 Not Too Good
1 Not Good At All

Source: Reprinted with permission from Catherine Palmer, PhD.

APPENDIX 16–I
SATISFACTION WITH AMPLIFICATION IN EVERYDAY LIFE

Name: _____ D/O/B: _____ Today's Date: _____

INSTRUCTIONS: Listed below are questions about your experiences with obtaining and using your current hearing aid(s). For each question, please circle the letter that best corresponds to your opinion about your current hearing aid(s). Use the list of words below to determine your answer.

A: Not at all   **B:** A little   **C:** Somewhat   **D:** Medium
E: Considerably   **F:** Greatly   **G:** Tremendously

Keep in mind that your answers should reflect your opinions about the hearing aids that *you are currently wearing or have most recently worn.*

While we would like you to answer every question, if you feel that a question cannot apply to your experiences, please write an "X" through the number in front of the question.

1. Compared to using no hearing aid at all, does your hearing aid(s) help you understand the people you speak with most frequently?   A B C D E F G

2. Are you frustrated when your hearing aid(s) picks up sounds that keep you from hearing what you want to hear?   A B C D E F G

3. Are you convinced that obtaining your hearing aid(s) was in your best interests?   A B C D E F G

4. Do people notice your hearing loss more when you wear your hearing aid(s)?   A B C D E F G

5. Does your hearing aid(s) reduce the number of times you have to ask people to repeat?   A B C D E F G

6. Do you think your hearing aid(s) is worth the trouble?   A B C D E F G

7. Are you bothered by an inability to turn your hearing aid(s) up loud enough without getting feedback (whistling)?   A B C D E F G

8. How content are you with the appearance of your hearing aid(s)?   A B C D E F G

9. Does wearing your hearing aid(s) improve your self-confidence?   A B C D E F G

Experience with Current Hearing Aids:
☐ Less than 6 weeks
☐ 6 weeks to 11 months
☐ 1 to 10 years
☐ Over 10 years

Total Hearing Aid Experience
☐ Less than 6 weeks
☐ 6 weeks to 11 months
☐ 1 to 10 years
☐ Over 10 years

Daily Hearing Aid Use
☐ Less than 1 hour
☐ 1 to 4 hours per day
☐ 4 to 8 hours per day
☐ 8 to 16 hours per day

Degree of Hearing Difficulties (without wearing a hearing aid)
None
☐ Mild
☐ Moderate
☐ Severe

10. How natural is the sound from your hearing aid?   A B C D E F G

11. How helpful is your hearing aid(s) on MOST telephones with NO amplifier or loudspeaker?   A B C D E F G

12. How competent was the person who provided you with your hearing aid(s)?   A B C D E F G

13. Do you think wearing your hearing aid(s) makes you seem less capable?   A B C D E F G

14. Does the cost of your hearing aid(s) seem reasonable to you?   A B C D E F G

15. How pleased are you with the dependability (how often it needs repairs) of your hearing aid(s)?   A B C D E F G

Additional Comments: _____

_____

_____

_____

_____

Back of SADL

FOR AUDIOLOGIST'S USE ONLY

Hearing Aid Fitting   Monaural   Binaural

Right ear   Left ear

Make _____   Make _____

Model _____   Model _____

Ser. No. _____   Ser. No. _____

Fitting Date _____   Fitting Date _____

Hearing aid type	Hearing Aid Features (all that apply)		
CIC	Directional mic	Peak clipping	Multiprogram
ITC	Output limiting	Multichannel	K-amp
ITE	T-coil	WDRC	FM
BTE	Curvilinear	DAI	BILL
	Vent	Other _____	

_____

Source: Reprinted with permission of Robyn L. Cox

APPENDIX 16–J
ARE YOU PROVIDING QUALITY SERVICE?

Check "Yes" or "No" for each question.

1. There is easy access for patients to my practice, including convenient parking, and they do not need to climb any stairs to get to my office.
   ☐ YES   ☐ NO

2. I send maps or other written instructions to help new patients get to my office.
   ☐ YES   ☐ NO

3. When a patient calls my office, there is someone knowledgeable available to help the person over the phone.
   ☐ YES   ☐ NO

4. My office is a comfortable, well-lighted, climate-controlled facility with adequate working space. Amenities include coffee and other beverages, reading materials, information booklets, and comfortable chairs with arms.
   ☐ YES   ☐ NO

5. Patients are not kept waiting if they arrive on time for their appointment.
   ☐ YES   ☐ NO

6. When a patient has a problem, prompt help is available.
   ☐ YES   ☐ NO

7. I use a "no pressure" sales approach.
   ☐ YES   ☐ NO

8. The atmosphere in my office is friendly, and patience abounds. I always take a patient, unhurried approach to patients, no matter how busy I am.
   ☐ YES   ☐ NO

9. For conducting hearing tests, I use a sound booth and a calibrated audiometer.
   ☐ YES   ☐ NO

10. I give patients word-recognition tests at more than one level, as needed.
    ☐ YES   ☐ NO

11. I use a fairly new, high-quality hearing aid test set.
    ☐ YES   ☐ NO

12. I give clear, simple explanations, both orally and in writing, of all available hearing aids, including their price.
    ☐ YES   ☐ NO

13. I have high-quality, informative, up-to-date booklets available for patients.

  ☐ YES   ☐ NO

14. I have a functioning telephone amplifier device in my office that is demonstrated for every new patient; information on getting one is given to the patient.

  ☐ YES   ☐ NO

15. There is an infrared TV system in my office that can be easily demonstrated to interested patients.

  ☐ YES   ☐ NO

16. I follow a well-thought-out program for cerumen management, using written instructions and appropriate products and equipment, and I have received training from an accredited national association or some other formal instruction.

  ☐ YES   ☐ NO

17. My practice has a facility for doing in-office minor repairs, including replacing broken battery doors, ear hooks, and tubing on earmolds (prebent tubing is mandatory), unplugging *deeply* impacted sound tubes, and using grinding/polishing equipment to adjust earmolds and shells.

  ☐ YES   ☐ NO

18. I have a good supply of loaner BTE hearing aids (about 40) available for patients to use when their own hearing aids need to be sent in for service.

  ☐ YES   ☐ NO

19. I have spare custom-made earmolds or high-quality universal earmolds. (If you only have one or two boxes of 10-year-old universal earmolds, you don't get credit on this one.)

  ☐ YES   ☐ NO

20. I provide batteries by mail.

  ☐ YES   ☐ NO

Give yourself a point for every YES answer. If you scored 17 to 19, you did well.

Source: Reprinted with permission from "Nuts and Bolts: Are You Providing Quality Service, by R. Martin, 1997. *The Hearing Journal, 50*(8), 66.

Audiology Services

Outcome Measures Questionnaire IOI-HA

Please select the best answer to each question in regards to your most recently issued hearing aids.

1. Think about how much you used your present hearing aid(s) over the last two weeks. On an average day, how many hours did you use the hearing aid(s)?

   None   Less than 1 hour   1–4 hours per day   4–8 hours per day
   More than 8 hours per day

2. Think about the situation where you most wanted to hear better, before you got your present hearing aid(s). Over the past two weeks, how much has the hearing aid helped in those situations?

   None at all   Slightly   Moderately   Quite a lot   Very much

3. Think again about the situation where you most wanted to hear better. When you use your present hearing aid(s), how much difficulty do you still have in that situation?

   Very much   Quite a lot   Moderate   Slight   None

4. Considering everything, do you think your present hearing aid(s) is worth the trouble?

   Not at all   Slightly   Moderately   Quite a lot   Very much

5. Over the past two weeks, with your present hearing aid(s), how much have your hearing difficulties affected the things you can do?

   Very much   Quite a lot   Moderately   Slightly   Not at all

6. Over the past two weeks, with your present hearing aid(s), how much do you think other people were bothered by your hearing difficulties?

   Very much   Quite a lot   Moderately   Slightly   Not at all

7. Considering everything, how much has your present hearing aid(s) changed your enjoyment of life?

   Worse   Not at all   Slightly better   Quite a lot better   Very much better

8. How much hearing difficulty do you have when you are not wearing a hearing aid?

   Severe   Moderate-severe   Moderate   Mild   None

Source: Robyn L. Cox. Copies in the standard format can be downloaded at http://www.HARLmemphis.org

APPENDIX 16–L
ABC HEARING, AUDIOLOGY SERVICES:
EVALUATION AND/OR TREATMENT

Read each item carefully and **circle** the one answer that is best for you.

SA = Strongly Agree   A = Agree   N = Neutral   D = Disagree
SD = Strongly Disagree   NA = Not Applicable

1. Did we see you in a timely manner?

    A. My appointment was scheduled in a reasonable period of time.   SA A N D SD NA

    B. I was seen on time for my scheduled appointment   SA A N D SD NA

2. Did you benefit from Audiology Services?

    A. I feel I gained valuable information from my visit.   SA A N D SD NA

    B. I feel I benefited from this appointment.   SA A N D SD NA

3. Were you and your needs important to us?

    A. The staff who serviced me was courteous and pleasant.   SA A N D SD NA

    B. Staff considered my special needs.   SA A N D SD NA

    C. Staff encouraged participation by my family/friends/aides.   SA A N D SD NA

4. Our staff are highly trained and qualified to serve you.

    A. My clinician(s) were prepared and organized.   SA A N D SD NA

    B. My clinician(s) were experienced and knowledgeable.   SA A N D SD NA

5. Was our office safe, acceptable, and accessible?

    A. Health and safety precautions were taken when serving me.   SA A N D SD NA

    B. The environment was clean and pleasant.   SA A N D SD NA

    C. Test and consultation rooms were quiet and free of distractions.   SA A N D SD NA

    D. The office was easily accessible.   SA A N D SD NA

6. Were your services and treatment efficient and comprehensive?

    A. The purpose and nature of the procedures were explained clearly.   SA A N D SD NA

    B. My clinician(s) planned ahead and provided sufficient   SA A N D SD NA
       instruction.

7. We respect and value your comments.

A. Overall, the program services were satisfactory. SA A N D SD NA

B. I would seek your services again if needed. SA A N D SD NA

C. I would recommend your services to others. SA A N D SD NA

My clinician(s) were: [ ] Ruth Smith [ ] Dan Owens [ ] Beverly Green [ ] Julie Carter

Comments: _____

_____

Thank you for your time. We will carefully review your comments to improve our practice!

Source: Reprinted with permission from ASHA Adaptation Office Survey, by American Speech-Language-Hearing Association.

APPENDIX 16–M
ARTICLES SUPPORTING THE APPLICATION
OF OUTCOME MEASURES IN DETERMINING
SUCCESSFUL HEARING AID USE

An excellent article was published by Mendel (2009) in which she mentions verification and validation. Validation is best defined as a process by which one can determine if the hearing aid is providing benefit. That is, is the instrument meeting it's required electroacoustic response to meet the patient needs?

The primary thrust of this article was to demonstrate the need to employ subjective and objective measures when evaluating the efficacy of a hearing aid programs. The authors reviewed a number of self-assessment inventories in defending the position relating to the use of subjective measures. Among other concepts, she reviews the importance of understanding the role played by validity and reliability. The relationship between validity and reliability is most important if one is to achieve a satisfactory program. One is cautioned that a program can be valid, but not reliable. Weinstein (1997), defines treatment efficacy in three specific areas.

1. Treatment effectiveness: Does the hearing aid provide improved speech discrimination (intelligibility) in quiet and in noise, or do they restore normal loudness function?
2. Treatment efficiency: Are certain hearing aid instrumental adjustments more efficient than others in improving speech understanding?
3. Treatment effects: Does the hearing aid improve the social and psychological well-being of the patient?

In general, the issue is whether a subjective or an objective approach should be utilized in measuring outcomes? It seems rather evident to the editors that each approach should be incorporated into any outcome assessment. There is no doubt that many instruments are rejected based solely on emotional (subjective) reasons.

For many years, elderly hearing-impaired persons have been compared with the younger hearing impaired population. Chang et al. reports a study involving a group of 59 subjects.

Group A subjects consisted of 32 individuals between 65 to 80 years of age. There were 27 subjects in Group B, all of whom were older than 80 years. Assessment tools were the Hearing Handicap Inventory for the Elderly Screening Version (HHIE-S) and the frequently used Client Oriented Scale of Improvement.

The results of the study revealed no significant differences relative to speech performance among the populations investigated. Somewhat unexpected were the findings that there were no significant differences in analysis of data from the HHIE-S and the COSI scores after 4 months use of digital hearing aids.

Chang concluded that "Age by itself is not a limiting factor for older patients to benefit with hearing impairment to benefit assessment."

It would appear that there is a growing interest in investigating the subjective side of hearing aid evaluation program relative to outcomes and conditions affecting successful hearing aid use. One would agree that assessing the subjective side of the hearing aid evaluation process would be most efficacious in developing or modifying patient management strategies.

For the experienced hearing instrument dispenser fitting high frequency, bilateral impairment can be a difficult task. The question often posed is whether a closed or open-canal is the best instrument of choice (Gnewikow & Moss, 2005). The authors are quick to remind us that many patients with bilateral high-frequency loss have little difficulty in understanding speech in a relatively quiet environment. However, in reviewing a series of instruments intended for high-frequency loss, none has proven to be superior in performance in all instances of comparison.

A chronic problem encountered in fitting high-frequency hearing loss is related to an open or closed canal fitting. In an open canal, there is little no occlusion effect. Incidentally, a uniquely appropriate name was introduced by Sweetow when discussing open-close canal fitting, *it* is ampclusion (Sweetow & Pirzansk, 2003).

They describe ampclusion as a phenomenon caused by low-frequency amplification and the standard occlusion caused by the inserted earmold into the external canal.

The dilemma encountered is that of determining what instrument to use for the patient with high-frequency loss. For most, the open mold is the more acceptable.

It doesn't take a background in rocket science to realize the benefits of measuring program outcomes in developing a patient management strategy. There are a large number of scales and other measuring instruments that one can employ in assessing outcomes in a number of different areas. It is somewhat difficult to understand why so many hearing health professionals fail to see the benefits of such a useful procedure.

The editors believe that some individuals may feel that measuring outcomes is time-consuming and interferes with financial growth. Some who fit hearing aids are satisfied if the patient says, "I like it." For some, failing to exercise a formal assessment program can be nothing more than professional laziness.

It is quite possible that the audiologist or hearing aid dispenser will be obligated to provide "proof of performance" before being compensated. This directive may never be written by federal or state agency. It may be a form of action best taken by some major HMO. It seems intuitively obvious that the more demands made on dispensing practices of the audiologists would—or should—result in a higher success rate from the use of amplification. There is just too much data available to ignore the value of assessing outcomes. One of the intriguing advantages of looking at outcomes is to assist the audiologist in fitting the best hearing aid(s).

Although audiology is an academic field of study, in part, it is truly clinical in nature. As such, audiology has yet to develop measurement and follow-up procedural protocols in the fitting and follow-up care. Perhaps it's time to start?

References

Chang, H. P., Ho, C. Y., Chou, P. (2009). The factors associated with a self-perceived hearing handicap in elderly people with hearing impairment—results from a community-based study. *Ear and Hearing, 30*(5), 576–583.

Gnewikow, D., & Moss, M. (2005). Hearing aid outcomes with open-and closed-canal fittings. *Hearing Journal, 59*(11), 66–72.

Mendel, L. L. (2009). Subjective and objective measures of hearing aid outcome. Retrieved from http://www.audiologyonline.com

Sweetow, R. W., & Pirzanski, C. Z. (2003). The occlusion effect and the ampclusion effect. *Seminars in Hearing,* 24(4), 333–334.

Weinstein, B. (1997). Customer satisfaction with hearing aids. *Seminars in Hearing,* 3–6.

CHAPTER 17

Assistive Technologies for the Hearing Impaired

JOSEPH J. SMALDINO
BRIAN M. KREISMAN
ANDREW B. JOHN

It is well-recognized that the major complaint of individuals with sensorineural hearing loss (SNHL) is communicative difficulty, particularly in noisy and reverberant listening environments (Cooper & Cutts, 1971; Crandell, 1991a; Crandell, Henoch, & Dunkerson, 1991; Crandell & Smaldino, 1996a, 1996b; Dirks, Morgan, & Dubno, 1982; Duquesnoy & Plomp, 1983; Finitzo-Hieber & Tillman, 1978; Humes, 1991; Nabelek, 1982; Nabelek & Pickett, 1974a, 1974b; Needleman & Crandell, 1996a, 1996b; Plomp, 1978, 1986; Ross, 1978; Suter, 1985). Because of the deleterious effects of SNHL on communication, additional research has indicated that hearing loss may detrimentally affect both psychosocial and physical health status (see Crandell, 1998, for a review of these studies). Unfortunately, many forms of hearing aid technology have been shown to offer minimal speech-recognition benefit to listeners with hearing impairment in adverse listening environments (Boothroyd, 1991; Crandell, 1991a, 1991b; Crandell & Smaldino, 1999; Crandell, Smaldino, & Flexer, 1995; Festen & Plomp, 1983; Moore, 1997; Plomp, 1978, 1986; Van Tassell, 1993). For example, Plomp (1986), reported that hearing aids offered limited improvements in speech recognition when background noise levels exceeded 50 dB(A), a noise level commonly encountered in everyday listening environments. With these considerations in mind, this chapter examines various rehabilitative technologies for improving communicative efficiency within commonly used noisy and reverberant listening environments. The terms rehabilitative technology or assistive technology are used to describe these technologies. These terms were selected over the more commonly used assistive listening devices (ALDs), as many of these technologies are not limited to simply improved listening ability.

EFFECTS OF REVERBERATION, NOISE, AND DISTANCE ON SPEECH RECOGNITION

The accurate transmission of speech in a room can be affected by the acoustic characteristics of the room, including reverberation time (RT), the intensity of ambient noise in comparison with the intensity of the desired signal, and the distance from the speaker to the listener. Prior to examining rehabilitative technologies that can improve speech recognition in adverse listening environments, it is first imperative to summarize some of the general effects of these variables on speech recognition. For more detailed information on the effects of noise, reverberation, and distance on speech recognition, the reader is directed to Crandell and Smaldino (1994, 1995, 1996a, 1996b, 1999); Siebein (1994); and Smaldino, Crandell, and Kreisman (2005).

Reverberation time refers to the amount of time it takes for a steady-state sound to decrease 60 dB from its peak amplitude. In a reverberant room, the reflected speech from the room surfaces reaches the ear of the listener temporally delayed and overlaps with the direct speech signal (the signal not reflected before reaching the listener's ear), which masks certain acoustic speech components (Bolt & MacDonald, 1949; Lochner & Burger, 1964; Siebein, Crandell, & Gold, 1997). Because vowels are more intense than consonants, reverberation tends to produce a prolongation of the spectral energy of vowel phonemes, which reduces consonant recognition. A reduction of consonant information can have a significant effect on speech recognition because the vast majority of the acoustic information that is important for speech recognition is provided by consonants (French & Steinberg, 1947; Licklider & Miller, 1951; Wang, Reed, & Bilger, 1978).

Speech recognition tends to decrease with increases in RT. Speech recognition in adults with normal hearing is not significantly degraded until the RT exceeds approximately 1 second (Gelfand & Silman, 1979; Houtgast, 1981; Kreisman, 2003; Moncur & Dirks, 1967; Nabelek & Pickett, 1974a, 1974b). Listeners with SNHL, however, need considerably shorter RTs (0.4 to 0.5 second) for optimal communication (ASHA, 1995; Crandell, 1991b; 1992; Crandell & Smaldino, 1994, 1995, 1996a, 1996b, 1999; Crandell et al., 1995; Finitzo-Hieber, 1988; Finitzo-Hieber & Tillman, 1978; Gengel, 1971; Neimoeller, 1968; Olsen, 1981, 1988). In addition to listeners with SNHL, there are a number of populations of individuals (primarily children) with "normal hearing" sensitivity that exhibit greater perceptual difficulties in reverberation (and noise) than young adults with normal hearing (Berg, 1993; Bess, 1985; Bess & Tharpe, 1986; Boney & Bess, 1984; Crandell, 1991b, 1992, 1993; Crandell & Bess, 1986; Crandell & Smaldino, 1992, 1994, 1995, 1996a, 1996b; Crandell et al., 1995; Flexer, 1992; Nabelek & Nabelek, 1994). A list of these "normal hearing" listeners is presented in Table 17–1. Because of this increased difficulty listening in noise, acoustical guidelines for hearing-impaired and "normal-hearing" populations suggest that RTs should not exceed 0.4 to 0.5 seconds in

Table 17–1. Populations of Listeners with "Normal Hearing" Who May Be Affected by Poor Room Acoustics

---

Elderly individuals with normal hearing sensitivity

Young children (less than 15 years)

Individuals with conductive hearing loss

Individuals with a history of otitis media

Individuals with articulation and/or language disorders

Individuals with learning disabilities

Individuals who speak English as a second language

Individuals diagnosed with central auditory processing deficits

Individuals with minimal or borderline degrees of SNHL (16–25 dB HL)

Individuals with unilateral hearing loss

Individuals with developmental delays

Individuals with attention deficits

Individuals with reading deficits (such as dyslexia)

---

communication environments frequented by these individuals.

Background noise in a room also reduces speech recognition by masking the acoustic/linguistic cues in the message. As with reverberation, background noise in a room tends to mask the weaker consonant phonemes significantly greater than the more intense vowel phonemes. The most important factor for accurate speech recognition is often the ratio of the intensity of the desired signal compared with the intensity of the undesired signal or noise. This ratio is referred to as the SNR and is reported as the decibel difference between the two intensities. Speech recognition is generally highest at advantageous SNRs and decreases as the SNR of the environment is reduced (Cooper & Cutts, 1971; Finitzo-Hieber & Tillman, 1978; Miller, 1974; Nabelek & Pickett, 1974a, 1974b). Speech-recognition ability in adults with normal hearing is not significantly reduced until the SNR is reduced below 0 dB. To obtain recognition scores equal to those of normal hearers, listeners with SNHL require the SNR to be improved by 4 to 12 dB (Crandell et al., 1995; Moore, 1997; Plomp, 1986) and by an additional 3 to 6 dB in rooms with moderate levels of reverberation (Hawkins & Yacullo, 1984). Based on these data, acoustical guidelines for hearing-impaired populations (and "normal hearers") suggest that SNRs should exceed +15 dB for maximal speech recognition (Crandell & Smaldino, 1995).

The acoustics of a speaker's voice also vary as a function of the distance to the listener. When the listener is relatively near to the speaker, the direct sound field dominates, and the listener receives the sound directly from the speaker unaffected by reflections from surfaces within the room. Direct sound pressure decreases 6 dB for every doubling of distance from the sound source, a phenomena referred to as the inverse square law. As speaker-listener distance increases, there is a point at which the direct sound energy and the intensity of sound reflected off room surfaces (reverberation) is equal. This point is called the critical distance of the room. Beyond the critical distance, the direct sound from the speaker arrives at the listener first (but at a decreased intensity) and is quickly followed by reflections of the direct sound from the walls, floor, and ceiling. Because there is a decrease in sound intensity with distance and because some frequencies will be absorbed more than others by the absorptive elements in the room (including the occupants), the reflected sound reaching the listener will have a different acoustic signature in the intensity, frequency, and temporal domains. Speech recognition tends to decrease until the critical distance (the point at which the direct and reverberant sound energy is equal) of the room is reached. The critical distance in most small rooms (such as classrooms) is approximately 3 to 6 feet from the speaker. Beyond the critical distance, recognition ability tends to remain essentially constant unless the room is very large (such as an auditorium). In larger rooms, speech recognition may continue to decrease as a function of increased distance. These findings suggest that speech recognition can only be improved by decreasing the distance between a speaker and listener within the critical distance of the room. Stated another way, the simple recommendation of preferential seating for a listener with hearing loss is often not adequate to ensure optimal communication.

Reverberation, background noise, and distance from the speaker synergistically interact in a room. That is, when these factors are combined (which is the case in virtually all real-world listening environments), they affect speech recognition more than any one of the factors alone. Finitzo-Hieber and Tillman (1978), for example, demonstrated that children with SNHL obtained speech-recognition scores of only 29% in typical classroom learning environments (RT = 0.4 second; SNR = 0 dB; distance of 12 feet). Leavitt and Flexer (1991), using the Rapid Speech Transmission Index (RASTI), demonstrated that 83% of the speech energy was available to the listener in the front row of a typical classroom-sized environment. In the back row of the classroom, however, only approximately 50% of the speech energy was available. Even less of the signal would be available if the listener has a hearing loss, attention difficulties, or reduced auditory/language processing. That is, add the loss of the speech signal due to the acoustical environment to the distortion imposed by a damaged auditory or linguistic system, and it becomes apparent why simply turning up the gain of a hearing aid is frequently not a satisfactory communicative solution.

HEARING ASSISTIVE DEVICES

Whether the goal is group communication or one-to-one communication, the initial approach for improving speech recognition in a room is modification of the acoustics within that environment. For a detailed review of acoustical modifications, the reader is directed to Crandell and Smaldino (1999). Unfortunately, due to cost factors, appropriate acoustical conditions for the hearing impaired are infrequently met with physical acoustical modification of the room. Consequently, assistive technologies must often be implemented. One well-recognized strategy for improving speech recognition in rooms is the utilization of group or personal room amplification systems. Often, these devices are called hearing assistive devices. As seen in Table 17–2, possible hearing assistive devices include hard wired, personal Frequency Modulation (FM), sound field FM, induction loop, and infrared systems. The goals of assistive systems are depicted in Table 17–3.

Table 17–2. Various Types of Hearing Assistive Devices

Hard-Wired
Personal FM
Audio Distribution System—FM
Induction Loop
Audio Distribution System—Infrared

Table 17–3. The Primary Goals of Hearing Assistive Devices

Maintain favorable SNR with minimal reverberation at the listener's ears
Allow the acoustic signal to be modified to meet the hearing needs of the individual
Provide wide frequency amplification with a minimal degree of distortion
Allow mobility for both speaker and listener
Allow the listener to hear not only the primary speaker, but also other speakers in the room and the listener's own voice
Accept auditory inputs such as from compact disc players, televisions, and digital audio devices

Source: Adapted from *Management of Hearing Handicap: Infants to Elderly*, by D. Sanders, 1993. Englewood Cliffs, NJ: Prentice-Hall.

Hard-Wired Systems

With hard-wired systems, a wire connects the microphone of the speaker to the amplifier and the amplifier is similarly wired to the receiver used by the listener. Thus, with hard-wired systems, there is a direct physical connection between the sound source and the individual. Because of the "hard wiring" involved in such systems, and consequently the reduced mobility for both the speaker and the listener, they are generally not recommended for most listening environments. It should be noted, however, that several investigators have reported that some small, inexpensive hard-wired systems may be beneficial for individuals who cannot manage a hearing aid due to conditions such as dementia or severe manual dexterity difficulties (Crandell & Smaldino, 1999; Weinstein & Amsel, 1986). A summary of the advantages and disadvantages of hard-wired systems are shown in Table 17–4.

Personal Frequency Modulation (FM) Amplification

With a personal FM system (often called an Auditory Trainer), the speaker's voice is picked up via an FM wireless microphone located 3 to 4 inches from the speaker's mouth (where the detrimental effects of reverberation and noise are minimal). The acoustic signal is converted to an electrical waveform and transmitted via an FM radio signal to a receiver (Figure 17–1).

Table 17–4. Potential Advantages and Disadvantages of Hard-Wired Systems

Advantages	Disadvantages
May be useful in some patients with hearing impairment who may not be able to use conventional amplification (cognitive declines, physical disabilities, and/or severe manual dexterity difficulties)	Hard-wired systems are not specified as medical devices by the Food and Drug Administration (FDA); therefore, there are no standards for the electroacoustic characteristics (gain, frequency response, SSPL90, harmonic distortion) of such devices
Not susceptible to electromagnetic interference	Limited mobility for the speaker and/or listener
Installation of such systems tends to be relatively easy	Installation costs can be high for systems used by more than one listener, particularly in already constructed buildings
Inexpensive	

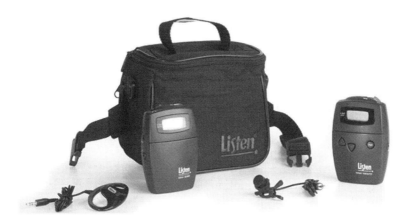

Figure 17–1. An example of a frequency modulation (FM) system. Image provided by Listen Technologies Corporation. © 2013. All rights reserved.

The electrical signal is then amplified, converted back to an acoustical waveform, and conveyed to one or more listeners in the room. Often, FM systems can improve the SNR of the listening environment by 20 to 30 dB. The Federal Communication Commission (FCC) has allocated the frequency region of 72 to 76 MHZ (and recently 216 to 217 MHZ) for FM devices utilized for the hearing impaired.

As noted in Table 17–5, there are several ways of coupling an FM system to the user. For a discussion of the advantages and disadvantages of various coupling strategies, the reader is directed to Lewis (1998). For listeners with hearing loss, the FM signal can be presented through headphones, earbuds coupled directly to the ear via a button or behind-the-ear transducer, or directly to hearing aids via induction loop or Direct Audio Input (DAI). For individuals with conductive or mixed hearing losses, the FM system can be coupled to a bone conduction transducer. For "normal-hearing" individuals, the signal can be presented through earbuds or small headphones. More recently, personal FM systems have become available for both individuals with SNHL and "normal hearing" in ear-level models. For listeners with SNHL, this type of FM system provides the user with a combination of *both* a hearing aid and an FM system in the same ear-level device. For individuals with "normal hearing," the FM system is simply located in a behind-the-ear

configuration with an open fitting. In both cases, these types of systems allow the user the freedom of not having to use the body-worn receivers required with traditional FM systems. Another current advancement in FM technology allows a personal FM receiver to be coupled to a hearing aid via an "audio boot" (Figure 17–2). This technology allows the user to convert his or her personal hearing aid into an FM system simply by attaching the audio boot. These FM systems may be

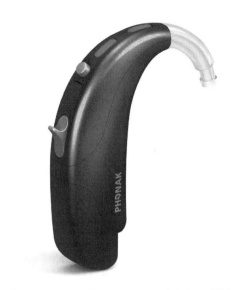

Figure 17–2. Frequency modulation (FM) system coupled to a hearing aid via a wireless "audio boot." Courtesy of Phonak, LLC.

Table 17–5. FM Coupling Strategies for Listeners with Hearing Loss and "Normal Hearing"

Individuals with Hearing Loss	Individuals with "Normal Hearing"
Headphones	Headphones
Earbuds	Earbuds
Direct to the ear via a button or behind-the-ear transducer	Ear level (behind-the-ear style device with an FM system integrated)
Direct to hearing aids via induction loop or Direct Auditory Input (DAI)	
Ear level (audio boot or behind-the-ear style device with hearing aid + FM system integrated)	
Bone conduction transducer	

particularly useful for individuals who may not want to utilize personal FM systems due to the potential negative stigma that may be associated with such devices.

Finally, prior to concluding this section, it should be noted that although FM systems are the most popular room amplification used in theaters, classroom, and therapy-room settings, they also can be beneficial in other settings. For example, FM systems can be used to provide important early auditory input to infants with hearing impairment, particularly when limited auditory information is available (Crandell & Smaldino, 1999). Advantages and disadvantages of personal FM systems are found in Table 17–6.

FM Audio Distribution Systems

An FM audio distribution system is similar to a personal FM system, but the speaker's voice is conveyed to all listeners in the room via one or more strategically placed loudspeakers (Figure 17–3). FM audio distribution systems are generally used to assist "normal-hearing" individuals, such as children in a classroom setting. The objectives when placing a FM audio distribution FM system in a classroom are to: (1) amplify the speaker's voice by approximately 8 to 10 dB, thus improving the SNR of the listening environment and (2) provide amplification uniformly throughout the classroom regardless

Table 17–6. Potential Advantages and Disadvantages of Personal FM Systems

Advantages	Disadvantages
High degree of portability	User often has to wear a body-worn receiver
Simple installation	Learning curve for use and maintenance
Not susceptible to electromagnetic interference	May be susceptible to FM interference from other sources
High degree of electroacoustic flexibility	
Buildings can have many rooms using FM systems as long as the transmission channels are selected to not interfere with one another	Relatively high unit cost
	Localization abilities may be limited if the device is not open fit
FM systems can be used in many communication situations (large rooms, small rooms, indoor, outdoors, field trips, broadcast media) that may not be practical for other forms of room amplification	
High mobility for speaker and listener	

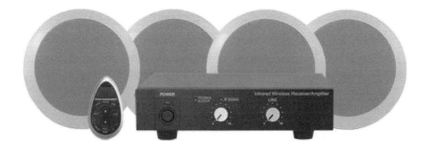

Figure 17–3. Components of a frequency modulation (FM) audio distribution system with mountable speakers. Courtesy of Audio Enhancements.

of teacher or student position. Audio distribution systems vary from compact, portable, battery-powered single-speaker units to more permanently placed, alternating-current (AC) powered speaker systems that utilize multiple (usually four) loudspeakers. New loudspeaker designs such as cylindrical wave and bending wave or new implementations of older speaker designs may provide adequate sound coverage with fewer speakers. Loudspeakers are generally placed on stands or mounted on the walls and strategically placed within the classroom. Several companies now sell loudspeakers that can be placed in the ceiling (Figure 17–4).

A number of studies have demonstrated that when sound distribution systems are correctly placed within learning settings (such as classrooms and lecture halls), speech recognition, psychoeducational, and psycho-

social improvements occur for listeners with "normal hearing" (see Berg, 1993, Crandell et al., 1995; Crandell & Smaldino, 1996b; Langlan, Sockalingam, Caissie, & Kreisman, 2009). At present, there remains limited data concerning the effects of FM audio distribution systems on individuals with moderate to severe degrees of SNHL. Advantages and disadvantages of sound-field FM systems are found in Table 17–7. For a detailed discussion on measuring efficacy of audio distribution placement, the reader is referred to Kreisman, Crandell, Smaldino, and Kreisman (2005).

Infrared Light Wave Systems

Infrared systems consist of a wireless microphone, infrared converter, and infrared receiver. The microphone converts the acoustical

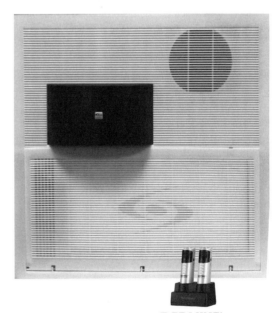

Media Connector

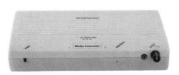

Figure 17–4. An audio distribution system loudspeaker in the ceiling. Courtesy of Lightspeed Technologies, Inc.

Table 17–7. Potential Advantages and Disadvantages of FM Cads Systems

Advantages	Disadvantages
Provides benefit to all "normal hearing" listeners in the room	May not provide adequate benefits in excessively noisy or reverberant listening environments
Can provide benefit to children with SNHL while malfunctioning hearing aids or auditory trainers are being repaired	Primarily used only for "normal hearers" and listeners with milder degrees of SNHL
Often the most inexpensive procedure of improving classroom acoustics	Loudspeaker arrangement and/or number of loudspeakers(s) must be appropriate
Audio distribution system does not stigmatize certain listeners	May not be feasible in smaller rooms due to feedback problems associated with the interactive effects of reflective surfaces and speaker closeness
Speakers/teachers overwhelmingly accept sound field amplification system once they receive an in-service on the instrumentation or utilize the equipment	May not benefit children with severe recruitment or hypersensitive hearing
Speakers/teachers report lessened stress and vocal strain during teaching activities	Audio distribution systems may not be portable (unless desktop units are used)
Parents and students overwhelmingly accept sound field amplification systems Audio distribution systems can be used to enhance the auditory signal from other instructional equipment (e.g., television, compact disc, and mp3 players)	
High mobility for speaker and listener	
Not susceptible to electromagnetic interference	

signal to an electrical signal, which is then transmitted to the converter. The converter transduces the electrical signal to an invisible infrared signal and transmits it to a receiver worn by the listener. The receiver (which often also has an amplifier) contains photo-detector diodes that pick up the infrared signal to transduce the infrared signal back into electrical energy. The electrical signal is then changed into acoustical energy and routed to the listener via an induction loop and hearing aid telecoil setup, through headphones or insert earphones or DAI. The majority of infrared systems designed for individuals with SNHL use a carrier frequency of 95 kHz. Infrared systems are often used in larger room settings, such as auditoriums, conference halls, theaters, and churches. For large rooms, such as theaters and auditori-

ums, arrays of transmitters must be utilized to ensure that all listeners are appropriately placed within the infrared light beam. In the clinical setting, infrared systems are often recommended for television and radio communication. An example of one such device is found in Figure 17–5. A summary of the advantages and disadvantages of infrared systems are found in Table 17–8.

Large Area Electromagnetic Induction Loop Systems

A large area induction loop system consists of a microphone connected via a hardwire or an FM transmitter to an amplifier. A length of wire, which is wound around a magnetic core under its installation, extends from the ampli-

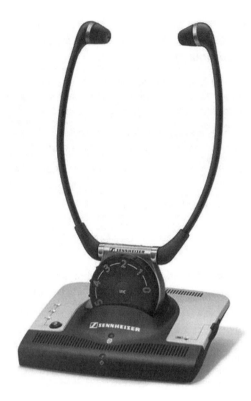

Figure 17–5. A personal infrared device. Courtesy of Seinnheisser USA.

fier. This wire is placed either around the head of an individual (neckloop) or around a designated area, such as a classroom or theater (Figure 17–6). When an electrical current flows through the wire loop, it creates a magnetic field, which can be picked up by any device utilizing telecoil technology (such as a hearing aid). Advantages and disadvantages of large area induction loop systems are presented in Table 17–9.

To avoid many of the difficulties associated with traditional induction loop systems, Hendricks and Lederman (1991) developed a three-dimensional induction loop system. In the three-dimensional induction loop system, a wireless microphone transmits the speaker's voice to an audio mixer, signal processor, and power amplifier. The amplified signal is then transmitted to specially designed induction loops that are placed within a floor mat that is placed under the room's carpet. Advantages of such systems over traditional induction loop systems include significantly-reduced "spillover" and a more uniform signal, thus providing a consistent signal to more listeners in the room.

Table 17–8. Potential Advantages and Disadvantages of Infrared Systems

Advantages	Disadvantages
Worldwide use is high	Because the infrared cannot penetrate solid barriers, listener must be in a direct line of sight with the transmitter
Not susceptible to electromagnetic interference	
Relatively inexpensive	
	Cannot be used outside, or in highly lit rooms, because infrared is susceptible to interference from sunlight

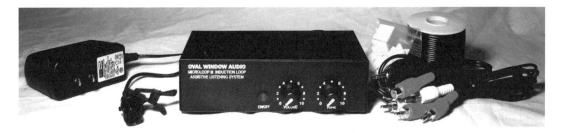

Figure 17–6. Components of a large area induction loop system. Courtesy of Oval Window.

Table 17–9. Potential Advantages and Disadvantages of Large Area Induction Loop Systems

Advantages	Disadvantages
Often least costly of the room amplification systems	Require functional telecoil that is sensitive enough to pick up the magnetic field throughout the room and/or incorporate a preamplifier
Installation, portability, troubleshooting, and maintenance of such systems tend to be relatively easy	Require hearing aids (or some device with telecoil) that limits use for "normal hearers"
Hearing aid users already have a receiver if their hearing aid contains a telecoil	Require hearing aids that contain telecoil option
High degree of electroacoustic flexibility (due to hearing aid telecoil)	Signal quality may decrease as the listener moves away from the induction loop
	Reduced portability; for example, it is not practical to move such systems to accommodate outdoor activities
	Number of rooms in a building that can be equipped with such technology may be limited, because "spillover" can occur across systems
	Signal quality may be reduced by additional devices in the room that produce electromagnetic fields (and 60 Hz hum), such as fluorescent lighting and electric power lines

IMPROVING TELEPHONE COMMUNICATION WITH REHABILITATIVE TECHNOLOGIES

In addition to communicative difficulties in rooms, another common complaint of individuals with SNHL is speech-recognition difficulties when communicating via the telephone. The present section examines various strategies for improving communication over the telephone.

Hearing Aid Telecoils and Telephone Use

A common procedure to improve telephone communication is through a hearing aid telephone induction pickup coil, or telecoil. A hearing aid telecoil picks up the electromagnetic leakage from the telephone receiver. The signal is then amplified, transduced into acoustical information, and delivered to the individual's ear. Improved telephone communication is obtained because: (1) the hearing aid microphone is turned off, reducing the level of the background noise and reverberation and (2) the frequency response of most telecoils tends to be smoother than when the hearing aid is acoustically coupled to the telephone. Unfortunately, due to the miniaturization of hearing aids, many hearing aids are not equipped with telecoils or are equipped with telecoils that produce inappropriate amounts of amplification. Often, amplified telecoils must be ordered to provide significant improvements in communication via the telephone. Certainly, whenever telecoil technology is implemented into a hearing aid, it is imperative that the patient is instructed properly concerning its use, particularly whether the telecoil is switched manually or if it is an automatic telecoil, and placement with the telephone. Most audiologists have had the experience of an individual with a hearing aid, attempting (with no success) to place the telephone receiver over his or her ear instead of near the telecoil. Moreover, patients should be warned that hearing aid telecoil technology may not be particularly beneficial within environments where electromagnetic interference (computers, fluorescent lights) may be high.

Rehabilitative Technologies and Telephone Use

A number of individual rehabilitative technologies can also be used with the telephone to improve communication for the individual with hearing loss. One device, for example, consists of a disk-shaped microphone that attaches to the telephone handset. The signal is then routed into the listener's personal hearing aid via DAI. Often, the use of an individual personal rehabilitative technology, particularly DAI, can be beneficial in environments where electromagnetic interference is high.

Acoustic Couplers

Acoustic couplers are foam or plastic cushions that fit on the receiver of the telephone handset. Such cushions are available in both square and round shapes to fit ear- and mouthpieces. In addition to providing comfort, these cushions allow the hearing aid user to utilize the telephone acoustically with reduced feedback, particularly when the telephone is equipped with amplification. Acoustic telepads may be particularly useful for those individuals with hearing aids that are too small to incorporate telecoil circuitry.

Telephone Amplifiers

There are several types of amplifiers for telephones (Table 17–10, Figures 17–7, and 17–8). Each of these amplifiers can be used with or without a hearing aid. If used with a hearing aid, such amplification systems may be used

Table 17–10. Various Types of Amplifiers for Telephones

Amplified telephones

Amplified telephone handsets

In-line amplifiers

Portable telephone amplifiers

Acoustic-induction loop amplifiers

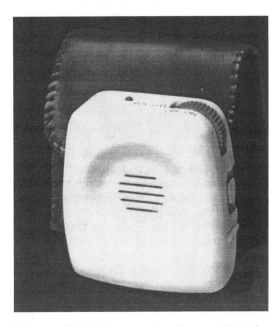

Figure 17–7. An example of a portable telephone amplifier. Courtesy of Ameriphone.

through acoustic coupling (through the microphone of the hearing aid) or inductive coupling (through the telecoil of the hearing aid).

Amplified telephones often provide adjustable gain characteristics, tone controls, and an enhanced dynamic range. Amplified telephones may also contain low-frequency, high-intensity ringers. Unfortunately, many of the more inexpensive, electronic-based telephones may not provide enough amplification to assist listeners who have more than a mild degree of hearing loss. In addition to amplified telephones, speaker telephones, with adjustable gain characteristics, may also be used by some individuals with hearing loss.

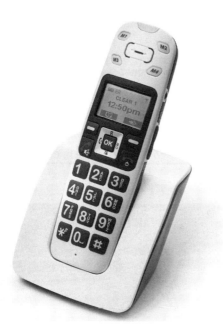

Figure 17–8. An amplified telephone with adjustable volume and tone controls. © 2013 Clear Sounds Communications, Inc. All rights reserved. ClearSounds, the logo design, Moving Beyond the Sound Barrier, A400, A500, and the trade dress are all registered trademarks of Clear Sounds Communications, Inc.

Another form of telephone amplification is amplified replacement handsets. Amplified handsets generally are available with volume control capabilities. In addition, several companies are now dispensing amplified handsets with mute switches, tone controls, and noise cancellation circuitry. Replacement handsets can be attached to most traditional modular telephones. Replacement handsets may not be compatible with many of the newer, more inexpensive, electronic telephone systems. To overcome this problem, amplified replacement handsets may be purchased with their own power supply. It should be noted that when placing a replacement handset on a telephone, the impedance characteristics of the replacement handset and telephone must be matched. Otherwise, the gain may not be maximized and the signal distorted. If such handsets are coupled to a hearing aid, it is imperative that the handset is hearing aid compatible. The Americans with Disabilities

Act (1990; PL 101-336) requires that all commercially used pay telephones have handsets with adjustable gain controls. Cell phone amplifiers are available that can be used with external headsets or earphones. The amplifier plugs into the 2.5-mm audio adapter of the cell phone and the external headset then plugs into the amplifier.

In-line telephone amplifiers are available only with modular telephones. In-line amplifiers come with variable gain controls, frequency response controls, or both. The most common placement of an in-line amplifier is between the base of the telephone and the cord of the handset. In-line amplifiers can either be externally or internally powered. Such amplifiers can also be used with personal rehabilitative technologies. For example, an in-line amplifier can be connected from the telephone base into a FM system. In this case, the individual would receive a high SNR through the FM system and would speak through the handset of the telephone. Most in-line amplifiers are relatively compact and portable.

Portable 20-dB telephone amplifiers can be coupled to the telephone acoustically, magnetically, or both. Portable amplifiers that are acoustically coupled to the telephone provide approximately 20 dB of gain and can be used with the vast majority of telephones (mobile and land line) on the market today. In the case of portable telephone amplifiers coupled magnetically, the user must switch the hearing aid to the telecoil setting. Magnetic coupling strategies, however, can only be used with hearing-aid-compatible telephones. As of 1991, all telephones manufactured or imported for use in the United States were required to be hearing aid compatible (Public Law 394, The Hearing Aid Compatibility Act, 1988).

In 2003, the FCC removed an exemption to this law referring to wireless telephony, making mobile telephones subject to hearing aid compatibility requirements as described in ANSI C63.19. Specifically, a digital wireless telephone is considered to be compatible for inductive coupling (via telecoil) if it has a T3 or T4 rating under the ANSI standard. A higher "T rating" indicates greater compatibility and likelihood of clearer communication via telecoil. Hearing aids with a microphone (M) rating of M3 or M4 under the ANSI standard have a microphone that will work well with wireless telephones. Again, the higher the "M rating," the better the signal quality through the hearing aid microphone is likely to be.

A good way to estimate compatibility between a phone and a hearing aid is to add the phone's T rating to the hearing aid's M rating. A total of six is considered to be excellent; a total of 5 is considered normal, and a total of 4 is considered minimally usable. Most new hearing aids and standard wireless telephones have a rating of M2/T2 (for a total of 4), which is not ideal for wireless communication. Hearing aid users should ask an audiologist about the M rating of hearing aids before fitting. T-ratings for wireless telephones are available from phone manufacturers and wireless telephone service providers; since 2009, both manufacturers and service providers have been required to post information about hearing-aid-compatible devices offerings on their websites. Other telephone features that a hearing aid user may consider for telephone communication include a volume control, vibrating alerts, adjustable ringer volume and tone, availability of text messaging, TTY compatibility, and video streaming. For smartphones, there are several third-party applications (or "apps") available to assist listeners with hearing loss while using the phone.

Bluetooth Telephone Devices

Options for phone use have expanded to include Bluetooth connective devices for the use with landlines and cell phones. Bluetooth is a proprietary wireless technology for data transmission and exchange over short distances. The landline phone connection device must be installed on the landline phone line, while cell phones must be Bluetooth compatible. These devices enable the audio output to be transmitted wirelessly via Bluetooth technology, so that the individual can receive the signal through his or her hearing aids. Most of these hearing aids require a gateway device that receives the Bluetooth signal and

transmits the signal via near-field magnetic induction (NFMI) to the hearing aids. However, manufacturers are beginning to release hearing aids that do not need require an intermediary device.

Telecommunication Devices for the Deaf (TDD)

Individuals with severe to profound hearing losses, poor speech recognition, or severe speech impairments may not be able to effectively use the telephone even with amplification devices. For these individuals, Telecommunication Devices for the Deaf (TDDs; also called teletypewriters [TTYs] or Text Telephones [TTs]) may be required (Figure 17–9). The TDD transmits a typed, visual message (in Baudot code) over standard telephone lines. The typed communication appears on either a light-emitting diode display, or it can be printed out. Braille TDDs are available to those with visual as well as hearing difficulties. For a TDD conversation to take place, both the sender and receiver must have TDD instrumentation that is compatible with each other. A TDD system can also be modified to communicate to a computer. To allow this type of communication, an interface option is required to process the

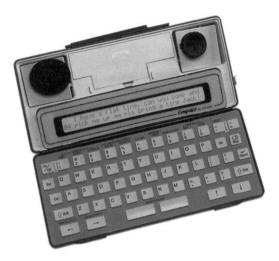

Figure 17–9. A portable Telecommunication Device for the Deaf (TDD). Courtesy of Ultratec.

slower transmission rate of the Baudot code of the TDD to the faster transmission speed (American Standard Code for Information Interchange—ASCII) of the computer. The ADA mandates that all emergency access services have TDD accessibility.

Telephone relay services (TRS) are available to the TDD user who needs to communicate with a non-TDD user. With the TRS, the individual using the TDD types a message to a state-designated telephone number that is picked up by a normal-hearing operator and transmitted verbally to the non-TDD user. The non-TDD user can then respond to the TDD user by verbally giving the message to the relay operator, who in turn, relays the message via written text to the TDD user. With TRSs, individuals with normal hearing can also telephone persons who use TDDs. As of 1993, the ADA mandated that all telephone companies provide within and across state telephone relay services.

Communication via Personal Computers and Other Digital Devices

In addition to computer-based TDD systems, several teletext computer programs have also become available over the past several years. These personal computer (PC) programs allow the user to communicate to TDD units, computers, or touch-tone telephones via typewritten messages or synthesized voice. In addition, email, real-time instant messaging, and "chat room" technologies offer communicative access for individuals with hearing or speech deficits.

Communication via Video Conferencing

Video-conferencing technology on computers is readily available and is used in a variety of settings, including businesses, education, and interpersonal communication. With such systems, a camera (Webcam) is connected to the PC. Both audio and video of the person being called are then presented through a computer monitor and speakers. With many of these systems, keyboard-produced text and TDD capabilities are also available options. Video conferencing is no longer limited to PC-based devices; smart phones, tablets, and other personal computing devices typically have built-in webcams and screen-in-screen pictures that allow for wireless video conferencing.

Video conferencing using more traditional telephone transmission has dramatically improved, but Internet- and satellite-based telephony is growing in use and will probably eclipse the use of traditional phone transmission.

Communication via Facsimile Transmission

An additional form of technology that may communicatively aid the individual with hearing or speech difficulties is facsimile (or fax) machines. The sending fax machine scans a hard-copy message, then encodes and compresses the message and transmits the information over telecommunication lines to the receiving fax machine. The receiving machine then decodes, decompresses, and prints the information. More recent technology enables faxing over the internet or sending documents via email attachments. With this method, a scanner and computer replace the standard fax machine. All-in-one printers with both traditional fax and scanners are also available for use with a computer.

IMPROVING RECEPTION OF BROADCAST MEDIA WITH REHABILITATIVE TECHNOLOGIES

Another communicative concern commonly reported by individuals with hearing loss is difficulty hearing and understanding the auditory signal that is broadcast over the television or radio. As was outlined in the first section of the chapter, distance from the sound source, noise, and reverberation can produce a distorted or inaudible signal to the hearing impaired individual. Hearing aids alone often do little to reduce the effects of such environmental disturbances and are often not a solution to improving the recognition (and enjoyment) of broadcast media. Rehabilitative devices such as hard-wired systems, induction loop, FM, and infrared systems can all be used to link the broadcast media to the individual with hearing loss, thus effectively improving the quality of the audio signal received. There are also television-band radios that can be tuned to the channel being watched and placed close to the individual so that the volume can be increased and the effects of distance from the signal reduced. Personal sound-field FM systems are new devices that may be useful as well. The transmitting microphone is placed close to the television or radio speaker, and the receiving speaker amplifier is placed close to the listener. The increased volume and reduction of the effects of room acoustics often significantly improve sound reception.

Bluetooth connective devices for the television and other broadcast media (such as MP3 players) have become a more popular option in recent years. These devices enable the audio output to be transmitted wirelessly via Bluetooth technology, so that the individual can receive the signal through his or her hearing aids. As previously mentioned, a gateway device that converts Bluetooth signal to NFMI may be necessary.

Closed Captioning

Television viewing can also be enhanced with a running-text subtitle of the audio program in the lower portion of the screen. This running-text subtitling of the broadcast, called closed captioning, is encoded in the television signal and must be decoded to appear on the screen. As a result of the Television Decoder Circuitry Act of 1990 (PL 101-431), all television sets of more than 13 inches must be equipped with a decoder chip, so that individuals can have access to closed captioning when available. Most closed captioning is done "off line" and added to the recorded television program before broadcast. Real-time captioning has become available for live broadcasts, such as the news, sporting events, and even meetings. A trained captioner follows the audio signal, and with a delay of 2 to 3 seconds converts it to text that appears on the television screen. Recently voice-to-text technology has become refined enough to use as a real-time captioning device. Using sophisticated voice identification technology, these devices hold promise of directly converting the speech signal into text that can be read by the individual with SNHL.

Two newer captioning technologies promise to significantly improve access for people who are deaf or hearing impaired. Discrete personal captioning uses state of the art electronic, optical, and voice recognition technologies to provide text in a "heads-up" display (similar to that found in fighter aircraft) that is built into a pair of glasses. A text readout seems to "float in the air" about 18 inches in front of the wearer. The second technology, called reflective captioning, uses a small handheld LED screen that follows the auditory signal by flashing captions of the signal on the screen. Both technologies are designed to provide equal access to public places by providing an inconspicuous and efficient translation and text display of ongoing auditory signals.

Another challenge for individuals with hearing loss is access to closed captioning for internet content. Several companies have released closed caption programs that use speech recognition software to generate captions for videos on websites that otherwise do not have captions. Currently there are limitations to this type of automatic captioning software, such as background noise and/or music in the video; however, it is anticipated that such technology will be improved (National Public Radio, 2010).

ALERTING SYSTEMS

Alerting devices help alert the individual with SNHL through visual, auditory, olfactory, or vibrotactile outputs (Table 17–11).

Alerting devices can be: (1) hard-wired or wireless and (2) attached to detect one or multiple environmental signals in the home, car, or office. Generally, alerting systems are considered to be beneficial only for individuals with profound degrees of hearing loss. Many alerting devices can also be helpful for individuals with milder degrees of SNHL, however. Persons with high frequency hearing loss, for example, may have difficulties hearing the microwave timer, the doorbell, knocking on the door, or the telephone ringer.

There are three ways that environmental signals can be detected via alerting technology: (1) direct electrical connection; (2) sound activated; and (3) induction based (Larose, Evans, & Larose, 1989). Several examples of alerting devices are found in Figures 17–10, 17–11, and 17–12. Direct electrical connect

Table 17–11. Sensory Modalities Used for Alerting Devices

Visual	Auditory	Vibrotactile
Turning on/off lamp	Amplified signal	Pocket pagers
		Bed shakers
Strobe light	Lowered pitch signal	Increases in airstream (such as a fan)
Bright incandescent light		

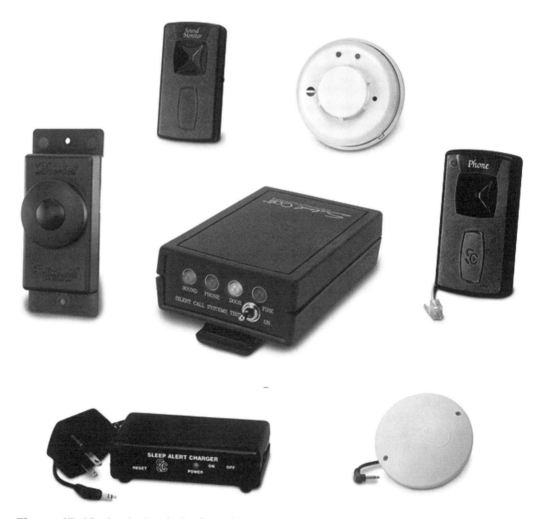

Figure 17–10. An alerting device for various sources with personal pager. Courtesy of Silent Call.

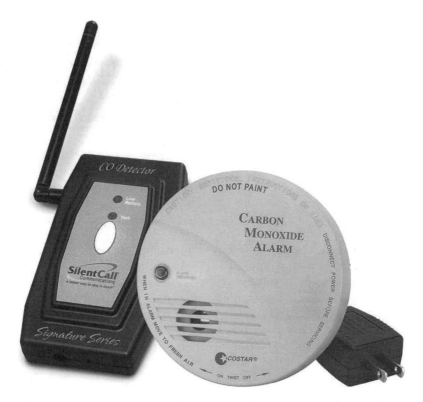

Figure 17–11. An example of an alerting device that uses flashing lights. Courtesy of Silent Call.

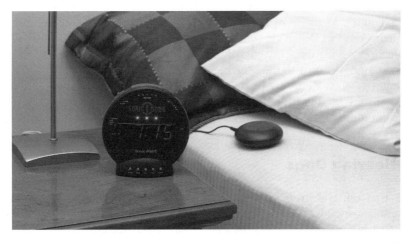

Figure 17–12. An alarm clock alerting device. Sonic Alert, Inc. Owner: Adam Kollin .

systems are permanently interfaced with, and directly activated by, the electrical system of the sound-activating device. In this case, the alerting device is directly connected to the telephone, alarm clock, microwave timer, or doorbell. When the device is activated, a visual, auditory, or tactile signal is presented to the individual. Direct electrical connected alerting devices, while highly reliable for alerting purposes, are not very portable. Sound-activated systems detect the presence of an environmental sound through the placement of a remote microphone system at or near that device. When the microphone detects the presence of a particular environmental sound, a signal is transmitted to the alerting system. For example, a remote microphone may be placed near the microwave or oven timer to inform the individual when the timer is activated. Another common example of such technology in use would be to place the sound-activated microphone near a baby crib so that the parents can be informed when the child cries or make noises. Sound-activated systems generally have sensitivity settings to reduce the possibility of other environmental sounds activating the system. Recently sound-activated technologies have been developed that allow the user with hearing impairment to monitor important traffic noises, such as emergency vehicle sirens or car horns. Sound-activated systems are generally portable. Induction-based systems use the electromagnetic field from electrical devices to send a signal to the alerting device. With such systems, a suction cup electromagnetic detection device is placed on the desired environmental sound-producing device. When the electromagnetic detection device detects activation of the system, a signal is sent to the alerting system. Although such systems are portable, signal detection may be negatively affected by incorrect placement of the suction cup.

Hearing Dogs

In addition to traditional alerting systems, an individual with hearing loss may also choose to use a dog that is professionally trained to attract the attention of the person with hearing loss when particular sounds occur in the environment (door bell, fire alarm, telephone ring, etc.) and to lead them to the source of the sound. In most states, restrictions on the use of hearing dogs in public places are similar to restrictions on guide dogs for individuals with loss of vision.

SELECTING REHABILITATIVE TECHNOLOGIES FOR INDIVIDUALS WITH HEARING LOSS AND "NORMAL HEARING"

As previously noted, rehabilitative technologies are designed to minimize the communication deficits caused by a hearing loss. The first step to determine an appropriate rehabilitative device is through a comprehensive evaluation of the audiological dimensions of the hearing loss. In addition to the usual comprehensive evaluative components of thresholds for pure tones and speech, speech recognition in quiet, and immittance measures, the evaluation should include speech-recognition measures in commonly encountered backgrounds of noise. Measures of the central auditory processing (CAP) capabilities of the subject should be conducted as research has demonstrated that some of these individuals do not receive as much benefit from personal hearing aids as persons with intact central auditory processing abilities (Crandell, 1999).

In addition to audiological measures, measures of communication disability and needs are a crucial component of the rehabilitative process. Forms such as the Client Oriented Scale of Improvement (COSI), Hearing Handicap Inventory for the Elderly/Adult (HHIE/HHIA), Abbreviated Profile of Hearing Aid Benefit (APHAB), and the Glasgow Scale of Communication function, as well as a detailed case history, have been shown to be useful in assessing such needs and disability. These scales are discussed in greater detail elsewhere in this book. On the basis of the audiological and communication assessments, the audiologist can recommend hearing aids, rehabilitative technologies, communication strategies, and therapies that will minimize the impact of the hearing loss on the client's everyday activities.

It must be noted that evaluating communication needs, and consequently, recommending appropriate rehabilitative technologies, can be a difficult task for a number of reasons (Tye-Murray, 2009). First, communication handicap varies as a function of the communication setting and communication partner. Second, hearing handicap varies with the topic of conversation. Third, handicap does not always happen during conversation; that is, a lack of miscommunication during the assessment process will provide the professional with an inaccurate assessment of the communication handicap the person has under more difficult listening circumstances. Fourth, communication handicap is a construct made up of many dimensions, thus no one assessment measure is likely to capture all of these dimensions. As a result, several assessment measures and a detailed case history should be taken on an individual and interpreted together. Finally, the technology requirements for effective communication for a particular individual will vary depending on location (home, work, travel, and so forth) and on the type of communication (face-to-face, through the media, over the telephone, or as an alerting communication; Tye-Murray, 2009).

Based on the transtheoretical model of behavioral change (DiClemente et al., 1991; McConnaughy, DiClemente, Prochaska, & Velicer, 1989; McConnaughy, Prochaska, & Velicer, 1983), Singer and Preece (1997) have suggested a five-stage model to assist patient compliance in these areas. The first stage of the model is called "precontemplative." This is the stage where the individual with hearing loss has not accepted that there are problems caused by the hearing loss. The authors suggest that helping the person become aware of the actual problems can be an effective intervention strategy. Hearing handicap scales, such as those previously mentioned, can be used to guide the individual through a discussion of situations that cause listening breakdowns in everyday communication environments. In the second stage, called "contemplation," the individual has become aware of listening problems and is considering ways to solve them. Singer and Preece (1997) suggested that the professional can help the individual at this stage by providing accurate information about available technol-

ogy and rehabilitative options, as well as a realistic assessment of how effective these options might be considering the individual's everyday listening environments. The third stage is referred to as "preparation," wherein the individual with hearing loss is essentially ready to take action to solve listening problems. Having the individual commit to change by signing up for rehabilitation following the fitting of assistive technology often solidifies the readiness of the individual to change. In the fourth or "action" stage, the individual makes tentative decision for change. Singer and Preece suggested that the emphasis should be on the tentative, in that without positive reinforcement for the decisions relating to change (such as the purchase of assistive technology), an individual can revert to an earlier stage in the process that can significantly delay change. The individual might return the assistive technology, for example. In the fifth or "maintenance" stage, the individual truly makes a change, and the benefits to the individual become manifest. During this stage, the individual requires support in the use of technology and specific rehabilitative strategy training. In the "termination" stage, the individual has fully accepted the hearing aid and assistive technology, which becomes integrated into his or her everyday listening environment.

In a similar model, Tye-Murray (2009) conceptualized essentially the same process in what she calls communication strategies training. Communication strategies training is composed of three stages. In the formal instruction stage, the client is provided with information about various types of communication strategies and appropriate listening and speaking behaviors. Included here are presentations that describe facilitative and receptive repair strategies and expressive repair strategies; also included are instructions in "clear speech," specific interventions to avoid a miscommunication, and information about how to recover from a miscommunication should one occur. The second stage is called guided learning, wherein the professional creates simulated real-life communication situations where the strategies acquired in the formal instruction stage can be practiced. The audiologist provides feedback and correction to the client as he or she progresses through the simulations. The last stage requires the client to engage in a prescribed real-world listening situation and to answer prepared questions regarding the effective use of information learned in stage one and practiced in stage two.

MEASURING EFFICACY FOR REHABILITATIVE TECHNOLOGIES

Whenever assistive technologies (or hearing aids) are recommended, it is imperative that efficacy be measured. Efficacy is a measure to demonstrate that an intervention was effective or ineffective and that a different intervention may be more appropriate. A number of procedures can be used to quantify the effectiveness of rehabilitative technology on a particular individual (Tye-Murray, 2009). One way of measuring efficacy is through the interview procedure. In this procedure, specific information about the effectiveness of rehabilitative technologies is elicited through the use of informal or formalized questions. One of the problems with the interview procedure, however, is that the patient's responses are hard to quantify. To circumvent these difficulties, forms such as the COSI could be utilized in the interview process. The COSI requires the interviewee to rank in order five handicaps that they perceive are a result of their hearing loss. This initial quantification of the person's problems before intervention can then be used as a measure of whether intervention was effective. A second procedure to measure efficacy is through the questionnaire. As noted above, many hearing handicap questionnaires have been developed and can be quite useful if the questions match the situation of the individual with hearing loss. If the match is not good, the questionnaire may not provide enough relevant informa-

tion about communication needs to be useful in the rehabilitative process. A well-matched hearing handicap scale can provide important information concerning the effectiveness of intervention. If after the intervention there is less hearing handicap, the intervention might be considered effective. One such questionnaire, the Hearing Function Profile (Singer & Preece, 1997) has been developed to determine why an individual is unsuccessful with assistive technology and provides a basis for recommending additional technologies or rehabilitation training.

A third procedure to evaluate efficacy is a daily log or diary, wherein the individual with hearing impairment provides qualitative information about communication difficulties with use of the rehabilitative technology over time. These logs provide an ongoing self-report analysis of changes that occur as a result of intervention and can be used to assess the effectiveness of an intervention. Logs can be reactive, however, in that the act of completing the log can affect communication handicap. This is not necessarily bad but lessens the usefulness of the log procedure to gauge the effectiveness of a specific intervention. Group discussion is another possible measure of efficacy. The interactions that occur during a group discussion of persons having hearing loss often force each individual discussant to introspect and reflect upon their communication problems and rehabilitative technology utilization. Over time, these group interactions can provide important information (and psychosocial support) about technology use.

The fifth procedure for measuring efficacy is referred to as structured communication interactions, wherein conversations between the person with hearing loss and the evaluator are simulated to reflect communication situations that are typical for the person. Situations are identified that produce communication handicap under more or less realistic situations. The effectiveness of intervention can be directly assessed by simulating difficult communication situations with and without the assistive technology in use.

INCREASING CONSUMER UTILIZATION OF ASSISTIVE TECHNOLOGIES

Unfortunately, although this chapter has addressed many advantages of having listeners with hearing loss utilize assistive technologies, research suggests that patients are often unaware of assistive technology and that relatively few audiologists are actively dispensing such technologies. It appears that individuals with hearing impairment are unaware of assistive technology due to two factors (Mahon, 1985). First, audiologists have been relatively indifferent to incorporating assistive technologies into their available product line; second, audiologists often have not had an adequate knowledge base to accurately inform their patients about such technologies. McCarthy, Culpepper, and Winstead (1983), for example, showed that a majority of 50 individuals with hearing loss were not familiar with assistive technologies despite the fact that they reported difficulties in most listening situations. Many of the subjects were interested in purchasing assistive technologies when informed about them. Hartley, Rochtchina, Newall, Golding, and Mitchell (2010) determined the prevalence of ALD and hearing aid use in a sample of 2,956 persons aged 49 to 99 years of age. While 33% of the sample had a hearing loss, only 4.4% had used an ALD in the past 12 months. A consumer survey by John, Marsh, and Kreisman (2013) found low familiarity with a range of hearing assistive technology, though respondents who were using HAT rated their own devices as very useful. Certainly, such data emphasize the need for greater training about assistive technologies for both audiologists and individuals with hearing loss.

It seems reasonable to speculate that, for consumers to accept assistive technologies, audiologists must be convinced first of the value of assistive technologies in the overall rehabilitative plan for an individual. Unfortunately, in audiology training programs, great emphasis has been placed on the proper fitting of hearing aids, but minimal attention has been given to the assistive technology and other rehabilitative needs of the person with hearing impairment (Crandell & Smaldino, 1999). Thus, it appears that the first step in creating consumer acceptance of these technologies is the development of a philosophy of rehabilitation that includes multidimensional assessment of the individual's auditory and communication capabilities and needs. Within the context of a comprehensive rehabilitative plan, the value of assistive technologies will be self-evident because these technologies are not "add-ons" but are an integral part of the services provided in the rehabilitative plan for an individual, along with hearing aids and communication strategies training. Ross (1994) eloquently discussed assistive technologies as necessities rather than as a luxury in the rehabilitation process.

In addition to a carefully constructed rehabilitation program, there is a need to engage in activities to enhance consumer acceptance of assistive technology. The same negative stigmas that are attached to hearing loss and hearing aids are attached to assistive devices and even to a greater extent because assistive technologies are typically more noticeable and intimidating than a hearing aid. Sutherland (1995) detailed the following strategies that hearing health care professionals can employ to increase consumer acceptance of assistive technologies: (1) educating consumers about assistive devices including strengths and limitations, (2) training consumers to use technical devices, (3) helping consumers make informed choices, (4) providing consumers with support, (5) encouraging more experienced consumers to help those who are learning about technical devices, (6) empowering consumers by working closely with them as part of a team or partnership, and (7) aligning with consumers to advocate for better laws and services, and for universal accessibility for people with hearing loss.

Today, many individuals with normal hearing can be seen wearing ear-level Bluetooth headsets. It is, therefore, anticipated that the stigma of ear-level hearing devices among the Millennial generation will be virtually nonexistent. Audiologists and hearing aid companies are making people more aware of the abilities of hearing aids to communicate with Bluetooth technologies for such purposes as television and hands-free cell- or land-line phone use. While these are positive developments in the potential acceptance of some assistive technologies, other technologies are less discussed with patients. Unfortunately, many audiologists still may not actively dispense or recommend other assistive technologies, such as alerting devices.

LEGISLATION FOR ASSISTIVE TECHNOLOGY

As previously discussed, several federal laws provide for the utilization of assistive technology; however, two laws are prominent. The first law is the Americans with Disabilities Act of 1990. The second law is the Education for All Handicapped Children Act of 1975, now codified as the Individuals with Disabilities Education Act, most recently amended by the Individuals with Disabilities Education Improvement Act (IDIEA) of 2004. Colloquially, the law is still referred to as the Individuals with Disabilities Education Act (IDEA). These legislative efforts demonstrate the sustained interest in removing barriers for persons with hearing loss and other disabilities. One of the ways that acoustic barriers to communication can be diminished is through the use of assistive listening technology, and these technologies are included as a reasonable accommodation that is required under all of these laws.

ILLUSTRATIVE CASE STUDIES

The following four cases serve as illustrative examples of the kind of patients that the authors have assisted through the use of rehabilitative technologies.

Case 1

Case History

Jamie was a college-aged student who was seen in the clinic because of the difficulty she was having understanding the professors in class and because she was unable to follow class discussions among other students, especially in large lecture halls. Although she wore hearing aids, she was frustrated because she had been able to get along in high school but now was experiencing great difficulty. The listening difficulties were leaving her fatigued at the end of the day with no energy to properly study or complete assignments. She was thinking of withdrawing from school.

Audiological Assessment

Jamie had moderate SNHL in both ears. Her hearing aids were properly fit and matched NAL targets for the type of aid. Although her aided speech identification was good in quiet, she experienced a loss in ability to hear in noise.

Hearing Aid Assessment

The original dispenser had chosen an ITE model with no telecoil, direct audio input (DAI), or wireless connectivity options.

Intervention

Although the hearing aids were only 2 years old, they did not have options that would have solved Jamie's main listening problem. New hearing aids were fit incorporating an FM receiver into the hearing aid (assistance for the new aids was obtained through a local vocational rehabilitation office). The use of the transmitting FM microphone nearly eliminated Jamie's trouble hearing in class. In tandem with the new hearing aids, Jamie received communication strategies training to help her cope more successfully in situations where even the new aids are not completely adequate for her listening needs.

Case 2

Case History

Frank was a 42-year-old male with a long history (since childhood) of severe-profound SNHL. The hearing loss was of uncertain etiology, but Frank reported a positive family history of hearing loss; thus, hereditary hearing loss was suspected. He was seen in the clinic because he noted a change in his hearing. He also noted that he was having increased difficulty in his home environment. Specifically, he complained of not always hearing the telephone, the doorbell, the microwave oven timer, or alarm clock. Frank had been fit with hearing aids at several other clinics but always reported that they offered limited to no benefit. He had returned the hearing aids to the dispenser in each case. His audiologist suggested that Frank be evaluated as a potential candidate for cochlear implantation, but Frank was not interested in surgery to correct his hearing.

Audiological Assessment

A complete audiological evaluation indicated a bilateral profound SNHL. These results suggested an approximate 10 to 20 dB change in his pure-tone sensitivity over the previous 2 years. Because of the extent of his hearing loss, speech recognition measures could not be conducted. Speech reading tests indicated that Frank was an excellent speech reader. He also had extensive sign language abilities. Frank normally used a TDD at home and at work.

Intervention

Frank was counseled regarding his change in hearing. In addition, the following recommendations were made. First, it was recommended that Frank use alerting devices in his apartment. Specifically, sound activated and electrically activated alerting devices were placed for the following: (1) door knocking, (2) doorbell, (3) microwave/oven timer, and (4) telephone ringer. The alerting devices were hooked up to several lamps, which turned on/off in response to a signal and were located in different rooms, and to a personal paging device that vibrated in response to a signal. His alarm clock was hooked up to a bed and pillow vibrator. He reported that these devices helped immensely. Second, Frank was recommended for additional auditory rehabilitation at the university and trial utilization of new hearing aids and an FM system. To date, he has not followed up on the hearing aid trial recommendation.

Case 3

Case History

Tommy was an 8-year-old boy who had a long history of recurrent otitis media. His parents were concerned because he did not pay attention at home and his teacher believed he is functioning below his capacity. The teacher was also concerned that he might have an attention deficit and a developing behavioral problem because he was disruptive in class. While the teacher was aware of his fluctuating hearing loss and tried preferential seating in the front of the classroom, this had not diminished the problem.

Audiological Assessment

Tommy had many hearing tests, and they often showed a mild conductive hearing loss due to either negative middle-ear pressure, fluid in the middle ear, or both. His physician treated him with antibiotics and antihistamines when the fluid was present. He never received PE tubes. While his hearing showed a mild conductive loss, there was also a mild sensorineural loss in the higher frequencies. The Listening Inventories for Education (LIFE); Anderson & Smaldino, 1998) were completed by the teacher, the parents, and Tommy confirming that listening and attention were problems. The Auditory Continuous Performance Test (ACPT; Keith,

1994) also showed that Tommy had an inability to attend to auditory stimuli.

Intervention

Although Tommy's teacher tried preferential seating, it was not successful because the teacher moved around the room during instruction. It was thought that Tommy was exhibiting inattentiveness, which often accompanies fluctuating hearing loss with the concomitant inconsistent auditory signal. To provide a consistent signal and to help him focus on important instructional speech, an FM audio distribution system was installed in the classroom. The system was designed to amplify the teacher's voice about 10 dB consistently throughout the classroom. In addition, Tommy received some listening training to help him better attend to sound. Almost immediately, the teacher noticed that Tommy was "on task" during classroom instruction and was less of a behavioral problem. A posttest LIFE was administered after a month of classroom amplification and showed improvement in all of the initial areas of concern.

Case 4

Case History

Bob was a 53-year-old male who went hunting with his shotgun almost every day as a teenager, without the use of hearing protection. His job as a teacher trainer takes him overseas to different countries. He was seen because he was having increased communication difficulties, especially in group settings or around individuals who speak different languages or have a strong accent when speaking English. Bob recently purchased one of the newest smart phones on the market.

Audiological Assessment

A complete audiological evaluation indicated a bilateral asymmetrical hearing loss. Bob had previously consulted an ear, nose, and throat (ENT) physician, who concluded that the asymmetry was consistent with the extended history of shooting guns. The right ear was worse, with a mild hearing loss through 1000 Hz, steeply sloping to profound at 3000 Hz; the left ear had normal hearing through 2000 Hz, with a mild-to-moderate notch from 3000 to 6000 Hz. Compared with his audiogram from 2 years ago, there was a 5- to 10-dB decrease in hearing sensitivity at most frequencies at and above 2000 Hz.

Intervention

Bob was counseled regarding his change in hearing. He was fit with a pair of bilateral, miniature open-fit receiver-in-canal hearing aids that were paired to a Bluetooth gateway device. He also decided to try Bluetooth connective devices for the landline telephone and the television. He listened to his smart phone mp3 player and said it was "awesome." He also reported that his wife was much happier with the volume of the television set, now that he was able to utilize the Bluetooth device to listen through his hearing aids.

SUMMARY

The deleterious influences of distance, background noise, and reverberation, particularly for listeners with SNHL, are well documented. Unfortunately, hearing aids often offer limited speech-recognition benefit in adverse listening environments. Conversely, many assistive listening technologies such as infrared assistive listening systems, personal FM amplification devices, induction loop, and FM audio distribution systems have been shown to enhance speech communication significantly in poor listening environments. Such technologies have also been shown to improve communication of broadcast media and telecommunications. For assistive technology to be accepted and used by an individual with hearing loss, however, the communication needs and proper selection of assistive devices must be conducted within the context of an overall rehabilitative plan. Assistive technology offers the hearing health care professional a challenge, but it also offers an opportunity to maximize communicative abilities for listeners with hearing impairment.

Acknowledgment. Carl Crandell and I composed the first edition of this chapter. Carl has passed away, but his thoughts are echoed in the words found in this revision. Brian and Andrew (both students of Carl's) and I know that Carl would smile on our collaboration and our improvements to the chapter. *Joseph Smaldino*

REVIEW QUESTIONS

1. Classroom acoustics are typically characterized in terms of:
   a. Standing waves
   b. SNR
   c. Harmonic distortion
   d. Transient distortion

2. Assistive listening devices can be grouped as:
   a. FM
   b. Alerting
   c. Inductance loop
   d. A, B, and C

3. Assistive listening devices:
   a. Should be considered separately from a hearing aid.
   b. Should be considered as part of the overall rehabilitation plan.
   c. Should never be considered with a hearing aid.
   d. Should be considered after acceptance of a hearing aid.

4. The three stages in communication strategies training are _____, _____, and _____.

5. Closed caption decoders are mandatory on all television sets with screens larger than 13 inches.
   a. True
   b. False

6. The advantage(s) of the 3D induction loop system as compared with the traditional induction loop system is/are:
   a. Easier for the listener to use.
   b. Spillover is significantly reduced.
   c. The signal tends to be more uniform.
   d. Both B and C.
   e. All of the above.

7. Speech-recognition ability is not significantly reduced in normal-hearing adults until the SNR is reduced to:
   a. +5 dB
   b. +3 dB
   c. 0 dB
   d. –2 dB

8. Many electronic-based amplified telephones are advantageous because they are inexpensive and can be used with all degrees of hearing loss.
   a. True
   b. False

9. When selecting rehabilitative technologies for a particular client, measures of central auditory processing should also be tested.
   a. True
   b. False

10. According to Singer and Preece's three-stage model of acceptance, "contemplation" is the stage where the individual has not accepted that there are problems caused by the hearing loss.
    a. True
    b. False

Answer Key

1. b
2. d
3. b
4. Formal Instruction, Guided Learning and Real World Practice
5. a
6. e
7. d

8. a
9. a
10. b

REFERENCES

American Speech-Language and Hearing Association. (1995). Guidelines for acoustics in educational environments. *American Speech and Hearing Association, 37*(Suppl. 14), 15–19.

Americans with Disabilities Act of 1990. (1990). Pub. L. No. 101–336, 104 Stat. 328.

Anderson, K., & Smaldino, J. (1998). *Listening inventories for education*. Tampa, FL: Educational Audiology Association.

Berg, F. (1993). *Acoustics and sound systems in schools*. Boston, MA: College-Hill Press.

Bess, F. (1985). The minimally hearing-impaired child. *Ear and Hearing, 6*, 43–47.

Bess, F., & Tharpe, A. (1986). An introduction to unilateral sensorineural hearing loss in children. *Ear and Hearing, 7*, 3–13.

Bolt, R., & MacDonald, A. (1949). Theory of speech masking by reverberation. *Journal of the Acoustical Society of America, 21*, 577–580.

Boney, S., & Bess, F. (1984). *Noise and reverberation effects in minimal bilateral sensorineural hearing loss*. Paper presented at the American Speech-Language-Hearing Association Convention, San Francisco, CA.

Boothroyd, A. (1991). Speech perception measures and their role in the evaluation of hearing aid performance in a pediatric population. In J. Feigin & P. Stelmachowicz (Eds.), *Pediatric amplification* (pp. 77–91). Omaha, NE: Boys Town National Research Hospital.

Cooper, J., & Cutts, B. (1971). Speech discrimination in noise. *Journal of Speech and Hearing Research, 14*, 332–337.

Crandell, C. (1991a). Individual differences in speech-recognition ability: Implications for hearing aid selection. *Ear and Hearing, 12*, 100–108.

Crandell, C. (1991b). Classroom acoustics for normal-hearing children: Implications for rehabilitation. *Educational Audiology Monographs, 2*, 18–38.

Crandell, C. (1992). Classroom acoustics for hearing-impaired children. *Journal of the Acoustical Society of America, 92*, 2470.

Crandell, C. (1993). Noise effects on the speech recognition of children with minimal hearing loss. *Ear and Hearing, 7*, 210–217.

Crandell, C. (1998). Hearing aids: Their effects on functional health status. *Hearing Journal, 51*, 22–30.

Crandell, C., & Bess, F. (1986). Speech recognition of children in a "typical" classroom setting. *Asha, 29*, 87.

Crandell, C., Henoch, M., & Dunkerson, K. (1991). A review of speech perception and aging: Some implications for aural rehabilitation. *Journal of the Academy for Rehabilitation Audiology, 24*, 121–132.

Crandell, C., & Smaldino, J. (1992). Sound-field amplification in the classroom. *American Journal of Audiology, 1*, 16–18.

Crandell, C., & Smaldino, J. (1994). The importance of room acoustics. In R. Tyler & D. Schum (Eds.), *Assistive listening devices for the hearing impaired* (pp. 142–164). Baltimore, MD: William and Wilkins.

Crandell, C., & Smaldino, J. (1995). An update on classroom acoustics for children with hearing impairment. *Volta Review, 1*, 4–12.

Crandell, C., & Smaldino, J. (1996a). The effects of noise on the speech perception of non-native English children. *American Journal of Audiology, 5*, 24–29.

Crandell, C., & Smaldino, J. (1996b). Sound field amplification in the classroom: Applied and theoretical issues. In F. Bess, J. Gravel, & A. Tharpe (Eds.), *Amplification for children with auditory deficits* (pp. 22–250). Nashville, TN: Bill Wilkerson Center Press.

Crandell, C., & Smaldino, J. (1999). Room acoustics and amplification. In M. Valente, R. Roeser, & H. Hosford-Dunn (Eds.), *Audiology treatment strategies*. New York, NY: Thieme Medical.

Crandell, C., Smaldino, J., & Flexer, C. (1995). *Sound field FM amplification: Theory and practical applications*. San Diego, CA: Singular.

DiClemente, C. C., Prochaska, J. O., Fairhurst, S. K., Velicer, W. F., Velasquez, M. M., & Rossi, J. S. (1991). The process of smoking cessation: An analysis of precontemplation, contemplation, and preparation stages of change. *Journal of Consulting and Clinical Psychology, 59*, 295–304.

Dirks, D., Morgan, D., & Dubno, J. (1982). A procedure for quantifying the effects of noise on speech recognition. *Journal of Speech and Hearing Disorders, 47*, 114–123.

Duquesnoy, A., & Plomp, R. (1983). The effect of a hearing aid on the speech-reception threshold of hearing-impaired listeners in quiet and in noise. *Journal of the Acoustical Society of America, 73*, 2166–2173.

Education of Handicapped Children Act of 1975. (1995). Pub. L. No. 94–142, 42 Stat. 163.

Festen, J., & Plomp, R. (1983). Relations between auditory functions in impaired hearing. *Journal of the Acoustical Society of America, 73*, 652–661.

Finitzo-Hieber, T. (1988). Classroom acoustics. In R. Roeser (Ed.), *Auditory disorders in school children* (2nd ed., pp. 221–233). New York, NY: Thieme.

Finitzo-Hieber, T., & Tillman, T. (1978). Room acoustics effects on monosyllabic word discrimination ability for normal and hearing-impaired children. *Journal of Speech and Hearing Research, 21*, 440–458.

Flexer, C. (1992). Classroom public address systems. In M. Ross (Ed.), *FM auditory training systems: Characteristics, selection and use* (pp. 189–209). Timonium, MD: York Press.

French, N., & Steinberg, J. (1947). Factors governing the intelligibility of speech sounds. *Journal of the Acoustical Society of America, 19*, 90–119.

Gelfand, S., & Silman, S. (1979). Effects of small room reverberation upon the recognition of some consonant features. *Journal of the Acoustical Society of America, 66*, 22–29.

Gengel, R. (1971). Acceptable signal-to-noise ratios for aided speech discrimination by the hearing impaired. *Journal of Audiology Research, 11*, 219–222.

Hartley, D., Rochtchina, E., Newall, P., Golding, M., & Mitchell, P. (2010). Use of hearing aids and assistive listening devices in an older Australian population. *Journal of the American Academy of Audiology, 21*(10), 642–653.

Hawkins, D., & Yacullo, W. (1984). Signal-to-noise ratio advantage of binaural hearing aids and directional microphones under different levels of reverberation. *Journal of Speech and Hearing Disorders, 49*, 278–286.

Hendricks, P., & Lederman, N. (1991). Development of a three-dimensional induction assistive listening system. *Hearing Instruments, 42*, 37–38.

Houtgast, T. (1981). The effect of ambient noise on speech intelligibility in classrooms. *Applied Acoustics, 14*, 15–25.

Humes, L. (1991). Understanding the speech-understanding problems of the hearing impaired. *Journal of the American Academy of Audiology, 2*, 59–69.

Individuals with Disabilities Education Improvement Act of 2004. (2004). (IDIEA), Pub. L. No. 108–446, 118 Stat. 2647.

John, A. B., Marsh, M., & Kreisman, B. (2013). *Consumers' perspectives on hearing assistive technology.* Poster presented at the 25th Annual American Academy of Audiology Conference, Anaheim, CA.

Keith, R. (1994). *Auditory continuous performance test.* San Antonio, TX: The Psychological Corporation.

Kreisman, B. (2003). *The effects of simulated reverberation on the speech-perception abilities of listeners with normal hearing* (Unpublished doctoral dissertation). University of Florida, Gainesville, FL.

Kreisman, B., Crandell, C., Smaldino, J., & Kreisman, N. (2005). Measuring efficacy of sound field placement. In J. Smaldino, C. Flexer, & C. Crandell (Eds.), *Sound field amplification: Applications to speech perception and classroom acoustics* (2nd ed., pp. 192–217). Clifton Park, NY: Thomson Delmar Learning.

Langlan, L., Sockalingam, R., Caissie, R., & Kreisman, B. (2009). The benefit of sound-field amplification in First Nations elementary school children in Nova Scotia, Canada. *Australian New Zealand Journal of Audiology, 31*(2), 55–71.

Larose, G., Evans, M., & Larose, R. (1989). Alerting devices: Available options. *Seminar on Hearing, 10*, 66–77.

Leavitt, R., & Flexer, C. (1991). Speech degradation as measured by the Rapid Speech Transmission Index (RASTI). *Ear and Hearing, 12*, 115–118.

Lewis, D. (1998). Classroom amplification. In F. Bess (Ed.), *Children with hearing loss: Contemporary trends* (pp. 277–298). Nashville, TN: Vanderbilt Bill Wilkerson Center Press.

Licklider, J., & Miller, G. (1951). The perception of speech. In S. Stevens (Ed.), *Handbook of experimental psychology.* New York, NY: Wiley.

Lochner, J., & Burger, J. (1964). The influence of reflections in auditorium acoustics. *Journal of Sound Vibrations, 4*, 426–454.

Mahon, W. (1985). Assistive devices and systems. *Hearing Journal, 38*, 7–14.

McCarthy, P., Culpepper, N., & Winstead, T. (1983). *Hearing-impaired consumers' awareness and attitudes regarding auditory assistive devices.* Paper presented at the annual meeting of the American Speech, Language, and Hearing Association Convention, Cincinnati, OH.

McConnaughy, E. A., DiClemente, C. C., Prochaska, J. O., & Velicer, W. F. (1989). Stages of change in psychotherapy: A follow-up report. *Psychotherapy: Theory, Research, and Practice, 26*, 494–503.

McConnaughy, E. A., Prochaska, J., & Velicer, W. (1983). Stages of change in psychotherapy: Measurement and sample profiles. *Psychotherapy: Theory, Research, and Practice, 20*, 368–375.

Miller, G. (1974). Effects of noise on people. *Journal of the Acoustical Society of America, 56*, 724–764.

Moncur, J., & Dirks, D. (1967). Binaural and monaural speech intelligibility in reverberation. *Journal of Speech and Hearing Research, 10*, 186–195.

Moore, B. (1997). *An introduction to the psychology of hearing.* San Diego, CA: Academic Press.

Nabelek, A. (1982). Temporal distortions and noise considerations. In G. Studebaker & F. Bess (Eds.), *The Vanderbilt hearing aid report: State of the art-research needs.* Upper Darby, PA: Monographs in Contemporary Audiology.

Nabelek, A., & Nabelek, I. (1994). Room acoustics and speech perception. In J. Katz (Ed.), *Handbook of clinical audiology* (4th ed., pp. 624–637). Baltimore, MD: Williams & Wilkins.

Nabelek, A., & Pickett, J. (1974a). Monaural and binaural speech perception through hearing aids under noise and reverberation with normal and hearing-impaired listeners. *Journal of Speech and Hearing Research, 17*, 724–739.

Nabelek, A., & Pickett, J. (1974b). Reception of consonants in a classroom as affected by monaural and binaural listening, noise, reverberation, and hearing aids. *Journal of the Acoustical Society of America, 56*, 628–639.

National Public Radio. (2010, March 9). *Google launches closed captioning for YouTube.* Retrieved from http://www.npr.org/templates/story/story.php?storyId=124501330

Needleman, A., & Crandell, C. (1996a). Speech perception in noise by hearing impaired and masked normal hearing listeners. *Journal of the American Academy of Audiology, 2*, 65–72.

Needleman, A., & Crandell, C. (1996b). Simulation of sensorineural hearing loss. In M. Jestadt (Ed.), *Modeling sensorineural hearing loss* (pp. 461–474). Boston, MA: Allyn & Bacon.

Neimoeller, A. (1968). Acoustical design of classrooms for the deaf. *American Annals of Deafness, 113,* 1040–1045.

Olsen, W. (1981). The effects of noise and reverberation on speech intelligibility. In F. Bess, B. Freeman, & J. Sinclair (Eds.), *Amplification in education* (pp. 151–163). Washington, DC: Alexander Graham Bell Association for the Deaf.

Olsen, W. (1988). Classroom acoustics for hearing-impaired children. In F. Bess (Ed.), *Hearing impairment in children* (pp. 266–267). Parkton, MD: York Press.

Plomp, R. (1978). Auditory handicap of hearing impairment and the limited benefit of hearing aids. *Journal of the Acoustical Society of America, 75,* 1253–1258.

Plomp, R. (1986). A signal-to-noise ratio model for the speech reception threshold for the hearing impaired. *Journal of Speech and Hearing Research, 29,* 146–154.

Ross, M. (1978). Classroom acoustics and speech intelligibility. In J. Katz (Ed.), *Handbook of clinical audiology* (2nd ed., pp. 469–478). Baltimore, MD: Williams and Wilkins.

Ross, M. (1994). Assistive devices: Luxury or necessity? *The Hearing Review, 13.*

Siebein, G. (1994). *Acoustics in buildings: A tutorial on architectural acoustics.* New York, NY: Acoustical Society of America.

Siebein, G., Crandell, C., & Gold, M. (1997). Principles of classroom acoustics: Reverberation. *Educational Audiology Monographs, 5,* 32–43.

Singer, J., & Preece, J. (1997). Hearing instruments: A psychological behavioral perspective. *Hearing Review, 1,* 23–27.

Smaldino, J., Crandell, C., & Kreisman, B. (2005). Classroom acoustic measurements. In C. Crandell, J. Smaldino, & C. Flexer (Eds.), *Sound-field amplification: Applications to speech perception and classroom acoustics* (2nd ed., pp. 115–131). Clifton Park, NY: Thomson Delmar Learning.

Suter, A. (1985). Speech recognition in noise by individuals with mild hearing impairments. *Journal of the Acoustical Society of America, 68,* 887–900.

Sutherland, G. (1995). Increasing consumer acceptance of assistive devices. In R. S. Tyler & D. J. Schum (Eds.), *Assistive devices for persons with hearing impairment* (pp. 251–256). Needham Heights, MD: Allyn & Bacon.

Tye-Murray, N. (2009). *Foundations of aural rehabilitation* (3rd ed.). San Diego, CA: Singular.

Van Tassell, D. (1993). Hearing loss, speech, and hearing aids. *Journal of Speech and Hearing Research, 36,* 228–244.

Wang, M., Reed, C., & Bilger, R. (1978). A comparison of the effects of filtering and sensorineural hearing loss on patterns of consonant confusions. *Journal of Speech and Hearing Research, 24,* 32–43.

Weinstein, B., & Amsel, L. (1986). The relationship between dementia and hearing impairment in the institutionalized elderly. *Clinical Gerontology, 4,* 3–15.

CHAPTER 18

Cochlear Implants

DAWN BURTON KOCH
MARY JO OSBERGER

OUTLINE

INTRODUCTION

A cochlear implant is a surgically implanted device that provides hearing sensation to individuals with severe-to-profound hearing loss who obtain limited benefit from hearing aids. By electrically stimulating the auditory nerve directly, a cochlear implant bypasses damaged or undeveloped sensory structures in the cochlea, thereby providing usable information about sound to the central auditory nervous system.

In the three decades since the introduction of cochlear implants to the United States, the devices have become the standard treatment for adults and children with profound bilateral sensorineural hearing loss. Bilateral implantation is becoming common practice, particularly in very young children who rely upon auditory input to develop oral speech and language. The benefits experienced by recipients of today's implant technology are remarkable. Adult recipients can be expected to hear speech well in quiet, to communicate in noise, and even to appreciate music. Pediatric recipients implanted early in life are developing speech and language skills commensurate with peers having normal hearing.

Cochlear implants are regulated in the U.S. by the Food and Drug Administration (FDA) as Class III medical devices. Prior to commercial distribution, they must be evaluated for safety and efficacy in clinical trials monitored by the FDA. Over the last 30 years, the information from clinical trials and from studies on approved devices have advanced the development of implant designs, provided longitudinal data on implant benefit, and sparked development of assessment tools that now have become standard in audiologic practice. Clinical trials also have shown the improvement in benefit experienced as technology has evolved, which has allowed implants to be made available to more individuals, including very young children, adults with residual hearing sensitivity, prelingually deafened adults, and individuals with auditory neuropathy.

This chapter serves as a general introduction to audiologists on how cochlear implants work, who may be a potential candidate for a cochlear implant, and the benefits that can be expected from contemporary devices. Specifically, it outlines the basic characteristics of cochlear implant systems available in the United States and briefly describes the important signal-processing steps used in electrical stimulation of the inner ear. Then, it discusses clinical applications, including evaluation procedures, candidacy criteria, and speech perception results in adults and children with cochlear implants. Finally, the chapter considers some of the issues that impact current and future uses of cochlear implant technology. Comprehensive reviews of cochlear implants appear in Cooper and Craddock (2006), Eisenberg (2009), Niparko (2009), and Zeng, Popper, and Fay (2004).

COCHLEAR IMPLANT TECHNOLOGY

The function of a cochlear implant is to provide hearing sensation to individuals with severe-to-profound hearing loss. Typically, people with that level of loss have absent or malfunctioning sensory cells in the cochlea. In a normal ear, sound energy is converted to mechanical energy by the middle ear, which then is converted to mechanical fluid motion in the cochlea. Within the cochlea, the sensory cells—the inner and outer hair cells—are sensitive transducers that convert that mechanical fluid motion into electrical impulses in the auditory nerve. Cochlear implants are designed to substitute for the function of the middle ear, cochlear mechanical motion, and sensory cells, transforming sound energy into electrical energy that will initiate impulses in the auditory nerve.

All cochlear implant systems comprise both internal and external components. The external components include: (1) a microphone, which converts sound into an electrical signal, (2) a sound processor, which manipulates and converts the signal into a special code (i.e., sound processing strategy), and (3) a transmitter, which sends the coded electrical signal to the internal components.

The internal components are those parts of the system that are surgically implanted under the skin behind the ear. They include: (1) a receiver/stimulator, which decodes the signal from the sound processor, and (2) an electrode array, which is inserted into the cochlea and delivers electrical current to the auditory nerve. The entire system is powered by batteries located in the sound processor.

Currently there are three cochlear implants available in the United States (January 2011)—the Harmony HiResolution Bionic Ear system (Advanced Bionics, USA), the Cochlear Nucleus 5 System (Cochlear, Australia), and the Maestro cochlear implant system (Medical Electronics/Med-el, Austria). The following sections briefly describe the fundamental components of these devices. However, because implant technology changes rapidly, detailed information about each contemporary system can be found online at advancedbionics.com, cochlearamericas.com, and medel.com

Sound Processor/ Headpiece/Receiver

The externally worn sound processor typically is a behind-the-ear device similar to a hearing aid, or a body-worn device that is worn off the ear in a pouch or clipped to clothing. The headpiece is worn on the head over the implant site and contains an antenna and a magnet. For individuals using some body-worn processors, the microphone is located in the headpiece or in an earpiece. For most users, the microphone is located on or attached to the sound processor (Figure 18–1). Together, the microphone and sound processor convert acoustic energy into an electrical code that is sent across the skin to the implanted receiver. In addition to microphone input, sound processors typically offer direct connection to audio devices as well as a telecoil or FM receiver. The system is powered by either rechargeable or disposable batteries.

In all current implant systems, data and power are sent via the headpiece to the implanted receiver through transcutaneous inductive coupling of radio frequency (RF) signals using forward telemetry. The receiver decodes the data and determines the stimulation pattern for the electrodes. Data also can be sent from the implant out to the sound processor using back telemetry. Contact impedances, electrical field spread, and local auditory nerve responses can be measured using the electrode contacts and sent back to the processor for analysis.

Electrode Array

Cochlear implant electrode arrays consist of either half-banded or flat platinum contacts arranged along a silicone carrier. The length of the array can range from 19 mm to 35 mm. The number of contacts varies between 12 and 22 depending on the manufacturer.

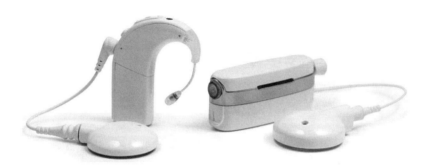

Figure 18–1. Naída CI Q70 behind-the-ear processor with T-mic (*left*) and swimmable Neptune processor with headpiece microphone (*right*). Images courtesy of Advanced Bionics LLC, Valencia, California.

The electrode array is inserted into the scala tympani of the cochlea longitudinally to take potential advantage of the place-frequency coding mechanism used by the normal cochlea. Information about low-frequency sound is sent to contacts at the apical end of the array, whereas information about high-frequency sounds is sent to contacts nearer the base of the cochlea. The ability to take advantage of the place-frequency code is limited by the number and pattern of surviving auditory neurons in an impaired ear, as well as the spread of current between the contacts.

The most commonly used electrodes fall into two categories, curved perimodiolar and straight (Figure 18–2). Curved perimodiolar electrodes are designed to hug the modiolus so contacts are near the spiral ganglion cells. Straight electrodes typically lie along the lateral wall of the cochlea with their contacts under the basilar membrane. For each implant system, the electrode used will be dependent on surgeon experience and preference, and upon the anatomy of the individual implant recipient. Manufacturers also may offer additional electrodes to accommodate ossified cochleas and common cavities, or to facilitate electroacoustic stimulation (see Future Directions).

Sound Processing Strategy

A sound processing strategy defines the way a cochlear implant system transforms sound into electrical stimulation of the auditory nerve. A cochlear implant must analyze and encode the frequency, amplitude, and timing parameters in the acoustic signal and convert the information into an electrode stimulation pattern. In general, frequency information is conveyed by the site of stimulation, amplitude is encoded by amplitude of the stimulus current, and temporal cues are conveyed by the rate and pattern of stimulation. However, there are different approaches for accomplishing each step in the sound processing algorithm (see also Wilson & Dorman, 2009).

Like a hearing aid, the input to the implant system is a miniature high-fidelity microphone. The microphone can be located above the ear, on the head, clipped to clothing, or at the entrance to the ear canal. Recent research indicates that microphone placement can have an effect on the ability to understand speech, especially in noise. Gifford and Revit (2010) compared sentence understanding in noise in Harmony implant users between a BTE microphone and the T-Mic Microphone, which is situated at the entrance to the ear canal. The within-subjects comparison showed that the T-Mic offered a mean improvement of +4 dB SNR compared with the BTE microphone (Figure 18–3). This significant advantage is a result of listeners' ability to make use of torso, head, and pinna reflections.

AGC circuits are used by all implant systems because the input sound signal varies over a wide dynamic range and must be accommodated to the narrow dynamic range of electrical hearing (Shannon, 1983; Zeng,

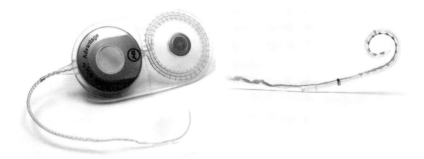

Figure 18–2. HiRes 90K Advantage implant with HiFocus 1j electrode (*left*) and close-up of HiFocus Mid Scala electrode (*right*). Images courtesy of Advanced Bionics LLC, Valencia, California.

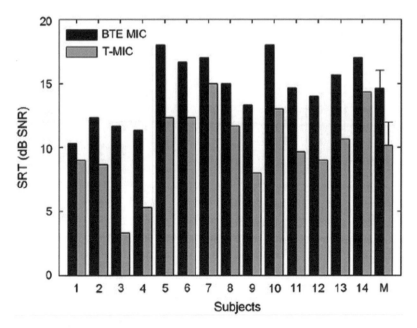

Figure 18–3. Individual and mean R-SPACE speech reception thresholds (SRTs) for 14 Advanced Bionics implant users (*error bars show ± 2 SE*). Black bars represent the SRTs obtained with the behind-the-ear microphone. Gray bars represent SRTs obtained with the T-Mic. A lower SRT is a better score. Republished with permission of American Academy of Audiology, from "Speech Perception for Adult Cochlear Implant Recipients in a Realistic Background Noise: Effectiveness fo Preprocessing Strategies and External Options for Improving Speech Recognition in Noise," by R. H. Gifford and L. Revit, *Journal of American Academy of Audiology*, *21*, Copyright 2010; permission conveyed through Copyright Clearance Center, Inc.

2004). An implant system uses a single-channel fast-acting AGC algorithm at the input processing stage in order to maximize audibility and make sure soft sounds are audible. Dual-action AGC circuits (Moore, Glasberg, & Stone, 1991; Stone, Moore, Alcantara, & Glasberg, 1999) have been implemented in the Advanced Bionics and Med-el systems. These AGC2 circuits implement a slow-acting compression circuit in combination with a fast-acting algorithm to protect listeners from loud transient sounds. The AGC2 offers listeners the opportunity to hear speech better in noise compared with the conventional AGC circuit (Figure 18–4). Another type of slow-acting AGC called adaptive dynamic range optimization (ADRO) is an option in the Nucleus system. ADRO is applied to each channel separately so that the gain is varied slowly and the signal remains within the electrical dynamic range of the listener. ADRO can provide some advantage over fixed-gain channels when listening to soft speech (James et al., 2002).

After the various front-end processing stages, the signal is split into a number of frequency bands or channels. The number of channels typically is aligned with the number of stimulating contacts in the cochlea. In the CIS strategy, which is the basis for most contemporary sound processing strategies, each channel involves a bandpass filter, envelope detection, and compression (Wilson et al., 1991). Envelope detection is accomplished with a rectifier followed by a low-pass filter. A logarithmic transformation is used to compress the relatively wide dynamic range of the derived envelope to the narrow dynamic range of electrical hearing. The resulting envelope is used to modulate a biphasic pulse

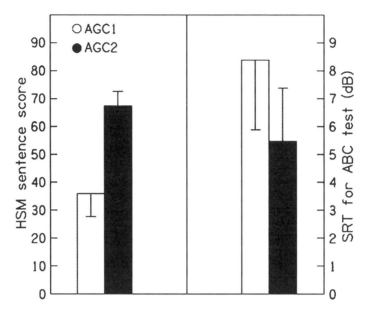

Figure 18–4. Group mean scores for 13 Advanced Bionics implant users following long-term experience with AGC1 and AGC2. The left pair of bars represents results (% correct) from the HSM sentence test. The right pair of bars represents results (dB) from the ABC sentence test, where lower numbers represent better outcomes. Error bars show ± 1 SE. Republished with permission of Taylor & Francis, Inc., from "Comparison of Dual-Time-Constant and Fast-Acting automatic gain control (AGC) systems in cochlear implants," by P. J. Boyle, A. Büchner, M. A. Stone, T. Lenarz, B. C. J. Moore, *International Journal of Audiology, 48*(4). Copyright 2009; permission conveyed through Copyright Clearance Center, Inc.

train that is delivered to the corresponding electrode contact. Outputs from the low-frequency channels are sent to apical contacts, and outputs from high-frequency channels are sent to basal contacts. The trains of biphasic pulses are delivered to the electrodes in an interleaved or nonoverlapping fashion to minimize electrical field interactions between stimulated electrodes. The rate at which the pulses are delivered to the electrodes is an important variable in the implementation of CIS strategies. High-rate stimulation typically results in better speech understanding than low-rate stimulation (Wilson, 1993).

Variations on the full-spectrum CIS strategy include n of m, SPEAK, and ACE, which present only a portion of the spectrum to the electrode array. For these strategies, a subset of electrodes is stimulated based on an analysis of the energy present in each channel. These strategies select the n highest-amplitude channels from a total of m analysis channels and stimulate only those electrodes associated with the n channels. More recent versions of the full-spectrum CIS strategy include the CIS+ strategy, a strategy similar to CIS except that the envelope information is extracted using a Hilbert transform rather than bandpass filters. The HiRes strategy is a variation on the full-spectrum CIS strategy without the low-pass filter stage and using a high stimulation rate to represent the envelope more accurately across all analysis channels.

Newer sound processing algorithms are designed to deliver a more complete representation of the acoustic signal to the implant user. The Fine Structure Processing (FSP) strategy is a variation of CIS in which fine frequency variations in low-frequency sounds are represented by delivering rapid pulse trains to the three most apical electrodes at the positive zero crossings of the outputs of the associated analysis channels. Conventional CIS stimulation is delivered to the other electrodes. FSP thus theoretically delivers a more accurate representation of pitch than classic CIS. Data suggest that some FSP users experience benefit for speech perception and when listening to music compared with CIS+ (Arnolder et al., 2007).

The HiRes 120 strategy uses current steering to create additional spectral bands, thereby increasing the number of stimulation sites beyond the number of physical electrode contacts. Because each contact has its own separate power source, current can be delivered to multiple contacts at the same time. Through simultaneous delivery of current to pairs of adjacent electrodes, the locus of stimulation theoretically can be steered to sites between the contacts by varying the proportion of current delivered to each electrode of the pair. Thus, many intermediate regions of stimulation can be created, with fine control over the proportion and amplitude of current delivered to each electrode (Noguiera et al., 2009). Studies in HiRes 120 users show that the majority of subjects perceive additional spectral channels other than those associated with stimulation of the fixed electrodes when current steering is implemented (Brendel et al., 2009; Donaldson, Kreft, & Litvak, 2005; Firszt, Koch, Downing, & Litvak, 2007; Koch, Downing, Osberger, & Litvak, 2007). The results suggest that the average cochlear implant user may have significantly more place-pitch capability than is exploited presently by cochlear implant systems.

Like hearing aid users, cochlear implant recipients still can have difficulty hearing in noise even though most implanted adults can understand speech remarkably well in quiet. Various techniques have been implemented to address that concern. For example, beam forming uses dual microphones to emphasize signals originating in front of the listener (Gifford, Dorman, Shallop, & Sydlowski, 2010). Directional microphones also can reduce noise coming from locations other than the front. Using a different approach, Advanced Bionics ClearVoice strategy is a HiRes 120 option that identifies frequency bands in which nonspeech energy is present and reduces the gain of those bands, thereby enhancing the desired speech signal. Clinical data show that users experience a significant improvement in the ability to understand speech in noise with ClearVoice (Figure 18–5). An additional advantage is that speech perception in quiet remains unaffected with ClearVoice.

CANDIDACY AND PREIMPLANT EVALUATION

Cochlear Implant Candidacy

The criteria for cochlear implant candidacy continue to evolve and can be different across device manufacturers depending upon the status of regulatory review. Table 18–1 summarizes the general criteria for cochlear implant referral and evaluation. It is important that individuals and their families have access to cochlear implant information as soon as possible, even if candidacy has not been clearly established. It usually takes many months for an individual to reach a decision regarding implantation. Moreover, securing reimbursement for the cochlear implant and associated costs may be a lengthy process.

Medical Evaluation

Experience with cochlear implants indicates that individuals with nearly all causes of severe and profound hearing loss deafness may be appropriate candidates for implantation. With few exceptions, stimulable auditory nerve fibers appear to be present even in profound deafness, irrespective of etiology (Nadol, 1984).

Medical and otologic evaluations are required before an individual is considered further as a cochlear implant candidate. The

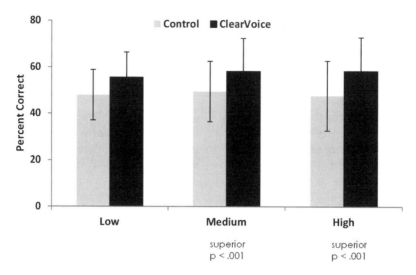

Figure 18–5. Group mean scores for AzBio sentences in speech-spectrum noise (*n* = 46) for HiRes Fidelity 120 without ClearVoice (control) and HiRes Fidelity 120 with ClearVoice (Low, Medium, and High gain settings). The SNR was adjusted for each subject to yield approximately 50% of their score in quiet using HiRes Fidelity 120 without ClearVoice. The same SNR was used in all subsequent testing in noise. ClearVoice provided significantly improved speech understanding in noise compared with the control. Adapted from images courtesy of Advanced Bionics LLC, Valencia, California.

Table 18–1. Cochlear Implant Referral Guidelines for Adults and Children

Adults

- 18 years of age or older
- Severe-to-profound bilateral sensorineural hearing loss (pure-tone average ≥70 dB HL)
- Limited benefit from appropriately fitted hearing aids (e.g., CNC word score ≤30%)
- Limited ability to converse interactively on the telephone, even with amplification devices
- Difficulty understanding conversations in groups or noisy places
- Relies heavily on speechreading in face-to-face communication
- Limits his or her social and business life as a result of severe-to-profound hearing loss

Children

- Profound bilateral sensorineural hearing loss (pure-tone average ≥90 dB HL)
- Plateau or limited progress in acquisition of auditory milestones (e.g., response to name or environmental sounds) with appropriate hearing aids and rehabilitation
- Delayed or lack of oral speech and language development

primary care physician's examination ensures that an individual is able to undergo surgery without risks to general health. The otolaryn- gologist's evaluation ensures that an individual is a suitable implant candidate and that no otologic conditions exist that contraindicate ear surgery (see also, Tucci & Pilkington, 2009). In addition, a radiographic evaluation consisting of high-resolution computed tomography (CT) evaluates the anatomical integrity of the cochlea. Usually, congenital malformations of the inner ear (e.g., Mondini deformity) do not preclude cochlear implantation. Anatomical contraindications to implantation are Michel deformity (complete absence of the cochlea) and small internal auditory canal syndrome in which the VIIIth nerve may be absent. Chronic otitis media must be resolved before implant surgery can take place.

CT scans also reveal cochlear ossification, a condition that frequently occurs following deafness from meningitis. Cochlear ossification may be partial or complete and may be localized to one or more cochlear turns. The obstructive intracochlear bone and soft tissue often requires modifications in implant surgical technique and, in some cases, a complete insertion of the electrode array cannot be achieved (Gantz, McCabe, & Tyler, 1988). Nonetheless, if the ossification process is identified in its early stages, a full electrode insertion often can be made, offering the individual the best potential for speech perception benefit. Clinical practice suggests that all individuals with profound hearing loss should have high-resolution CT scanning of the cochleae within the first 2 months following the onset of meningitis. If early signs of ossification are detected, and there is no evidence of hearing recovery, implantation is recommended as soon as possible (Novak, Fifer, Barkmeier, & Firszt, 1990).

Magnetic resonance imaging (MRI) also is helpful adjunct to CT, especially for children (Adunka et al., 2006; Parry, Booth, & Roland, 2005). MRI can reveal the presence of absence of fluid in the cochlear turns, as well as showing the size of the cochlear/vestibular nerve within the internal auditory canal (Seitz et al., 2001).

Before surgery, it is recommended that all patients undergo age-appropriate vaccination for organisms associated with meningitis, including *Streptococcus pneumoniae* and *Haemophilus influenzae*. Recommended vacci- nations and immunization schedules can be found at http://www.cdc.gov, using a search for "cochlear implant."

Audiologic Evaluation

A comprehensive audiologic evaluation is performed to establish the degree and type of hearing loss, and to assess functional hearing aid benefit. Air and bone conduction thresholds are measured in each ear under earphones. All candidates must demonstrate a severe-to-profound sensorineural hearing loss bilaterally. Impedance testing is conducted to rule out middle ear infections, and to demonstrate absent stapedius reflexes. Auditory brain stem response (ABR) testing is performed in young children to verify the presence of a profound hearing loss bilaterally. Routine speech audiometry is conducted under earphones. Implant candidacy, however, is determined by speech recognition performance with appropriately fitted hearing aids rather than on results obtained under earphones. The procedures used to assess speech perception performance are discussed below.

SPEECH PERCEPTION ASSESSMENT AND PERFORMANCE

Adult Procedures

Early cochlear implant investigations assessed speech understanding with sentences because most cochlear implant recipients scored near zero on traditional tests of word recognition. Although moderate-to-high levels of mono-syllabic word recognition are observed in today's cochlear implant users, most audiologists still administer a sentence test in quiet and in background noise to simulate real-world listening. Testing is typically conducted with recorded materials presented at the level of conversational speech (approximately 60 dB SPL).

During the preimplant evaluation, monosyllabic word testing is performed with each ear monaurally and in the binaural condition. The results of the word testing are used to identify the "best-aided" condition for assessment of sentence recognition in quiet and in noise. The preimplant speech perception results, together with the unaided and aided thresholds and imaging data, are used to determine candidacy and the ear to be implanted. Post-implant assessments are recommended at 1, 3, 6, and 12 months following device activation, and annually thereafter (Fabry, Firszt, Gifford, Holden, & Koch, 2009). Aided sound-field thresholds (with warble tones or narrowband noise) are usually assessed at each visit (preimplant with hearing aids and postimplant).

The specific tests used to assess speech understanding have evolved over time with advances in technology, improved outcomes, and changes in candidacy. For example, in 1996, a committee composed of representatives from the American Academy of Audiology (AAA), the American Academy of Otolaryngology-Head and Neck Surgery (AAO-HNS), and cochlear implant manufacturers convened to identify a set of materials to be used clinically and in research studies to assess the performance of adults with cochlear implants. At that time, the committee recommended the Consonant-Nucleus-Consonant (CNC) test (Peterson & Lehiste, 1962) to assess open-set word recognition and the Hearing in Noise Test (HINT; Nilsson, Soli, & Sullivan, 1994) to assess open-set sentence recognition in quiet and in speech-spectrum noise.

Contemporary performance data indicate that the CNC test is still an appropriate measure (Bassim et al., 2005; Firszt et al., 2004; Gifford, Shallop, & Peterson, 2008; Koch et al., 2004). In contrast, study results and clinical experience indicate that the HINT is too easy and that more difficult sentence tests should be used to determine candidacy and assess benefit. For example, Gifford et al. (2008) reported that as many as 71% of implanted subjects scored 85% or higher on the HINT.

Consequently, the current trend is to assess performance with CNC words and a more difficult sentence test such as the AzBio sentence test (Spahr & Dorman, 2004) or the Bamford-Kowal-Bamford Speech-in-Noise test (BKB-SIN) (Etymotic Research, 2005; see Appendix 18-A). The AzBio test is more sensitive than the HINT because the sentences are spoken by different talkers (male and female) in a conversational manner rather than by a single-talker with a slower, more deliberate speaking style. Moreover, the AzBio sentences have limited contextual cues that the listener can use to predict or "fill in" unintelligible words. The sentences can be presented in quiet or in multitalker babble. Testing in multitalker babble is conducted with both the speech and noise at fixed levels. Fabry et al. (2009) recommend a SNR of +5 dB although this might be too difficult for some patients and/or during the early months of implant use.

The BKB-SIN test uses a modified adaptive approach wherein sentences are presented at a fixed level and four-talker babble is presented at different SNRs. Performance is expressed as the SNR loss, defined as the increased SNR required by a subject to understand speech in noise compared with the SNR required by individuals with normal hearing. Although this is not a true adaptive procedure, it can be used easily in a clinical setting.

Gifford and colleagues (2008) suggested that a combination of CNC words, AzBio sentences in quiet, and the BKB-SIN test, for which scores are closely correlated, provides the most useful clinical information. This battery also provides the headroom for tracking changes in speech perception benefits that occur over time or with changes in program parameters. Similar recommendations were made by Fabry et al. (2009), including a timetable and a regimen that is intended to maximize information about performance within a clinically reasonable time frame (Table 18–2). Each test takes approximately 5 to 7 minutes to administer for each condition.

A recent study by Gifford and colleagues (2010) demonstrated the high level of benefit that can be realized by adult cochlear implant recipients. Figure 18–6 shows the best-aided preimplant CNC word scores along with the

Table 18–2. Recommended Speech Perception Test Battery for Cochlear Implant Candidates and Recipients

	Monosyllabic Words (CNC Test*)	Sentences in Quiet (AzBio Test*)	Sentences in Noise (AzBio or BKB-SIN**)
Preimplant with hearing aids	Right ear alone Left ear alone Both ears together	Best-aided condition	Best-aided condition
Unilateral implant	Implant ear	Implant ear	Implant ear
Bilateral implants	Right implant alone Left implant alone Both implants	Both implants together	Both implants together
Bimodal (implant plus hearing aid)	Implant ear alone Hearing-aided ear alone Both ears together	Both ears together	Both ears together

*1 list per condition.   ** 2 lists per condition.
Source: Adapted from Fabry et al., 2009, with permission.

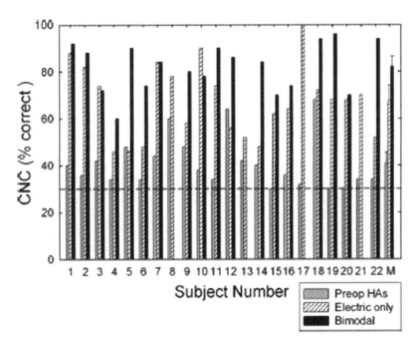

Figure 18–6. Individual and mean performance for CNC monosyllabic words for 22 adult cochlear implant recipients. The shaded bars represent the best-aided preoperative score, the hatched bars represent the implant-only score, and the filled bars represent the bimodal score (implant plus hearing aid). Reprinted with permission from Gifford, Dorman, Shallop, and Sydlowski, 2010. Republished with permission of Lippincott, Williams & Wilkins, from "Evidence for the Expansion of Adult Cochlear Implant Candidacy," by R. H. Gifford, M. F. Dorman, J. K. Shallop, and S. A. Sydlowski, *Ear and Hearing*, *31*(2). Copyright 2010; permission conveyed through Copyright Clearance Center, Inc.

postoperative scores for listening with the implant alone, and for listening with the implant plus a contralateral hearing aid for 22 subjects. The mean improvement for using the implant alone compared with preimplantation with hearing aids was 27%. When a contralateral hearing aid was used in combination with the implant, the mean improvement reached a remarkable 41%.

These data should be of great interest to audiologists who fit and assess hearing aids. Many adults with some residual hearing who have limited open-set speech recognition with conventional amplification may have the potential for better hearing with an implant. That better hearing, in turn, may be associated with improved quality of life, a reduction in depression and social isolation, and emotional benefits (see, e.g., Francis, Chee, Yeagle, Cheng, & Niparko, 2002). Gifford's study also indicates the use of a hearing aid in the ear contralateral to the implant can provide considerable additional benefit (see also, Ching, Incerti, & Hill, 2004; Gifford, Dorman, McKarns, & Spahr, 2007; Kong, Stickney, & Zeng, 2005; Mok, Grayden, Dowell, & Lawrence, 2006; Potts, Skinner, Litovsky, Strube, & Kuk, 2009).

Pediatric Procedures

Appendix 18-B describes the tests that are used most frequently with children. Because most pediatric recipients are very young (3 years of age and younger) at the time of implantation, they lack the skills required for traditional measures of speech recognition. Therefore, detection tasks using nonspeech (warble tones or narrowband noise) and speech stimuli must be used. The Ling Six Sounds test (Ling, 1976, 1989) consists of sounds with low-, mid-, and high-frequency components of speech. Another tool, developed to document the acquisition of auditory milestones in young children with implants, is the Infant-Toddler Meaningful Auditory Integration Scale (IT-MAIS; Zimmerman-Phillips, Robbins, & Osberger, 2001). The IT-MAIS is a criteria-referenced measure that employs a structured parent interview to assess the frequency of occurrence of targeted auditory behaviors in everyday situations. An advantage of the IT-MAIS is that it taps auditory behaviors that are universal and independent of the child's native language. Consequently, it has been translated into many languages. Kishon-Rabin and colleagues (2001) evaluated the IT-MAIS with normal-hearing children, aged 2 to 40 months, whose parents spoke Arabic or Hebrew. The children with normal hearing showed rapid progress in auditory skill acquisition, attaining a score of 80% by approximately 12 months of age.

Studies have shown performance differences on the IT-MAIS as a function of age at implant. Specifically, children implanted at a younger age showed a more rapid rate of auditory skill acquisition than children implanted at an older age (Osberger, Zimmerman-Phillips, & Koch, 2002; Robbins et al., 2004) and children using a more advanced sound processing strategy attained higher scores than children using previous-generation technology (Osberger & Koch, 2004).

An example of IT-MAIS scores over time is illustrated by the data in Figure 18–7. The results were collected during the clinical trial of HiResolution sound processing children. The children were 12 months to 2 years of age at time of implant (n = 35). The data show that the largest increase in scores occurred during the first 3 months of implant use with smaller increases after that time. Most of the children were near the test ceiling at the 12-month visit.

Although most children are too young to be tested with word and sentence tests prior to implantation, they are ultimately assessed with these measures as they mature and their auditory skills develop. Currently, there is no standardized test battery for children although there are numerous pediatric measures used clinically. Figure 18–8 shows a proposed test hierarchy for clinical use based on recommendations from a panel of audiology advisors (Cowdrey et al., 2009). The hierarchy is similar to the ones developed and evaluated by Eisenberg et al. (2006) and Wang et al. (2008).

The Early Speech Perception Test (ESP; Moog & Geers, 1990) is the first measure used

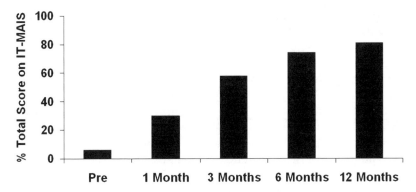

Figure 18–7. IT-MAIS scores over time for 35 children implanted with the Harmony cochlear implant.

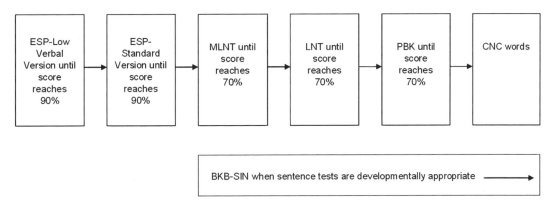

Figure 18–8. Hierarchy of tests recommended for use with pediatric cochlear implant recipients.

to assess emerging speech recognition skills. This closed-set word identification test has been formatted for younger (Low Verbal version) and older (Standard version) children. Testing with the Low Verbal Version usually begins around age 2, assuming the child has the cognitive skills to choose between two alternatives. The Standard version is introduced once the child scores near the test ceiling on the Low Verbal version. The ESP most often is administered via monitored live-voice, although testing also can be conducted with recorded stimuli. The Multisyllabic Lexical Neighborhood Test (MLNT) (Iler-Kirk, Pisoni, & Osberger, 1995) is introduced once the child scores near the ceiling of the Standard version of the ESP and is able to imitate words. This measure and its companion test, the Lexical Neighborhood Test (LNT), are

open-set measures that control for the lexical properties of words (Iler-Kirk et al., 1995). Although the tests were standardized with recorded materials, they often are administered via monitored live voice depending on the developmental skills of the child. Some clinicians also use the closed-set Word Intelligibility by Picture Identification (WIPI; Ross & Lerman, 1970) and Northwestern University Children's Perception of Speech (NU-CHIPS; Elliott & Katz, 1980) tests prior to proceeding to open-set word tests (Madell, 2007).

The Phonetically Balanced Kindergarten (PBK; Haskins, 1949) continues to be used as an open-set word test even though some of its vocabulary is out of date. The advantage of this test is that it is more difficult than the MLNT and LNT tests, and thereby avoids ceiling effects. The adult CNC word test is introduced as soon as the child can repeat the items on the test even though the child may not have command of the test vocabulary. In this context, performance is assessed based on recognition rather than comprehension. The advantage of the CNC test is that there are more lists available, and the test is more difficult than the pediatric measures.

Sentence tests are introduced later because children have more difficulty with sentences than words because of their limited language abilities. The BKB-SIN test is recommended once the child is able to perform a sentence repetition task. The children's version of the HINT, the HINT-C, also can be used to assess sentence recognition in quiet or in fixed-level noise (Nilsson, Soli, & Gelnett, 1996).

The recommended evaluation schedule is 3 months following device activation, and every 6 months thereafter until the child is 5 or 6 years of age, followed by annual evaluations. Generally, performance is assessed with both ears until the child can be tested with the PBK or CNC test. Once these measures are appropriate, individual ear testing is conducted with words while sentence testing continues to be conducted with both ears. Ideally, open-set word and sentence testing is performed with recorded materials presented at 60 dB SPL. In all cases, auditory and speech perception skills are assessed using tools that are deemed to be most appropriate for the developmental level of each child. Auditory skills develop over time, with rate of progress and overall benefit affected by variables such as age at implant, preimplant residual hearing, socioeconomic status, and communication mode (Fryauf-Bertschy et al., 1997; Osberger & Fisher, 2000; Robbins et al., 2004; Waltzman & Cohen, 1998).

Bilateral Cochlear Implants

Bilateral cochlear implantation has become common in both adults and children (Balkany et al., 2008; Craddock, Brinton, Saeed, & Balkany, 2008; Murphy & O'Donoghue, 2007). Many of the bilateral hearing advantages experienced by listeners with normal hearing are regained at least in part when individu-als use two devices. For example, almost all adult recipients of two implants experience a head shadow effect. Some bilateral users also exhibit binaural squelch and binaural summation. Typically, bilaterally implanted adults hear better in noise and demonstrate an improved ability to localize sounds compared with unilateral implant recipients (see, e.g., Dunn et al., 2010; Dunn, Tyler, Oakley, Gantz, & Nobel, 2008; Gantz et al., 2002; Koch, Soli, Downing, & Osberger, 2009; Litovsky, Parkinson, Arcaroli, & Sammeth, 2006a; Litovsky, Parkinson, & Arcaroli, 2009; Müller, Schön, & Helms, 2002; Nopp, Schleich, & D'Haese, 2004; Neuman, Haravon, Sislian, & Waltzman, 2007; Schleich, Nopp, & D'Haese, 2004). Adults also report improved quality of life with two implants (Bichey & Miyamoto, 2008; Laske et al., 2009). Moreover, bilateral benefit improves over time as listeners gain experience with two devices (Buss et al., 2008; Chang et al., 2010; Eapen, Buss, Adunka, Pillsbury, & Buchman, 2009).

Similar bilateral advantages have been reported for children (e.g., Litovsky, Johnstone, & Godar, 2006; Litovsky et al., 2006b; Peters et al., 2007; Wolfe et al., 2007). Moreover, for very young deaf children, providing sound input to both ears assures that sound is processed on both sides of the brain, thereby enabling the right and left auditory cortices to develop in a more normal sequence. The developmental advantages realized with bilateral implants in young deaf children have important implications for language acquisition, academic success, and educational and occupational opportunities. Preliminary results from children implanted simultaneously with two devices suggest that there may be a trend for faster auditory skill development in younger children with bilateral implants compared with younger children using only one implant (Gifford, 2009).

FUTURE DIRECTIONS

Cochlear implants have become an accepted medical treatment for severe-to-profound sensorineural hearing loss in children and adults. Today's cochlear implant recipients understand speech remarkably well in quiet, and recent advances in sound processing have improved speech understanding in noise. Moreover, the introduction of sound processing strategies that provide more spectral or pitch information (e.g., HiRes 120 and FSP) allow implant users access to greater spectral resolution and the potential to improve their music perception and appreciation (Limb, 2006). Studies with early generation technology showed that music perception and enjoyment were poor (e.g., Gfeller et al., 2000; McDermott, 2004; Mirza, Douglas, Lindsey, Hildreth, & Hawthorne, 2003). The limited spectral resolution delivered by older implant technology precluded music enjoyment in most implant users because music perception requires as many as 100 channels of spectral (frequency) resolution, even in subjects with normal hearing (Oxenham, Bernstein, & Penagos, 2004; Shannon, 2005). In contrast, a recent study conducted with adult users of HiRes 120 showed that the majority of subjects enjoyed listening to music (Osberger, Quick, Arnold, & Boyle, 2010).

Based on the increasing ability of implant recipients to listen to and enjoy music, several music tests have been developed to evaluate these abilities. Currently, these procedures have been used in research studies and are not commonly employed in the clinical evaluation of cochlear implant performance. These tests include the Appreciation of Music by Cochlear Implantees (AMICI) (Spitzer, Mancuso, & Cheng, 2008), which uses real music samples to evaluate instrument identification and melody recognition, the University of Washington-Clinical Assessment of Music Perception (UW-CAMP; Kang et al., 2009), a computer-based test battery that evaluates pitch discrimination, melody recognition, and instrument identification (timbre), and the Montreal Battery for Evaluation of Amusica (MBEA; Cooper, Tobey, & Loizou, 2008; Peretz, Champod, & Hyde, 2003), a test battery used as a diagnostic tool to identify amusia in normal and brain-damaged individuals recently applied to evaluate music perception in cochlear implant users.

The combination of electrical and acoustic stimulation may provide hearing benefits to an ever expanding number of people with hearing loss. For individuals with some residual low-frequency acoustic hearing, electro-acoustic stimulation (EAS) may prove helpful. In EAS, electrical stimulation is delivered to the basal end of the cochlea, often using a short electrode, in order to minimize damage to the apical part of the cochlea where some hair cells still may be functional. Presenting low-frequency pitch information acoustically may complement the high-frequency information delivered by the cochlear implant. Studies have shown that EAS provides better speech perception in quiet and noise, and improved music perception compared with using either acoustic or electrical stimulation alone (Dorman et al., 2008; Gantz, Turner, Gfeller, & Lowder, 2005; Gfeller, Olszewski, Turner, Gantz, & Oleson, 2006; Gstoettner et al., 2006). Devices designed for EAS are not approved by the FDA. However, many of the same benefits are seen in individuals who use a cochlear implant in one ear and a hearing aid in the other ear (bimodal stimulation; Ching, Incerti, & Hill, 2004; Gifford et al., 2007; Kong et al., 2005; Potts et al., 2009). For individuals with some residual acoustic hearing, this bimodal advantage is important because an implanted ear, even with an EAS-targeted electrode, typically loses any residual acoustic hearing over time.

In summary, cochlear implants enable deafened adults to reconnect with the world of sound—ranging from understanding speech to appreciating music. For young deaf children, cochlear implants provide new access to the world of sound, where they can develop oral speech and language similar to children with normal hearing. The future of cochlear implants is limited only by technological imagination. Digital signal processing advances should lead to improved implant reliability and enhanced speech perception benefit. New miniaturization processes should result in smaller processors for both adults and children. It is conceivable that future cochlear prostheses will allow individuals to function like people with normal hearing, with bilateral invisible devices that adjust automatically to the acoustic environment and that are tailored in real time to their individual hearing needs.

REFERENCES

Books

Cooper, H. R., & Craddock L. C. (Eds). (2006). *Cochlear implants: A practical guide* (2nd ed.). London, UK: Whurr.

Eisenberg, L. (Ed). (2009). *Clinical management of children with cochlear implants*. San Diego, CA: Plural.

Niparko, J. K. (Ed). (2009). *Cochlear implants: Principles and practices* (2nd ed.). Philadephia, PA: Lippincott, Williams & Wilkins.

Zeng, F. G., Popper, A. N., & Fay, R. R. (Eds). (2004). *Cochlear implants: Auditory prostheses and electric hearing*. New York, NY: Springer-Verlag.

Original Research Articles and Other Readings

Adunka, O., Rousch P. A.,Teagle, H., Brown, C. J., Zdanski, C. J., Jewells, V., & Buchman, C. A. (2006). Internal auditory canal morphology in children with cochlear nerve deficiency. *Otology and Neurotology, 27*, 793–801.

Advanced Bionics. (2009). *HiRes with Fidelity 120 clinical results*. Advanced Bionics: Valencia, CA.

Arnoldner, C., Baumgartner, W. D., Gstoettner, W., & Hamzavi, J. (2005). Surgical considerations in cochlear implantation in children and adults: A review of 342 cases in Vienna. *Acta Otolaryngologica, 125*, 228–234.

Arnoldner, C., Riss, D., Brunner, M., Durisin, M., Baumgartner, W. D., & Hamzavi, J. S. (2007). Speech and music perception with the new fine structure speech coding strategy: Preliminary results. *Acta Otolaryngologica, 127*, 1298–1303.

Balkany, T., Hodges, A., Telischi, F., Hoffman, R., Madell, J., Parisier, S., . . . Litovsky, R. (2008). William House cochlear implant study group: Position statement on bilateral cochlear implantation. *Otology and Neurotology, 29*(2), 107–108.

Bassim, M. K., Buss, E., Clark, M. S., Kolln, K. A., Pillsbury, C. H., Pillsbury, H. C., & Buchman, C. A. (2005). MED-EL Combi40+ cochlear implantation in adults. *Laryngoscope, 115*(9), 1568–1573.

Bhatia, K., Gibbin, K. P., Nikolopoulos, T. P., & O'Donoghue, G. M. (2004). Surgical complications and their management in a series of 300 consecutive pediatric cochlear implantations. *Otology and Neurotology, 25*, 730–739.

Bichey, B. G., & Miyamoto, R. T. (2008). Outcomes in bilateral cochlear implantation. *Otolaryngology-Head and Neck Surgery, 138*, 655–661.

Boyle, P. J., Büchner, A., Stone, M. A., Lenarz, T., & Moore, B. C. J. (2009). Comparison of dual-time-constant and fast-acting automatic gain control (AGC) systems in cochlear implants. *International Journal of Audiology, 48*(4), 211–221.

Brendel, M., Büchner, A., Saalfeld, H., Frohne-Büchner, C., & Lenarz, T. (2009). *A signal enhancement algorithm for cochlear implant users: First results of a pilot study with HiRes 120*. Poster presentation at 2009 Conference on Implantable Auditory Prostheses, Lake Tahoe, CA.

Brendel, M., Frohne-Büchner, C., Stöver, T., Lenarz, T., & Büchner, A. (2009). Investigation of pitch discrimination and the effect of learning for virtual channels realized by current steering. *Acta Otolaryngologica, 129*(12), 1425–1433.

Brown, C. J., Abbas, P. J., Frayauf-Bertschy, H., Kelsay, D., & Gantz, B. J. (1994). Intraoperative and postoperative electrically evoked auditory brainstem responses in nucleus cochlear implant users: Implications for the fitting process. *Ear and Hearing, 15*, 168–176.

Brown, C. J., Abbas, P. J., & Gantz, B. J. (1998). Preliminary experience with neural response telemetry in the Nucleus CI24M cochlear implant. *American Journal of Otology, 19*, 320–327.

Brown, C. J., Hughes, M. L., Lopez, S. M., & Abbas, P. J. (1999). Relationship between EABR thresholds and levels used to program the clarion speech processor. *Annals of Otology, Rhinology, and Laryngology, 108*(Suppl. 177), 50–57.

Buss, E., Pillsbury, H. C., Buchman, C. A., Pillsbury, C. H., Clark, M. S., Haynes, D. S., . . . Barco, A. L. (2008). Multicenter US bilateral MED-EL cochlear implantation study: Speech perception over the first year of use. *Ear and Hearing, 29*(1), 20–32.

Chang, S. A., Tyler, R. S., Dunn, C. C., Ji, H., Witt, S. A., Gantz, B., & Hansen, M. (2010). Performance over time on adults with simultaneous bilateral cochlear implants. *Journal of the American Academy of Audiology, 21*(1), 35–43.

Ching, T. Y., Incerti, P., & Hill, M. (2004). Binaural benefits for adults who use hearing aids and cochlear implants in opposite ears. *Ear and Hearing, 25*, 9–21.

Cohen N. L., & Hoffman, R. A. (1991). Complications of cochlear implant surgery in adults and children. *Annals of Otology, Rhinology, and Laryngology, 100*, 131–136.

Cooper, W. B., Tobey, E., & Loizou, P. (2008). Music perception by cochlear implant and normal hearing listeners as measured by the Montreal Battery for Evaluation of Amusia. *Ear and Hearing, 29*(4), 618–626.

Cowdrey, L., Madell, J., Osberger, M. J., Teagle, H., Staller S., Zimmerman-Phillips, S., & Koch, D. B. (2009). *Meeting of the audiological advisory sub-*

committee on assessing speech perception benefits in children. Sponsored by Advanced Bionics LLC, Chicago, IL.

Craddock, L., Brinton, L., Saeed, S., & Balkany, T. (2008). Bilateral cochlear implantation: The British cochlear implant group position. *Cochlear Implants International, 9*(2), 65–69.

de Jong, A. L., Nedzelski, J., & Papsin, B. C. (1998). Surgical outcomes of paediatric cochlear implantation: The Hospital for Sick Children's experience. *Journal of Otolaryngology, 27*, 26–30.

Dodson, K. M., Maiberger, P. G., & Sismanis, A. (2007). Intracranial complications of cochlear implantation. *Otology and Neurotology, 28*, 459–462.

Donaldson, G. S., Kreft, H. A., & Litvak, L. (2005). Place-pitch discrimination of single-versus dual-electrode stimuli by cochlear implant users. *Journal of the Acoustical Society of America, 118*(2), 623–626.

Dorman, M. F., Gifford, R. H., Spahr, A. J., & McKarns, S. A. (2008). The benefits of combining acoustic and electric stimulation for the recognition of speech, voice and melodies. *Audiology and Neurotology, 13*, 105–112.

Dunn, C. C., Noble, W., Tyler, R. S., Kordus, M., Gantz, B. J., & Ji, H. (2010). Bilateral and unilateral cochlear implant users compared on speech perception in noise. *Ear and Hearing, 31*(2), 296–298.

Dunn, C. C., Tyler, R. S., Oakley, S., Gantz, B. J., & Noble, W. (2008). Comparison of speech recognition and localization performance in bilateral and unilateral cochlear implant users matched on duration of deafness and age at implantation. *Ear and Hearing, 29*(3), 352–359.

Dutt, S. N., Ray, J., Hadjihannas, E., Cooper, H., Donaldson, I., & Proops, D. W. (2005). Medical and surgical complications of the second 100 adult cochlear implant patients in Birmingham. *Journal of Laryngology and Otology, 119*, 759–764.

Eapen, R. J., Buss, E., Adunka, M. C., Pillsbury, H. C., & Buchman, C. A. (2009). Hearing-in-noise benefits after bilateral simultaneous cochlear implantation continue to improve 4 years after implantation. *Otology and Neurotology, 30*(2), 153–159.

Eisenberg, L. S., Johnson, K. C., Martinez, A. S., Cokely, C. G., Tobey, E. A., Quittner, A. L., . . . CDaCI Invstgative Team. (2006). Speech recognition at 1-year follow-up in the childhood development after cochlear implantation (CDaCI) study. *Audiology and Neurotology, 11*, 259–268.

Elliott, L., & Katz, D. (1980). *Development of a new children's test of speech discrimination.* St. Louis, MO: Auditec.

Etymotic Research, Inc. (2005). *BKB-SIN test. Speech-in-Noise Test Version 1.03.* Retrieved from http://www.etymotic.com

Fabry, D., Firszt, J. B., Gifford, R. H., Holden, L. K., & Koch, D. B. (2009, May–June). Evaluating speech perception benefit in adult cochlear implant recipients. *Audiology Today,* pp. 36–43.

Firszt, J. B., Holden, L. K., Skinner, M. W., Tobey, E. A., Peterson, A., Gaggl, W., . . . Wackym, P. A. (2004). Recognition of speech presented at soft to loud levels by adult cochlear implant recipients of three cochlear implant systems. *Ear and Hearing, 25*, 375–387

Firszt, J. B., Koch, D. B., Downing, M., & Litvak, L. (2007). Current steering creates additional pitch percepts in adult cochlear implant recipients. *Otology and Neurotology, 28*(5), 629–636.

Firszt, J. B., Rotz, L. A., Chambers, R. D., & Novak, M. A. (1999). Electrically evoked potentials recorded in adult and pediatric clarion implant users. *Annals of Otology, Rhinology, and Laryngology, 108*(Suppl. 177), 58–63.

Francis, H. W., Buchman, C. A., Visaya, J. M., Wang, N. Y., Zwolan, T. A., Fink, N. E., & Niparko, J. K. (2008). Surgical factors in pediatric cochlear implantation and their early effects on electrode activation and functional outcomes. *Otology and Neurotology, 29*, 502–508.

Francis, H. W., Chee, N., Yeagle, J., Cheng, A., & Niparko, J. K. (2002). Impact of cochlear implants on the functional health status of older adults. *Laryngoscope, 112*, 1482–1488.

Fryauf-Berschy, H., Tyler, R., Kelsay, D., Gantz, B. J., & Woodworth, G. G. (1997). Cochlear implant use by prelingually deafened children: The influences of age at implant and length of device use. *Journal of Speech and Hearing Research, 40*, 183–199.

Gantz, B. J., McCabe, B. F., & Tyler, R. S. (1988). Use of multichannel cochlear implants in obstructed and obliterated cochleas. *Otolaryngology-Head and Neck Surgery, 98*(1), 72–81.

Gantz, B. J., Turner, C., Gfeller, K., & Lowder, M. W. (2005). Preservation of hearing in cochlear implant surgery: Advantages of combined electrical and acoustical speech processing. *Laryngoscope, 115*, 796–802.

Gantz, B. J., Tyler, R. S., Rubinstein, J. T., Wolaver, A., Lowder, M., Abbas, P., . . . Preece, J. P. (2002). Binaural cochlear implants placed during the same operation. *Otology and Neurotology, 23*(2), 169–180.

Gfeller, K., Christ, A., Knutson, J. F., Witt, S., Murray, K. T., & Tyler, R. S. (2000). Musical backgrounds, listening habits, and aesthetic enjoyment of adult cochlear implant recipients. *Journal of the American Academy of Audiology, 11*, 390–406.

Gfeller, K., Olszewski, C., Turner, C., Gantz, B., & Oleson, J. (2006). Music perception with cochlear implants and residual hearing. *Audiology and Neurotology, 11*(Supplement 1), 12–15.

Gibbin, K. P., Raine, C. H., & Summerfield, A. Q. (2003). Cochlear implantation—United Kingdom and Ireland surgical survey. *Cochlear Implants International, 4*, 11–21.

Gifford, R. (2009). *Development of auditory skills in young deaf children with bilateral cochlear implants.* Presentation at the 12th Symposium on Cochlear Implants in Children, Seattle, WA.

Gifford, R. H., Dorman, M. F., McKarns, S. A., & Spahr, A. J. (2007). Combined electric and contra-lateral acoustic hearing: Word and sentence recognition with bimodal hearing. *Journal of Speech, Language, and Hearing Research, 50*, 835–843.

Gifford, R. H., Dorman, M. F., Shallop, J. K., & Sydlowski, S. A. (2010). Evidence for the expansion of adult cochlear implant candidacy. *Ear and Hearing, 31*(2), 186–194.

Gifford, R. H., & Revit, L. (2010). Speech perception for adult cochlear implant recipients in a realistic background noise: Effectiveness of preprocessing strategies and external options for improving speech recognition in noise. *Journal of the American Academy of Audiology, 21*, 441–451.

Gifford, R. H., Shallop, J. K., & Peterson A. (2008). Speech recognition materials and ceiling effects: Considerations for cochlear implant programs. *Audiology and Neurotology, 13*(3), 193–205.

Green, K. M., Bhatt, Y. M., Saeed, S. R., & Ramsden, R. T. (2004). Complications following adult cochlear implantation: Experience in Manchester. *Journal of Laryngology and Otology, 118*, 417–420.

Gstoettner, W. K., Helbig, S., Maier, N., Kiefer, J., Radeloff, A., & Adunka, O. F. (2006). Ipsilateral electric acoustic stimulation of the auditory system: results of long-term hearing preservation. *Audiology and Neurotology, 11*(Suppl. 1), 49–56.

Haskins, H. (1949). *A phonetically balanced speech discrimination test for children* (Master's thesis). Northwestern University, Evanston, IL.

Hehar, S. S., Nikolopoulos, T. P., Gibbin, K. P., & O'Donoghue, G. M. (2002). Surgery and functional outcomes in deaf children receiving cochlear implants before age 2 years. *Archives of Otolaryngology-Head and Neck Surgery, 128*, 11–14.

Hodges, A. V., Butts, S., Dolan-Ash, S., & Balkany, T. J. (1999). Using electrically evoked auditory reflex thresholds to fit the CLARION cochlear implant. *Annals of Otology Rhinology, and Laryngology,* Suppl. 177, 64–68.

Iler-Kirk, K., Pisoni, D. B., & Osberger, M. J. (1995). Lexical effects on spoken word recognition by pediatric cochlear implant users. *Ear and Hearing, 16*, 470–481.

James, C. J., Blamey, P. J., Martin, L., Swanson, B., Just, Y., & Macfarlane, D. (2002). Adaptive dynamic range optimization for cochlear implants: A preliminary study. *Ear and Hearing, S23*, 49S–58S.

Kang, R., Nimmons, G. L., Drennan, W., Longnion, J., Ruffin, C., Nie, K., . . . Rubinstein, J. (2009). Development and validation of the University of Washington clinical assessment of music perception test. *Ear and Hearing, 30*(4), 411–418.

Kishon-Rabin, L., Taitelbaum, R., Elichai, O., Maimon, D., Debyiat, D., & Chazan, N. (2001). Developmental aspects of the IT-MAIS in normal-hearing babies. *Israeli Journal of Speech and Hearing, 23*, 12–22.

Koch, D. B., Osberger, M. J., Segel, P., & Kessler, D. (2004). HiResolutionTM and conventional sound processing in the HiResolutionTM bionic ear: Using appropriate outcome measures to assess speech recognition ability. *Audiology and Neurotology, 9*(4), 214–223.

Koch, D. B., Downing, M., Osberger, M. J., & Litvak, L. (2007). Using current steering to increase spectral resolution in CII and HiRes 90K users. *Ear and Hearing, 28*, 38S–41S.

Koch, D. B., Soli, S., Downing, M., & Osberger, M. J. (2009). Simultaneous bilateral cochlear implantation: Prospective study in adults. *Cochlear Implants International*.

Kong, Y. Y., Stickney, G. S., & Zeng, F. G. (2005). Speech and melody recognition in binaurally combined acoustic and electric hearing. *Journal of the Acoustical Society of America, 117*, 1351–1361.

Krüger, B., Joseph, G., Rost, U., Strauss-Schier, A., Lenarz, T., & Büchner, A. (2008). Performance groups in adult cochlear implant users: Speech perception results from 1984 until today. *Otology and Neurotology, 29*(4), 509–512.

Laske, R. D., Veraguth, D., Dillier, N., Binkert, A., Holzmann, D., & Huber, A. M. (2009). Subjective and objective results after bilateral cochlear implantation in adults. *Otology and Neurotology, 30*(3), 313–318.

Limb, C. J. (2006). Cochlear implant-mediated perception of music. *Current Opinion in Otolaryngology-Head and Neck Surgery, 14*, 337–340.

Ling, D. (1976). *Speech and the hearing-impaired child: Theory and practice.* Washington, DC: Alexander Graham Bell Association for the Deaf.

Ling, D. (1989). *Foundations of spoken language for the hearing-impaired child.* Washington, DC: Alexander Graham Bell Association for the Deaf.

Litovsky, R. Y., Johstonc, P. M., & Godar, S. P. (2006). Benefits of bilateral cochlear implants and/or hearing aids in children. *International Journal of Audiology, 45*(Suppl. 1), 78–91.

Litovsky, R. Y., Johnstone, P. M., Godar, S., Agrawal, S., Parkinson, A., Peters, R., & Lake, J. (2006). Bilateral cochlear implants in children: Localization acuity measured with minimum audible angle. *Ear and Hearing, 27*(1), 43–59.

Litovsky, R. Y., Parkinson, A., & Arcaroli, J. (2009). Spatial hearing and speech intelligibility in bilateral cochlear implant users. *Ear and Hearing, 30*(4), 418–431.

Litovsky, R., Parkinson, A., Arcaroli, J., & Sammeth, C. (2006). Simultaneous bilateral cochlear implantation in adults: A multicenter clinical study. *Ear and Hearing, 27*(6), 714–731.

Madell, J. R. (2007). *Developing a speech perception test protocol for children.* Poster presentation at 2009 Conference on Implantable Auditory Prostheses, Lake Tahoe, CA.

McDermott, H. J. (2004). Music perception with cochlear implants: A review. *Trends in Amplification, 8*(2), 49–82.

Migirov, L., Carmel, E., & Kronenberg, J. (2008). Cochlear implantation in infants: Special surgical and medical aspects. *Laryngoscope, 118*, 2024–2027.

Migirov, L., Muchnik, C., Kaplan-Neeman, R., & Kronenberg, J. (2006). Surgical and medical complications in paediatric cochlear implantation: A review of 300 cases. *Cochlear Implants International, 7*, 194–201.

Mirza, S., Douglas, S. A., Lindsey, P., Hildreth, T., & Hawthorne, M. (2003). Appreciation of music in adult patients with cochlear implants: A patient questionnaire. *Cochlear Implants International, 4*, 85–95.

Mok, M., Grayden, D., Dowell, R. C., & Lawrence, D. (2006). Speech perception for adults who use hearing aids in conjunction with cochlear implants in opposite ears. *Journal of Speech, Language, and Hearing Research, 49*(2), 338–351.

Moog, J. S., & Geers, A. E. (1990). *Early speech perception test.* St. Louis, MO: Central Institute for the Deaf.

Moore, B. C. J., Glasberg, B. R., & Stone, M. A. (1991). Optimization of a slow-acting automatic gain control system for use in hearing aids. *British Journal of Audiology, 25*, 171–182.

Müller, J., Schön, F., & Helms, J. (2002). Speech understanding in quiet and noise in bilateral users of the MED-EL COMBI 40/40+ cochlear implant system. *Ear and Hearing, 23*, 198–206.

Murphy, J., & O'Donoghue, G. (2007). Bilateral cochlear implantation: An evidence-based medicine evaluation. *Laryngoscope, 17*(8), 1412–1418.

Nadol, J. (1984). Histological considerations in implant patients. *Archives of Otolaryngology, 110*, 160–163.

Neuman, A. C., Haravon, A., Sislian, N., & Waltzman, S. B. (2007). Sound-direction identification with bilateral cochlear implants. *Ear and Hearing, 28*(1), 73–82.

Nilsson, M. J., McCaw, V. M., & Soli, S. (1996). *Minimum speech test battery for adult cochlear implant users.* Los Angeles, CA: House Ear Institute.

Nilsson, M. J., Soli, S., & Gelnett, D. J. (1996). *Development of the hearing in noise test for children (HINT-C).* Los Angeles, CA: House Ear Institute.

Nilsson, M. J., Soli, S., & Sullivan, J. (1994). Development of the hearing in noise test for the measurement of speech reception thresholds in quiet and in noise. *Journal of the Acoustical Society of America, 95*, 1085–1099.

Nilsson, M. J., Soli, S., & Sumida, A. (1995). *Development of norms and percent intelligibility functions for the HINT.* Los Angeles, CA: House Ear Institute.

Nogueira, W., Litvak, L., Edler, B., Ostermann, J., & Büchner, A. (2009). Signal processing strategies for cochlear implants using current steering. *EURASIP Journal on Advances in Signal Processing.*

Nopp, P., Schleich, P., & D'Haese, P. (2004). Sound localization in bilateral users of MED-EL Combi 40/40+ cochlear implants. *Ear and Hearing, 25*, 205–214.

Novak, M. A., Fifer, R. C., Barkmeier, J. C., & Firszt, J. B. (1990). Labyrinthine ossification after meningitis: Its implications for cochlear implantation. *Otolaryngology-Head and Neck Surgery, 103*, 351–356.

Osberger, M. J., & Fisher, L. (2000). Preoperative predictors of postoperative implant performance in children. *Annals of Otology, Rhinology, and Laryngology, 209*(Suppl. 185), 44–45.

Osberger, M. J., & Koch, D. B. (2004). Effect of sound processing on performance of young children with cochlear implants. In R. T. Miyamoto (Ed.), *Cochlear implants: Proceedings of the VIIth International Cochlear Implant Conference* (pp. 7–10). Amsterdam: Elsevier B. V. International Congress Series 1273.

Osberger, M. J., Quick, A., Arnold, L., & Boyle, P. (2010). Music benefits with HiRes Fidelity 120 sound processing. *Cochlear Implants International, 11*(Suppl. 1), 352–354.

Osberger, M. J., Zimmerman-Phillips, S., & Koch, D. B. (2002). Cochlear implant candidacy and performance trends in children. *Annals of Otology, Rhinology, and Laryngology, 189*(Suppl. 189), 62–65.

Oxenham, A. J., Bernstein, J. G. W., & Penagos, H. (2004). Correct tonotopic representation is necessary for complex pitch perception. *Proceedings of the National Academy of Sciences, 10*, 1421–1425.

Parry, D. A., Booth, T., & Roland, P. S. (2005). Advantages of magnetic resonance imaging over computed tomography in preoperative evaluation of pediatric cochlear implant candidates. *Otology and Neurotology, 26*, 976–982.

Peretz, I., Champod, A., & Hyde, K. (2003). Varieties of musical disorders: The Montreal battery of evaluation of amusia. *Annals of the New York Academy of Sciences, 999*, 58–75.

Peters, B. R., Litovsky, R., Parkinson, A., & Lake, J. (2007). Importance of age and postimplantation experience on speech perception measures in children with sequential bilateral cochlear implants. *Otology and Neurotology, 28*(5), 649–657.

Peterson, G. E., & Lehiste, I. (1962). Revised CNC lists for auditory tests. *Journal of Speech and Hearing Disorders, 27*, 62–70.

Potts, L. G., Skinner, M. W., Litovsky, R. A., Strube, M. J., & Kuk, F. (2009). Recognition and localization of speech by adult cochlear implant recipients wearing a digital hearing aid in the nonimplanted ear (bimodal hearing). *Journal of the American Academy of Audiology, 20*(6), 353–373.

Proops, D. W., Stoddart, R. L., & Donaldson, I. (1999). Medical, surgical and audiological complications of the first 100 adult cochlear implant patients in Birmingham. *Journal of Laryngology and Otology,* Suppl. 24, 14–17.

Robbins, A. M., Koch, D. B., Osberger, M. J., Zimmerman-Phillips, S., & Kishon-Rabin, L. (2004). Effect of age at implantation on auditory skill development in infants and toddlers. *Archives of Otolaryngology-Head and Neck Surgery, 130*(5), 570–574.

Ross, M., & Lerman, J. (1970). A picture identification test for hearing-impaired children. *Journal of Speech and Hearing Research, 13*, 44–53.

Schleich, P., Nopp, P., & D'Haese, P. (2004). Head shadow, squelch, and summation effects in bilateral users of the MED-EL Combi 40/40+ cochlear implant. *Ear and Hearing, 25*, 197–204.

Seitz, J., Held, P., Waldeck, A., Strotzer, M., Völk, M., Strutz, J., & Feuerbach, S. (2001). Value of high-resolution MR in patients scheduled for cochlear implantation. *Acta Radiologica, 42*(6), 568–573.

Shallop, J. K., Van Dyke, L., Goin, D. W., & Mischke, R. E. (1991). Prediction of behavioral threshold and comfort values for Nucleus 22-channel implant patients from electrical auditory brainstem response test results. *Annals of Otology, Rhinology, and Laryngology, 100*, 896–898.

Shannon, R. V. (1983). Multichannel electrical stimulation of the auditory nerve in man. I. Basic psychophysics. *Hearing Research, 11*(2), 157–189.

Shannon, R. V. (2005). Speech and music have different requirements for spectral resolution. *Review of Neurobiology, 70*, 121–134.

Shannon, R. V., Fu, Q. J., & Galvin, J. (2004). The number of spectral channels required for speech recognition depends on the difficulty of the listening situation. *Acta Otolaryngologica,* (Suppl. 552), 1–5.

Spahr, A., & Dorman, M. F. (2004). Performance of subjects fit with the Advanced Bionics CII and Nucleus 3G cochlear implant devices. *Archives of Otolaryngology-Head and Neck Surgery, 130*, 624–628.

Spitzer, J. B., Mancuso, D., & Cheng, M. Y. (2008). Development of a clinical test of musical perception: Appreciation of music in cochlear implantees (AMICI). *Journal of the American Academy of Audiology, 19*(1), 56–81.

Stone, M. A., Moore, B. C. J., Alcantara, J. I., & Glasberg, B. R. (1999). Comparison of different forms of compression using wearable digital hearing aids. *Journal of the Acoustical Society of America, 106*, 3603–3619.

Tucci, D. L., & Pilkington, T. M. (2009). Medical and surgical aspects of cochlear implantation. In J. K. Niparko (Ed.), *Cochlear implants: Principles and practices* (pp. 161–186). Philadelphia, PA: Lippincott Williams & Wilkins.

Venail, F., Sicard, M., Piron, J. P., Levi, A., Artieres, F., Uziel, A., & Mondain, M. (2008). Reliability and complications of 500 consecutive cochlear implantations. *Archives of Otolaryngology-Head and Neck Surgery, 134*, 1276–1281.

Waltzman, S. B., & Cohen, N. L. (1998). Cochlear implantation in children younger than 2 years old. *American Journal of Otology, 19*, 158–162.

Wang, N. Y., Eisenberg, L. S., Johnson, K. C., Fink, N. E., Tobey, E. A., Quittner A. L., . . . the CDaCI Investigative Team. (2008). Tracking development of speech recognition: Longitudinal data from hierarchical assessments in the childhood development after cochlear implantation study. *Otology and Neurotology, 29*, 240–245.

Wilson, B. E. (1993). Signal processing. In R. S. Tyler (Ed.), *Cochlear implants: Audiological foundations* (pp. 35–85). San Diego, CA: Singular.

Wilson, B. E., & Dorman, M. (2009). The design of cochlear implants. In J. K. Niparko (Ed.), *Cochlear implants: Principles and practices* (2nd ed., pp. 95–135). Philadelphia, PA: Lippincott, Williams & Wilkins.

Wilson, B. E., Finley, C. C., Lawson, D. T., Wolford, R. D., Eddington, D. K., & Rabinowitz, W. M. (1991). Better speech recognition with cochlear implants. *Nature, 352*, 236–238.

Wolfe, J., Baker, S., Caraway, T., Kasulis, H., Mears, A., Smith, J., . . . & Wood M. (2007). 1-year postactivation results for sequentially implanted bilateral cochlear implant users. *Otology and Neurotology, 28*(5), 589–596.

Zeng, F. G. (2004). Trends in cochlear implants. *Trends in Amplification, 8*(1), 1–34.

Zimmerman-Phillips, S., Robbins, A. M., & Osberger, M. J. (2001). *Infant-toddler meaningful auditory integration scale (IT-MAIS)*. Valencia, CA: Advanced Bionics.

APPENDIX 18–A
ADULT SPEECH TESTS

Arranged in alphabetical order

The **AzBio Sentence Test** (Spahr & Dorman, 2004) was developed at Arizona State University and consists of lists of sentences (6 to 10 words per sentence) that have been equated for intelligibility. Each list contains sentences spoken by two male and two female talkers in a conversational style. The sentence materials are available on an audio CD designed specifically for use with a clinical audiometer. Each CD contains 15 lists of 20 sentences, a soundfield calibration noise, and a 1000-Hz calibration tone. A 10-talker babble noise runs continuously on the second track of the CD. Score sheets are available for download as a printable document (pdf) and as an Excel spreadsheet that tracks patient information, sentence scores, and notes. Auditory Potential, LLC is an authorized distributor of the AzBio sentences (http://www.auditorypotential.com).

The **Bamford-Kowal-Bench Speech in Noise Test (BKB-SIN**; Etymotic Research, 2005) consists of sentences recorded in a background of four-talker babble. It employs an adaptive procedure with 10 different SNRs that are decreased in 3 dB steps from +21 to −6 dB. There are 18 list pairs that are equated for intelligibility. Both lists of a pair (A & B) must be administered for valid scoring. Each list contains one sentence with each of the 10 SNRs (10 sentences per list; 20 sentences per list pair). The BKB-SIN can be used to estimate SNR loss in children and adults by comparing results with normative data. The test can be purchased from Etymotic Research (http://www.etymotic.com).

The **CNC Monosyllabic Word Test** (Petersen & Lehiste, 1962) consists of 10 lists of phonemically balanced monosyllabic words in a consonant-nucleus-consonant format (50 words per list). Performance is scored as the number of words or phonemes correctly understood. The recorded version of the test that is used most often by cochlear implant clinicians is on the *Minimum Speech Test Battery for Adult Cochlear Implant Patients* CD (Nilsson, McCaw & Soli, 1996).

The **Hearing in Noise Test (HINT**; Nilsson, Soli, & Sullivan, 1994; Nilsson, Soli, & Sumida, 1995) consists of 25 equivalent 10-sentence lists (which also can be presented as 12 equivalent 20-sentence lists) and speech-spectrum noise that matches the long-term average spectrum of the sentences. The HINT was designed to determine the reception threshold for sentences (RTS) with an adaptive procedure in which noise is presented at a fixed level, and the sentence levels are varied depending on the accuracy of the listener's responses. The HINT was modified for cochlear implant patients to allow administration of the sentences with a fixed presentation level in quiet or with a fixed SNR in noise. The fixed-level HINT was originally distributed on the *Minimum Speech Test Battery for Adult Cochlear Implant Patients* CD (Nilsson, McCaw, & Soli, 1996) but is now distributed by Bio-Logic (HINT Pro) (http://www.bio-logic.com).

Arranged in order of difficulty

The **Ling Six Sounds Test** (Ling, 1976, 1989) consists of sounds that represent low-, mid-, and high-frequency components of speech: /ah/, /oo/, /ee/, /m/, /s/, and /sh/. The stimuli are presented live voice as a detection, discrimination, or identification task, depending on the skills of the child.

The **Infant-Toddler Meaningful Integration Scale (IT-MAIS**; Zimmerman-Phillips, Robbins, & Osberger, 2001) employs a structured interview schedule that assesses a child's spontaneous response to sound in everyday situations as observed by the parents (or primary caregiver). A rating is assigned to each of 10 target behaviors based on frequency of occurrence: 0 = never (i.e., the behavior is never observed); 1 = rarely; 2 = occasionally; 3 = frequently; 4 = always. Three areas of behavior are assessed: vocalization, alerting to sounds, and deriving meaning from sound.

The **Early Speech Perception (ESP) Test** (Moog & Geers, 1990) consists of a *Standard Version* for older children and a *Low Verbal Version* for younger children. The *Standard Version* consists of three subtests: Pattern Perception, Spondee Word Identification, and Monosyllable Word Identification. For each subtest, the child is shown a picture plate with 12 items and is asked to point to the picture representing the spoken word. Each item is presented two times in random order (36 trials). Ideally, the test is presented in recorded format. The *Low Verbal Version* employs the same subtests as the Standard Version, but it is designed to be used with younger children. A four-alternative response format is used with objects rather than pictured representations of the stimuli. The test can be administered in recorded format or live voice.

The **Multisyllabic Lexical Neighborhood Test (MLNT**; Iler-Kirk, Pisoni, & Osberger, 1995) was developed based upon the same design principles as the Lexical Neighborhood Test (LNT), described below, except that multisyllabic words are used to make the task easier. The MLNT is an open-set test consisting of lists of lexically "easy" and "hard" words. Each list contains 24 words that are scored for the number of phonemes and words correctly understood. The test is administered in recorded format and can be obtained from Auditec (http://www.auditec.com).

The **Lexical Neighborhood Test (LNT**; Iler-Kirk, Pisoni, & Osberger, 1995) assesses speech recognition in children while controlling for lexical properties of the stimulus words. The LNT equates words for the number of phonemes shared by other words and for the frequency of occurrence of the words in spoken English. For example, the word "cat" is considered to have many lexical "neighbors" or words that rhyme (e.g., hat, bat, mat, etc.). It also is a high-frequency word. In contrast, the word "juice" has few lexical neighbors (i.e., few words that rhyme with it) and occurs less infrequently in spoken English. The LNT consists of monosyllabic words, arranged in lists of "easy" and "hard" words. There are 25 words in each list that are scored for the number of phonemes and words correctly understood. The test is administered in recorded format and can be obtained from Auditec (http://www.auditec.com).

The **Phonetically Balanced Kindergarten test (PBK**; Haskins, 1949) consists of three lists of phonetically balanced monosyllabic words (four different randomizations of 50 words each). This older test is commonly used even though some of the vocabulary items are out of date. It is a more difficult test of open-set speech recognition than the LNT and MLNT, and a precursor to the use of adult word tests. The child is instructed to repeat what is heard. Performance is scored by the number of phonemes and words correctly understood. A recorded version of the test should be used and can be obtained from Auditec (http://www.auditec.com).

The **Hearing-In-Noise Test for Children (HINT-C**; Nilsson, Soli, & Gelnett, 1996) is a pediatric version of the HINT test developed for children ages 6 to 12 years. The sentences are presented at a fixed level in recorded format. Performance also can be assessed in the presence of speech-spectrum noise presented a fixed level. The HINT-C is part of the HINT Pro system distributed by Bio-Logic (http://www.bio-logic.com).

CHAPTER 19

Fitting Options for Adult Patients with Unilateral Hearing Loss

MICHAEL VALENTE
L. MAUREEN VALENTE

INTRODUCTION

Patients with unilateral hearing loss (UHL) typically experience difficulty in (a) localizing sounds, (b) recognizing speech when the signal arrives on the side of the poorer ear, and (c) recognizing speech in background noise (especially if the noise is arriving on the side of the better ear). These patients also want to know:

a. What caused the hearing loss in his or her one ear?
b. If the hearing will return to normal?
c. What are the chances this will occur for the opposite ear?
d. If the hearing will not return by itself, what can done medically or surgically to restore the hearing?
e. What will the treatment cost?
f. Will the cost be covered by his or her insurance?

It is clear that patients with UHL can present a challenge to the audiologist. The audiologist can follow a traditional dispensing model that provides extensive counseling on the communication problems associated with UHL, and/or recommend Contralateral Routing of the Signal (CROS) or Bilateral Contralateral Routing of the Signal (CROS) amplification to the better ear. On the other hand, the audiologist could explore CROS and BICROS options as well as other current alternative fitting options.

This chapter focuses on information that may prove beneficial for audiologists who want to explore current fitting options for patients with UHL.

DEFINING UHL

For the purpose of this chapter, UHL is defined as unaidable hearing in one ear and normal hearing (≤15 dB HL at 250–8000 Hz) in the opposite ear. It has been estimated that there are about 200 new cases of SSD per million individuals (http://www.singlesided-deafness.com/) or about 60,000 new cases a year in the United States. Unaidable hearing is demonstrated in an ear having one or more of the following characteristics:

1. Profound sensorineural hearing loss, so that amplified sound cannot be heard with any degree of usefulness
2. Very poor word recognition
3. Marked intolerance for amplified sounds

PROBLEMS ASSOCIATED WITH UHL

The patient with UHL can no longer enjoy the advantages of binaural hearing. These binaural advantages include:

1. Eliminating the head shadow effect
2. Preserving the squelch effect
3. Preserving localization
4. Preserving binaural summation

Head Shadow Effect

The "head shadow effect" was described by Tillman, Kasten, and Horner (1963), who reported that, as a spondee word arrives from one side of the head (near ear or monaural direct condition), the intensity of the signal is attenuated around the head by an average overall level of 6.4 dB before the signal reaches the opposite ear (far ear or monaural indirect condition). Furthermore, the head shadow effect increases as a function of frequency. For example, at frequencies above 2000 Hz, the intensity level of the signal to the far ear can be as great as 15 to 20 dB lower than the level of the signal at the near ear (Hodgson, 1986).

The reduction in signal level in the higher frequencies at the far ear can have a significant impact on speech recognition. For example, if speech is delivered to the impaired ear and noise is directed to the better ear (monaural indirect) at the same input level, the patient can experience great difficulties in communicating. In this situation, the overall speech signal is reduced by 6.4 dB to the better ear due to the head shadow effect. The noise delivered to the better ear is not attenuated, however, resulting in a –6.4 dB SNR at the better ear. Furthermore, a +6.4 dB SNR is present at the impaired ear (monaural direct) because the noise is attenuated by 6.4 dB, but the signal is unattenuated. In essence, the unilaterally impaired patient has a 13 dB interaural deficit compared with the same listening situation for a normal hearing patient. Clearly, if this listening situation is reversed, then the unilaterally impaired patient is not at a disadvantage relative to the normal listener. Valente (1982) summarized a series of studies concerning speech recognition for monaural direct versus monaural indirect listening. The advantage of monaural direct to monaural indirect word recognition can be as high as 20% to 50% depending on the type of signal, noise, azimuth, and SNR (Valente, 1982).

Squelch Effect

Gulick, Gescheider, and Frisina (1989) have described the advantages of binaural hearing to "squelch" or reduce the deleterious effects of background noise and/or reverberation on speech recognition abilities. Gulick et al. (1989) reported improved binaural "release from masking," particularly when time, intensity, or phase differences of the signal are present (i.e., signal presented at any azimuth in a sound field other than 0°), and these differences are not present for the masker (i.e., masker presented at 0° azimuth). That is, the presence of differences in time, intensity, and/or phase of the speech signal between the two ears will result in improved performance compared with the situation in which these differences are not present between the two ears. Obviously, these interaural differences could not be present or capitalized upon in a patient with UHL.

Localization

Gulick et al. (1989) devoted a section of their text to sound localization, describing various studies that have contributed to the profession's knowledge. Explanations of directional hearing have centered about differences in stimulation between the two ears in time and intensity (i.e., duplex theory of localization) and the integration of this information for improved sound localization. In particular, the normal listener uses interaural time (low-frequency cue) and intensity differences (high-frequency cue) for improved localization in the horizontal plane. Obviously, if there is a large difference in hearing between the ears, localization skills are significantly reduced. One of the first questions patients with UHL ask is if hearing aids will restore his or her ability to localize. In this situation, the authors counsel the patient that it is highly unlikely that he or she will ever be able to localize, but that some patients can localize by perceiving differences in sound quality between the ears. If he or she perceives "normal" sound quality, then the sound must have arrived on the side of his or her better ear. On the other hand, if he or she perceives a "tinny" sound quality in the better ear, then the sound must have arrived from the poorer ear where the microphone resides and sent the amplified signal to the better ear.

Binaural Summation

Brookhouser, Worthington, and Kelly (1991) reminded the reader that patients with binaural hearing demonstrate improved thresholds for pure-tone and speech stimuli presented binaurally. Gulick et al. (1989) described this binaural summation phenomenon as an advantage in processing information (specifically, detecting threshold) with two ears over listening with one ear. They stated that if the ears are equally sensitive, the binaural threshold is about 3 dB better than the monaural threshold and the binaural advantage increases to 6 dB during suprathreshold listening (i.e., most comfortable loudness) and 10 dB sensation level (SL re: threshold). This additional advantage may have significant effects on improved word recognition scores when listening binaurally in comparison with monaural listening. That is, if speech recognition increases at a rate of 5%–10% per each additional decibel (i.e., articulation function), then the binaural advantage at suprathreshold levels could be 30% to 60% better (6 dB × 5% to 10%/dB).

HEARING AID FITTING PROCESS FOR UHL

Case History and Referral

When providing audiologic care for patients with UHL, the audiologist should seek answers to some important questions prior to considering amplification. Information should include the age of the patient, occupation, demands on listening, typical listening environments, and indications of motivation toward amplification. The patient history should also include as much detail as possible regarding the duration and etiology of the UHL and any related symptoms such as tinnitus or dizziness. Like any other hearing aid fitting, the audiologist should require medical clearance prior to dispensing hearing aids and an audiogram completed within 6 months of the time the hearing aid is dispensed. This is especially true in cases of UHL because the hearing loss may be the result of a space-occupying lesion. If the hearing loss is sudden, waiting several weeks before pursuing amplification is suggested because approximately 65% of patients with sudden hearing loss report complete or partial recovery (Stachler et al., 2012).

Fitting Options

There are numerous fitting options available for patients with UHL that include:

a. CROS or BICROS
b. Transcranial CROS
c. Auditory Osseointegrated Implant System (AOIS)
d. TransEar
e. SoundBite
f. Cochlear Implant

CROS

Potential Problems with CROS or BICROS Fittings from the Authors' Perspective

When fitting any CROS or BICROS device and considering any treatment plan, the audiologist should consider the communication strategies the adult patient may have developed over time. Typically, many adult patients have been communicating with one normal and one unaidable ear for some time. Over the years, these patients have likely developed strategies to situate themselves, so the "wanted" signal is on their better side. When able to stage and manage advantageously, they perform quite well. On the other hand, these patients try to avoid situations where the noise is on their better ear side, and the signal is on the side of their poorer ear side. As one can imagine, constantly having to "scan" the listening environment, so the better ear is toward the signal, and the poorer ear is toward the noise may be fatiguing and in many listening situations, impossible. In addition, patient judgments in this regard may not always be accurate. These patients have invested much effort to determine how to effectively communicate, and for the most part, seem to be doing quite well.

At this point, the audiologist enters the picture, with the best of intentions, suggesting some type of CROS or BICROS fitting by placing a transmitting microphone behind or in the poorer ear to "capture" the wanted signal at the side of the poorer ear. The goal is to simply regain the clues the patient was missing all those years. There is, however, the likelihood that noise will also be on that side. In the past, this noise was attenuated by the patient's poorer hearing. With the CROS or BICROS hearing aid, the noise is now amplified and sent to the better ear and mixed with the signal directed to that ear. Thus, what has the well-intentioned audiologist really accomplished? He or she has potentially reversed the patient's unaided world. What was "difficult" without amplification becomes easier (i.e., speech on the poorer side), but what was "easy" without amplification (i.e., noise on the poorer side) now becomes more difficult. Thus, amplification has reversed the patient's world as easy becomes difficult and difficult becomes easy. Still, the question remains, what has the audiologist really done to significantly improve the patient's listening environment between the unaided and aided condition? The answer is "probably little." This may explain, in at least the authors' experience, the high rate of dissatisfaction typically seen when patients are fit with CROS or BICROS amplification in comparison with other types of hearing aid fittings. This dissatisfaction, as will be examined later in this chapter, has been fairly recently been reversed somewhat by the recent introduction of new CROS and BICROS technologies by Unitron and Phonak. Some of these anticipated problems (i.e., the "reversed listening world") can be addressed upfront with extensive counseling, but in many cases, patients still remain dissatisfied.

Solutions to address this potential problem can be resolved in at least two ways. First, the audiologist may consider dispensing a BICROS configuration with a volume control on the transmitting microphone side and a volume control, microphone, amplifier, and receiver to an open earmold to the better ear. Typically, a CROS fitting is fit with an open mold to the better ear and a BICROS is fit with a more closed mold in the better ear, but in many CROS devices a volume control is not available on the transmitter side. By using a BICROS fitting, the audiologist would want a device having volume controls on both sides, microphones on both sides, and use of an open mold due to the normal hearing in the better ear. This arrangement at

least allows the patient to reduce amplification via the use of a volume control from the transmitting microphone on the poorer side if the patient perceives the presence of noise. This fitting still achieves the benefits of the open earmold fit to the normal ear. A similar outcome may be achieved with an on/off switch to reduce the deleterious impact of the noise from the poorer side. Another option is for the patient to use a remote control to accomplish the same goal (i.e., reducing the volume on the transmitter side or turning off the transmitter side). A second solution is to use noise reduction (NR) that is now available in DSP hearing aids. For example, the reader is encouraged to consider a CROS/BICROS hearing aid where NR within the hearing aid containing the transmitting microphone on the poorer ear would shut the aid off (or significantly attenuate amplification) if an unmodulated signal (noise) is detected. This strategy might resolve the problem addressed above because the offside transmitting microphone on the poorer ear would only be active if the processor detects a modulated signal (speech). In this manner, what was "easier" in an unaided condition remains easier in an aided condition (signal on the better side; noise on the poorer side). What was difficult in an unaided condition (noise on the poorer side) becomes easier in an aided condition because the noise is not being amplified as occurs with most current CROS/BICROS aids.

This suggestion achieved reality with the recent introduction of the Tandem 4 (four channels/four bands) and 16 (sixteen channels/16 bands) wireless CROS/BICROS hearing aid from Unitron (Figure 19–1). This hearing aid provides programmable multichannel NR on the transmitter (poorer ear side; left side of Figure 19–1) and receiver (better ear side; right side of Figure 19–1) hearing aids and includes a volume control on both sides. The Tandem 16 has four programmable settings of NR that can be programmed for the receiver *and* transmitter. These settings include no NR, mild (~ –3 dB SPL), moderate (~ –5 to 6 dB SPL), and maximum NR (~ –8 to 9 dB SPL). The amount of

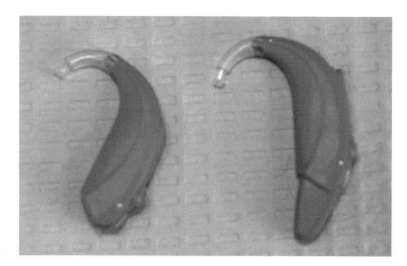

Figure 19–1. Uniron Tandem 16 BICROS hearing aid. Hearing aid to the left is the transmitting hearing aid, and the hearing aid to the right is the receiver hearing aid. Both hearing aids have volume controls.

NR does not vary by input level and is based upon the estimated SNR in a particular frequency channel, and activation of NR begins at an input level of approximately 40 dB SPL. In a recent study, Oeding and Valente (2013) assessed the performance of the NR of the Tandem 16 on 21 participants using an eight-loudspeaker array where restaurant noise, held constant at 65 dB SPL, surrounded the participant. Results of the study revealed no statistically significant differences in the Reception Threshold for Sentences (RTS in dB) between unaided, no NR, mild NR, and maximum NR. This finding may be clinically significant because many of the prior studies on differences in performance between CROS and BICROS reported unaided performance to be better than aided performance when the noise was on the side of the poorer ear. Subjective impressions using a subjective questionnaire, however, revealed statistically and clinically significant benefit with the Tandem 16 BICROS and the subject's own BICROS compared with unaided.

On a related note, the authors have experienced some confusion within the professional community with the nomenclature used for CROS/BICROS fittings. To provide some standardization, when the aided sig- *aided* nal is routed to the *left* ear, it is important to remember that this is a *Left CROS or BICROS*. On the other hand, a *Right CROS or BICROS* suggests that the aided signal is routed to the *right* ear.

One final point must be emphasized regarding CROS amplification. In the original report by Harford and Barry (1965) and subsequent reports by Harford (1969), and Harford and Dodds (1966), there is a clear recommendation that acceptance of CROS amplification is related to the magnitude of hearing loss in the better ear. If hearing in the better ear is within normal limits, then the probability of acceptance with CROS amplification is reduced. On the other hand, if a mild hearing loss is present above 1500 Hz, then a greater probability of patient acceptance will be achieved.

Different Types of CROS Arrangements

Wired-Analog

One of the earliest attempts to improve communication for UHL patients was the CROS hearing aid (Harford, 1969; Harford & Barry,

1965; Harford & Dodds, 1966; Hayes, Pumford, & Dorscher, 2005; Hill, 2006). In the earliest version, CROS amplification consisted of a microphone placed over or near the unaidable ear to pick up signals arriving at that side. The output from the microphone was wired to an amplifier, receiver, and volume control via headband. The amplified signal was delivered via tubing gently placed in the open ear canal of the better ear. Due to the presence of the open earmold in the better ear, no gain was provided below 800 Hz, and only marginal gain was provided between 800 and 1500 Hz. The greatest amount of gain was provided above 1500 Hz. As mentioned earlier, patients most likely to receive the greatest acceptance from CROS amplification were patients with normal hearing in the better ear through 1500 Hz and a slight to mild hearing loss above 1500 Hz. Problems with using a wire to transfer the signal from the transmitter to the receiver side included selecting the correct length of the wire that was manufactured in discrete sizes, breakage of the wire, deterioration of the connection of the wire to the transmitter and receiver sides, and the cosmetics related to the presence of the wire running along the back of the neck.

Wired-Programmable with Directional Microphone

The wired-analog aid gave way to wired programmable CROS and BICROS hearing aids with omnidirectional and directional microphones. It is important to note that the directional microphone was available only for use on the receiver side when the transmitter side was not communicating with the receiver side. In some of these CROS or BICROS aids, the buttons on a remote control were programmed such that pressing one button would activate omnidirectional performance for listening in quiet, while a second button could be programmed to activate the directional microphone (again, only if the transmitter was not communicating with the receiver side) for better performance in noisy listening situations. A third button could acti-

vate a telecoil for improved listening over the telephone or assistive listening device. The remaining buttons served as a volume control, as well as an on/off switch. The presence of a directional microphone provides the possibility for greater speech recognition in noise than the omnidirectional microphone available in all current wireless models (Valente, Fabry, & Potts, 1995a).

While CROS or BICROS amplification effectively eliminates the head shadow effect by amplifying signals from the poorer side, localization and speech recognition in noise still remain a problem. Some CROS or BICROS users have reported improved localization based on differences in sound quality perceived from the two ears. If the signal appears "natural," it may be judged to be arriving from the better side. If the sound appears "tinny" or "metallic," it may be judged to be arriving from the impaired side (Harford, 1969). Also, if the level of ambient noise is high, few users of CROS or BICROS amplification report any significant benefit regardless of the side from which the signal or noise may be arising. In these environments, it may be best to counsel the patient to reduce the volume control setting or remove the hearing aids (Harford, 1969; Hodgson, 1986).

Wireless-Analog

As mentioned earlier, one of the major drawbacks of the earlier CROS or BICROS systems was the need for a wire connecting the output from the transmitting microphone on the impaired ear to the receiver on the better ear. To solve this problem, one manufacturer (i.e., Telex) introduced a wireless BTE to ITE CROS and BICROS. Other models included a BTE to BTE version. This wireless CROS and BICROS used an amplitude-modulated (AM) carrier frequency to transmit signals from the microphone on the side of the impaired ear to the receiver placed in the better ear. Distance between the transmitter and receiver is critical (approximately 6.5 inches). For every half-inch increase in distance between the transmitter and receiver, there is a 3 to 4 dB decrease in gain.

Clinically, a major drawback of this wireless CROS or BICROS system was the limited ability to shape the frequency-gain response to provide the prescribed gain to the aided ear. These models were manufactured with only a low-frequency tone control or low- and high-frequency tone controls as a way to shape the frequency response.

Wireless-Digital

With the next generation of CROS/BICROS options, several manufacturers introduced wireless BTE to BTE, BTE to custom, and custom to custom CROS aids with multichannel digital signal processing (DSP). Because of significant advances in DSP over the past decade, these models have eliminated most of the shortcomings cited above for the original wireless models.

As mentioned earlier, Unitron recently introduced the Tandem 4 and 16 (sixteen channels/16 bands) wireless CROS/BICROS hearing aid (see Figure 19–1). This hearing aid provides programmable multichannel NR on the transmitter (poorer ear side; left side of Figure 19–1) and receiver (better ear side; right side of Figure 19–1) hearing aids and includes a volume control on both sides. The Tandem 16 has four programmable settings of NR that can be programmed for the receiver *and* transmitter. These settings include no NR, mild (~ −3 dB SPL), moderate (~ −5 to 6 dB SPL), and maximum NR (~ −8 to 9 dB SPL). The amount of NR does not vary by input level and is based on the estimated SNR in a particular frequency channel and activation of NR begins at an input level of approximately 40 dB SPL.

Another recent advancement is the introduction, for the first time, of the patient having directional microphone technology available in a CROS or BICROS hearing aid. Phonak recently introduced their Quest or Spice hearing instruments containing an automatic adaptive multichannel directional microphone on the receiver side while the transmitter is active. The hearing aid on the receiver side can have as few as 8 channels/bands signal processing to as many as 20 channels/bands of signal processing depending upon the model that is paired to communicate with the wireless transmitter (hearing instrument to the left in Figure 19–2). In Figure 19–2, the upper right is the Bolero Q9 (20 channels), and the lower right is the Audeo Q9 (20 channels). The transmitter can be an ITE or BTE model, and the receiver side hearing aid can also be a BTE or an ITE. Two recent studies (Linnebjerg & Wetke, 2013; Williams, McArdle, & Chisolm, 2012) reported positive reports of this new BICROS hearing aid system when compared with the participant's own BICROS system.

Transcranial CROS

A different approach in providing amplification to UHL patients has been advocated by several authors (Fagelson, Noe, Mumane, & Blevins, 2003; Sullivan, 1988; Valente, Potts, Valente, & Goebel, 1995b). These authors have suggested placing a conventional high gain/high output air conduction CIC, ITE, or BTE hearing aid in the impaired ear to take advantage of the fact that the cochleas for each ear, contained within the temporal bones, are not acoustically isolated. If an air conducted signal of sufficiently high enough output is presented to the cochlea of an impaired ear, the signal will eventually be heard in the cochlea of the better ear because it will be intense enough to overcome the acoustic isolation (interaural attenuation or IA) between the cochleas. Because the signal picked up by a microphone placed in the impaired ear is transferred to the cochlea of the better ear through the cranial structures of the temporal bone, the authors cited above referred to this type of fitting as a transcranial CROS.

The concept behind transcranial CROS is apparent to any audiologist having experience testing a patient via air conduction (earphone or insert receiver) with normal hearing in one ear and moderate-severe to severe hearing loss in the opposite ear. The initial unmasked air conduction thresholds for the impaired ear represent the magnitude of interaural attenuation (IA) sometimes referred to as the "shadow curve." For this patient,

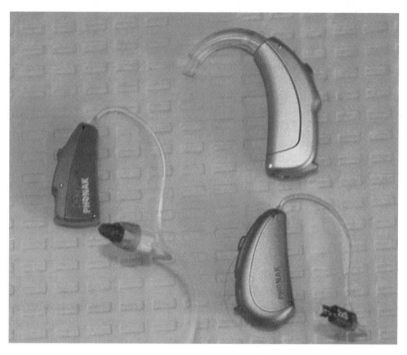

Figure 19–2. Phonak CROS transmitter (*left*). Bolero Q90 (*upper right*) and Audeo Q90 (*lower right*) as two of the many options for the hearing aid on the receiver side.

this unmasked threshold represents the lowest intensity at which stimuli (nonspeech or speech) will pass through the temporal bone and around the head by air conduction and is heard by the cochlea of the normal ear. In much the same way, the output (input signal plus the gain of the hearing aid) from a power BTE or custom hearing aid placed on the impaired ear can deliver amplified sound to the cochlea of the normal ear via air and bone conduction (AC and BC). Signals picked up by the microphone of a hearing aid placed over or in the impaired ear can be amplified and eventually cross through the head and be heard by the cochlea of the normal ear via BC.

In an effort to determine if transcranial fittings had merit, Valente et al. (1995b) evaluated 12 patients with an unaidable ear in one ear and normal hearing in the opposite ear. For each patient, a power ITE hearing aid (maximum saturation sound pressure level of 120 dB; full-on gain of 55–65 dB) with a

long canal and pressure vent was fitted to the impaired ear. Four patients were experienced users of CROS amplification. Two patients had experience with an eyeglass BC hearing aid placed on the mastoid process of the impaired ear. Five patients had no experience with amplification, and one patient had experience with a mild ITE hearing aid coupled to the better ear. At the end of 4 weeks, one half of the patients felt the ITE transcranial CROS provided significant benefit, while the other half noted little additional benefit and decided to continue to utilize their current hearing aids or not pursue amplification at all. For the interested reader, the Valente et al. (1995b) manuscript provides a method whereby real measures can be used to measure the transcranial thresholds (in dB SPL) of the poorer ear by placing a probe microphone in the poor ear while measuring thresholds at 250 to 8000 Hz. This value (in dB SPL) has been coined "transcranial threshold (TCT)." The TCT represents the lowest level of which the real ear aided response (REAR) in the poorer ear must exceed in order to verify that the output from the hearing aid provides sufficient amplification to be heard in the cochlea of the better ear.

It is important to note that user acceptance at Washington University at that time for conventional CROS fittings for this population (normal hearing in the better ear) was approximately 10%, while the acceptance rate for the transcranial CROS was 50%. The reasons for rejection of the transcranial CROS by many subjects were related to feedback or to a sensation of vibration generated from the hearing aid. The results of this study were encouraging. Interestingly, and perhaps of some clinical value, was that subjects preferring the transcranial fit were those subjects with the lowest IA values (i.e., greater ease for the amplified signal to reach the normal ear).

Revisiting Transcranial via DSP

The authors have recently revisited transcranial CROS due to the advances in DSP. The greatest potential advantage of DSP is the availability of NR and feedback management. The reader may recall that one of the limiting factors preventing success with the analog version of transcranial CROS was the presence of feedback. This would not allow sufficient gain/output to allow the measured REAR (dB SPL) to exceed the individually measured TCT measured in dB SPL in the poor ear using probe microphone measures.

Auditory Osseointegrated Implant System

In 2002, the Food and Drug Administration approved the Auditory Osseointegrated Implant System (AOIS) to be fit to patients with UHL (Andersen, Schroder, & Bonding; 2006; Bosman, Hol, Snik, Mylanus, & Cremers, 2003; Bosman, Snik, Hol, & Mylanus, 2013; Hol, Bosman, Snik, Mylanus, & Cremers, 2004; Lin et at., 2006; Linstrom, Silverman, & Yu, 2009; Newman, Sandridge, & Wodzisz, 2008; Niparko, Cox, & Lustig, 2003; Oeding, Valente, & Kerckhoff, 2010; Stenfelt,

2005; Vaneecloo, Ruzza, & Hanson, 2001; Wazen et al., 2003; Wazen, Spitzer, Ghossaini, Kacker, & Zschommler, 2001; Yuen, Bodmer, Smilsky, Nedzelski, & Chen, 2009). In January of 2005, Medicare provided coverage for the AOIS. It is important to note that Medicare reimburses the surgical procedure and processor, but does not reimburse the audiologist for his or her professional services. In order for the audiologist to receive payment for his or her services, the patient is required to sign an ABN (Advanced Beneficiary Notice) that clearly states that the patient has been counseled and that audiological services (hearing aid evaluation, hearing aid selection, hearing aid fitting, counseling, and all follow-up care relative to the processor) are not covered by Medicare. Via this avenue, the patient agrees to pay for these services at the fitting. In addition, there are private insurers that will follow the Medicare model and do not reimburse the audiologist for his or her services. In these cases, the authors counsel these patients in the same manner as they do Medicare patients and require the patient to sign a ABN-like form, so the audiologist is paid by the patient at the time of the fitting.

With the AOIS, the patient typically undergoes outpatient surgery where a titanium fixture (screw) is anchored into the skull, and a percutaneous titanium abutment is attached to the titanium fixture and penetrates the skin. With the AOIS processor coupled onto the abutment, these titanium components transmit amplified sound directly to the skull without interference from the intermediate tissue. In the adult, it takes approximately 3 months for the implant to osseointegrate with the mastoid bone before the AOIS processor is coupled to the abutment and fit. In the authors' experience, if the BC thresholds in the better ear are ≤20 dB HL at 500 to 3000 Hz, there is a high probability that the patient will have a high level of benefit and satisfaction with the AOIS. This is very important because the authors are aware of several patients fit with the AOIS where the BC thresholds in the better ear exceeded these guidelines, and the patient was not satisfied with the AOIS.

Currently, the AOIS is available from Cochlear Americas in the Baha 3 (BP100), Baha 3 Power (BP110; Figure 19–3), and Cordelle II. The figure to the left in Figure 19–3 illustrates the front of the Baha 3 Power (BP110), whereas the figure to the right illustrates the side of the Baha 3 Power (BP110) revealing the snap connector that couples the Baha 3 Power (BP110) to the abutment. Features of this AOIS device include:

a. Ability to measure BC thresholds directly through the AOIS
b. Availability of three programs
c. 12 channel signal processing
d. Wide dynamic range compression (WDRC)
e. Automatic adaptive multiband directional microphone
f. Automatic noise management
g. Automatic feedback cancellation
h. Programmability through NOAH
i. Program indicators and low-battery warning signals
j. Direct audio input

Another manufacturer offering AOIS technology is Oticon Medical, who introduced the Ponto Pro (Figure 19–4) and Ponto Pro Power. The figure to the left in Figure 19–4 illustrates the front of the Ponto Pro, while the figure to the right illustrates the side of the Ponto Pro revealing the snap connector that couples the Ponto Pro to the abutment. The Ponto Pro offers:

a. Linear signal processing
b. Ten channel DSP
c. Automatic multichannel adaptive directional microphones
d. Tri-state noise reduction
e. Data logging
f. Self-learning volume control
g. Programmability via NOAH
h. Four programs
i. Direct auditory input
j. Program indicators and low-battery warning signals

These latter two AOIS devices from Oticon Medical can be coupled to the Cochlear Americas abutment, and a slightly different abutment configuration is available through Oticon Medical. The BP-100, however, cannot be connected to the Oticon Medical abutment. It is suspected that in the not too distant future that wireless technology that is available currently in conventional hearing aids will become available with AOIS devices. This will allow users of these devices the opportunity to wirelessly communicate

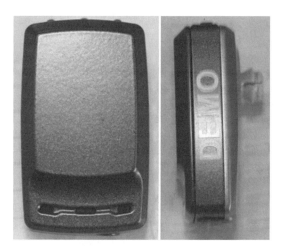

Figure 19–3. Cochlear Americas BP3 (BP110) AIOS device. The left side illustrates the front and the right side illustrates the snap connector.

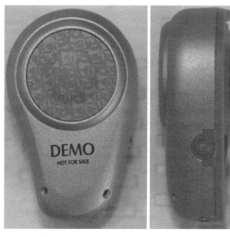

Figure 19–4. Oticon Medical Ponto Pro AIOS device. The left side illustrates the front and the right side illustrated the snap connector.

with telephones, televisions, mp3 players, and computers.

Audiologic Criteria for the AOIS for UHL

Patients for whom no better alternative treatment exists may be considered candidates for the AOIS if he or she:

1. Has a better ear BC pure-tone average (BC$_{PTA}$) at 500, 1000, 2000, and 3000 of ≤20 dB HL (the closer to 0 dB HL the better).
2. Is free from a generalized disease process that could result in poor wound healing.
3. Is unable to use conventional AC or BC hearing aids.
4. Is strongly motivated toward this surgical procedure.
5. Is able to understand the objectives and expectations of this method of amplification.
6. Is psychoemotionally stable to maintain the hygiene of the percutaneous titanium abutment.
7. Is at least 5 years old.

TransEar

A fitting option that became available in 2008 for UHL patients is the TransEar from Ear Technology (Figure 19–5). With this device, acoustical signals are amplified and processed by the BTE and transferred to a small BC vibrator encased in an earmold-like transfer unit via an appropriately sized connecting wire. This device is placed in the ear canal of the poorer ear and transferred to the cochlea of the better ear via BC. The technology of the TransEar is ever changing, and each device is currently shipped with two earpieces where one device has a BC vibrator whose primary peak is at 630 Hz (TE270), and a second earpiece where the BC vibrator has a resonant peak at 2200 Hz (TE380). An internal study using five subjects reported a mean improvement of 11 dB in Speech Recognition Thresholds (SRT), 43% improvement in Word Recognition Scores (WRS), and significant improvement in aided sound-field thresholds

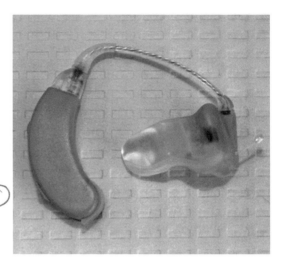

Figure 19–5. Illustration of the TransEar.

at 1000 to 3000 Hz using the TE380 vibrator when compared with the performance of the TE270 vibrator. The TransEar has:

a. Four-channel digital signal processing for each program.
b. Twelve (12) graphic equalizers for each program.
c. Programmability via a stand-alone Noah module.
d. Has two programs (quiet listening in the first program and noisy listening in the second program that is similar to the first program with NR added). Two additional memories can be added.
e. High power output stage.
f. Program indicators and battery warning.

SoundBite

Sonitus Medical (http://www.sonitusmedi cal.com) recently introduced a new approach to UHL (Moore & Popelka, 2013; Popelka, Derebery, Blevins, Murray, & Moore, 2009). The system, SoundBite Hearing System, consists of the two components illustrated in Figure 19–6. The first component is a BTE microphone unit (upper BTE in Figure 19–6). The BTE microphone component is similar in size to an open-fit BTE hearing aid and

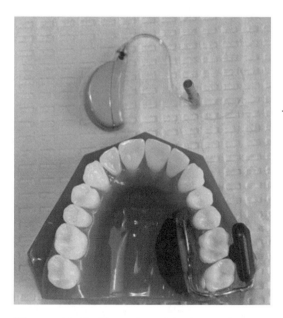

Figure 19–6. Illustration of the Sound Bite with the BTE component in the upper segment and the ITM component attached to the molars in the lower segment.

placed over the poorer ear. In addition, a microphone can be placed in the ear canal of the poorer hearing ear and is held in place with an open earmold. The BTE also has a second microphone in the BTE case to help improve the SNR. The BTE component includes a rechargeable battery that provides ~12 to 15 hours of use between recharging and provides wireless communication to the ITM and other wireless devices. The second component is a removable in-the-mouth (ITM) hearing device (lower, Figure 19–6) not requiring surgery, but delivering a BC signal directly to the skull with substantial high frequency output by using the teeth (lower, Figure 19–6). The ITM component contains a BC transducer applying a signal to the teeth. Applying a BC transducer against the surface of the tooth provides a bone-conducted signal that is transmitted to the cochlea of the better ear. The ITM component, held in place against the molars, contains an embedded BC transducer, rechargeable battery, digital electronics, and wireless capability for communicating with the BTE microphone

component on the poorer ear. All these components are sealed within an acrylic that is safe and appropriate for long-term use and easily inserted and removed by the patient.

External exposure to the electronic components in the ITM component could be a safety consideration. To addresses this concern, systems have been engineered into the internal components to detect any breach of the ITM component case and send an alarm to alert the patient to remove the device.

All BC systems promoted for patients with UHL use a transducer similar to the transducer used on audiometers. These transducers have limited bandwidth and are bulky and too large to embed into an ITM component. To address this issue, a flat piezoelectric transducer was developed to solve the physical size and bandwidth limitations of other devices. The transducer used in the SoundBite is flat and better suited to the limited space available in the mouth. Because this transducer has a higher frequency output than past BC transducers, the transducer used in the SoundBite provides a wider bandwidth than available in other BC devices used for patients with UHL.

Cochlear Implant

A more recent advance in fitting options for patients with UHL is a number of recent investigations on the utility of a cochlear implant (CI) implanted to the poorer ear to provide added binaural advantages that may not be able to be achieved with the other fitting options presented in this chapter. Initially, the CI implanted on the poorer ear in patients with UHL was investigated as an option for patients reporting severe tinnitus (Punte et al., 2011). As a result of those initial investigations, it was discovered that these patients also reported improved localization and to a lesser degree, improved ability to recognize speech in noise. Although still in the investigational stage and not approved by the FDA for use with UHL, several investigations (Firszt, Holden, Reeder, Waltzman, & Arndt, 2012; Kamal, Robinson, & Diaz, 2012; Punte et al., 2011; Stelzig, Jacob, & Mueller, 2011) reported, using small sample sizes, improved localization in UHL patients fit with a CI on the poor ear. In time, if these investigations continue to report improved performance in localization and/or speech recognition in noise when compared with some or all of the other fitting options described in the chapter, it may be feasible that the FDA may approve the CI as another fitting option for patients with UHL.

CONCLUSION

The primary goal of this chapter has been to reinforce the idea that several fitting options are available for UHL. Hopefully, the information conveyed within this chapter instills the concept that UHL patients experience significant communication problems. Suggestions of "turning your head to the desired signal" or pursuing CROS or BICROS amplification to the better ear should not be the exclusive rehabilitative options for these patients.

The authors have gained considerable experience with the fitting strategies outlined in this chapter and urge the readers to also consider transcranial CROS, TransEar, AOIS, SoundBite, or perhaps soon, a Cochlear Implant, for UHL patients. The authors believe, and have demonstrated on numerous patients, that one or more of these "nontraditional" fittings may be more beneficial in many cases than "traditional" fittings.

Finally, fitting adult patients with UHL has recently caught the attention of the American Academy of Audiology (AAA). AAA recently created a Task Force whose charge is to create an evidence-based best practice guideline for adult patients with severe-to-profound unilateral sensorineural hearing loss. It is hoped that the guideline will be published in 2015. This guideline will cover:

a. Auditory assessment
b. Self-perception of communication needs, performance, and goals for rehabilitation
c. Nonauditory needs assessment
d. Hearing device selection
e. Quality control upon receipt of the device(s)
f. Fitting and verification
g. Hearing assistive technology
h. Device orientation
i. Counseling and follow-up audiologic rehabilitation
j. Validation or assessment of outcomes

REFERENCES

Andersen, H. T., Schroder, S. A., & Bonding, P. (2006). Unilateral deafness after acoustic neuroma surgery: Subjective hearing handicap and the effect of the bone-anchored hearing aid. *Otology Neurotology, 27*(6), 809–814.

Bosman, A. J., Hol, M. K., Snik, A. F., Mylanus, E. A., & Cremers, C. W. (2003). Bone-anchored hearing aids in unilateral inner ear deafness. *Acta Otolaryngology, 123*(1), 258–260.

Bosman, A. J., Snik, A. F., Hol, M. K. S., & Mylanus, E. A. (2013). Evaluation of a bone-anchored hearing system: A comparison study. *Journal of the American Academy of Audiology, 24*, 505–513.

Brookhouser, P., Worthington, D., & Kelly, W. (1991). UHL in children. *Laryngoscope, 101*, 1264–1272.

Fagelson, M., Noe, C., Mumane, O., & Blevins, J. (2003). Predicted gain and functional gain with transcranial routing of signal completely-in-the-canal hearing aids. *American Journal of Audiology, 12*, 84–90.

Firszt, J. B., Holden, L. K., Reeder, R. M., Waltzman, S. B., & Arndt, S. (2012). Auditory abilities after cochlear implantation in adults with unilateral deafness: A pilot study. *Otology and Neurotology, 33*, 1339–1346.

Gulick, W., Gescheider, G., & Frisina, R. D. (1989). *Hearing*. New York, NY: Oxford University Press.

Harford, E. (1969). Is a hearing aid ever justified in UHL? *Otolaryngology Clinics of North America*, 153–173.

Harford, E., & Barry, J. (1965). A rehabilitative approach to the problem of unilateral hearing impairment: Contralateral routing of signals (CROS). *Journal of Speech and Hearing Disorders, 30*, 121–138.

Harford, E., & Dodds, E. (1966). The clinical application of CROS. *Archives of Otolaryngology, 83*, 73–82.

Hayes, D., Pumford, J., & Dorscher, M. (2005). Advantages of DSP instruments for wireless CROS fittings. *Hearing Journal, 3*, 44–46.

Hill, S. (2006). Assessment of patient satisfaction with various configurations of digital CROS and

BICROS hearing aids. *Ear Nose and Throat Journal, 7*, 427–430.

Hodgson, W. R. (1986). Special cases of hearing aid assessment. In W. R. Hodgson (Ed.), *Hearing aid assessment and use in audiologic habilitation* (3rd ed., pp. 191–216). Baltimore, MD: Williams and Wilkins.

Hol, M., Bosman, A., Snik, A., Mylanus, E., & Cremers, C. (2004). Bone-anchored hearing aid in unilateral inner ear deafness: A study of 20 patients. *Audiology Neurotology and Otology, 9*, 274–281.

Kamal, S. M., Robinson, A. D., & Diaz, R. C. (2012). Cochlear implantation in single-sided deafness for enhancement of sound localization and speech perception. *Current Opinion in Otolaryngology Head-Neck Surgery, 20*, 393–397.

Lin, L. M., Bowditch, S., Anderson, M. J., May, B., Cox, K. M., & Niparko, J. K. (2006). Amplification in the rehabilitation of unilateral deafness: Speech in noise and directional hearing effects with bone-anchored hearing and contralateral routing of signal amplification. *Otolology Neurotology, 27*(2), 172–182.

Linnebjerg, L. B., & Wetke, R. (2013). The benefits of CROS aids for individuals with unilateral sensorineural hearing loss. *Hearing, Balance and Communication.* Early online 1–5.

Linstrom, C. J., Silverman, C. A., & Yu, G. P. (2009). Efficacy of the bone-anchored hearing aid for single-sided deafness. *Laryngoscope, 119*(4), 713–720.

Moore, B. C. J., & Popelka, G. R. (2013). Preliminary comparison of bone-anchored hearing instruments and a dental device as treatments for unilateral hearing loss. *International Journal of Audiology,* Early online 1–9.

Newman, C. W., Sandridge, S. A., & Wodzisz, L. M. (2008). Longitudinal benefit from and Satisfaction with the AOIS system for patients with acquired unilateral sensorineural hearing loss. *Otolology Neurotology, 29*, 1123–1131.

Niparko, J., Cox, K., & Lustig, L. (2003). Comparison of the bone anchored hearing aid implantable hearing device with contralateral routing of offside signal amplification in the rehabilitation of unilateral deafness. *Otolology Neurotology, 24*, 73–78.

Oeding, K., & Valente, M. (in press). Sentence recognition in noise and perceived benefit of noise reduction in the receiver and transmitter side of a BICROS hearing aid. *Journal of the American Academy of Audiology.*

Oeding, K., Valente, M., & Kerckhoff, J. (2010). Effectiveness of the directional microphone in the AOIS Divino. *Journal of the American Academy of Audiology, 21*, 546–557.

Popelka, G. R., Derebery, J., Blevins, N. H., Murray, M., & Moore, B. C. J. (2009). Preliminary evaluation of a novel bone-conduction device for single-sided deafness. *Otology and Neurotology, 31*, 492–497.

Punte, A. K., Vermeire, K., Hofkens, A., De Bolt, M., De Ridder, D., & de Heyning, P. V. (2011). Cochlear implantation as a durable tinnitus treatment in single sided deafness. *Cochlear Implants International, 12*, S26–S29.

Stachler, R. J., Chandrasekhar, S. S., Archer, S. M., Rosenfeld, R. M., Schwartz, S. R., Barrs, D. M., . . . Robertson, P. G. (2012). Clinical practice guideline: Sudden hearing loss. *Archives of Otolaryngology-Head and Neck Surgery, 141*, S1–S45.

Stelzig, Y., Jacob, R., & Mueller, J. (2011). Preliminary speech recognition results after cochlear implantation in patients with unilateral hearing loss: A case series. *Journal of Medical Care Reports, 5*, 1–6.

Stenfelt, S. (2005). Bilateral fitting of AOISs and AOIS fitted in unilateral deaf persons: Acoustical aspects. *International Journal of Audiology, 44*, 178–189.

Sullivan, R. (1988). Transcranial ITE CROS. *Hearing Instruments, 39*, 11–12, 54.

Tillman, T., Kasten, R., & Horner, I. (1963). Effect of head shadow on reception of speech. *American Speech Language and Hearing Association*, 778–779.

Valente, M. (1982). Binaural amplification. *Audiology Journal of Continuing Education, 7*, 79–93.

Valente, M., Fabry, D., & Potts, L. (1995a). Recognition of speech in noise using a hearing aid with dual microphones. *Journal of the American Academy of Audiology*, 440–449.

Valente, M., Potts, L., Valente, M., & Goebel, J. (1995b). Wireless CROS versus transcranial CROS for UHL. *Journal of the American Academy of Audiology*, 52–59.

Vaneecloo, F. M., Ruzza, I., & Hanson, J. N. (2001). The monaural pseudo-stereophonic Hearing aid (AOIS) in unilateral total deafness: A study of 29 patients. *Laryngology, Otology and Rhinology, 122*(5), 343–350.

Wazen, J., Spitzer, J., Ghossaini, S., Fayad, J., Niparko, J., Cox, K., . . . Soli S. (2003). Transcranial contralateral cochlear stimulation in unilateral deafness. *Otolaryngology Head-Neck Surgery, 129*(3), 248–254.

Williams, V. A., McArdle, R. A., & Chisolm, T. H. (2012). Subjective and objective outcomes from new BiCROS technology in a veteran sample. *Journal of the American Academy of Audiology, 23*, 789–806.

Yuen, H. W., Bodmer, D., Smilsky, K., Nedzelski, J. M., & Chen, J. M. (2009). Management of single-sided deafness with the bone-anchored hearing aid. *Otolaryngology Head-Neck Surgery, 41*(1), 16–23.

CHAPTER 20

Future Considerations

MICHAEL J. METZ
ROBERT E. SANDLIN

OUTLINE

INTRODUCTION

Perhaps it would have been better to title this chapter "Discussions with Sandy" as many of the ideas and items discussed were the result of our conversations over a number of years. Even so, putting predictions of the future into writing sounds like a risky thing to undertake. If one were correct, there would be a really high "up side." However, it is much more likely that one will fail to predict the future, and thus the "down side" is a lot more likely. After all, if one could predict the future, it might be best to keep it to one-self or at least make some opportune investments. And, no one likes to make predictions that don't come true, even if they were fun to discuss.

Although the thought of a personal down side hangs over this chapter, it is nonetheless too tempting to resist, even if it were not interesting, to use such a forum to speculate, wish, criticize, and look toward a brighter, dimmer, or at least different, tomorrow. For the most part, these speculations about the future are the products of both of us and were conceived and discussed without the use of mind-altering substances. When Bob decided to do a third edition of this text in 2009, he asked me to help. He was 82 years old at the time. We had had many conversations about the field as we traveled across California for many years while organizing and offering continuing education courses. We had different views on many topics, and it will come as no surprise to anyone who knew Bob, his views were dignified, somewhat conservative, and not always the same as mine to say the least.

During the planning of this text revision, we decided to include many of these topics, and the essence of those discussions, warnings, and predictions follow. As such, there are few, if any, references that will substantiate these views. Some opinions or ideas come from others who would talk with us, from friends who share opinions both in favor of these predictions, and even from those who

would opine against these statements. In the parlance of the day, this chapter would rate a 5/6D (Joint Committee on Clinical Practice Algorithms and Statements, 2000) and it should be read with that low rating in mind. We would ask that readers consider these topics in this less than optimal form with an open mind. With those caveats, here are the products of our discussions, which may include a couple of things that may come to pass, or at least generate a little discussion among those so inclined.

HEARING INSTRUMENT TECHNOLOGY

During the past 30 years or more, the major (and perhaps the only widespread) advancement in the use of hearing aids for hearing loss has been in the area of increased, heightened, or modified technologies. Starting with the concept of compression in the 1970s, and moving through any number of fitting formulae that attempted to define the amount of amplitude gain per frequency, multiple controls (usually manipulated in the beginning with a small screwdriver, furnished by the manufacturer), and independent channels allowing for the patient to select from different amplification paradigms in attempt to suit patient's listening needs of various situations. The person overseeing the fitting of the instrument did most all of these manipulations at the request of the user.

And then, along came the digital circuits —instruments incorporating a digital processing chip that promised alterations of the hearing aid response that were never dreamed by patients or hearing care clinicians. These instruments allowed for changing not only the compression aspects of the amplifier, for example, but also allowed for reversing the compression (expansion), making more channels than were represented on the audiogram of any patient, biasing toward the front, side, or rear of multiple-microphone, directional instruments, and even "learning" if a volume setting or specific frequency emphasis was judged "satisfactory" by the patient and adjusting automatically thereafter.

During these years, pundits, clinicians, statisticians, and even an occasional consumer group, consistently sampled patient satisfaction with these wonderful low-voltage, low-drain digital circuits, and were hard pressed to find satisfaction levels that rose commensurate with the huge changes in signal processing. Nevertheless, the industry has forged ahead with many improvements that likely were overlooked by many, but have perhaps set a stage for the "killer-app" technology that will enable more people to use these devices more successfully. Essentially, the technology made huge strides in the past 20 years, while the application of this technology in the clinic has not kept up very well.

No doubt, by the time many read this text, the technology will have produced more innovations, and perhaps some of these will prove to be more beneficial than those in the past. After all, progress is typically measured in small steps and only seldom in giant leaps. So, what would be the changes most likely to occur, both from a technology standpoint as well as from a clinical or diagnostic perspective? For the most part, if history is any predictor, the technology will produce devices that continue to astound and perhaps confuse the clinician. These changes appear annually in the new products from many manufacturers. They may even prove useful to some hearing-impaired patients.

1. Hearing aid communicating with other devices such as phones, TV, and other things to make communication easier and more comfortable. Not only does this sort of application help significantly in adverse signal-to-noise situations, there may also be benefit to be had in situations such as those that occur in times when the "outside world" is not so demanding. Such situations as are encountered in listening to music come to mind.
2. Hearing instruments most likely will "learn" and make adjustments to vari-

ous parameters that enhance the communication experience. The industry has not attempted to utilize this "getting smart" aspect nearly as much as one might expect. Instruments that "learn" to amplify in a manner most consistent with the patient's appreciation of "good" might be helpful in cases of patients who cannot adequately describe just what is "good" and "bad." For example, what if a patient was instructed to "touch the hearing aid" each time they like or don't like the sound. Could an algorithm be developed that would gradually set the circuit to more readily accommodate to a sound or a set of sounds with these simple types of patient input? A little imagination is all that is needed to construct a couple of interesting scenarios. Imagination and a lot of engineering.

3. More instruments will "communicate" with each other while paired on the same patient, so that listening in extreme situations is better. A simple way to think about this application is to consider the manner in which the brain or neural structures "apply squelch" to noises that interfere with desired sounds. If the central nervous systems can "squelch" noise, can similar algorithms be employed to do similar things in the hearing aid? A beginning took place with algorithms that define "bad" sound—noise—as opposed to "good" sound and then amplify each with a different set of rules.

4. RIC/RITE aids that are easy to fit to limited types of hearing loss and perhaps other styles will also make hearing aids easier and more comfortable to wear, and also more available to patients. If one could employ a suitable "learning" circuit, then a simply-fit hearing aid, available outside the medical model, may be possible also. Although this application poses serious sales threats to the fields of audiology and dispensing, the larger good for a greater number of hearing impaired patients may trump the financial damage to the profession. And, although

this change likely will not come from the field of audiology itself, this "improvement" is certainly within possibility from the technical, engineering standpoint.

5. Cochlear and other ear implants combined with hearing aids pose an interesting prospect for the future. We may tend to think of these devices as being useful only in certain cases of extreme impairment or when other forms of amplification are counterindicated. But, when one recalls that the first use of cochlear implants was with patients who were severely hearing impaired and now are common and successful in much less impaired patients, one can hypothesize a future with surgical implantation of various types of devices that might provide a more permanent solution to many types of less dramatic hearing losses.

6. Prevention and therapeutic reversal of hearing loss has received considerable attention of late. This one might seem to be a bit of a stretch at present, but is certainly in the realm of the possible. This last decade has seen the mapping of the human genome as well as the beginnings of genetic manipulation and stem cell regenerations. To think that this direction of research will not proceed for the benefit of hearing impaired patients is naïve. There are already the beginnings of treatments after the fact for noise exposures and for countering the effects of ototoxic medications.

These "drawing board" items have a couple of things in common. Most obviously, they are all technologically oriented. If the past has any predictive value in any field, then it might be prudent to use the past to predict that the future changes in technology will solve many or most of the problems faced in our field by the hearing-impaired patient today. That commonality is likely obvious to most readers. What may not be as obvious is the lack of the clinician participation in this prediction of future treatment of hearing loss. Or, that may be the most serious object of focus to the exclusion of potential benefits.

This observation was not made without hesitation, as there are certainly clinicians who may take great umbrage with the idea that technology alone will solve hearing loss in many or most of its form. However if the past 20 to 30 years are even remotely predictive of the future treatment of hearing loss, one is at a significant disadvantage in quoting rehabilitative literature to support the participation of hearing therapy in the treatment of hearing loss in the future. Audiologists have been reluctant at worst and slow at best to accept the need for services beyond the simplest application of technology (hearing aids) to the complaints of the hearing impaired. And, this reluctance is not just recent, but has been the norm for the past 30 years or more.

The field would seem to have consistently ignored the need for anything other than the most basic diagnostic evaluation to support the application of amplification. The "92557" combination billing—air and bone threshold testing, coupled with threshold speech tests and speech or word understanding in quiet—has been the standard, and most of the time, the only test of hearing function. It seems like many clinicians take little note of patient histories in making decisions about hearing aids except in the hope that one or more technologies will provide some additional benefit for the complaint. Very few clinicians test with prediction of success in mind. Even fewer seem to test with intentions of doing little more than ruling out a sale. While this might seem a little harsh, can the disagreeing reader cite peer-reviewed literature that demonstrates a different position for any but a minority of the practicing clinicians involved in the fitting of hearing aids?

While one might argue that there are no tests that are capable of predicting a successful hearing aid fitting, there are certainly a number of questionnaires that help a clinician determine the personal needs of a hearing impaired user. There are also tests that help define the integrity of the cochlear structures—not to the point of definitive diagnosis but certainly to the point of making a determination of the extent of the damage to the system beyond that portrayed by a pure-tone audiogram. As for speech in quiet, there were few patients who appeared before us in our clinical careers who complained that they could not hear when only two people were in the room. Wouldn't it be expected that we know more about how hearing functions as we attempt to supplement the loss of hearing?

WHAT DO WE REALLY KNOW ABOUT HEARING LOSS?

This brings up the question that seems to hold the most cogent predictor of what audiology will most likely bring to the future treatment of hearing loss. What does a clinician need to know about any individual's hearing loss, and what will future therapies or treatments do to fix what the clinician finds? This may be the pivotal question of the future, for, if it was known just what specifically went wrong with a person's hearing, there would seem to be a much better chance of fixing, supplementing, engineering, or otherwise helping to alleviate the problem(s). For example, audiology seems to be at a place where the field now understands that if the outer hair cells do not function correctly, then the amplifying effect of these structures is lost. This "loss" shows up on the pure-tone audiogram in the same manner that it has appeared since the 1950s or so. Most clinicians fit hearing aids to try and account only for this loss of sensitivity. Speculatively, if it were determined that malfunctions of the inner hair cells were in part responsible for a decrease in understanding speech in noise, perhaps a hearing aid algorithm could be constructed that would compensate in such a manner as to minimize the impact of this dysfunction. Such would seem to be the case for a common complaint of hearing-impaired patients—inability to hear as well as a normal-hearing person in the presence of background noise.

For the past 40 years, the major, and for the most part, the only two aspects of almost any given hearing loss that is universally used in fitting hearing aids are pure-tone threshold changes and the loss of speech discrimination in quiet. Although some clinicians who use hearing aids in their practice will measure other psychoacoustic aspects of the hearing loss such as most comfortable and uncomfortable levels, use of any other aspect of the diagnostic information is not only uncommon but most often not even investigated.

The American Academy of Audiology has published a "best practices" protocol for fitting hearing aids to adults. It can be found on the academy's website, and all clinicians are encouraged to adhere to the suggestions contained in the protocols. If all clinicians were to do the recommended diagnostic, verification, and outcome measures, it is likely that the degree of user satisfaction would rise at least a little bit. If that improvement is not the case, what does that say about the efficacy of the profession and its approach to treatment? Moreover, if more diagnostic information from the impaired ears were sought, clinicians may be in a better position to investigate auditory measures that would make the application of hearing aids more successful.

One needs to note at this point that in looking for an increase in patient satisfaction via the use of all these measures, there may be revealed a lack of benefit to all the measures. If that were the case, it may be best to not investigate it fully. If the use of advanced clinical measures does nothing more than that, which is accomplished by "self-fitting" (over-the-counter hearing aids) or by the old "how does it sound now?" tests, the field needs to beat a hasty retreat to the drawing table.

Almost all hearing aids fit in the decades from 1960 to 2010 were fit relative to a pure-tone audiogram. While it is known that pure tones do not delineate or define a hearing loss to a very accurate extent, it seems as if the field is reluctant to use other measures to define the fitting needs of the hearing loss. For example, while hearing quiet speech is one of the most common complaints of hearing impaired patients (references), hearing music for many of these patients is a common additional complaint. When speech is clear, music sounds "funny." Very few clinicians routinely use methods to determine the best amplifying protocol that enables a hearing-impaired patient to hear music in a fashion that pleases the user. Furthermore, it appears as if most clinicians simply assume that the outer hair cells in any hearing-impaired patient all "go wrong" in the same manner with all hearing losses. Very little thought is apparently given to such measures as preferred listening levels, maximum tolerable sound levels, ability to hear in noise, ability to appreciate music, inner versus outer hair cell function, and so on.

The growth of hearing aid sales in audiology practices seems to have led to a majority of emphasis on the sale of the instrument rather than the definition of the problem presented by the patient. Otoacoustic emissions appeared in the early 1980s, and hearing-in-noise tests in the 1990s. Yet, through the first decade of the 2000s, neither of these tests seem to be used routinely in the fitting of hearing aids, even though there is ample evidence of their diagnostic or descriptive utility. But, as most clinicians will hasten to add, there is no data to show when or if knowledge of these functions can help anyone's hearing loss. Perhaps because there is little data that would support conclusions regarding the usefulness or worthlessness of such tests in a predictive sense, the field appears to have stopped looking. Some would likely argue that no data exist because there is no relationship between these psychophysical systems and their predictive functions, and to that argument, one could answer that it is not convincing to ignore the universal biological rule of "Form Follows Function" and to conclude that is absent in the auditory system. That is, the intact auditory system acts in a manner that allows this organ to do its job remarkably well when it is whole. Is it reasonable to believe that the loss of these functions does not in some manner affect audition? (Additionally, it is pretty universally accepted that it is difficult to prove a negative, so demonstrating that these functions and tests have no value would seem to imply that the profession has not investigated sufficiently.)

In a way, these data are not nearly as important as would be the generation of any data that would predict and, therefore, demonstrate the usefulness of any of the technologies used in the application of modern hearing aids to any type of hearing loss. The lack of substantiating data, and therefore the lack of verification and validation measures of the typical fitting technologies, is at the heart of the success (or lack thereof) that these devices provide to the hearing impaired public. As of the date of this text (2013), there is little evidence that much of the technology in hearing aids is of much benefit to many with hearing loss. It is almost as if, when hearing aid design engineers are asked why they designed processing algorithms to function as they do, they answered "because we can," not "because the hearing-impaired ear will hear more normally, or clearer, or better." That is to say, if there were an underlying reason for the ear functioning as it does in cases of hearing loss, the least the clinician should do involves resolving those issues with technology designed for this decrease in function. Instead, the industry seems to function by designing an approach, and then seeing if the approach has benefit after the new technology reaches the market.

This sort of backward approach is largely the fault of audiology. If the field knew more about how the ears and hearing work, it might have developed a better method of treating hearing deficits. There seems to be so much attention given to the technology and sale of these devices, determining what was necessary to provide the most help in the best fashion has been neglected.

Specifically, if the problem of hearing loss is to be "solved" by the application of an external contrivance, it would surely behoove clinicians to produce the kinds of measures that quantify the deficit as precisely as possible in order to justify the treatment, first of all, to the patient, but equally important, to the payer. It would seem intuitive, as above, that to fix any given problem, one should first define it as succinctly as possible. As definitive descriptions of the peculiarities of any given hearing loss are known, the treatments for these deficits may become a great deal more obvious. And, if the problem can be described adequately, the engineers devising algorithms can likely build one to solve it.

DISTRIBUTION

During the past 50 or 60 years, hearing instruments have been sold to patients and customers primarily through a system of independent offices. The sales model has been typical of many systems that sell to retail customers. And, like many historical sales models, it is likely that this hearing aid model will change significantly in the future.

As protective patents on any pharmaceutical expires, and if the medication has shown to be of benefit to the consumer with little or no contraindications, the manufacturing and distribution of the drug is undertaken by companies not holding any patent rights and who essentially compound and supply the medication at lesser cost under its generic name. A good drug has at least two lives—one during its patented lifespan and one that follows the expiration of the patent. Similarly, as many consumer devices achieve large-scale acceptance by users, and/or the patents on these devices expire, competition in manufacturing and/or distribution change, and increased supply generally cause device prices to decrease. Digital watches, calculators, mobile phones, computers, and (potentially) hearing aids come to mind as examples of the financial consumer benefits due to advancing technology and expanding markets.

Why would we not expect the same course of events with the hearing aid industry? Are the concepts, technologies, and especially the clinical participants as necessary as they have been in the past, or as necessary as we would like to think? Are there alternatives to the current distribution models that would provide more benefits to more people that the current models? And, if the same or better benefits accrue to the end user, what is

left to impede the adaptation of those alternatives? That is, who stands to benefit the most from changes in the hearing aid industry? Questions such as these deserve attention and speculation if the field of audiology wishes to maintain its position in the hearing health industry. And, these questions need to be addressed in a manner that best benefits those we serve. A difficult task and the limited professional history of inability to accept these alternatives is not very good. Consider the personal sound amplifying devices such as PSAPs, the Songbird device, and those devices over which the field has little control or influence. Up until now, those clinicians dealing with the fitting and sale of hearing instruments have not readily or widely accepted these devices. More importantly, most of these "aids" have been dismissed out of hand with vitriol more appropriate for home remedies and potions. It would seem that people seeking help for hearing loss better not seek it beyond the manner in which it was offered 50 years ago, technology notwithstanding.

The first consideration pertaining to distribution ought to focus itself on the benefits to the hearing-impaired patient. During the past 30 years or so, the wholesale cost of hearing instruments has risen by a factor of approximately 10. During this period, the costs to the patient have also risen by a factor of about 10. Hearing instruments that cost $100 wholesale in the 1970s now wholesale at a cost well over $1000. Retail costs of $300 to $400 per instrument in the 1970s now also stand at 10 times these costs. Granted, these costs exist primarily in the offices of clinicians—audiologists and physicians—and traditional dispensers. Nontraditional sales outlets (read "big-box" stores, manufacturer-owned offices, some publically funded institutions, etc.) routinely offer hearing instruments at lesser costs. And, these nontraditional offices many times pay a handsome cost for their reduced pricing policies in terms of professional criticism. There is no reasonable data that would suggest that these nontraditional outlets are any less successful in helping the hearing-impaired public than are the traditional, clinician-based offices. With very little differentiating data, one wonders how the traditionalists will argue their "case" to third-party payers, the general medical community, the government, or, of greatest importance, to their patients.

As mentioned earlier, it may not be in the best interest of professional organizations to investigate the success rate of the various distribution or sales methods. What would be the consequences if it were learned that the rate of success and/or acceptance did not differ significantly no matter where or how a hearing-impaired consumer sought help? It would seem that, professionally, there would be little to gain in such an investigation and a great deal to lose.

With no proof of outstanding benefit for type of intervention, and with the presence of increasing levels of technology, it is not apparent that there exists any distribution model that supports the concept of retail costs of hearing instruments continuing to rise forever. The absence of demonstrative proof of the benefits of clinical approaches and therapies places the burden of benefit in the realm of technological improvements. And, when one recalls the other examples of consumer electronics, devices, services, and so on, it is difficult to construct a scenario in which costs of hearing aids continue to rise beyond a critical point. It is much easier to read from history and predict that retail —consumer—costs will decrease. And this decrease may be caused by any number of factors coming into play.

As the potential benefits from hearing instruments increase—and all the data accumulated by most manufacturers and independent investigators suggests this trend—more hearing-impaired people will seek amplification to help their hearing loss. Technology will increasingly drive the market in spite of price, but only to a similar degree as we have witnessed in the past 20 or so years. As the number of buyers (users) increases, it is reasonable to predict that the prices of these devices will come under pressure to decrease. Such are the economics of a free market. But

there are other factors that may also influence distribution and price.

If it can be shown that the use of hearing aids constitutes no hazard to most consumers, and, if the perceived benefits of hearing aid use continue to rise, how long before a distribution model will arise that allows these devices to be sold "over-the-counter"—that is, without the input of any licensed professional or even from a sales person in a "big box" store? After all, if the "down sides" to the use of hearing aids can, for the most part, be eliminated by technology, and the "upside" benefits due to this technology are real, wouldn't the expectation be that the regulating agencies governing the sale of hearing aids would evolve to allow more people the unrestricted or unregulated use of these devices? They become even less of a medical device than they are currently. If hearing aids are of real help, if PSAPs also provide significant benefit, and if either don't hurt anyone, why do any of them need regulation? If hearing aids provide benefit and only very rarely cause a health problem, wouldn't lowering the price help more people? As an example, consider the sale of eyeglasses in many situations that do not require a prescription, medical visit, or any other clinical intervention prior to their sale over many counters. Or, one might consider why aspirin is not a "regulated" drug.

INSURANCE PARTICIPATION

On the other hand, most clinicians argue that "There are many times when patients require medical intervention prior to the use of hearing aids." Following the application of hearing instruments, there still exist the need to set or program the instruments correctly, granted, not to the degree that is required by cochlear implants, but still, a significant rehabilitative effort is helpful to many patients. Furthermore, there needs to be instruction, follow-up, and counseling that will assure that the patient gets the maximum benefit from the devices. And, some verification and validation would also prove helpful. While it should be apparent that much of this postfitting discussion would not constitute "therapy," most traditional dispensers and clinicians would all likely agree with the position that, in many situations, hearing aids should be classified as a part of medical rehabilitation or treatment. And if the verification tests were not considered a "therapy," but rather a required documentation that demonstrated the outcome of a solution to a health problem wouldn't that constitute a better argument for these procedures being included in health care coverage?

If you believe that clinical methods, including verification and validations, are a necessary part of the application of hearing aids to hearing loss, then you have made a reasonably good argument for placing the determination, application, and benefit verification of hearing aids in the medical-audiological arena. In other words, you would advocate that hearing aids be treated as durable medical goods or equipment. The placement of hearing aids in the "medical" or "audiological" arena requires this "durable medical goods" classification. (Perhaps this is not exactly as the audiologic community would wish, but this decision likely resides entirely in the provenance of the government, third-party payers, and/or the medical community in general.) This is the point at which the third-party payers get into the picture; to wit, the insurance companies.

At this time in the new century, the beginnings of this other "payer player" in the hearing aid industry are already visible. There are probably many reasons why insurers and other third-party payers are beginning to participate in the patient's purchase and use of hearing aids. The first reason involves the insurer being able to make money from dealing with another health problem, or, in their words, their "health product." The money involves the pricing of hearing aids. Having an insurer pay at least part of the cost of amplification would seem to be of great benefit to most patients. After all, most of

us want our health problems and costs to be "covered" by our insurer and, if hearing loss were truly a health problem, why would any patient refuse the participation of any third party insurer helping to pay for this help? So, at this point, most patients would likely be in favor of third-party participation in any manner and to any degree. Furthermore, if insurers participate in the hearing health care of those whom they insure, wouldn't the logical assumption be that these insurers would attempt to control as many aspects of the pricing of these devices as they can? That's how insurers function in the provision of all the products and services they approve. As insurance companies participate more in the hearing health of their insured, that participation in the supplying of hearing aids certainly will not result in them paying higher prices for these devices. The control of these devices in a "semidistributional" manner would certainly seem of potential benefit to these third-party payers and perhaps to their customers as well.

So, both above arguments—hearing aids as nonregulated "listening helpers" and hearing aids as part of hearing health care—would equally lead one to the conclusion that, as these devices get better and/or are more appreciated and used by consumers (or patients, depending on your point of view), the distribution pressures and management by third parties ought to drive consumer pricing downward. There are few if any obvious examples that would persuade otherwise.

WHO WILL FIT AND SELL HEARING AIDS?

Historically, there has been little to differentiate between audiologists, typically having obtained an advanced degree in order to be licensed, and hearing aid dispensers, for whom there is usually no advanced degree requirement. Audiologists, by virtue of training and license, can participate in the testing and rehabilitation of patients by applying to and being "accepted" as providers by insurers and other third-party payers. They may then bill for various services and procedures by using a series of "billing codes." It is typical that these billing codes contain provisions for the billing and reimbursement of durable medical devices and/or equipment. So, under a medical-based distribution system, audiologists in most states would be able to participate and be reimbursed by third parties for the testing, fitting, and even perhaps the rehabilitation surrounding hearing aid use while hearing aid dispensers would be denied this reimbursement from insurers. That is not to say that hearing aid dispensers would lose this potential billing avenue permanently, but it would certainly imply that they would have to take some sort of legal or political action to obtain this privilege. Such participation in the reimbursement system would seem to overwhelmingly favor the audiologist over the traditional retail dispenser.

On the other hand, if the advance of technology continues and the "downsides" of hearing aid use can be adequately disproven, one might expect that a usual retail "sales model" might prevail. In this model, sales and use of hearing aids are essentially devoid of professional input (like the sale and use of nonprescription eyeglasses and over-the-counter drugs) and subject to the typical sales avenues and methods of the marketplace. Neither audiologists, nor physicians, nor hearing aid dispensers are treated differently under this sales model. All are treated as retailers of a nonregulated appliance.

It is suspected that, faced with the choice between the two opposite distribution models above, most clinicians, audiologists, and dispensers today would opt for today's status quo rather than either alternative. One would like to argue in support of the higher educational degree being able to provide better results, but in a purely retail model, that outcome may not result. One thing would seem certain: Most consumer markets are highly fluctuant, and the hearing health care market does not show any reason why it would not be subject to the same influences as observed in other retail arenas. Therefore, the field of

hearing aid dispensing should anticipate a gradual change of the present model in the direction of one of the above alternatives. Or, perhaps there will be some other factors that effectively differentiate between a hearing instrument being a medical device versus one which is considered a "nonmedical" device. As a patient, which would you choose if your insurance would help you pay for the medical device? Or, would you rather have hearing aids be treated solely as a retail product? In the long run, it will be the consumer who decides.

WHOLESALE COST OF INSTRUMENTS FROM MANUFACTURERS

As mentioned previously, when audiologists entered into the field of hearing aid dispensing in the 1970s, wholesale costs of hearing aids seldom exceeded $100 per instrument. Typical retail costs were in the $300 to $400 range. Over the last 35 or 40 years, costs, both on the wholesale and the retail sides, have increased 10-fold. During that time span, the use of hearing instruments has risen slightly and in-step with the increase in population, sometimes nicely influenced by other factors such as a U.S. presidents being fit for hearing aid use, the arrival of ITC instruments, digital hearing aids, economic downturns, and the like. But, overall, the "penetration" of the hearing-impaired market has remained remarkably stable over these years. There are probably a lot of reasons for this lack of penetration. Lots of people have speculated about factors that do or do not influence the use of hearing aids, but it is difficult to minimize cost as one of the most, if not the most significant impediment.

One might argue that the wholesale cost of instruments really reflects quite nicely the percentage of the population that can afford to use hearing aids. That is, it is not far-fetched to base the wholesale cost of a hearing aid almost entirely on a decision of the manufacturer to maintain the same profit ratio per instrument that existed 40 years ago. The wholesale cost, apparently yielding ample profit to the manufacturer, as well as the retail cost to the consumer and perhaps beyond the reach of many hearing impaired patients, seem to assure that only a limited number of the hearing impaired population can afford hearing aids. The "lower" end of the financial spectrum may get hearing help from special government, veteran, or indigent programs. The "high" end of the money spectrum can generally afford to purchase repairs on their faulty hearing mechanisms. Those in the middle—by far the statistical majority of all hearing-impaired U.S. citizens—seem to be unconvinced of the benefits of private-purchased hearing aid help.

Indeed, inspection into costs will generally find many justifications for the cost of hearing aids as they are offered in today's dispensing offices. Many reasons are given for this pricing. Likely the most commonly blamed costs are in the areas of research and development of the digital algorithms used in these instruments. A second reason for high cost might be the costs of maintaining a sales force across the country in order to "detail" sales offices—another example of sales methods from the medical world.

One has a difficult time finding data from any manufacturer that adequately expresses true costs of research and development, manufacturing, distribution, and so on. But, we can certainly deduce that the manufacturing cost of hearing aids is substantially less than the single-unit wholesale cost, even though we cannot easily determine how much gross or net profit comes from each sale, as it is obvious that many units sell at a wholesale cost much less that the single-unit cost. Further, we can draw some logical conclusions about the real, wholesale cost of research and development involved as each hearing aid sold contains essentially the same digital chip that is used in a multitude of instruments, albeit with some of the "routines" or algorithms locked out of the "active" circuit. If, in fact, manufacturers use the same chip in various models of hearing aids and simply "lock out" some of the "premium" features of the algorithm, at least some of the cost arguments in the "R&D" column need to be revisited. That is, if the lowest level model of the hearing aid has the same chipset as the highest level model, it might be concluded that even the sale of the lowest level model is profitable for the manufacturer, and it would not cost much to "unlock" the chip for higher model use, thus increasing significantly the gross profit in the sale of a "higher" level instrument.

Furthermore, it should be obvious with even the most casual observation by a hearing aid retail provider that there exist in the marketplace many methods of purchasing hearing aids on the wholesale and retail sides at costs that are significantly reduced from the "normal" or the "published" wholesale or retail price, or those prices charged to other, likely smaller providers. This observation supports the previous observation. Volume, for one thing, would seem quite important in determining cost, not so much on the retail side of things, but certainly on the wholesale aspect. As in all buying situations, if you purchase more, you get a lower cost per unit. It is, therefore, reasonable to conclude that the manufacturer maintains a "reasonable" profit margin per unit, even on the most basic iteration of the hearing instrument.

Similar volume discounting has been available to almost any retail provider of hearing aids for many years. Some clinicians or dispensers may argue against such practices, but in reality, increased profits will be served in most situations despite many reasonable arguments to the contrary. Purchasing, either wholesale or retail, through various groups can decrease wholesale pricing, can decrease the need for detailing, can consolidate billing issues, and can be of value to the consumer. After all, there exist many different types of distributors in most industries. While the ethical or legal issues of volume purchasing may cause some clinicians (or the ethical committees of some professional organizations) to question some buying situations, group purchasing of one type or another will likely grow over the next few years.

This "maximization" or maintenance of profit is also certainly at the root of group formation at the manufacturing level, as the "volume discount" concepts work well in almost all aspects of the hearing aid business. If you can build more, sell more, do more by increasing volume, it sometimes becomes advantageous to purchase or otherwise obligate your manufacturing competition. Thus, we have seen some larger hearing aid manufacturers incorporate smaller manufacturers into their companies, either by outright purchase or by other contractual obligation. Just as with group purchasing, some may argue that this consolidation is good for business, while others rue the loss of smaller companies who are seemingly more capable or willing to provide individual or special products and customized and personal services. Larger scales of operation benefit larger companies to the exclusion of smaller companies at almost every level, all other things being equal. And, sometimes, these larger scales may result in lower consumer prices. More often than not, larger scales provide a more stable platform for pricing at the manufacturing level and the maintenance of profit at the wholesale level. This is not necessarily a bad thing if the acquiring company maintains the profit per unit that enables them to advance both technologically and financially. However, carried to the extreme, this consolidation may approach levels that impede or impact in a negative manner such as is encountered in decreases in competition, unjustifiably higher pricing, and other "negative" market or price manipulations. If consolidation results in a lower profit per unit to the manufacturer, and if this lower cost is passed along to the consumer, who would stand to lose? And, who would be the most likely "winner"?

An example of a potential negative resulting from "industry consolidation" is seen in the rise of retail offices owned by manufacturers. It is suspected or at least hypothesized that hearing aid manufacturing companies who have in the past and continue today to purchase retail offices do so primarily in order to protect their present and future distribution channels. At least, this would seem to be the most palatable argument. What other argument would be more accepted by those retail offices with whom the company-owned offices compete? In a distribution system that is so loosely built on patient benefit that is unproven for the most part, this protection of distribution may be in the best interests of the manufacturer, but may not be in the best interests of patients. That it is not in the best interests of independent clinicians in independent offices is hardly arguable. It is likely that this type of absorption of small dispensing offices will continue for some time, especially as many of the current, larger manufacturers seem to have an exceptionally large amount of money available for such purchases. How it may affect the future distribution of hearing instruments is probably not open to much debate.

FUTURE DISTRIBUTION

There are a number of obvious "pseudo facts" that anyone having access to any industry trade journal or Web-based blog can eventually determine for themselves.

1. The number of hearing aids sold in the United States in past years has not varied much but rather seems pinned to the overall growth in U.S. population.
2. While the exact information is not available, reasonable estimates of the number of retail outlets for hearing aids is certainly below 10,000 and more likely in the range of 7000 to 8000.
3. Data indicating number of units sold or distributed in 2013 will likely show that while the Veterans' Administration is the largest distributor, a "big box" chain will come in second place.
4. There are a growing number of insurance plans offering full or partial coverage for hearing aids.
5. Internet-based companies appear to be popping up at a rapid rate and, while there are no financial reports, would appear to be at least profitable if not prospering.

There is certainly no abundance of references to these pseudofacts, and readers can choose to ignore them, sort of believe them, look them up for themselves, or whatever. It would seem prudent that these indicators and others be discussed in professional groups at every level as they may be at least somewhat indicative of where the industry is going.

It would seem that the most likely scenario involves the continued growth of manufacturer consolidation, if for no other reason than they can do this without disturbing and perhaps enhancing their present sales figures. It is also easy to speculate that at the very minimum, some retail offices will become tied financially in some manner to one or more manufacturers. These types of arrangements—reduced pricing for increased volumes—with retail offices have occurred with regularity in the past and will likely continue despite the potential for ethical and legal issues.

As more retail offices become "attached" to manufacturers, there ought to be pressure on retail pricing. That is, following the consolidation of offices, there is generally a consolidation and increase in marketing and advertising in an effort to "harvest" the benefits of the consolidation. Office specials, "open houses," limited-time offers, and other retail, advertising programs have a tendency to boost pricing, but the rebound is that "normal" pricing tends to fall following such campaigns. Couple this tendency with consolidated wholesale purchasing, competition from internet-based sales, and the "big box" chains, and the overall pressure on hearing aid pricing should increase due to all that competition.

Additional factors affecting the tendency for pricing to consumers to decrease include the increase of well-informed patients or customers. No one will disagree that the internet is a grand place for the dissemination of information, and we think that more and more, potential users of hearing instruments will seek information on the world wide web. "Neutral" sites on the web often discuss the pricing of hearing aids, and many are not reluctant to give recommendations for patients seeking good products as well as lower pricing. Likely many of these people, after reading opinions, letters from users, and company ads, will appear in their local retail clinic or office prepared to discuss prices with the idea of lowering them. That discussion has certainly been a part of both our clinical experiences.

The influence of third-party reimbursement has already been discussed, and if the reader is not yet convinced that these "payers" do not wish to do much "paying," we can only warn that the influence of third parties will only increase in the future. This is good news for consumers, as third-party reimbursement is as good for hearing aids as it is for medical treatment, dental examinations, and eyeglasses. Patients seem to place more faith in the benefits of any treatment if a third party is willing to bear some of the cost. This rather universal consumer benefit has had little effect on the hearing aid industry in the past which, in our opinion, makes it all the more fertile for such participation in the future. We also believe that in the same manner as many in the medical services field—physicians—dislike the intrusion of insurers in their reimbursement, those of us in the hearing services field will come to the same position of dislike, if we aren't there already. It is unreasonable to expect that any professional group can easily isolate themselves from these reimbursement arguments, especially if that group is attempting to operate in the medical arena. It may be much easier to learn to work within that system. And, to top it all off, what would be the likely impact of the federal government getting more involved in the treatment of hearing loss. It is also unreasonable to think that Medicare involvement in the provision of hearing aids would do much to increase reimbursement levels.

Future distribution will likely involve lower wholesale and retail pricing as well as more consolidation occurs at all levels. Coupled with the participation of third-party reimbursement at varying levels of benefit, it would seem that the small private office may be in danger of losing some advantage.

At a recent lecture and discussion, one of us (MJM) was accused of being really pessimistic about the field in general and hearing aids in particular, and the help these instruments can provide hearing impaired patients. Lest the reader draw the same conclusion from the above discussion, let me be clear that it seems likely that the dispensing of hearing aids will change rather dramatically in the future. That does not necessarily imply that the future of audiology is similarly going to change in the same manner. While a discussion of audiology's future would be fascinating, it is beyond the scope of this chapter. That does not mean that the reader should ignore the potential futures of audiology, it just means that careful thought should be taken to ensure that audiology as a field will persist no matter what course the distribution of hearing instruments takes.

WILL TECHNOLOGY REPLACE THE CLINICIAN?

Nearly everyone is every field will almost always be in consensus on this question, and the short answer will always be "Yes." Technology is a very powerful force and drives the progress of all fields. It has transformed all of humanity and will continue to do so despite any well-intentioned protests about maintaining a status quo. How soon will technology replace the good clinician is always a question that is more difficult to answer. That technology will eventually triumph over hearing loss seems to be quite probable. The major hurdle at present appears to be that the field does not know just what should be fixed. Our clinical understanding of hearing loss seemed to have been limited to the very basics for so very long. Just an audiogram was all that was necessary to surgically or prosthetically "fix" a hearing loss—that plus a little "therapy" in some situations. It seems that recently we have come to a conclusion that there might be more to hearing loss than a simple loss of sensitivity. The more precise the tests that define the hearing loss, the more

likely it will be that a solution to overcome that problem will result. Of course, more information will likely also result in more complications and lead to a higher degree of complexity that we must come to understand. But, no one should argue that better measurements will lead to better treatment. The more we know, the better the fix. Then, before we know it, technology will find a way to do the testing too. It's happened before in audiology and other professional fields, and it is likely something like these changes will happen again.

But, it would also seem that even some of the hearing-impaired patients of the not-so-near future would need the help of therapists who understand the concepts and problems of dealing with hearing loss, despite the manner in which their prostheses were delivered. However, even the most optimistic of clinicians would have hesitations in predicting that a full patient schedule is in the future for a hearing therapist. Technological progress in science will develop methods for restoring "normal" to many impaired ears, with or without our help. Although this restoration is most likely far in the future, it is not as far away as it was when any of us entered this field.

Will audiology and dispensing be ready to supplement the technological changes that might take place? Unless these changes occur with unprecedented speed and from way on the outside, the answer is that the field will likely morph to fit the needs of the patients and consumers that are being served. Of course, knowledge will increase to fill the void in what the field does for patients. The rise of advanced audiology educational programs will gradually change into a "needs-driven" number of programs, graduating a sufficient number of clinicians to meet the supply of patients. The emphasis in clinical education and preparation will change to reflect the technological advances and the reimbursement patterns in place. Hearing science will come closer to medicine.

It is only reasonable to conclude that the practice of selection, fitting, and verifying and validating hearing aid use will bend gradually, but inevitably toward the more scientific.

Not only will these practice changes result from necessity within the profession, but will also be part of the mandate of the consumers served. That they have been advocated for at least a decade is not in question (Audiology Clinical Practice Algorithms and Statements, 2000). The field's general acceptance and use of these practices could have been better. There are likely many reasons for this slow lack of adaptation, but that discussion is certainly better left to those clinicians who are directly involved with clinical practice on a daily basis. Suffice to say that a field based on services to patients, that which does not adequately service those patients to the extent expected by those very patients, will either disappear or the profession will change into something less than a service-oriented field.

Bob used to quote J. Donald Harris who, at one of his International Hearing Aid Society meetings in the 1970s, stated to the audience of dispensers and audiologists that "what you do is not science." Professor Harris was referring to the methods by which the field fit hearing aids to patients. Forty years later, best practices for the application of hearing aid amplification are still in early stages. Gradually, the knowledge, skills, and application of such practices are being incorporated in every clinic. In the past, many people fitting hearing aids to patients used the patient's beginning and downstream self-evaluations as the only element of benefit. The field is gradually retreating from this position of using patient judgments of quality as the sole method of justifying hearing aid fittings. Some clinicians use objective tests to determine the features of the hearing aids they will recommend. Some even predict the benefits that will be realized from the instruments. More clinicians verify and validate their hearing instrument fittings with tests that are valid and reliable. As this "how does it sound" method of validation slips into its appropriate place, the frequency of patient use and appreciation of the technology involved can only improve.

While many audiologists claim to perform "therapy" following the fitting of hearing instruments, there is little documentation to verify that stance. One of us (MJM) recently reviewed 145 clinical cases that were submitted to third-party payers for reimbursement. One of the cases, out of the 145 submitted, asked for the insurer to cover the costs of hearing therapy. While all of the 145 were asked to submit audiological testing, questionnaires, and a complete patient history to justify their hearing aid selections, only six of the 145 submitted any sort of hearing-in-noise scores. Of those few submitting any type of patient history supporting their recommendations, there were no submissions of "standard" test results such as the Client Oriented Scale of Improvement (indicative of patient problems), or any other standardized tests. Every submission consisted of just an audiogram, sometimes omitting bone conduction and sometimes even omitting speech-in-quiet scores. One might argue that these 145 cases do not represent what is typically found in most clinics, and one can certainly hope that such is a very valid argument. However, the types of information submitted in requesting payment for "top-tier" hearing instruments did not do much to differentiate these audiologists from any salesperson, nor did they offer any evidence of the accumulation of clinical information that would justify the use of "this year's newest and best hearing aids." In these situations where third-party reimbursement and coverage for therapeutic follow-up was available for the asking, only one clinician of the 145 sought prior authorization for this coverage.

Most audiologists with whom we talked about this replied that insurers and third parties did not reimburse for therapy. The billing codes are in place for such billing. Educational and licensing requirements include training and knowledge for such, and yet it is not billed, either to the patient or the insurer. It is hard to justify the necessity for such skill and time spent with patients if it never shows up on invoices. One does not like to consider a conclusion of both patients and third parties that may result—if it is not reimbursed, then it is not necessary. Although that conclusion may be another part of the reason that all audiologists who engage in dispensing hearing instruments need to consider both the professional and the business aspects of their clinical time.

So, perhaps the most important future consideration for audiology and the use of hearing aids may be "With the field's present state of understanding, if there were a complete audiological evaluation that determined the extent and the needs of the patient, what would it encompass?" What information is necessary to determine what features of a hearing aid are essential and will be helpful for the patient? Can any set of clinical tests predict patient benefit to any degree? Is there any benefit in predicting amplification benefits and then demonstrating these outcomes following the hearing aid fitting? Is there value in the patient knowing that no technology will replace many aspects of hearing loss? Can a clinician evaluate when a new algorithm or technology will actually help a patient and be noticeable in that patient's life and thus be worth the expense?

We leave discussion and determination of these questions to those of you who practice every day with hearing-impaired patients. We would remind you that you owe these patients the very best you can deliver in terms of goods and services. To do less than your best may produce consequences even more grave than we all can imagine.

REFERENCES

Audiology Clinical Practice Algorithms and Statements. (2000, August). Special issue, *Audiology Today.*

Brent, E. (2007). The future of hearing aid technology. *Trends in Amplification, 11*(1), 31–46.

Joint Committee on Clinical Practice Algorithms and Statements. (2000, August). Audiology clinical practice algorithms and statements. Special issue, *Audiology Today, 12.*

American Academy of Audiology Ethical Practice Guideline for Relationships with Industry

USED BY PERMISSION OF THE
AMERICAN ACADEMY OF AUDIOLOGY

The Code of Ethics of the American Academy of Audiology (AAA) is a set of principles intended to specify "professional standards that allow for the proper discharge of audiologists' responsibilities to those served, and that protect the integrity of the profession" (American Academy of Audiology, 2006, p. xv). Membership in the Academy requires that the member agree to provide services in a manner that does not violate principles of the Code. This requirement is important to establish the Academy as a professional society dedicated to the highest standards of patient care, and positions Audiologists among health care professionals who subscribe to such standards. Apart from raising the standard of audiology practice, self-governed

ethical behavior may obviate costly external scrutiny and regulation.

Principle 4 Rule 4c of the Code of Ethics provides that "Individuals shall not participate in activities that constitute a conflict of professional interest (COI)" (American Academy of Audiology, 2006, p. xvi). In 2003, AAA and the Academy of Dispensing Audiologists jointly adopted *Ethical Practice Guidelines on Financial Incentives from Hearing Instrument Manufacturers* to define acceptable relationships with industry and specify those relationships that violate Rule 4c. Since then, public scrutiny regarding professional COIs has increased, for healthcare and other professions. Scientific studies have revealed influences on human behavior resulting from the exchange of gifts. This body of evidence has fostered a sweeping trend toward more restrictive policies and more transparency in relationships between healthcare professionals and industry. The United States legislature has increasingly become concerned about this issue and has inserted into legislation monitoring and reporting requirements for a variety of professions including but not limited to medicine and higher education. In response, many professional organizations have clarified their approach to management of COIs. The need to update the guidelines for the American Academy of Audiology became apparent from this greater awareness that activities previously thought to be benign may actually not be in the best interests of patients or may be so perceived by the public.

Guidelines are provided by the Academy to assist the professional with interpreting and applying the principles of the Code of Ethics. A guideline is a defined set of recommended actions or procedures based on available scientific evidence, best practice, and/or expert opinion that has been developed to guide member decision making when certain conditions exist. These guidelines may serve as an ethical compass for the profession that is in line with current legislative policies and ethical guidelines of related professional organizations. Such an ethical compass is effective only to the extent to which it unites the membership in a clear vision of the greater good. It is recognized that while all gifts have the ability to influence, other factors also affect clinical decisions, including product pricing, durability, features, customer service, patient needs, etc. The practitioner weighs many variables, and thus may feel immune to the "gift effect." These guidelines are provided to help the practitioner keep the "gift effect" in mind while making clinical decisions. In combination with evidence-based design of products and evidence-based practice in audiology, such guidelines provide supporting evidence of the commitment of the members of the American Academy of Audiology to uphold-

ing the highest values in patient care in the practice of audiology.

The guidelines provided in this document supersede the previous AAA document *Ethical Practice Guidelines on Financial Incentives from Hearing Instrument Manufacturers (approved by the Board of Directors July 2003)* and provides guidance for relationships between audiologists and industry. Each ethical guideline defines areas of professional conduct that are inconsistent with Rule 4c. Although these represent the Academy's guidelines, they may be less stringent than those developed by an audiologist's place of business.

CONFLICT OF INTEREST

Conflict of interest (COI) exists when a person or entity in a position of trust has a financial or personal interest that could unduly influence or could appear to influence, decisions related to a primary interest such as patient care, student education or validity of research. COI is inevitable in professional life and should be avoided, but when unavoidable must be managed in an ethical manner. The goal of COI management is not to eliminate or reduce financial gain, but rather to keep those interests from influencing or appearing to influence professional decisions. Ideally, COI is best managed by avoiding the situation that produces the conflict. When avoidance is not possible, the conflict must be managed by placing priority on the best interest of the patient, such as through evidence-based practice and transparent documentation of services and reason for services. Failure to avoid or manage a COI is a violation of Rule 4c of the Code of Ethics and in some cases may be illegal.

COI may stem from financial incentives offered by industry and may take a variety of forms. This document provides guidance for avoiding and managing conflicts that may result from a relationship between an audiologist and industry.

GUIDELINES

1. Gifts

For the purpose of this guideline, "gifts" are defined as anything of monetary value given to individuals by industry for personal use and/or personal profit. These "gifts" would include (but are not limited to) material goods, personal entertainment such as tickets to a play or private social event, scholarships, and personal rebates. Meals and travel deemed as rewards are also considered gifts; however, provisions for necessary and modest meals and travel associated with valid and necessary educational/training experiences are not prohibited, and are covered in Guideline 3c.

Gifts represent a conflict of interest because of the real or apparent influence they may have on audiologists' clinical decisions. Considerable evidence from social sciences suggests that gifts of even negligible value can influence the behavior of recipients in ways the recipient does not always realize (Katz & Merz, 2003). Individual behavior is powerfully impacted by the impulse to reciprocate for even small gifts, and those receiving gifts often lose objectivity (Brennan et al., 2006). Furthermore, a systematic review of gift-giving literature in medicine revealed that the interactions had a negative impact on clinical care in an overwhelming majority of cases (Wazana, 2000).

A special problem is the *Quid Pro Quo* arrangement, which is receiving or accepting remuneration in exchange for a purchase, referral, or recommendation. In audiology, this presents in numerous ways including, but not limited to gifts, trips, tuition reimbursement, business support programs, advertising and other marketing efforts, and gifts that are tied directly or indirectly to purchases of hearing and balance products. *Quid Pro Quo* arrangements are not only unethical, but are prohibited by the Federal Anti-Kickback Statute (AKS). AKS prohibits "any person to knowingly and willfully solicit or receive any remuneration, directly or indirectly, overtly or covertly, in cash or in kind, in return for purchasing, leasing or ordering (or recommending the purchase, lease or ordering) of any item or service reimbursable in whole or in part under a federal health care program (except the Federal Employee Health Benefit Program)" (Hahn et al., 2005, p. 34).

Ethical Guideline #1

Acceptance of gifts of any value by a member of the American Academy of Audiology from any company that manufactures or supplies products that he or she dispenses, sells, or recommends , may compromise the audiologist's ability to make ethical decisions, and should be avoided. A provision for modest and necessary meals and travel associated with valid educational/training experiences are covered in Guideline 3c.

2. Commercial Interest

An audiologist has a conflict of interest when he or she, or a member of his/her immediate family, has ownership in, or owns stock in, a company that an audiologist uses in professional business. The commercial interest may influence or appear to influence the audiologist's professional judgment. The conflict arises from the real or perceived increase in value of the stock or ownership that may result from the audiologist's professional use or recommendation of that company's products. In some cases, this type of conflict is managed by disclosing the commercial interest to the patient. However, recent research indicates that disclosure does not eliminate the behavior or potential negative impact of the conflict of interest (Dana & Loewenstein, 2003; Kassirer, 2004; Surowiecki, 2002).

Ethical Guideline #2

A member of the American Academy of Audiology should avoid ownership interests in a company that supplies or manufactures products that he or she dispenses, sells, or recommends. It is unethical for an audiologist who does not follow this guideline to fail to provide patient with written and oral disclosure of the conflict of interest. The disclosure must also offer patients the option of obtaining a second opinion from an audiologist who does not have this form of conflict of interest. Exceptions to this guideline are (a) receiving equity in a company as part of his or her compensation package for selling that company's products to audiologists (e.g., a sales representative to a manufacturer), and (b) owning shares in the company that are part of a managed portfolio (e.g., a mutual fund).

3. Industry-Sponsored Education

Educational events conducted by industry at industry expense may pose ethical dilemmas for members who attend the event and for members who teach at the event. When a member receives payment, travel expenses, lodging, and meals in association with a company-sponsored event, a potential conflict of interest exists if he or she dispenses, sells, or recommends products sold by the company. In addition, a conflict may exist between the manufacturer and the participant when participants receive incentives to sell products manufactured or sold by the sponsor.

Audiologists must make a distinction between necessary and cost-effective educational offerings and those that contain incentives that are not necessary or required for product training, and should not participate in the latter. Receiving travel, lodging and/or meals that is not necessary because training could be obtained otherwise constitutes the acceptance of gifts, and is covered under Guideline #1. Although necessary and modest arrangements for training are acceptable, whenever possible members are encouraged to pay for their own training-related expenses because others may view the provision of training-related expenses as a form of a gift.

When members are hired by industry to teach material that is related to equipment/products manufactured or supplied by the sponsor of the educational program, a real or apparent conflict of interest may occur in two contexts. If the audiologist uses the product clinically, the objectivity of the audiologist's recommendations may be questioned. Additionally, objectivity in the presentation of the educational material may be questioned because of the financial relationship. Audiologists attending the educational event must be made aware of the potential conflict of interest so that they can evaluate the objectivity of the presenter, and patients of the presenter should similarly be made aware of the dual relationship.

In audiology, industry supports a wide range of educational events to the substantial benefit of clinicians, students and their present or future patients. However, the potential or perceived conflict created by the relationship between the company and faculty should be managed by full disclosure to create transparency for the audience attending the event.

Ethical Guideline #3

a. *Members should distinguish between educationally necessary events and those that contain elements that are not necessary for their education, and only attend or present at the former type of offerings.*

b. *Members should not attend or participate in educational events whereby participants are rewarded for conducting business with a specific manufacturer and/or where a Quid Pro Quo relationship exists between attendees and that manufacturer.*

c. *Attendees should not accept anything that is beyond modest travel expenses, meals, and lodging. Members are encouraged to pay for their own education-related expenses.*

d. *Members participating as presenters in educational activities should provide participants with a full disclosure of the relationship between themselves and the industry sponsor. Full disclosure should include a general description of the relationship and the nature of the remuneration for their participation in the educational event (honorarium, travel expenses, gifts, stock options, etc.);*

e. *It is unethical for a member to knowingly present information that is not accurate and complete because such information could lead attendees to deviate from evidence-based practice.*

f. *Members who receive remuneration or travel compensation for presenting at company-sponsored educational events in the last 12 months[1] and who utilize that company's products should disclose the relationship to their patients. The disclosure must also offer patients the option of obtaining a second opinion from an audiologist who does not have this form of conflict of interest.*

4. Consulting

Consulting relationships between industry and audiologists have been important in influencing product development to achieve better clinical outcomes. When a clinician is a paid consultant for a company whose products the clinician dispenses, sells, or recommends, a real or apparent conflict of interest exists, and in certain circumstances could violate the Federal Anti-kickback Statute (AKS).

If the company pays the audiologist above-market rates for the work performed, then there is the appearance of a conflict of interest; the remuneration can be viewed as a reward for the relationship with the company. When a consulting relationship exists, it should be managed in a manner that informs and protects patients. To avoid a violation of AKS, work performed under such a relationship should be specified in a written agreement and compensation should be consistent with the fair market value of the work performed. The consulting relationship should be disclosed to patients for whom products manufactured or distributed by the contractor are sold, dispensed, or recommended. Written disclosure is best but when disclosure is provided orally, documentation of the disclosure should be entered into the patient record.

Ethical Guideline #4

a. *It should be considered unethical for a member to serve as a paid consultant when the consulting services are not specified in a contract and/or if the compensation is not based on the fair market value of the work provided.*

b. *If an audiologist sells, dispenses, or recommends a product manufactured by a company while serving as a paid consultant for that company within the past 12-months, the audiologist should disclose the consulting relationship to the patient in writing.*

5. Research

Research relationships between industry and investigators are increasingly prevalent and create real or apparent COI (DeAngelis et al., 2001). Scientific discovery is essential to the profession. Without industry-funded research, many important advances and discoveries might not occur. However, the integrity of the knowledge base must be ensured. The active involvement in and control of research data and subsequent publication (or a decision to not publish) by companies whose products are being evaluated and who have a financial interest in the study represents a clear conflict of interest. Grants that are given without a specific research plan are considered to be gifts and conflicts of interest, and may constitute a violation of the AKS (Brennan et al., 2006; Chimonas et al., 2004).

For the purpose of this policy there is a distinction between research which is conducted to reveal new scientific knowledge and product evaluation which is conducted to obtain proprietary information about devices.

Ethical Guideline #5

a. *Members should disclose financial relationships between the researcher and the sponsor in all written and verbal research reports.*

---

[1]Some states stipulate that non-compete clauses must be limited in scope and time line. 12 months is a standard time line used for non-compete clauses and was thus adopted for the purposes of the guideline.

b. *Members should disclose any financial relationships between the researcher and the sponsor in any public written or verbal reports of product evaluation activities.*

c. *It should be considered unethical for a member to conduct research in a manner that does not provide an honest, fair, accurate and complete evaluation of the product, device, or procedure.*

d. *Members should avoid agreements with industry sponsors that limit the dissemination of research results.*

e. *Members should only enter into explicit research contracts with specific deliverables restricted to scientific issues and should not accept "no strings attached" grants and gifts.*

f. *Members who conduct industry-sponsored research and who also utilize that company's products clinically should disclose that relationship to their patients in writing.*

CONCLUDING COMMENTS

In the general marketplace, sales and profits are accepted as the natural result of a free-market society and buyers are expected to look out for themselves (*caveat emptor*). But there is a different set of expectations in healthcare. Health professionals are expected to hold paramount the interests of patients before profit motive. There are a variety of professional and legal sanctions that enforce that expectation. A heightened awareness of real and perceived conflicts of interest that may result from an audiologist's relations with industry has created the impetus for these revised guidelines. Acceptance of and adherence to these guidelines will benefit patients and, thereby, benefit the profession of audiology.

These guidelines were based on current understanding and experience regarding relations between audiologists and industry. Obviously, not all pitfalls potentially resulting in a conflict of interest can be detailed here; therefore, professional judgment and prudence should be exercised in all circumstances. As professionals, audiologists should endeavor to avoid real, apparent, or potential conflicts of interest whether or not they are presented in this document. In contemplating their relationships with industry, the audiologist may want to consider some guiding questions:

1. *How might my patients feel about my relationship with industry?*
2. *How might clients view my receiving gifts from industry?*
3. *How would independent colleagues view my association with industry?*
4. *Would I be willing to publicize the details of my involvement with industry?*
5. *Could my relationship with industry be viewed as one which may influence my professional judgment in patient care in compromised ways?*

Partnerships between audiologists and industry in the interest of enhancing patient care have and will continue to benefit our profession and our patients. The American Academy of Audiology encourages our industry partners to join us in ensuring that our clinical practices follow ethical guidelines and help us provide the best possible care for our patients.

REFERENCES

American Academy of Audiology. (2006). *Ethics in Audiology: Guidelines for ethical conduct in clinical, educational, and research settings.* Reston, VA: Author.

Brennan, T., Rothman, D., Blank, L., Blumenthal, D., Chimonas, S., Cohen, J., . . . Smelser, N. (2006). Health industry practices that create conflicts of interest: A policy proposal for academic medical centers. *JAMA, 295*(4), 429–433.

Chimonas, S., & Rothman, D. (2005). New Federal guidelines for physician-pharmaceutical industry relations: The politics of policy formation. *Health AFF, 24,* 949–960.

Dana, J., & Loewenstein, G. (2003). A social science perspective on gifts to physicians from industry. *JAMA, 290,* 252–255.

DeAngelis, C. D., Fontanarosa, P., & Flanagin, A. (2001). Reporting financial conflicts of interest and relationships between investigators and research sponsors. *JAMA, 286*(1), 89–91.

Hahn, R., Abel, D., & Kukula, J. (2005). Audiologists beware! . . . And be aware of conflicts of interest. *Audiology Today, 17*(4), 34–35.

Kassirer, J. (2004). *On the take: How medicine's complicity with big business can endanger your health.* New York, NY: Oxford Press.

Katz, D. C., & Merz, J. (2003). All gifts large and small: Toward an understanding of the ethics of pharma-ceutical gift giving. *American Journal of Bioethics, 3*(3), 39–36.

Surowiecki, J. (2002, December 9). The talking cure. *The New Yorker,* p. 54.

Wazana, A. (2000). Physicians and the pharmaceutical industry: Is a gift ever just a gift? *JAMA, 283,* 373–380.

Index

Note: Page numbers in **bold** reference non-text material.